THE ROUTLEDGE HANDBOOK OF PHILOSOPHY OF PAIN

The phenomenon of pain presents problems and puzzles for philosophers who want to understand its nature. Though pain might seem simple, there has been disagreement since Aristotle about whether pain is an emotion, sensation, perception, or disturbed state of the body. Despite advances in psychology, neuroscience, and medicine, pain is still poorly understood and multiple theories of pain abound.

The Routledge Handbook of Philosophy of Pain is an outstanding reference source to the key topics, problems, and debates in this exciting and interdisciplinary subject and is the first collection of its kind. Comprising over 30 chapters by a team of international contributors, the *Handbook* is divided into nine clear parts:

- Modeling pain in philosophy
- Modeling pain in neuroscience
- Modeling pain in psychology
- Pain in philosophy of mind
- Pain in epistemology
- Pain in philosophy of religion
- Pain in ethics
- Pain in medicine
- Pain in law.

As well as fundamental topics in the philosophy of pain such as the nature, role, and value of pain, many other important topics are covered including the neurological pathways involved in pain processing; biopsychosocial and cognitive-behavioral models of pain; chronic pain; pain and non-human animals; pain and knowledge; controlled substances for pain; pain and placebo effects; and pain and physician-assisted suicide.

The Routledge Handbook of Philosophy of Pain is essential reading for students and researchers in philosophy of mind, philosophy of psychology, and ethics. It will also be very useful to researchers of pain from any field, especially those in psychology, medicine, and health studies.

Jennifer Corns is Lecturer in Philosophy at the University of Glasgow, UK. Her published research focuses on pain and affect. She aims to use philosophical tools and evaluate empirical research to make progress on topics that matter within and beyond the academy. She is currently revising a monograph, *Pain is Not a Natural Kind*.

ROUTLEDGE HANDBOOKS IN PHILOSOPHY

Routledge Handbooks in Philosophy are state-of-the-art surveys of emerging, newly refreshed, and important fields in philosophy, providing accessible yet thorough assessments of key problems, themes, thinkers, and recent developments in research.

All chapters for each volume are specially commissioned, and written by leading scholars in the field. Carefully edited and organized, *Routledge Handbooks in Philosophy* provide indispensable reference tools for students and researchers seeking a comprehensive overview of new and exciting topics in philosophy. They are also valuable teaching resources as accompaniments to textbooks, anthologies, and research-orientated publications.

Also available:

THE ROUTLEDGE HANDBOOK OF PHILOSOPHY OF PAIN

Edited by Jennifer Corns

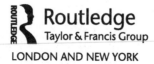

LONDON AND NEW YORK

First published 2017
by Routledge
2 Park Square, Milton Park, Abingdon, Oxon OX14 4RN

and by Routledge
52 Vanderbilt Avenue, New York, NY 10017

First issued in paperback 2020

Routledge is an imprint of the Taylor & Francis Group, an informa business

British Library Cataloguing-in-Publication Data
A catalogue record for this book is available from the British Library

Library of Congress Cataloging-in-Publication Data
Names: Corns, Jennifer, editor.
Title: The Routledge handbook of philosophy of pain /
edited by Jennifer Corns.
Description: 1 [edition]. | New York : Routledge, 2017. | Series: Routledge handbooks in philosophy | Includes bibliographical references and index.
Identifiers: LCCN 2016040765 | ISBN 9781138823181 (hardback : alk. paper) |
ISBN 9781315742205 (e-book)
Subjects: LCSH: Pain--Philosophy.
Classification: LCC BJ1409 .R58 2017 | DDC 128/.4--dc23
LC record available at https://lccn.loc.gov/2016040765

ISBN 13: 978-0-367-57342-3 (pbk)
ISBN 13: 978-1-138-82318-1 (hbk)

Typeset in Bembo
by Taylor & Francis Books

For David and Michael, steadfast partners in pain and suffering

CONTENTS

Contents

Contents

Contents

ILLUSTRATIONS

Figures

Tables

CONTRIBUTORS

Sunil Kumar Aggarwal, MD, PhD, FAAPMR, is a hospice and palliative medicine physician and medical geographer. He practices privately and with Tacoma, Washington-based MultiCare Health System where he is a Consulting Physician and an Associate Hospice Medical Director. He is an Affiliate Assistant Professor of Geography and Clinical Instructor in the School of Medicine at the University of Washington. Read more of his work at Cannabinologist.org.

Vania Apkarian is a Professor of Physiology, Anesthesia, and Physical Medicine and Rehabilitation at Northwestern University Medical School in Chicago. He has been studying brain mechanisms of acute and chronic pain in humans using neuroimaging technology, and in rodent models using electrophysiology, pharmacology, and more recently optogenetic and chemogenetic techniques combined with neuroimaging technology. His prime interest is expanding knowledge regarding brain physiology and perception.

Murat Aydede is Professor of Philosophy at the University of British Columbia. He works in the areas of philosophy of mind, psychology, and perception.

David Bain is Reader in Philosophy at the University of Glasgow. He was Principal Investigator of the Pain Project (2012–13) and the Value of Suffering Project (2013–16) and has published on the philosophy of language, color, perception, and especially pain.

Brianna Beck is a Research Associate in the Action and Body group at the Institute of Cognitive Neuroscience at University College London.

Carolyn Berryman is a physiotherapist and a Postdoctoral Fellow in the Body in Mind research group. She has over twenty years' experience as a clinician, a clinical educator, and senior lecturer in pain sciences, primarily for physiotherapy students.

Mark Catley is a Lecturer at the University of South Australia, a physiotherapist, and a member of the Body in Mind research group. He coordinates the Pain Sciences curricula in the School of Health Sciences.

Jonathan Cohen is a Professor of Philosophy at the University of California, San Diego. He works principally in the philosophy of mind, language, and perception, and is the author of *The Red and the Real: An Essay on Color Ontology* (Oxford, 2009).

Robert Cowan is a Lecturer in Philosophy at the University of Glasgow. His research is focused on the intersection between ethics, epistemology, and the philosophy of mind.

Arthur D. ("Bud") Craig is Atkinson Research Professor (Emeritus) at the Barrow Neurological Institute in Phoenix, Arizona, and Professor (Emeritus) of Psychology at Arizona State University in Tempe.

Brian Cutter is an Assistant Professor in the Department of Philosophy at the University of Notre Dame. His research is primarily in metaphysics and the philosophy of mind, with a focus on the metaphysics of consciousness and intentionality.

Michael Davis is Senior Fellow at the Center for the Study of Ethics in the Professions, and Professor of Philosophy, Illinois Institute of Technology, Chicago, Illinois. Among his recent publications are: *Profession, Code, and Ethics* (2002), *Engineering Ethics* (2005), and *Ethics and the Legal Profession* (2009).

Stuart W.G. Derbyshire is faculty in the Psychology Department at the National University of Singapore and at the A*-STAR Clinical Imaging Research Centre. His work involves theoretical and empirical research on the nature of pain, especially pertaining to pain that occurs without identifiable pathology.

Frédérique de Vignemont is a CNRS Researcher in Philosophy, leader of the BoSS (Body, Space and the Self) team at the Institut Jean Nicod in Paris. Her main research interests are in philosophy of mind, philosophy of cognitive science, and philosophy of psychopathology. She has a forthcoming book, *Mind the Body* (Oxford).

Trent Dougherty is Associate Professor of Philosophy at Baylor University in Waco, Texas. His main research interest is the normativity of rationality, especially the relationship between conceptions of epistemic rationality and pragmatic rationality.

Paula Droege is currently a Fellow at the Institute for Advanced Study/*Wissenschaftskolleg* in Berlin, Germany, where she is part of an interdisciplinary Focus Group on Animal Pain. Her home institution is in the Philosophy Department at Pennsylvania State University. She is the author of *Caging the Beast: A Theory of Sensory Consciousness* and articles on the role of consciousness in memory, free will, and delusions such as confabulation. Her research proposes a temporal representation theory of consciousness.

Owen Flanagan is James B. Duke Professor of Philosophy and Co-director of the Center for Comparative Philosophy at Duke University, Durham, North Carolina. He is the author of *The Geography of Morals: Varieties of Moral Possibility* (Oxford, 2017).

Matthew Fulkerson is an Associate Professor of Philosophy at the University of California, San Diego. He is interested in perception, pain, reasons, motivation, and justification. He is the author of *The First Sense: A Philosophical Study of Human Touch* (MIT Press, 2014).

Ariel Glucklich is Professor of Theology at Georgetown University in Washington, DC. He specializes in Hindu normative traditions and contemporary folk rituals and in the psychology of religion. Among his works are *Sacred Pain* (2001) and *Dying for Heaven* (2009), which deal with the religious psychology of pain and pleasure respectively. He is currently completing a project on the psychology of a spiritual community in Israel – *Everyday Mysticism* (Yale, 2016).

Palden Gyal is a Master of Theological Studies student at Harvard Divinity School, where he concentrates in Buddhist studies and philosophy of religion. Palden holds a BA in philosophy and history from Duke University, where he studied under Owen Flanagan. Palden's research interests lie at the intersection of political philosophy, ethics, and religion. He plans to continue his studies in comparative or cross-cultural philosophy.

Thomas Hadjistavropoulos, PhD, FCAHS, is Professor of Psychology at the University of Regina, Canada. His work, summarized in over 160 peer-reviewed articles and chapters, focuses primarily on pain behavior and on psychosocial influences on the pain experience.

Patrick Haggard is a professor at the Institute of Cognitive Neuroscience at University College London. He leads the Action and Body group.

Valerie Gray Hardcastle is Professor of Philosophy, Psychology, and Psychiatry and Behavioral Neuroscience at University of Cincinnati. Her research has focused primarily on developing a philosophical framework for understanding conscious phenomena, including pain, responsive to neuroscientific, psychiatric, and psychological data.

Christopher S. Hill is Faunce Professor of Philosophy at Brown University in the United States. He is the author of four books, including *Thought and World* (Cambridge, 2002), *Consciousness* (Cambridge, 2009), and *Meaning, Mind, and Knowledge* (Oxford, 2014).

Hilla Jacobson is a philosopher of mind and cognitive science. She is an Associate Professor at the Philosophy and the Cognitive Science Departments, the Hebrew University of Jerusalem, Israel.

Colin Klein is affiliated with Macquarie University (Sydney, Australia) where he is a Senior Lecturer in Philosophy and an Associate Investigator in the ARC Centre of Excellence in Cognition and Its Disorders. He is also an Australian Research Council Future Fellow.

Peter Langland-Hassan is Assistant Professor of Philosophy at the University of Cincinnati. His research topics include imagination, inner speech, consciousness, and introspection.

Steve Layman is Professor of Philosophy at Seattle Pacific University. His books include *The Shape of the Good* (Notre Dame, 1991), *Letters to Doubting Thomas* (Oxford, 2007), and *Philosophical Approaches to Atonement, Incarnation, and the Trinity* (Palgrave Macmillan, 2016).

Pete Mandik is a Professor in the Department of Philosophy, William Paterson University, Wayne, New Jersey. He is the author of *This Is Philosophy of Mind: An Introduction* (2013) and *Key Terms in Philosophy of Mind* (2010), and is the co-host of the podcast SpaceTimeMind.

Olivier Massin is a Lecturer at the Department of Philosophy of the University of Geneva. He wrote a first PhD dissertation on the objectivity of tactile perception; and a second one on the nature and value of pleasure. He has published several papers in metaphysics, philosophy of mind, and value theory.

Avi I. Mintz is an Associate Professor in the University of Tulsa's Department of Educational Studies. Much of his work focuses on the history of educational philosophy. He has been particularly interested in debates – both contemporary and historical – about the value of pain in learning.

Daniel E. Moerman, William E. Stirton Professor Emeritus of Anthropology at the University of Michigan, Dearborn, has been interested in the meaning response ("placebo effect") for many years and has published widely on the subject. He has a dog, Peche, and two cats, Click and Clack.

Lorimer Moseley is a physiotherapist, a Principal Research Fellow with Australia's National Health and Medical Research Council, Professor of Clinical Neurosciences, and Foundation Chair in Physiotherapy at the University of South Australia. He leads the Body in Mind research group.

David Pereplyotchik received his PhD in philosophy, with a concentration in cognitive science, from the City University of New York, Graduate Center. He is currently an Assistant Professor at Kent State University, Ohio.

Katherine Pettus, PhD, is the Advocacy Officer for Human Rights and Palliative Care at the International Association for Hospice and Palliative Care. She was appointed to the Civil Society Task Force for UNGASS 2016 (UN General Assembly Special Session on the World Drug Problem) as representative of "affected populations" with no access to internationally controlled essential medicines.

Donald D. Price received his PhD in neurophysiology from the University of California, Davis, in 1969, and received postdoctoral training at the Brain Research Institute at UCLA (1970). He was Professor of neurophysiology and psychology at Virginia Commonwealth University (Medical College of Virginia, Physiology and Anesthesiology Departments, 1971–74, 1980–97), Psychologist and Neurobiologist at National Institutes of Health (NIDR, 1974–79), and Professor at the University of Florida (Oral Surgery and Neuroscience Departments, 1997–present). He has combined the disciplines of neuroscience, psychology, and experiential science to increase understanding of the neural and psychological basis of pain and emotions. His work has also focused on integrating experiential science, neurobiology, and philosophy to increase understanding of consciousness.

Ben A. Rich received his JD degree from Washington University School of Law in St. Louis, Missouri (1973), and his PhD in philosophy from the University of Colorado at Boulder (1995). His legal practice specialized in civil litigation, health-care and higher education law. He has taught health-care law and bioethics at the University of Colorado and the University of California, Davis. From 2007 to 2015 he was the UC Davis School of Medicine Alumni Association Endowed Chair of Bioethics. He is currently Emeritus

Professor of Internal Medicine (Bioethics) at UC Davis. He has published extensively on the legal and ethical aspects of pain management and palliative care.

Mathieu Roy is Assistant Professor of Psychology at McGill University. He received his PhD in neuropsychology at the University of Montreal in 2009 and completed a post-doctoral fellowship in the Psychology and Neuroscience Department at Columbia University and at the University of Colorado in Boulder. His research focuses on the cerebral mechanisms underlying the generation of painful experiences and pain-related behaviors, such as escape and avoidance.

Irina A. Strigo is Associate Professor at the University of California, San Francisco, and Research Physiologist at the San Francisco VA Medical Center.

Mark D. Sullivan received his MD and his PhD in philosophy from Vanderbilt University. He is Professor of Psychiatry and Behavioral Sciences as well as Adjunct Professor of Anesthesiology and Pain Medicine and of Bioethics and Humanities at the University of Washington. He has served as attending physician in the UW Center for Pain Relief for over twenty-five years, where he is Co-director of Behavioral Health Services. He has published over 230 peer-reviewed articles, many on chronic pain. He is currently participating in NIMH-, NIDA-, CDC-, PCORI-, and VA-funded studies on opioid therapy for chronic pain. He has been chair of the Ethics Committee of the American Pain Society and on the editorial board of *Pain*. He has just completed a book titled, *The Patient as Agent of Health and Health Care*.

Mick Thacker is Senior Lecturer in Pain Neuroscience at King's College London and Senior Consultant AHP in Pain at Guy's and St. Thomas NHS Trust. He has a PhD in pain neuroscience and is currently collaborating with Professor Andy Clark investigating Predictive Processing as a model of Pain.

Tor D. Wager is a Professor of Psychology and Neuroscience and the Institute of Cognitive Science at the University of Colorado, Boulder. Since 2010, he has directed Boulder's Cognitive and Affective Neuroscience laboratory. Much of the lab's work focuses on the neurophysiology of pain and emotion, and multiple types of cognitive regulation. Prof. Wager is particularly interested in how thinking influences affective experiences, affective learning, and brain–body communication.

Daniel Weinstock is the James McGill Professor in the Faculty of Law at McGill University. He is also the Director of McGill's *Institute for Health and Social Policy*. He has written on a wide array of issues in moral, political, and legal philosophy, and is a regular contributor to public policy debates in Canada. He recently co-authored a report for the Royal Society of Canada on end-of-life decision-making, that has been cited in court cases on medically assisted death in several jurisdictions. He is currently working on a project on the ethics and law of harm reduction.

Amanda C. de C. Williams, PhD CPsychol, is an academic and clinical psychologist at University College London and the Pain Management Centre, National Hospital for Neurology and Neurosurgery (University College London Hospitals). She also works as a research consultant for the International Centre for Health and Human Rights. She has been active in research and clinical work in persistent pain for thirty years, with particular interests in evaluation of psychologically based treatments for pain; in expression of pain and its interpretation by clinicians; in evolutionary understanding of pain behavior; and in pain from torture. Dr. Williams has written over 170 papers and chapters, presents at national and international pain meetings, and is on the editorial boards of several major pain journals.

Andrew Wright was a physiotherapist. After twenty years in the profession, he took a sabbatical to further his understanding of chronic pain. He completed his doctorate in philosophy at the University of Birmingham in 2015 and has no plans to return to physiotherapy practice. His broad interests lie in the philosophy of medicine, biology, and mind. He is currently researching affectively neutral experience and advantageous behavioral change.

ACKNOWLEDGEMENTS

Thanks first to the editors at Routledge, Tony Bruce, and especially Adam Johnson, for their work throughout the development of this volume. Many thanks are also due to Michael Brady who suggested me for the project and provided invaluable support and advice along the way. My sincere thanks to all the contributors both for their willingness to share their time and expertise, and also their patience with my questions, suggestions, and prodding. Thanks finally to Robert Cowan for his good sense and calming influence in dealing with each and every bump and hurdle. Much of this work was completed through the Value of Suffering project, funded by the John Templeton Foundation and, I gratefully acknowledge their support.

INTRODUCTION

Pain research: where we are and why it matters

Jennifer Corns

1 Controversy

What is pain? Despite its ubiquity in our lives, there is no consensus about the nature of pain in either the sciences or the humanities – including philosophy.

To begin to see why, imagine the following:

(1) Merrily making your way to the office, you hear a lovely birdsong and look up. Engrossed and distracted, you trip on a pothole and wrench your ankle.

What happens next?

Here is a typical trajectory:

(A) You wince, lean down and massage the ankle, and continue walking. You limp for a few steps, concerned about the damage. Gradually, you increase the pressure and reach the office twenty minutes later, walking normally and focused on the day's work ahead.

Here is another:

(B) You laugh and continue on to work.

Here is a less typical, but nonetheless common, trajectory:

(C) You limp for a few steps, concerned about the damage. The ankle seems to be throbbing and each step becomes harder. You begin to sweat. You reach the office slightly shaken and distracted. You begin to stay off the ankle as much as possible and wear your most supportive tennis shoes. After a few days, you slip back into your regular shoes, continuing to step gingerly. When a friend asks about it a week later, you realize that you've forgotten all about your ankle.

Here is a less common, but regrettably frequent, trajectory:

(D) You limp for a few steps, concerned about the damage. The ankle seems to be throbbing and each step becomes harder. You begin to sweat. You reach the office slightly shaken and distracted. You begin to stay off the ankle as much as possible and to wear your most supportive tennis shoes. After a few days, your back begins to hurt from the limping and you develop a blister on your compensating foot. As walking becomes increasingly difficult, you begin to take the bus to work. After two weeks, you make an appointment with your general practitioner. She asks you to wait and see. After two more weeks without improvement and with increasing concern, you return and she refers you to a specialist. Questions are asked. Forms are completed. Scans are taken. They do not know what is wrong, but your suffering continues. Indeed, you begin to believe that there is nothing wrong with your ankle, but it still hurts.

In contrast, consider the following distinct case:

(2) Merrily making your way to the office, you hear a lovely birdsong. You stop to look up when you are distracted by a sudden, shooting, and unpleasant sensation in your ankle.

Note that cases beginning as in (2) may also follow the typical, common, and regrettably frequent trajectories (A)–(D): you may limp a few steps and forget all about it (A), laugh it off (B), take a few days to recover (C), or embark on a prolonged journey of dysfunction and suffering (D).

It is, of course, not only ankle pain which exhibits the causal variations, as in (1) and (2), or the variations in trajectories, as in (A)–(D). Headaches, toothaches, stomach aches, and backaches and all other types of pain are likewise variable. A herniated disc is a minor inconvenience for some, and a harrowing life-changing event for others. A broken leg may, variably, result in pain for weeks, months, or years. For many injuries, no pain or extremely transient pain is felt. For many reported pains, no identifiable injurious cause is ever identified.

Any answer to the question about pain's nature must be consistent with all these cases, and in thinking about what consistency requires we might begin to see why there is so much disagreement about the nature of pain.

As we say things like "there is a pain in your ankle," we might begin by identifying pain with some kind of damage to the body. Something, in the above cases, that is in your ankle. Now we must be consistent. If pain just is damage, then if there is no damage to your ankle – as in cases (2A)–(2D) – then there is no pain. So too, if pain is just damage, then there sometimes is pain – as in case (1B) – even if you don't feel anything unpleasant.

Concerned with whether this is plausible, we might instead think that pain is not a kind of damage to the body, but is instead a kind of mental episode of the person (perhaps in the brain). After all, we might say, pain is something that you, and not your ankle, feel and experience. But what kind of experience is it?

We might try identifying pain with a mental episode that registers that damage, or anyway that something bad or disturbing, has occurred in the body. After all, in the cases above, it seems like the problem with your ankle is what your pain is about. Again, we must be consistent. If we make this identification, then are cases like (2A)–(2D) hallucinations; are those pains simply registrations of damage occurring in your ankle when there isn't any? And why are (1A)–(1D) so different if they both involve registering the same damage: do three out of the four cases involve an illusion that registers the damage as being worse (or better) than it really is? If so, which one is the non-illusory one? Could so many of our pains really be hallucinations or illusions?

Such questions might lead us to doubt that pains can be accurate or inaccurate in these ways. Maybe pain experiences are instead just nasty feelings that can't be inaccurate about anything, because they simply aren't about anything. Pains, on this view, are identified with a certain kind of brute, unpleasant feeling. But even if we give up the idea that the pain is *about* your ankle, it might seem that the pain and your ankle must be connected in some way. It is, after all, an ankle pain and not a stomach ache. The relationship between the pain and the ankle might also seem important to explain the actions that we take when we are in pain. In cases (1) and (2) (A), (C), and (D), you do things about your ankle *because,* we might say, your ankle hurts. But how can your pain play this kind of role in getting you to do something about your ankle unless it tells you something about your ankle?

If we focus on the sorts of actions that we take in response to pain, we might begin to think that rather than telling us something about what is happening *to* our bodies, pains are experiences that tell us about something that we need to do *for* our bodies. Pains, on this kind of view, would be identified with those mental episodes that tell us to protect or take care of some part of our bodies. Again and finally, we must be consistent. What might we consistently say is happening in cases like (1B)? Is there just no pain despite the damage and its registration? Or, perhaps, is there a command that you don't hear or ignore? And what about cases like (2A)–(2D)? Why should our bodies so frequently tell us to protect places where there is no damage and when it doesn't seem clear whether or what kind of protective action to take?

A paradigmatic pain involves (a) damage to the body; (b) registration of that damage; (c) an unpleasant feeling; (d) the motivation to do something about both the unpleasant feeling and the damage; and (e) an action in response to the unpleasant feeling and the damage. Questions about which of (a)–(e) are causes, constituents, or consequences of pain are not easy. Given the presence of all five features in paradigmatic cases, it is perhaps not surprising that philosophical theories of pain have focused on all five – singly and in combination – when accounting for the nature of pain. As discussed further below, the theories currently dominating philosophy are presented in Part I-I.

Answers about the nature of pain that one gives in philosophy purport to tell us what pain is at a rather general, personal level of description. But pains are, of course, not merely of interest to philosophers, and there are other levels of description at which we might want to account for pain. The doctor doesn't just want to know whether pain is a type of bodily damage, a mental episode that registers that damage, an unpleasant feeling, or anything at this level of description: he wants to be able to effectively relieve your pain. Our answer to the question "what is pain?" might focus on a level of description appropriate for identifying treatment targets, i.e., the physical mechanisms that might be appropriately targeted for treatment. So too, if we are naturalistic philosophers, then we'll want our philosophical theory about pain to harmonize with our best scientific theories. Perhaps questions about the nature of pain can be settled – or at least advanced – by looking at the science of pain.

Here too, however, we find controversy. The scientific study of pain has changed dramatically in the last sixty years. For some time, the idea of a dedicated, linear pain system held sway: we believed in pain-specific receptors and pain-specific pathways across which pain-specific information was propagated and received by the pain-specific areas in the brain that we were, admittedly, still struggling to identify. Melzack and Wall's gate-control theory of the 1960s, however, convinced researchers that pain was more complicated – mechanistically and conceptually – than had previously been believed. This influential theory, and the ways it revolutionized pain science, is discussed in more detail within this volume. For now, note that Melzack and Wall's groundbreaking theory conjoined with technological advances have inspired a profundity of new models and approaches to the scientific study of pain. In both neuroscience and psychology, new models of pain, and indeed new models of different types of pain, are flourishing.

These theoretical and technological advances have, however, also led to the controversies that currently remain: no one model or approach to pain is either universally accepted within a discipline or dominant across the sciences. The dominant and contrasting views from neuroscience and psychology are presented in Parts I-II and I-III. In neuroscience, some maintain that there is a kind of neural, pain signature realized by activation across a "pain neuromatrix." Subregions of the matrix are sometimes taken to be well-correlated with the different components of pain discussed above. There is disagreement, however, about whether and which of the areas usually taken to be included in the neuromatrix are specific for pain and whether we should instead think of the identified network as a general purpose "body–self neuromatrix." Moreover, which neural areas, pathways, and chemicals we take to be central in our neuroscientific modeling of pain is not independent from the questions above concerning which components we take pain to have. Some leading neuroscientists in pain research hold that pain should be modeled as an interoceptive, homeostatic system that monitors the body and motivates responses when appropriate, while others maintain that pain serves not only interoceptive self-monitoring functions, but also exteroceptive functions that monitor the world and identify external threats. These are just two examples of distinct approaches that accordingly involve identifying pain with activities and components in distinct areas and pathways. There is, if anything, even more disagreement in psychology, where the role of cognition, behavior, and society in generating, constituting, and maintaining pain are all contested. It was, we learn, the perceived failures of the medical models of pain, focused on pathologies, which gave rise to the wide range of psychological models of pain that have been developed – highlighting that across the sciences we find parallel disagreements about the relationship between pain and damage that we saw in philosophy. Contemporary pain science will not settle our questions about the nature of pain in any straightforward way.

There are thus today a diversity of scientific and philosophical models of pain, leaving anyone interested in the nature of pain with a daunting task. They must identify and decode conflicting theories and studies from across the disciplines to cobble together an overarching view of the multidisciplinary landscape.

The difficult task of charting the terrain is only increased for those interested not only in the nature of pain, but some additional inquiry for which pain is important. These additional inquiries are plentiful. There are, for instance, inquiries in the philosophy of mind, epistemology, and the philosophy of religion for which an accurate understanding of pain is potentially crucial, e.g., whether there is a plausible solution to the problem of evil, whether we are infallible about any of our experiences, and whether every experience represents something in the world. Similarly, pain is integral for many practical inquiries and endeavors. An accurate understanding of pain can potentially illuminate many important questions and decisions in ethics, medicine, and the law, e.g., what is the appropriate use of pain in education, what role does pain play in the development of our moral character, and whether pain ever morally or legally either justifies or prohibits abortion or physician-assisted death.

Moreover, these inquiries not only rely on an understanding of the nature of pain, but are themselves informative of it. Even as a better understanding of the science of pain illuminates pain's nature, so too does a better understanding of the role that pains play in ethics, philosophy of religion, epistemology, and so on. Likewise, the pain researcher at work in neuroscience or psychology is benefited by understanding the different ways in which pains are modeled in philosophy, the important role that pain plays in legal and ethical theorizing, and so on. An overall understanding of the role of pain in multiple inquiries is, in short, of use for even the most specialized of pain researchers.

The present volume thus brings together experts from multiple disciplines, with both theoretical and practical concerns, to address the questions of pain's nature and its importance for additional practical and theoretical inquiries. While primarily focused on philosophical inquiries and aimed at philosophers interested in pain, it is hoped that it will also be of use to researchers of pain from all fields and philosophers of any subdiscipline.

What follows is an overview of the volume's contents and a brief, reflective conclusion on pain's nature.

2 Contents

The volume is organized around three broad questions:

1   What is pain?
2   Why does pain matter, theoretically?
3   Why does pain matter, practically?

As above, however, note that answers to these questions rightly inform each other, and the organization is not meant to suggest that "theoretical" and "practical" inquiries are independent. Each chapter concludes with a Related Topics section explicitly marking connections between chapters and across sections and parts that are likewise explicitly drawn by the authors in the text. The reader is invited to further consider the ways in which discussions from across the volume inform, extend, and challenge others.

Section I: The nature of pain – what is pain?

This section serves as an overview of the different views on the nature of pain that are currently dominant in philosophy, psychology, and neuroscience.

It is thus divided into three parts:

Modeling pain in philosophy
Modeling pain in neuroscience
Modeling pain in psychology.

The first part begins with Valerie Gray Hardcastle's overview (Chapter 1) of philosophical views of pain. The chapter is shaped around a purported puzzle that arises in various guises throughout the volume: "How is it that pain is both a sort of experience, but also the object of our experience?" She considers and rejects a range of historical and contemporary answers, before arguing that the puzzle dissolves if we accept a view of pain as a "neurobiological process" akin to other perceptual processes. In Chapter 2, Brian Cutter provides an overview to representationalism about pain: the idea, roughly, that pains represent the world to be a certain way. He defends the view from something akin to Hardcastle's puzzle: if pain is representational, then there should be an appearance/reality gap for pains, but there allegedly isn't. His advocated solution relies on disambiguating pain as an object (a bodily disturbance) and pain as an experience (a representation of the bodily disturbance). Two versions of representationalism, evaluativism and imperativism, are presented as possible avenues to solving remaining problems for the representationalist concerning qualities and affect. The next two chapters focus on these avenues. In Chapter 3, David Bain presents and defends an evaluative account of pain's unpleasantness. On this view, pains are unpleasant when bodily conditions are represented *as bad* for the subject. This evaluative account of the negative affective dimension of pain is compared and contrasted with others, most notably desire accounts and imperativism. In Chapter 4, Colin Klein defends the imperativist alternative. He begins by drawing a contrast between pain and other sensations: other sensations are indicative and motivate only indirectly, whereas pains motivate directly and are "remarkably uninformative." Imperativism is argued to be tailor-made to explain this contrast: according to imperativism, pains have a content that commands one to do certain things. Further motivations and possible versions of the view are presented, worries are diffused, and future directions are identified. The part ends with Christopher Hill (Chapter 5) arguing that there are two well-supported but inconsistent models of pain: *the bodily disturbance model* and *the central state model*. According to the latter, pains are higher-level perceptual states, while according to the former, they are located bodily disturbances. This final chapter, then, may be read as an extended and earnest return to Hardcastle's opening puzzle about how pains can be both experiences and the objects of experiences. Hill's advocated reconciliation, like Cutter's, is a disambiguation. Any monolithic conception of pain that we might have should be replaced with "a bevy of new ones." As a start, we ought to disambiguate *peripheral pain* (bodily disturbances of the relevant sort) and *central state pain* (the perceptual representation of the bodily disturbances of the relevant sort).

The reader will note that these opening chapters, along with many later chapters, are riddled with empirical claims. It is valuable for the philosopher interested in pain to see for themselves which models, methods, and assumptions are at play in contemporary empirical investigations into the nature of pain. It is thus appropriate that considerable space is given to the dominant empirical models of pain.

Part I-II is comprised of five chapters from leaders in the neuroscience of pain. As initially noted by Vania Apkarian, there has been a "veritable revolution" in the science of pain. In his Chapter 6, he offers a wide range of the resultant advances. He first distinguishes sharply between nociception, acute pain, and chronic pain, before discussing what he takes to be our best evidence concerning the neural circuitry underlying each and the transformations from one to the next. The evidence, by Apkarian's lights, is limited such that there is still no "convincing scientific data or palatable theories of underlying mechanisms" (p. 79). Nonetheless, there are advances, and having covered some of these he closes with optimism about the future of pain science. In their Chapter 7, Mathieu Roy and Tor Wager likewise confront the difficulty of identifying the mechanisms which turn nociceptive sensory signals into pain. The double-dissociation between nociception and pain suggests to them some "intermediate layer" of neural activity. The body–self neuromatrix originally presented by Ronald Melzack is presented as a possible model of this layer, and they argue that it is best understood as a general-purpose network. They discuss historical and contemporary attempts to identify distinct subregions or activity within this network as pain-specific – including work from Wager's own lab concerning a "pain signature." Against this, they support a "paradigm shift" towards thinking of pain as a family resemblance category for which there is not one, but instead a "palette of [neural] signatures." In the following two chapters, Irina A. Strigo and Arthur D. "Bud" Craig (Chapter 8) and Donald D. Price (Chapter 9) nonetheless argue for two influential, evidence-based definitions and models of pain. According to Strigo and

Craig, "pain in humans consists of a feeling and a motivation that reflects an adverse condition in the body which the homeostatic spinal and brainstem mechanisms can't rectify automatically and which urgently demands a behavioral response" (p. 104). They present evidence for a general-purpose homeostatic sensory system which, crucially, is interoceptive and not exteroceptive. Elements of this system are argued to "generate" pain along with all other bodily feelings and, indeed, all emotions. In explicit contrast, Price takes himself to offer a "more inclusive" understanding of pain which serves both interoceptive and exteroceptive functions. He presents his evidence and his contrasting understanding of the relevant neural architecture to argue for a "three-factor definition" of pain, according to which pains (necessarily and only jointly sufficiently) involve (1) particular sensations, (2) meanings of threat and intrusion attached to those sensations, and (3) unpleasant emotions resulting from those meaningful sensations. We shift gears as we proceed to Chapter 10 wherein Mick Thacker and Lorimer Moseley focus on chronic pain. After sketching the somatosensory system, the chapter discusses five pathophysiological mechanisms of chronic pain. Structural and functional neuroplasticity are identified as the keys to unlocking both what causes chronic pain and why it persists.

The distinction between neuroscientific and psychological models of pain is not sharp, and the relationship between these disciplines, and their approaches to pain, is undoubtedly deserving of a chapter (indeed, a volume) of its own. Nonetheless, these differences are exemplified by the differences in focus, aims, and models provided in Part I-III as against those offered in Part I-II.

Part I-III begins with Amanda C. de C. Williams' overview (Chapter 11) of the dominant psychotherapeutic models of pain, including their histories and their weaknesses. On Williams' telling, as initially noted above, psychological models of pain have arisen and developed largely in contrast to the failed "medical model" of pain, according to which pain is fully explained by tissue damage or pathology. Williams discusses three broad types of alternative models: behavioral; cognitive and combined cognitive–behavioral; and Third Wave (including Acceptance and Commitment Therapy and Mindfulness). She highlights the paucity of evidence for any one model and the difficulties in measuring pain outcomes. In the face of treatment inadequacy, she urges an evolutionary framework that better integrates the biological and social. Thomas Hadjistavropoulos focuses directly on biopsychosocial models in his Chapter 12. His overview involves highlighting both how these models are rooted in the gate-control theory of pain specifically and how they are related to biopsychosocial approaches to health and illness more generally. He provides a rich discussion of the evidence, applications, challenges, and possible developments of biopsychosocial models of pain, along with particular aspects of pain and related functioning. Both Willliams and Hadjistavropoulos, along with many others throughout the volume, decry dualistic assumptions as unduly complicating empirical investigations into pain; e.g., the assumption that there is a strict separation between the physical and mental or between the physiological and the psychological. Nowhere in the volume are dualistic assumptions such as these more directly criticized than by Mark D. Sullivan (Chapter 13), who urges a reconsideration of psychogenic pain that is freed of them. He provides a critical history of psychogenic pain and the current diagnostic situation wherein, he argues, diagnoses of psychogenic pain often merely stigmatize. Though other approaches (like those discussed in Williams' chapter) are argued to inadequately recognize or utilize the notion of psychogenic pain, Sullivan argues that the Explain Pain Program (further discussed in Chapter 33) is an example of an approach to pain and its treatment that has moved past dualistic thinking in the way that he is recommending. Potential for improved treatment likewise underlies Brianna Beck and Patrick Haggard's discussion (Chapter 14) of the causal interactions between (a) pain perception and processing; (b) voluntary action (where this includes the intention to act); and (c) the sense of agency, i.e., the feeling of control over one's actions and their sensory consequences. The authors discuss advances in our understanding of how these interact and, returning to a theme of Williams', relevant challenges for measuring outcomes. They raise a number of interesting questions and conclude with an explicit discussion of the possible implications of the interactive effects between (a)–(c) for the treatment of pain.

Section II: Theoretical implications – why does pain matter, theoretically?

This section provides the reader with a sample of pain-related inquiries in paradigmatically theoretical areas of philosophy.

The section is divided into three parts:

II-I Pain in philosophy of mind
II-II Pain in epistemology
II-III Pain in philosophy of religion.

As many of the views in Section I model pain as at least involving a mental episode, the relevance of pain for inquiries in the philosophy of mind is perhaps the most obvious. Part II-I begins with Paula Droege (Chapter 15) taking up questions of pain in non-human animals. To answer these questions, she offers a functionalist approach which she applies to pain, responses to pain, and the consciousness of pain across the animal kingdom. She argues that ethical questions about the pains of non-human animals should likewise be answered through functionalist considerations. In continuing to think about the possible pains of non-humans, in Chapter 16 Pete Mandik takes up the question of whether robots (broadly understood) can feel pain, i.e., consciously suffer pain from the first-person perspective. He adapts classic thought experiments from the philosophy of mind to argue, respectively, for both a negative and positive answer. These he evaluates before siding with the positive answer and the argument for it. His evaluations turn on considerations of what we can conclude about how things *are* on the basis of how they *seem* from the first person (and vice versa). His considerations are bolstered by his reading of higher-order thought theories of consciousness, leading us into David Pereplyotchik's Chapter 17 where the relationship between pain and consciousness is taken up directly. Pereplyotchik argues that pains can occur non-consciously. He canvasses different theories of consciousness, honing in on the two which he considers to be most plausible: global workspace and higher-order theories. These are compared and contrasted by their adequacy in accounting for cases involving mistakes or misrepresentations of pain that Pereplyotchik takes to support the case for non-conscious pains. Murat Aydede, in seeming contrast, argues in Chapter 18 that to feel a pain is always to introspect. Reminiscent again of Hardcastle's opening puzzle (Chapter 1) but now not just for pain but for *feeling* pain, Aydede asks: "Am I perceiving something in my elbow when I feel a pain there? Or am I engaged in some form of introspection about my awareness of something there?" (p. 221) While the perceptual view is supported by our practice of locating pains in bodily parts, Aydede argues that epistemic considerations decisively support the introspection view. In particular, Aydede argues that one is not wrong about whether they feel a pain in their elbow even if there is no damage there, but if to feel a pain was to perceive a pain, then one *would* be wrong in such a case. Our practice of locating pains remains to be explained, and he offers such an explanation by appeal to the ways in which pain experiences involve sensory attributions.

In Section II-II we turn to face epistemological questions squarely. Jonathan Cohen and Matthew Fulkerson (Chapter 19) begin with a focus on pain and rationality, considering the ways in which pains might either provide or be responsive to reasons. They raise some potential problems for pains' reason-providing role and ultimately argue that pains are "sticky" in the face of countervailing evidence in ways that other reason-providing states are not. They offer a discussion of the rational evaluability of pain, concluding that the available evidence is suggestive but insufficient to settle the matter. In continuing comparison of the epistemology of pain as against other types of mental states, Peter Langland-Hassan begins his chapter (Chapter 20) by noting that despite his skepticism about incorrigibility in general, he has concluded that it is not straightforward whether or not we are incorrigible about our pains in particular. By "incorrigible" Langland-Hassan means infallible, such that (a) whenever we believe we are in pain, we are in pain and (b) whenever we believe we are not in pain, we are not in pain. He considers and refutes a number of arguments for and against incorrigibility, before concluding by discussing the possibility that pains are incorrigible because they are assessment-dependent. On this view, it is necessary and sufficient for one being in pain that one believes they are in an unpleasant sensory state. In Chapter 21 we move from beliefs about our own pains, to beliefs about the pains of others. Frédérique de Vignemont here considers whether we can have perceptual knowledge of another's pain and, if so, how. She develops and defends an evaluative model of third-person pain perception, explicitly inspired by evaluative accounts of unpleasant pain (as in Chapter 3). De Vignemont argues that we directly perceive "warning properties": "properties of objects or events that occur either in personal or peripersonal space, to which the perceptual system ascribes a negative value because they indicate the high probability of something bad happening to the body." On her offered model, these perceptions of warning properties ground the direct epistemic awareness that something bad is happening to the person perceived, which in turn grounds the indirect epistemic awareness that a person is (or will be) in pain. Hilla Jacobson's Chapter 22 shifts the focus to pain and cognitive penetrability, i.e., to the question of whether the phenomenal character of pain may be influenced by cognitive states in particularly interesting ways, as further specified. After characterizing cognitive penetrability and applying it to pain, Jacobson provides some initial considerations for an affirmative answer, but leaves the question open. Pain is then yet again compared with sensory perception (in particular, visual perception) to yield a rich discussion of the epistemic and practical implications that would follow if pain is cognitively penetrable.

In our final theoretical part, Section II-III, we consider pain in the context of the philosophy of religion. In Chapter 23, Ariel Glucklich provides an overview, spanning multiple religious traditions, of the various ways in which pains (both voluntary and non-voluntary) are evaluated and modeled as positive. His discussion encompasses historical and contemporary cases, with a particular focus on pains that are self-inflicted during religious rituals. In Palden Gyal and Owen Flanagan's Chapter 24, we focus on the role of pain in Buddhism. The authors provide an account of existential suffering in the Buddhist world view, where it is taken to play a fundamental role, and the proposed method for alleviating it. Some implications for ethics are then identified, including a resultant notion of compassion. Turning from human pain and suffering as understood by religion, we turn to consider whether the divine reality, as posited by religion, is capable of feeling pain. In taking up this question (Chapter 25), Trent Dougherty canvasses a range of religious traditions, before focusing on the Christian tradition. It is the Christian tradition for which an answer to the question of whether the divine reality feels pain is most ambiguous, since the divine reality is there taken also to be both personal and human. Structuring the debate around recent work by Linda Zagzebski on omnisubjectivity (omniscience concerning "what it is like" for other creatures), Dougherty considers arguments both for and against the Christian divinity feeling pain, before ending with an injunction for further work. In the context of pain, the omniscience of the Christian divinity is more traditionally associated with the problem of evil, and in Chapter 26 Steve Layman offers a rich discussion of this traditional problem. Layman explains how the very existence of pain has been construed as an objection to traditional monotheism. After discussing other responses to this problem and their weaknesses, he advocates what he calls a "comparative response," according to which traditional monotheism is not explanatorily worse off than its philosophical rivals. Taking philosophical naturalism to be its dominant rival, Layman pursues this strategy, arguing that the naturalist has inadequate resources for explaining mental causation in general, and the causal role of pain in particular. After rebutting the objection that the traditional monotheist cannot adequately explain mental causation either, he concludes by noting that while pain is often considered a problem for the traditional monotheist, it is thus likewise a significant problem for the philosophical naturalist.

Section III: Practical implications – why does pain matter, practically?

This section provides the reader with a sample of pain-related inquiries in paradigmatically practical areas of philosophy.

This section is also divided into three parts:

III-I Pain in ethics
III-II Pain in medicine
III-III Pain in law

Part III-I focuses on the role of pain in a wide range of ethical topics. Two themes unite the part: considering the ethical relevance of pain as against some wider range of negative experiences and consideration of the badness of pain. Olivier Massin takes up both of these themes in his Chapter 27 when arguing for what he calls an *axiological theory of pain*. On this view, pains are bodily episodes that are bad in some way, as further specified. The view is contrasted with dominant positions (explicitly including evaluativism, as in Chapter 3) that take pain to be mental and non-axiological; on the current view, pain is instead non-mental and axiological. Massin argues that this axiological view provides additional resources for addressing – yet again – a puzzle akin to Hardcastle's (Chapter 1): whether pain is a perception or an object of perception. While pain is firmly held by Massin to be an object of perception, its perception-like features are argued to be explicable by its axiological features. Further explanatory gains are argued to be made by distinguishing pain (non-mental) from suffering (mental). In Michael Davis's Chapter 28, this distinction comes to the fore in his argument that an adequate understanding of torture requires focusing on suffering and not merely physical pain. He proceeds to defend an agent-centered definition of torture that emphasizes (a) the torturer's power over the tortured and (b) the torturer's intention to make the tortured suffer. He contrasts his approach and definition with their rivals, while identifying similarities and differences between torture and punishment. This latter contrast is thrown into yet sharper relief when in the next chapter (Chapter 29) we focus on those pains inflicted by authorities that are incurred during learning and education. Avi I. Mintz dubs these "educational pains" or the "pains of learning" and takes them to encompass a wide range of negative experiences. After reviewing different cultural and philosophical ideas about educational pains, Mintz discusses how to distinguish the "necessary, valuable or inevitable" educational pains and the role that both teachers and parents can play in fostering "productive responses" to them. We continue to consider the relationship between pains and learning, but from a different angle, when Robert Cowan asks whether pains can immediately justify evaluative beliefs (Chapter 30), i.e., whether and how pains could be the source of our justification for believing things about values, without any inferential support from other beliefs. He explicitly considers this question through the lens of evaluative approaches to pain (again, as in Chapter 3), with a nuanced consideration of the kind of evaluative content that pains may have and the epistemologies according to which they may then immediately justify evaluative beliefs. Inspired by Hutcheson, he closes by considering the possibility and candidate epistemologies of "moral pains" using this evaluativist framework.

While there is a sense in which every chapter in the volume concerns pain in medicine, Section III-II offers a brief but direct focus on pain in medical practice. We begin (Chapter 31) by looking at the definition of pain offered by the International Association for the Study of Pain (IASP), which Andrew Wright reminds us was explicitly intended for use in the clinic. He provides an introduction to the history, utility, and meaning of this influential and important definition and its controversial accompanying note. He argues that these (the definition and its note) are inadequate for taxonomic purposes – purposes which he explicitly characterizes as distinct from clinical purposes. In particular, Wright argues that the definition fails to pick out all and only pains, and it is likewise for this reason that he notes that philosophers should be "very wary" of drawing conclusions from it about pain's nature. He argues that it was the IASP's attempt to offer a definition of pain appropriate for *both* taxonomic and clinical purposes that underwrites its taxonomic failings, and that its endurance despite these failings is explained by its clinical utility. In continuing to think about the realities of the clinic, Chapter 32 focuses on placebo analgesia. With special focus on pain, Daniel E. Moerman argues that it is the *meaning* of an otherwise inert treatment that can best explain so-called "placebo effects," which are thus best understood as "meaning responses." Numerous examples of the target effects, both historical and contemporary, are provided. Moerman stresses that his meaning approach circumvents some of the ethical questions surrounding the administration of so-called placebos: since all administered treatments mean something to the patient, meaning is relevant to all treatment outcomes. The part ends with an overview of pain management (Chapter 33) offered by Carolyn Berryman, Mark Catley, and Lorimer Moseley. They begin by noting that despite pain's evident complexity, the clinical management of pain nonetheless requires a framework. They thus provide a rich and wide-ranging introductory assessment of the measures, screening tools, and strategies currently available. The chapter admirably highlights the practical realities, challenges, and importance of managing pain.

The volume concludes in Part III-III with a focus on pain in the law. Ben A. Rich first offers us an overview (Chapter 34); more specifically, an overview of the role of pain and suffering in tort law in the Anglo-American juridical tradition. It is a broad topic and Rich provides a wide survey, with three main issues receiving particular attention: pain and suffering as the basis for non-economic damages in tort law; laws related to opioid prescription and use; and the role of law in end of life care. Laws surrounding pain-relieving substances, such as opioids, are the focus of the following chapter (Chapter 35). Sunil Kumar Aggarwal and Katherine Pettus there discuss not only the legal practices as such, but the related social, political, and clinical practices. They argue that historical and current regulations are contributors to the "global pandemic of untreated pain." The chapter as a whole presents a sustained argument in favor of a "paradigm shift" on drug control policy that is argued to be already under way: from an old paradigm involving unduly restrictive regulations to a new paradigm that facilitates pain-relieving substances becoming more available to the people who need them. In continuing to think about the relationship between laws and norms, Stuart W.G. Derbyshire next argues (Chapter 36) that settling the issue of fetal pain will resolve neither the moral nor legal questions concerning abortion. Derbyshire presents a history of abortion laws in the United States and the United Kingdom and contrasts their differential relationships to the science of fetal pain. He provides an introduction to the relevant science, highlighting the ways in which the empirical facts require, and receive, interpretation for application to legal and moral questions. We conclude by thinking about the role of pain in end of life care through Daniel Weinstock's chapter (Chapter 37) on physician-assisted death. Weinstock begins by noting that the discussion has been moving from the general question of its ethical permissibility to specific questions concerning its best regulatory frameworks. His chapter accordingly focuses on the distinctive role that pain and suffering may play in these frameworks in both qualifying and disqualifying agents to request physician-assisted death.

3 Conclusion

This volume thus first provides an overview of advances and current controversies about the nature of pain in philosophy, neuroscience, and psychology, followed by chapters that exemplify pain's relevance for additional theoretical and practical inquiries. It is my hope that bringing these chapters together will contribute to the interdisciplinary and multidisciplinary work needed to advance our understanding of pain in philosophy, across the academy, and in the "real world."

In compiling this volume and in my own study of pains, it is not their similarities which strike me, but their differences. As in the cases initially offered and as attested in the following chapters: pains vary widely in how they are caused and what they cause. How a pain is felt and reported differs across people, times, places, and circumstances. For most of us, most of the time, getting chili powder in your eye will involve pain. But, sometimes it doesn't. Why? For most of us, a wrenched ankle will heal. But, sometimes it doesn't. Why? For most of us, aspirin will help a headache. But: sometimes it doesn't. And so on. An adequate theory of pain, it seems to me, needs to do justice to this variation.

The reader perusing the following chapters will perhaps be similarly struck not only by the wide variation in pains, but by the variation in the theories of pain's nature that are currently on offer. The present volume is a testament to the fact that philosophers do not agree whether pain is a type of bodily episode or a mental episode – much less do they agree about which type of bodily or mental episode it might be or the role that pains play in epistemology, ethics, and so on. While one may expect philosophers to be a contentious bunch, the evidenced disagreement across the sciences may perhaps be more surprising. As presented in Parts I-II and I-III, pains are modeled as being massively complex, involving multiple parallel lines of processing. Beyond that agreement, however, disagreement continues; there is disagreement about how pain is best conceptualized and which pathways, areas, and neurochemicals may be either necessary or sufficient for pain. A wide range of scientific models thus remain offered and disputed.

Of course, there are some similarities across pains and the dominant models and theories of them, and a good theoretician will make much of these. The progress we are making, and the things about which we currently agree, are important. These, too, are in evidence. But notice that similarities across pains and our models thereof are what we should expect. If there are pains, then we should expect – at least eventually – to be able to figure out what they are. We should expect – at least eventually – to be able to explain and predict them and to understand their role in our overall mental and physical economies. We should also expect this understanding to – at least eventually – yield adequate treatment.

As acknowledged and lamented time and again throughout this volume, pain treatment remains woefully inadequate.

Improving pain treatment is a crucial reason that it matters whether we arrive at an understanding of pain that does justice not only to the similarities across its instances, but the differences. It is individual people that arrive at the clinic presenting with pain. Adequate treatment requires recognizing not only the ways in which their pain is paradigmatic, but the ways in which it is idiosyncratic.

While all treatment is arguably appropriately individually tailored, pain is unique in being the only medical problem for which the diagnostic gold standard is the report. Doctors are thus advised to take pain to be whatever and however the patient says it is. This makes pain *unlike* other conditions for which treatment needs to be individually tailored, e.g., diabetes, cancer, or schizophrenia. Indeed, it makes pain unlike any other medical condition. Unlike these other conditions and despite thousands of years of research, we collectively remain without a valid, biological marker in the body or brain for pain. Nothing has yet been correlated with pain reports that will serve as an effective treatment target. We are left with the report and the sufferer.

In thinking about the advances and the similarities, we may optimistically hold that our understanding of pain, informed by both theoretical and practical inquiries, will progress such that we identify something which we can target for adequate treatment. We may expect that we will ultimately arrive at an identification of pain that involves general identifications of its causes and consequences, providing increasingly accurate predictions and explanations. Because pains are real, one might take for granted that such an understanding – at least eventually – is forthcoming.

Perhaps.

In my own view, however, we now know enough about the variation in pain experiences to make *this kind* of identification unlikely. Though I do not argue for it here, my own position is that each pain results from the convergent activity of multiple mechanisms and that the remarkable idiosyncrasy of this convergence undermines prediction and explanation across all pains that is useful for treatment. As initially noted, multiple components make up a paradigmatic pain: damage, registration of that damage, an unpleasant feeling, and the motivations and actions in response to both the feeling and the damage. I maintain that the mechanistic activities involved in each of these components combine so idiosyncratically on different occasions that our best explanations and predictions – in particular, for treatment purposes – will involve differentially targeting the particular mechanisms which may be involved in any particular case.

Anton Chekhov wrote, "When a lot of remedies are suggested for a disease, that means it can't be cured." I submit that we may never find a universal panacea for all pain. Not because pain is spooky, but because in attempting to cure pain as such we have perhaps set our sights in the wrong place. Pain, as such, may not be a disease entity.

In closing, then, I draw the readers' attention to (a) the profound variation across pains; (b) the profound variation in the theories of the nature of pain; and (c) the profound inadequacies of pain treatment. While I do not here argue for my own explanation of these, I ask that as the reader encounters evidence of (a)–(c) in this volume, they consider whether it may be best explained by the fact that a one-size-fits-all identification of the nature of pain is unlikely to be forthcoming. Whatever one makes of this idea, it should be agreed on all sides that our theories of the nature of pain need to be consistent with the realities of pains as we find them.

It is against this background that I invite the reader to peruse the following chapters and come to their own conclusion about what pain is and to ever consider this question in the light of the theoretical and practical realities for which pains matter. As we continue to collaborate to better understand pain, let us remember that it is real people who suffer from it.

SECTION I

THE NATURE OF PAIN

What is pain?

PART I-I

Modeling pain in philosophy

1

A BRIEF AND POTTED OVERVIEW ON THE PHILOSOPHICAL THEORIES OF PAIN

Valerie Gray Hardcastle

Common-sense views of pain analogize it to perception (Aydede 2005b). We see the face of a loved one, or a sprig of basil in the market, and we recognize them as such by their color, size, shape, arrangement of features, and so on. Our perceptual system interacts with our memory and other cognitive systems so that we can readily name and understand our percepts as being about things in the world. So too with pain, or so we normally think. We feel a twinge in our left shoulder, and we interpret it as indicating damage to our tissues where the pain is felt. In both cases, we perceive sensible qualities that, in collaboration with our cognitive systems, tell us about the state of the world. Our assertion that we see basil there on the display table depends upon our perceiving it as such. But what about the case of pain? What makes our assertion that we feel pain true? It turns out that the answer is complicated.

Pain is a weird phenomenon. We can often feel pain where there is (apparently) no injury. The pain in our left shoulder could be due to a shoulder injury, but it could also be a heart attack, in which case our pain is being referred from the chest to another location. Intuitively, we perhaps think that the pain is in our hearts – that is where the tissue damage is – but the sensation of pain locates the dysfunction in our shoulder. Readers are probably familiar by now with instances of phantom limb pain, an extreme example of this case. Folks missing a limb, an arm or a leg, often feel pain that seems to be located in the missing extremity. Obviously, there is no pain there, but the felt pain seems real nonetheless. (It isn't a delusion, for example.)

What makes these examples challenging is not their weirdness, but that the sensation of pain also appears, to some anyway, to be completely private, subjective, and incorrigible (cf. Kripke 1980; Chapter 20, this volume). If we are unsure about whether we are seeing basil, we can always ask our neighbor to take a look and confirm our suspicions. But we cannot do that with pain. I cannot ask my neighbor to perceive my pain and let me know whether it is referred or not. In addition, there does not seem to be any way to have a pain yet not feel it. To be in pain is to feel pain. Finally, we are each our own authority on whether we are in pain. If I think I am in pain, then I am in pain. There is no appearance/ reality distinction. Pain and the sensation of pain is the same thing. But if this is true, then how do we explain referred pains, cases in which our sensation of pain is misleading? How can we be wrong about something that is essentially subjective and private?

And this puzzle is one reason why philosophy is interested in pain. What sort of thing is pain such that it can seem private, subjective, and infallible, on the one hand, yet refer to things in the world about which we can be mistaken, on the other? How is it that pain is both a sort of experience, but also the object of our experience? Philosophers want to sort this out.[1]

1 Representationalism

The most common response by philosophers by far has been to accept that pain represents something in the world; it is not just a free-floating sensation. Modern conceptions of this view date back to Franz Brentano (1874, 1907), who held that pain is an emotion, which is intentionally directed to a sensed content. By asserting that pain is an emotion, a complex internal perception of sorts that gives rise to aversion, he believed that it would not fall prey to the difficulty of explaining how it could be incorrigible – we could not be wrong about feeling a pain any more than we could be wrong about feeling sad. In contrast to external experiences, which ascribe perceptions of external "sense-qualities" like color to intentional objects, pain is an internal affective experience, which, according to Brentano, just is an indubitable internal perception (Brentano 1907: 121; see also discussion in Geniusas 2014).

Following the science of the day (cf. Titchener 1973/1908), Brentano also believed that pain was psychical in nature, not physical. Of course, Brentano's views on intentionality qua psychical phenomenon[2] raise many of the well-known difficulties attached to sense-data views of mentality, which I shall not rehearse here. Suffice it to say, it becomes very difficult to attach a mental object to the physical body in a principled fashion, which is what one needs for pain to be aligned with damage to the person. Consequently, contemporary representationalists generally opt for physicalist interpretations of pain.

Armstrong (1962, 1968) and Pitcher (1970) were early proponents of contemporary versions of this view and advocated a form of perceptualism (see also Newton 1989; Wilkes 1977).[3] In contrast to Brentano's view of pain as an indubitable emotion, Armstrong and Pitcher held that pain tells us that a part of our body is in a "damaged, bruised, irritated, or pathological state" (Armstrong 1968: 371). What is essential about this perspective is that pain is, or is analogous to, perception. It gives us information about our world, just as our (other) perceptual systems do.

Contemporary representationalism comes in many flavors. More recent accounts include Bain (2003), Byrne (2001), Davis (1982), Dretske (1995, 1999, 2003), Hall (1989), Harman (1990), Kahane (2007), Lycan (1981), O'Sullivan and Schroer (2012), Seager (2002), Shoemaker (1975a, 1975b, 1981), and Tye (1996, 1997). They all start by accepting the perceptual nature of pain, but then (in its purest form) go on to claim that the informational content of the perception exhausts its phenomenal content. Or, put another way, they start with the view that the qualitative character of pain is nothing over and above the content, "Damaged tissue here!" They are, as Tye (1997) puts it, "*sensory* representations of tissue damage" (333, italics his). That is, a pain is a feeling, which might engender dislike for the feeling, as well as telling us that something is potentially wrong in a particular bodily region. Proponents of these accounts generally just flatly deny that knowledge of pain is incorrigible, despite how it might intuitively seem. We can misrepresent pain – we can miss its location; we could mistake it for another type of experience; we could even have unconscious pains, and so there is nothing fundamentally subjective or private about this type of experience at all.

One can then branch off from the basic structure of a representationalist account of pain, arguing, for example, that the content includes more than just a location for tissue damage; it might also include in its content that such damage is bad (e.g., Bain 2011; Cutter and Tye 2011; see also Chapter 3, this volume), or that the region needs to be protected (e.g., Hall 2008; Klein 2007, 2015; Martínez 2011; see also Chapter 4, this volume), or that it is part of a larger intensity-indicating system (Gray 2014). It might even deny that damage per se is part of the content. But in each instance, the fundamental touchstone is that pain sensation is an information-bearing state. One way to understand these variations is in terms of where one draws the line around the states of affairs associated with pain. We have tissue damage, its possibility, and its aftermath; a negative reaction to the events; and an impulse to protect or nurse the damaged area. Different philosophers include different permutations or subsets of these states under their definition of pain; the remainder then becomes a reaction or response to the primary event.

Objections to this view are numerous and strong (see also Chapter 2, this volume). Most of them boil down to the contention that, while pain may or may not be representational, there is also a phenomenal character to pain that exists over and above any content. It is a sensation as much as, or more than, it is a representation. McGinn (1997) puts this sentiment in stark terms: "Bodily sensations do not have an intentional object in the way perceptual experiences do. We distinguish between a visual experience and what it is an experience of; but we do not make this distinction in respect of pains" (8), as does Rorty (1980): Pains "do not represent, they are not *about* anything" (22, italics his).

Of course, McGinn and Rorty are expressing their opinion here and not giving an actual argument. But this does demonstrate the clash of intuitions here: one side believes that pains are *about* things; the other does not. To be fair, McGinn's and others' (cf. Block 1995: 234; Gillett 1991; Grahek 1991; Jacobson 2013; Kripke 1980; O'Shaughnessy 1980; Searle 1992) intuitions are that the sensation of pain is what itself hurts or is bad; the hurtiness is not some cognitive reaction to a sensation. In contrast, a representationalist view denies that there can be a sensation of pain beyond the representational content. The representation just is the sensation of pain.

There is an additional challenge that at least some representationalists need to confront. If the phenomenal character of pain just is representational content then it seems that in order to be aware of pain, one has to appreciate what it represents. For if there is nothing to pain over and above its representational content, then there is no pain in any meaningful sense without having the concepts that pain represents available. Either those contents are innate (cf. Tye 2005), which is unlikely, given what we know about cognitive development, or we cannot have the phenomenal experience of pain prior to our having knowledge of what it represents. This too seems unlikely to some (cf. Allen 2004). (To others, it might not seem so improbable. Small children, for example, are often unsure how much it hurts when injured.)

2 The phenomenology of pain

That representationalism means that we cannot experience pain without knowing or being aware of some content raises some phenomenological difficulties. For example, if something like the representational view is true, then how is it that a pain can wake you up while you are soundly asleep? This is an experience I assume most of the readers have had (if not by now, then you will before old age, I can practically guarantee). However, if you have no awareness of tissue damage while you are sleeping (because you are asleep) and hence cannot represent contents to yourself about your environment, how is it that a pain can intrude upon your slumber, as they apparently sometimes do? It would seem that we would have to know and not know that we are in pain at the same time.

Dartnell (2001) argues that this can only happen because we can have a sensation and yet not know that we are having that sensation. The pain was there while you were asleep, even though you were not aware of it. He explains it thus: "Being present *in* consciousness is not the same as being present *to* consciousness. The pain sensation that woke you up was *in* your consciousness but not present *to* your consciousness" (96, italics his). In other words, Dartnell denies representational views of pain, in which to be in pain is to know that you have tissue damage (and maybe that such damage hurts or that you should nurse it), and supports a traditional sense-data sort of empiricism that identifies basic knowledge with experience itself. This phenomenological view of pain (and other bodily sensations) appears to support the old Myth of the Given (Sellars 1963), that pain is just a raw feel, a quale. But, as a further step, to know that we are in pain, to feel the pain qua pain, means that we have cloaked that raw feel in a conceptualization of pain, and that conceptualization has made it into our conscious awareness and we have recognized it as such. But the pain itself, the thing that wakes us up, is just the bare sensation.

This view of pain as (conscious) sensation traces its roots back to the phenomenological movement and Husserl's *Logical Investigations* (Husserl 1984/1901), which provides the first explicit discussion of pain in the phenomenological literature (cf. Geniusas 2014). In contrast to his teacher and mentor Brentano, Husserl believed that there could be feelings without intentionality. Following Stumpf (1907), he called these "feeling-sensations." Pain was a prime example of such a phenomenon. Feeling-sensations are feelings that we do not ascribe to an object of experience, as we might the feeling of pleasure to seeing a sunset, but to the subject of experience, the person feeling the pain. In that sense, pains lack intentionality.

At the same time, Husserl also believed that pain was intentional – it has a dual nature. We can transform feeling-sensations into something contentful by interpreting it, by conceptualizing it as a pain with a particular location, for example:

> our sensations here receive an objective "interpretation" … . They themselves are not acts, but acts are constituted through them, wherever, that is, intentional char-acters like a perceptual interpretation lay hold of them, and as it were animate them. In just this manner it seems that a burning, piercing, boring pain, fused as it is from the start with certain tactual sensations, must itself count as a sensation. It functions at least as other sensations do, in providing a foothold for empirical, objective interpretations.
>
> *(Husserl 1984/1901: 406, as quoted in Geniusas 2014: 12)*

Pain then is a complex experience, both a simple feeling-sensation and an intentional object of experience.

Other philosophers have not ignored the importance of characterizing the complexity inherent in our pain experiences correctly (Aydede and Güzeldere 2002; see also Savage 1970), nor have pain researchers (Fields 1999; Price 1988, 2000). As Aydede and Güzeldere comment:

> In the case of pain experience, it is most often the experience itself that we are most immediately "presented with" and concerned about. That is, our immediate epistemic and practical focus is different in ordinary perception and in pain. Notice

that this is true even if we construe pain experiences in entirely representational or intentional terms ... . Our immediate interest remains focused on the experience itself as indicated by the fact that we name the experience itself "pain," and talk about it when we talk about our pains, rather than apply "pain" to the objects of the pain experience – if it has one.

(S269)

If we are going to understand pain with any depth, whether philosophically or scientifically, then we are going to have to understand its subjective elements. The International Association for the Study of Pain's definition of pain recognizes this fact as well: "Pain is always subjective. ... [It is] always a subjective state" (IASP 1986: 250; see also Chapter 31). A successful analysis of pain has to be sensitive to the phenomenological feel of pain, in all its multifarious glory, as well as perhaps the objective states associated with pain. The challenge, of course, is how to do this without falling prey to the Myth of the Given, without making pain qualia into something either inefficacious or mysterious.

3 Eliminativism

As you can see, there are several things philosophers have attributed to pain: the pure sensation (albeit a complex subjective experience), the realization of tissue damage, the awfulness of the hurt, and the tendency to nurse. Different philosophers put different collections of these items into the bucket labeled pain. The question is: which ones really belong and which ones do not? Despite lots of effort, philosophical analyses and argumentation do not seem to answer this query definitively. Indeed, they do not even seem to be coming into reflective equilibrium around a constellation of ideas or proposals.

The diagnosis that some give for why philosophy has failed so spectacularly is that there just is no such thing as pain as philosophers (or the common folk) conceive of it (Averill 1990; Dennett 1978; Hardcastle 1997, 1999; see also Corns 2014). Our intuitions are simply confused: we apparently simultaneously believe that pain is private, subjective, and incorrigible, and that we can be mistaken about it.[4] Something has to give. A potent suggestion is that the concept itself must go.

This is not to say that there is no such thing as being in pain or feeling pain or having an unpleasant reaction to tissue damage, or any other descriptor that one might attach to the idea of pain. Rather, it is that our folk concept of pain, like many of our folk concepts, is vague and fragile. It is good enough to get the job done in everyday life, but if you push on it very hard, it crumples quite easily (though see the section below for a discussion of recent empirical research into exactly what our folk concept of pain amounts to).

So what do we replace the folk concept with, if we accept that all the component pieces philosophers have associated with pain exist? Hardcastle advocates understanding pain as a neurobiological process, on analogy with our perceptual systems. We can readily agree that shape, motion, and color are processed in different areas of the brain and that sometimes we can be mistaken about any one of these or any combination of them (cf. Treisman and Gelade 1980). We simply take these facts to indicate that vision is complicated and is processed in many areas of the brain. Indeed, scientists have identified more than twenty areas associated with processing visual stimuli (of course, how many areas we think we have depends a great deal on how we think an area should be defined). Moreover, if we lose our ability to process color, for example, we do not then conclude that we cannot see or that vision is located in our eyeballs or even that philosophers need to wade in to explain what is wrong with our concept of vision. Instead, we recognize vision as a perceptual process that begins at the periphery in our retinas, travels via our thalamus to V1, then V2, then V4 or V6, and so on, until it culminates in our frontal areas as we use the processed stimuli to shape our decisions and our actions. As all this is going on, our brain is also feeding relevant information back into our visual processing system as well as siphoning information off as it travels around. At this point in the twenty-first century, we do not find any of these descriptions about our visual processes very shocking, nor do we find them confusing. Why should pain processing be any different?

We know now that incoming nociceptive information activates many different areas of the brain – much more than the original sensory-discriminative/affective dichotomy (cf. Part I–II of this volume) would suggest. Major regions of the nervous system that react to pain information include the dorsal horn, reticular formation, thalamus, amygdala, insula, anterior cingulate gyrus, posterior cingulate cortex, posterior parietal cortex, supplemental motor cortex, prefrontal cortex, and the cerebellum. Moreover, just as information is fed back into our visual system as information moves up it, so too is it in our pain processing system. We have a pain inhibitory system that can override our conscious sensations of or affective reactions to pain. This system includes at least the frontal cortex, hypothalamus, periaqueductal gray region, and dorsal raphe nuclei. (The pain inhibitory system explains why athletes can continue to play and soldiers can continue to fight even when injured; they do not notice that they are hurt because their pain responses are damped down.) I list all these areas to illustrate that pain processing is indeed very complicated, just as visual processing is. Perhaps, just as scientists use the word "vision" to refer to the entire neurophysiological and neuropsychological processing system for visual stimuli, so too perhaps should philosophers use the word "pain" to refer to the entire neurophysiological and neuropsychological system used to process nociceptive stimuli. The conscious percept or the quale of pain then becomes only a tiny subset of our pain processing system; it is not even the most important component of pain processing.

This sort of eliminativism of folk notions of pain has as its intellectual neighbors philosophers who advocate for psychofunctionalist views of pain, who may or may not consider themselves eliminativists (Aydede and Fulkerson submitted; Connee 1984; Graham and Stephens 1985; Kaufman 1985; Nelkin 1986, 1994). Psychofunctionalists about pain capitalize on the fact that pain seems inextricably linked to a group of behaviors and psychological reactions: we jerk our hand off the hot stove; we protect our wounds; we dislike pain and wish it would stop – and so on. This suite of causal roles connected to pain would then define what pain is. Pain is just the thing that causes all the typical reactions to pain. But, perhaps unlike traditional functionalist accounts in philosophy of mind, these psychofunctionalists are content to let the empirical sciences outline what the true causal (or other) connections are between pain and other physical and mental states and whether they are at a personal level (wishing pain would stop) or the subpersonal level (increased firing in the anterior cingulate). The model of pain described by our best science also describes pain's nature. Beyond that, psychofunctionalists believe, philosophers need not worry.

Of course, taking this approach means that the original concerns that brought pain to philosophy's attention are essentially ignored, for we have no guarantee that science will answer the question regarding how it is that pain can be incorrigible, subjective, and private, yet we can be mistaken about whether we are in pain, where the pain is located, why the pain is there, or what the pain is like. Indeed, we have no guarantee that science would even recognize the question as something deserving of an answer. Perhaps there should remain a place at the table for philosophers after all.

4 Folk conceptions of pain

Of course, all the above philosophical arguments rest on the assumption that folk views of pain are problematic in that we believe a person who feels a pain really is in pain, so it seems a mental phenomenon, and that pain is located somewhere in the body, where tissue is damaged, so it seems something external to the mind. However, a recent ingenious analysis of how people actually use the word pain suggests that the "folk" are not as incoherent as it may appear at first blush. Reuter (2011) ran a statistical analysis of online searches that showed that the intensity of pain people feel has a significant effect on whether they say that they "feel a pain" (lower intensities) or "have a pain" (higher intensities). We can perhaps index "feeling pain" with an introspective report of a mental state and "having pain" as an objective statement about bodily harm. One word, but with two different uses, depending on circumstance.

Reuter argues that the intensity that we experience properties as having, such as saltiness, loudness, or color, affects how confident we are in judging whether objects really have these properties (see also Lund 1926). "A low degree of confidence will often lead people to make introspective statements, making claims about the way things appear to them ('the shirt looks blue') rather than ascribing it to non-mental objects ('the shirt is blue')" (2). If the soup is mildly salty, then we politely note that, "it tastes salty to me." In other words, we make a comment about our mental state. However, if the soup is extremely salty, then we declare with confidence, "the soup is salty." Here, we comment upon an objective fact about the external world. The more confidence we have in a putative fact, the more likely we are to ascribe it as a property of an object instead of as an appearance of an object (cf. Quinton 1956).[5] Reuter suggests that this correlation between low signal intensity and introspection pervades all sensory modalities, as well as our pain processing system, and he has amassed some data to support this hypothesis. Looking at what it is that we search for on the Internet, he shows that we are much more likely to pair "feel" with a little, small, slight, or minor pain and "have" with severe, major, bad, or big pain.

Perhaps, our common folk expressions of pain do account for its complex nature. It is interesting to note that this more sophisticated (and empirically based) view of what we mean by our pain expressions dovetails fairly well with the biological complexity we find in pain processing, as adumbrated by Hardcastle. Perhaps the original problem that drove philosophers to contemplate the nature of pain was not actually a real problem – the folk already had a way to manage the apparent inconsistencies in their notions of pain as something both subjective and objective. It might be that philosophers invented their own problem of pain to solve, and have now conceptually come full circle.

Related topics

Acknowledgements

My sincere thanks to my research assistant Vincente Raja Galian for all his work in helping me collect and organize the references and to Jennifer Corns for her advice on how to make this chapter manageable.

Notes

1 Descartes himself gave a response to this puzzle in his *Principles* (Descartes 1983/1644). He suggested that the experience of pain was clear but not distinct. As a clear experience, it was indubitable, but as an experience that could be indistinct, one could confuse it with sensations in other parts of the body. Hence, we could never be wrong that we are in pain even though we might be mistaken about the pain's bodily location.

2 "Every mental phenomenon is characterized by what the Scholastics of the Middle Ages called the intentional (or mental) inexistence of an object, and what we might call, though not wholly unambiguously, reference to a content, direction toward an object (which is not to be understood here as meaning a thing), or immanent objectivity. Every mental phenomenon includes something as object within itself" (Brentano 1874: 88).

3 Evans (2007) argues persuasively that Plato anticipated these views in the *Philebus*.

4 This is ignoring the other problems associated with our concept of pain, discussed elsewhere in chapters throughout this book, in which we apparently can be in pain but not have it hurt or we can damage our tissues severely and not notice, and so on. But these problems too should give us pause in accepting our folk notion of pain as something coherent.

5 In contrast, Wilfred Sellars (1956) argues that our language for perceptible qualities cannot be reduced to or replaced by descriptors of physical objects and their interactions. Secondary qualities, in particular, exist only as subjective states.

References

Allen, C. (2004) Animal pain. *Noûs* 38: 617–643.

Armstrong, D.M. (1962) *Bodily Sensations*. London: Routledge & Kegan Paul.

Armstrong, D.M. (1968) *A Materialist Theory of Mind*. New York: Humanities Press.

Averill, E.W. (1990) Functionalism, the absent qualia objection, and eliminativism. *Southern Journal of Philosophy* 28: 449–467.

Aydede, M. (2005a) Cognitive architecture, concepts, and introspection: an information-theoretic solution to the problem of phenomenal consciousness. *Noûs* 39: 197–255.

Aydede, M. (2005b) A critical and quasi-historical essay on theories of pain. In M. Aydede (ed.), *Pain: New Essays on Its Nature and the Methodology of Its Study*. Cambridge, MA: MIT Press, pp. 1–58.

Aydede, M. and Güzeldere, G. (2002) Some foundational problems in the scientific study of pain. *Philosophy of Science* 69 (suppl. 3): S265–S283.

Aydede, M. and Fulkerson, M. (Submitted) Reasons and theories of sensory affect. In D. Bain, M. Brady, and J. Corns (eds.), *The Nature of Pain*.

Bain, D. (2003) Intentionalism and pain. *Philosophical Quarterly* 53: 502–523.

Bain, D. (2011) The imperative view of pain. *Journal of Consciousness Studies* 18: 164–185.

Block, B. (1995) On a confusion about a function of consciousness. *Behavioral and Brain Sciences* 18: 227–247.

Brentano, F. (1874) *Psychologie vom empirischen Standpunkt*, vol. 1. Leipzig: Verlag von Duncker & Humblot.

Brentano, F. (1907) *Untersuchungen zur Sinnespsychologie*. Leipzig: Verlag von Duncker & Humblot.

Byrne, A. (2001) Intentionalism defended. *Philosophical Review* 110: 199–240.

Connee, E. (1984) A defense of pain. *Philosophical Studies* 64: 239–248.

Corns, J. (2014) The inadequacy of unitary characterizations of pain. *Philosophical Studies* 169: 355–378.

Cutter, B. and Tye, M. (2011) Tracking representationalism and the painfulness of pain. *Philosophical Issues* 21: 90–109.

Dandy, W.E. (1933) Treatment of hemicrania (migraine) by removal of the inferior cervical and first thoracic sympathetic ganglion. *Bulletin from Johns Hopkins Hospital* 48: 357–361.

Dartnell, T. (2001) The pain problem. *Philosophical Psychology* 14: 95–102.

Davis, L. (1982) Functionalism and absent qualia. *Philosophical Studies* 41: 231–249.

Dennett, D. (1978) Why you can't make a computer that feels pain. *Synthese* 38: 449.

Descartes, R. (1983/1644) *Principia philosophiae (Principles of Philosophy)*, trans. V. Rodger and R.P. Miller. Dordrecht: Reidel.

Dretske, F. (1995) *Nauralizing the Mind*. Cambridge, MA: MIT Press.

Dretske, F. (1999) The mind's awareness of itself. *Philosophical Studies* 95: 103–124.

Dretske, F. (2003) How do you know that you are not a zombie? In B. Gertler (ed.), *Privileged Access: Philosophical Accounts of Self-Knowledge*. Hampshire: Ashgate, pp. 1–13.

Evans, M. (2007) Plato and the meaning of pain. *Apeiron* 40(1): 70–94.

Fields, H.L. (1999) Pain: an unpleasant topic. *Pain* 6 (suppl.): S61–S69.

Geniusas, S. (2014) The origins of the phenomenology of pain: Brentano, Stumpf, and Husserl. *Continental Philosophy Review* 47: 1–17.

Gillett, G.R. (1991) The neurophilosophy of pain. *Philosophy* 67: 191–206.

Graham, G. and Stephens, G.L. (1985) Are qualia a pain in the neck for functionalists? *American Philosophical Quarterly* 22: 73–80.

Grahek, N. (1991) Objective and subjective aspects of pain. *Philosophical Psychology* 4: 249–266.

Gray, R. (2014) Pain, perception, and the sensory modalities: Revisiting the intensive theory. *Review of Philosophical Psychology* 5: 87–101.

Hall, R.J. (1989) Are pains necessarily unpleasant? *Philosophy and Phenomenological Research* 49: 643–659.

Hall, R.J. (2008) If it itches, scratch! *Australasian Journal of Philosophy* 86: 525–535.

Hardcastle, V.G. (1997) When a pain is not. *Journal of Philosophy* 94: 381–409.

Hardcastle, V.G. (1999) *The Myth of Pain*. Cambridge, MA: MIT Press.

Harman, G. (1990) The intrinsic quality of experience. In E. Vallanueva (ed.), *Philosophical Perspectives: Action Theory and Philosophy of Mind*. Atascadero, CA: Ridgeview, pp. 31–52.

Husserl, E. (1984/1901) *Logische Untersuchungen: Zweiter Teil; Untersuchungen zur Phänomenologie und Theorie der Erkenntnis*, ed. U. Panzer. The Hague: Martinus Nijhoff.

IASP (International Association for the Study of Pain) (1986) Pain terms: a list with definitions and notes on usage. *Pain* 3 (suppl.): S216–S221.

Jacobson, H. (2013) Killing the messenger: representationalism and the painfulness of pain. *Philosophical Quarterly* 63: 509–519.

Kahane, G. (2007) Pain, dislike, and experience. *Utilitas* 21: 327–336.

Kaufman, R. (1985) Is the concept of pain incoherent? *Southern Journal of Philosophy* 23: 279–283.

Klein, C. (2007) An imperative theory of pain. *Journal of Philosophy* 104: 517–532.

Klein, C. (2015) *What the Body Commands: The Imperative Theory of Pain*. Oxford: Oxford University Press.

Kripke, S.A. (1980) *Naming and Necessity*. Cambridge, MA: Harvard University Press.

Lund, F.H. (1926) The criteria of confidence. *American Journal of Psychology* 37: 372–381.

Lycan, W.G. (1981) Form, function, and feel. *Journal of Philosophy* 78: 24–50.

McGinn, C. (1997) *The Character of Mind: An Introduction to the Philosophy of Mind*. Oxford: Oxford University Press.

Martínez, M. (2011) Imperative content and the painfulness of pain. *Phenomenology and the Cognitive Sciences* 10: 67–90.

Nelkin, N. (1986) Pain and pain sensations. *Journal of Philosophy* 93: 129–148.

Nelkin, N. (1994) Reconsidering pain. *Philosophical Psychology* 7: 325–343.

Newton, N. (1989) On viewing pain as a secondary quality. *Noûs* 28: 569–598.

O'Shaughnessy, B. (1980) *The Will*. Cambridge: Cambridge University Press.

O'Sullivan, B. and Schroer, R. (2012) Painful reasons: representationalism as a theory of pain. *Philosophical Quarterly* 62: 737–758.

Pitcher, G. (1970) Pain perception. *Philosophical Review* 79: 368–393.

Price, D.D. (1988) *Psychological and Neural Mechanisms of Pain*. New York: Raven Press.

Price, D.D. (2000) Psychological and neural mechanisms of the affective dimension of pain. *Science* 288: 1769–1772.

Putnam, P. (1992) *Renewing Philosophy*. Cambridge, MA: Harvard University Press.

Quinton, A.M. (1956) The problem of perception. *Mind* 64: 28–51.

Reuter, K. (2011) Distinguishing the appearance from the reality of pain. *Journal of Consciousness Studies* 19(9–10): 94–109.

Rorty, R. (1980) *Philosophy and the Mirror of Nature*. Oxford: Blackwell.

Savage, W. (1970) *The Measurement of Sensation: A Critique of Perceptual Psychophysics*. Berkeley: University of California Press.

Seager, W. (2002) Emotional introspection. *Consciousness and Cognition* 11: 666–687.

Searle, J. (1992) *The Rediscovery of the Mind*. Cambridge, MA: MIT Press.

Sellars, W. (1956) Empiricism and the philosophy of mind. In H. Feigl and M. Scriven (eds.), *Minnesota Studies in the Philosophy of Science*, vol. 1. Minneapolis: University of Minnesota Press, pp. 253–329.

Sellars, W. (1963) *Science, Perception, and Reality*. New York: Routledge & Kegan Paul.

Shoemaker, S. (1975a) Phenomenal similarity. *Critica* 7: 3–37.

Shoemaker, S. (1975b) Functionalism and qualia. *Philosophical Studies* 27: 291–315.

Shoemaker, S. (1981) Absent qualia are impossible. *Philosophical Review* 90: 581–599.

Stumpf, Carl. (1907) Über Gefuhlsempfindungen. *Zeitschrift für Psychologie und Physiologie der Sinnesorgane* 44: 1–49.

Titchener, E. (1973/1908) *Lectures on the Elementary Psychology of Feelings and Attention*. New York: Arno Press.

Treisman, A.M. and Gelade, G. (1980) A feature integration theory of attention. *Cognitive Psychology* 12: 97–136.

Tye, M. (1996) *Ten Problems of Consciousness: A Representational Theory of the Phenomenal Mind*. Cambridge, MA: MIT Press.

Tye, M. (1997) A representational theory of pains and their phenomenal character. In N. Block, O. Flanagan, and G. Güzeldere (eds.), *The Nature of Consciousness: Philosophical Debates*. Cambridge, MA: MIT Press.

Tye, M. (2005) Another look at representationalism about pain. In M. Aydede (ed.), *Pain: New Essays on Its Nature and the Methodology of Its Study*. Cambridge, MA: MIT Press.

Wilkes, K. (1977) *Physicalism*. London: Routledge.

2

PAIN AND REPRESENTATION

Brian Cutter

1 Introduction

Many mental states represent things as being a certain way. For example, my belief that snow is white represents snow as having the property of whiteness. My visual experience of the pen on my desk represents the presence of a black, elongated object at a short distance in front of me resting on a white matte surface. The way a mental state represents the world to be is its *representational content*. (Hereafter I shall use "representational content" and "content" interchangeably.) For example, the content of my belief that it's raining is *that it's raining*. That's how things are according to the belief in question. The content of my visual experience as of a red and cubical object before me is, at least roughly, *that there is something red and cubical before me*. That's how things are according to the testimony of my visual experience. Focusing specifically on *experiences*, as opposed to mental states generally, we can think of the representational content of an experience E roughly as the way things *seem* or *appear* to be in having E – in other words, the way things are presented (or ostensibly presented) to the subject, or the way the subject experiences things to be in undergoing E (cf. Byrne 2001: 201; McGinn 1989: 58; Siegel 2006: 363).[1]

It is not obvious that all experiences have content. For example, it's not obvious that a sensation of dizziness or a feeling of elation represent the world as being any particular way. More relevant to our purposes: it is sometimes alleged that *bodily sensations* – which include pains, itches, tickles, tingles, and so forth – lack representational content. This chapter focuses specifically on the case of *pain*. I examine two questions about pain and representational content. First, does pain have representational content? In Section 2, I review and evaluate the main considerations on each side of this question. Second, assuming pain does have content, is the phenomenal character of pain wholly determined by its content? According to one popular view in the philosophy of mind, the phenomenal character of every experience is wholly determined by its representational content (Tye 1995; Dretske 1995; Lycan 1996; Byrne 2001; Chalmers 2006). As we shall see, however, pain presents significant difficulties for this general thesis. In Section 3, I discuss some of these difficulties and consider strategies for addressing them.

2 Does pain have representational content?

Call the thesis that pain has representational content the *representational thesis*. Tradition has it that the representational thesis is false. Pain is not *about* anything. It does not represent things as being a certain way (Reid 1997/1785; Davidson 1980: 211; Searle 1983: 39; Peacocke 1983; Strawson 1994: 177; Lowe 2000: 102). As McGinn writes,

> Bodily sensations do not have an intentional object in the way perceptual experiences do. We distinguish between a visual experience and what it is an experience of; but we do not make this distinction in respect of pains. Or again, visual experiences represent the world as being a certain way, but pains have no such representational content.
>
> (*McGinn 1982: 8*)

The most common reason cited for the traditional view that pain lacks representational content is that pain does not admit of an appearance/reality distinction (McGinn 1982; Searle 1992; cf. Armstrong 1968: 313–317). Consider visual experience: a visual experience as of a red and cubical object before me plausibly has as its representational content *that there is something red and cubical before me*. Here there can be a disassociation between appearance – the way things are represented to be – and reality. It is possible for me to have an experience with this content even if there is nothing red and cubical before me, and it is possible for there to be something red and cubical before me without my having any such experience. Similarly, a feeling of pressure on my back plausibly represents the presence of pressure on my back. Here, again, representation and reality can come apart. It is possible to have a feeling of pressure in the absence of any physical pressure, and it is possible for there to be physical pressure without any feeling of pressure. But things seem different in the case of pain. It is not possible for there to be a feeling of pain in the absence of pain, or a pain in the absence of a feeling of pain. So pain seems to lack a characteristic mark of a representational state: the possibility of disassociation between representation and reality.

In order to evaluate this argument against the representational thesis, it will be helpful to formulate it more carefully. Say that a proposition *p* is *fallible* iff it's possible for *p* to be the content of an experience while *p* is false. Say that a proposition *p* is *experience-independent* iff it's possible for *p* to be true while *p* is not the content of any experience. The assumption above that any experience with representational content should admit of the possibility of disassociation between representation and reality can be formulated more precisely as follows: if an experience has representational content, then its content should be fallible and experience-independent. Beginning with a restricted version of this principle, the argument proceeds as follows:

1 If experiences of pain have representational content, then their contents should be fallible and experience-independent.
2 If experiences of pain have contents that are fallible and experience-independent, then it should be possible for there to be an experience of pain in the absence of pain (by fallibility) and pain in the absence of an experience of pain (by experience-independence).
3 But it is not possible for there to be an experience of pain in the absence of pain, or pain in the absence of an experience of pain.
4 Therefore, experiences of pain do not have representational content.

The argument is valid, and each premise is at least somewhat plausible. The denial of (1) amounts to the claim that a given experience of pain has a content p such that *either* (i) necessarily, if p is the content of an experience, then p is true, *or* (ii) necessarily, if p is true, then p is the content of an experience. Could any content satisfy either of these conditions? Well, any necessary truth trivially satisfies (i), but it's not plausible that experiences of pain have necessary truths as their contents. Alternatively, we might suppose that any given token pain experience E has a self-referential content to the effect that E is occurring. If this suggestion is correct, then the content of pain plausibly satisfies (i), in which case premise (1) is false. However, this seems to be a bizarre model of the content of pain, and (perhaps partly for this reason) it is not popular among proponents of the representational thesis. Another way to resist premise (1) is to hold that experiences of pain have contents that are necessarily false or non-veridical. After all, any necessary falsehood trivially satisfies condition (ii). Chalmers (2006) and Pautz (2010) endorse such a view, holding that an experience of pain attributes a necessarily uninstantiated pain quality to a certain bodily region. Many will find this option unattractive, however. It's commonly held that experiences in a given modality, if they have representational content, are at least *sometimes* veridical.

As for premise (2): given the meanings of "fallible" and "experience-independent," this premise says, in effect, that if the experience of pain has content, then its content is something like: *there is a pain*. This premise might be motivated by analogy to other experiences. Just as an experience of pressure plausibly has as its content *that there is pressure (at such-and-such location)*, it's natural to suppose that an experience of pain would have as its content *that there is a pain (at such-and-such location)*. Nonetheless, many proponents of the representational thesis would reject (2), holding (on one common approach) that the content of an experience of pain is not *that there is a pain*, but rather something along the lines of: *there is a bodily disturbance of so-and-so kind at such-and-such location* (Armstrong 1962, 1968; Pitcher 1970, 1971; Tye 1995).

As for premise (3): this is arguably a conceptual truth governing the concepts *pain* and *experience of pain*. Nonetheless, it might be denied. Hill (2009) argues that our concept *pain* picks out the peripheral bodily disturbances represented by the experience of pain.[2] In that case, there would be a distinction between pains and experiences of pain, since experiences of pain are obviously not peripheral bodily disturbances. On this view, there could be disassociations between pain and experiences of pain, rendering (3) false. A related response to (3) would be to distinguish pains-as-experiences from pains-as-objects, where the latter are understood as the bodily disturbances which serve as the intentional objects of the former (cf. Harman 1990; Byrne 2001; Tye 2005a, 2005b). It's plausible that the English word "pain" can be used to pick out either pains-as-experiences or pains-as-objects. Using "$pain_e$" to pick out the former and "$pain_o$" to pick out the latter, we can distinguish two possible readings of premise (3):

> (3-E) It is not possible for there to be an experience of pain in the absence of $pain_e$, or $pain_e$ in the absence of an experience of pain.
> (3-O) It is not possible for there to be an experience of pain in the absence of $pain_o$, or $pain_o$ in the absence of an experience of pain.

Reading (3) as (3-E), the premise is true, but the corresponding reading of (2) can be plausibly denied. On the other hand, if we read (3) as (3-O), then the premise is false.[3] Either way, the argument fails.

Despite traditional opposition to the representational thesis, the latter has won widespread assent over the past half century. The most important early proponents of the representational thesis were David Armstrong (1962, 1968) and George Pitcher (1970, 1971), both of whom held that pain is a form of *perception*. Specifically, pain is a form of *interoception* (internal perception), whose purpose is to inform us about the condition of our bodies. On Armstrong's account, to feel a pain in one's hand (say) is a matter of having a perception of a certain sort of physical disturbance in one's hand, "using the word 'perception' in the neutral sense that is compatible with failure to correspond to physical reality" (306). Pitcher (1970) similarly holds that "to feel a pain is to indulge in a form of [...] *bodily* sense perception" (371–372). What a person perceives, when he feels a pain, is a certain objective state of affairs – namely, a "disordered state of a part of his body" (377).

Among contemporary philosophers, a common motivation for accepting the representational thesis comes from a prior commitment to *intentionalism*, the thesis that the phenomenal character of an experience is exhausted by, or wholly determined by, its representational content (Tye 1995; Dretske 1995; Byrne 2001; Chalmers 2006). Given that pain has phenomenal character, it follows from intentionalism that its phenomenal character is determined by its representational content, from which it follows that pain at least *has* representational content. Intentionalism is an attractive thesis. If we consider visual experience, for example, it's intuitively plausible that there is a tight, constitutive connection between the representational content of an experience – the way things *look* or *appear* to the subject in undergoing the experience – and what it's like subjectively to undergo the experience (cf. Harman 1990; Byrne 2001; Shoemaker 2001). A closely related motivation for intentionalism comes from the "transparency thesis" (Harman 1990; Tye 1992). According to the latter, when one tries to introspect an experience of blue, for example, "one cannot help but see right through [the experience] so that what one actually ends up attending to is the real color blue" – that is, the quality *represented by* the experience (Tye 1992: 160). For those with reductionist leanings, intentionalism is attractive in part because it lends itself nicely to the project of giving a reductive account of phenomenal character (Tye 1995; Dretske 1995). If phenomenal character is determined by representational content, then if we can give a reductive theory of representational content, we will have gone some way toward giving a reductive account of phenomenal character.

Another motivation for the representational thesis derives from the *felt location* of pains. When I experience a pain in my leg, I seem to be presented with something going on *in my leg*. It arguably follows that my experience has a content according to which something is occurring, or certain qualities are present, in my leg. As Byrne (2001) writes,

> When one stubs a toe, the pain seems to be in the toe. But if stubbing a toe merely results in a non-intentional sensation, there should be no seeming at all – in particular, no seeming to be in the toe. So pain sensations are intentional after all.
>
> *(227)*

Besides location, we also experience pains as having such properties as shape, spatial extent, intensity, temporal duration, as well as various qualitative features, such as those which differentiate burning pains from stinging pains, aching pains from smarting pains, jabbing pains from shocking pains, and so forth. These qualities are not plausibly construed merely as intrinsic, non-representational features of our experience, for we experience these properties to be present at the apparent location of the felt disturbance. As Tye (1995) writes,

Consider, for example, a pricking pain in the leg. Here, it seems phenomenologically undeniable that pricking is experienced *as* a feature tokened within the leg, and not as an intrinsic feature of the experience itself. What is experienced as being pricked is a part of the surface of the leg.

(113)

We might offer the following argument as a succinct summary of the considerations above in favor of the representational thesis:

1   In having an experience of (bodily) pain, it seems to one that certain qualities (e.g., burning, aching, pricking, and stinging qualities, in addition to various spatio-temporal features) are present or instantiated in a certain bodily region. In other words, one experiences those qualities as present or instantiated in a certain bodily region.
2   If (1), then one's experience of pain represents those qualities as present/instantiated in that bodily region.
3   If the experience of pain represents certain qualities as present/instantiated in a certain bodily region, then one's experience of pain has representational content.
4   Therefore, the experience of pain has representational content.

Premise (1) is supposed to be a phenomenological datum supported by introspection. Premise (2) asserts a link between the notion of its *seeming* to one that such-and-such is the case and the notion of having an experience that *represents* that such-and-such is the case. Given the way the notion of experiential content is introduced (see, e.g., Byrne 2001: 201; McGinn 1989: 58; Siegel 2006: 363), this should be taken as something like a conceptual truth. It is largely through this link that we come to have a grip on the notion of experiential content in the first place. Finally, premise (3) relies on the principle that if a state S represents F as instantiated, then S has representational content (in particular, a representational content which entails that F is instantiated). This principle is likewise something akin to a conceptual truth governing the notions of representation and representational content.

3 The intentionalist view of pain

In Section 2, we saw that one motivation for the representational thesis comes from the (logically stronger) thesis of intentionalism, according to which the phenomenal character of any experience is wholly determined by its content. But as critics of intentionalism have pointed out, pain presents significant challenges for intentionalism, or at any rate for certain popular versions of intentionalism. In this section, I consider two challenges to intentionalism associated with the experience of pain, which I shall call the *problem of pain qualities* and the *problem of pain-affect*.

3.1 Intentionalism and the problem of pain qualities

Following Armstrong and Pitcher, intentionalists have traditionally held that the experience of pain has a content with roughly the following form: *there is a disturbance with such-and-such features at location* L (Tye 1995; Dretske 1995; Byrne 2001; Cutter and Tye 2011; Hill 2012). "Such-and-such" features include spatio-temporal features, such as shape, spatial extent, and temporal duration, as well as the qualitative aspects mentioned above – those which distinguish, for example, burning pains, racking pains, stinging pains, and so on. Call these qualitative aspects *pain qualities*. Some philosophers have argued that reflection on the nature of pain qualities reveals serious difficulties for one popular form of intentionalism, specifically a reductive externalist form of intentionalism, which is sometimes called *tracking intentionalism* (Tye 1995; Dretske 1995). Tracking intentionalism is the conjunction of the intentionalist thesis that phenomenal character is determined by representational content, together with an externalist "tracking" theory of intentionality. The latter holds (very roughly, and ignoring variations among different versions of the theory) that the properties represented by experience are the extra-cranial properties that our internal states "track" – that is, the properties with which these internal states causally covary under optimal conditions.

Since the internal states associated with the experience of pain arguably track local physical properties of disturbances, it seems that the tracking intentionalist must identify the pain qualities represented by pain experience with these physical properties. But there are at least two important objections to the identification of pain qualities with local physical properties of disturbances. The first we may call the *structural mismatch* objection. This objection begins with the observation from psychophysics that the perceived intensity of a pain doesn't correspond well to any physical magnitude of the relevant bodily disturbances, such as peripheral stimulation levels (Pautz 2010; Hill 2012). For example, when a subject reports that one pain feels twice as intense as another, it is generally not the case that the one disturbance is twice as great as the other in respect of any interesting physical magnitude (Price 1999). This is a special case of a more general problem for tracking intentionalism, namely the problem of structural mismatch between the sensible qualities and the physical properties causally involved in the production of the corresponding sensory experiences. For example, as many have observed, the resemblance structure of color space, as well as the unitary/binary division among the hues, does not correspond to any structural features of the space of external physical properties causally involved in color perception (Hardin 1988). Similar points can be made about the experience of pitch, loudness, taste, and smell (Pautz 2010).

This objection to tracking intentionalism is an important one. Although the issues involved are too complex to deal with adequately in this short survey, let it suffice to mention two possible strategies for responding to the structural mismatch objection as it applies to pain. One strategy, which may handle at least some cases of structural mismatch, is to say that pain experience represents (perhaps *inter alia*) the level of (actual or potential) *harm* associated with a peripheral disturbance. It might then be argued that although the perceived intensity of pain does not correspond well to physical stimulation levels, it does correspond well (in normal, non-illusory cases) to levels of (actual or potential) harm (Cutter and Tye 2011; Hill 2012). Another strategy, suggested by Hill (ibid.), is inspired by the observation that perceived pain intensity correlates well with nociceptive activity in the spinal cord. Hill suggests that the intensities represented by pain experience might therefore be identified with certain *relational* properties of peripheral disturbances – in particular, "relational properties that disturbances have in virtue of contributing to nociceptive activity in the spinal cord."

The second objection to identifying pain qualities with physical properties of disturbances is the *percipi objection*. This objection depends on the intuition that, for pain qualities, *esse est percipi*. More precisely:

> *Percipi* Intuition: For any pain quality Q, necessarily, if Q is instantiated, then Q is experienced.

Pinch your arm and focus on the pain quality you experience to be present at the location of the pinch. Could *that quality* be instantiated without being experienced (say, in the arm of a corpse or an anesthetized patient)? According to the *Percipi* Intuition, it could not. Note that the claim here is related to, but importantly different from, the claim that there could not be an unexperienced pain. One might account for the truth of the latter (assuming it is true) by saying that this is because pains *are* experiences, so it is trivially true that there cannot be unexperienced pains, just as it is trivially true that there cannot be unlaughed laughs (Tye 1995). But we cannot account for the truth of the *Percipi* Intuition (if it is true) in the same way, since by stipulation we are concerned not with pain *experiences* but with the qualities that pain experiences are supposed to represent.

If the *Percipi* Intuition is correct, there is a problem for the tracking intentionalist. As we saw earlier, the tracking intentionalist is arguably committed to the claim that pain qualities are local physical properties of disturbances. But any such property can be instantiated in the absence of experience. Given the *Percipi* Intuition, it follows by Leibniz's law that pain qualities are not local physical properties, from which it follows that tracking intentionalism is false (cf. Chalmers 2006; Block 2005; Pautz 2010).

There are a number of reactions one might have to this argument. A tracking intentionalist will likely opt to reject the *Percipi* Intuition. The *Percipi* Intuition makes a substantive claim about the nature of pain qualities, and it might be said that we should not expect deep facts about the natures of sensible qualities to be revealed to us in ordinary experience (Tye 2005b; Armstrong 1968: 314–315). Alternatively, an intentionalist might accept the conclusion, rejecting the reductive "tracking" version of intentionalism in favor of some non-reductive version of intentionalism. For example, we might embrace something like the non-reductive intentionalism of Shoemaker (2001). Consider some pain quality Q, and let P be the phenomenal property characteristic of an experience that represents Q. On the Shoemaker-inspired view I have in mind, the pain quality Q is identical to the property of causing (in an appropriate way) an experience with phenomenal property P. Properties of this kind – properties of the form *causing (in an appropriate way) an experience with such-and-such phenomenal property* – are what Shoemaker calls "occurrent appearance properties." If we assume that, necessarily, any experience with P represents this occurrent appearance property, then (the relevant instance of) the *Percipi* Intuition follows (cf. Block 2005). This version of intentionalism is *non-reductive* because it explains the pain qualities represented by pain experience in terms of the phenomenal properties of pain experience. It therefore cannot give a reductive explanation of the phenomenal properties of pain experience in terms of the representation of pain qualities, on pain of circularity.

Another way the intentionalist might respect the *Percipi* Intuition is by maintaining that pain qualities are primitive, non-physical qualities that are necessarily uninstantiated. If pain qualities cannot be instantiated, then *a fortiori* they cannot be instantiated without being experienced. This is the lesson drawn from the *Percipi* Intuition by Chalmers (2006) and Pautz (2010), both of whom accept a non-reductive version of intentionalism according to which having an experience with a certain phenomenal character is a matter of having an experience that represents an appropriate cluster of primitive "Edenic" qualities, qualities that aren't instantiated in reality. Of course, any intentionalist who responds to the *percipi* objection by adopting this version of intentionalism, or the Shoemaker-inspired intentionalist view described above, will have to abandon the reductive program that motivates many intentionalists.

3.2 Intentionalism and the problem of pain-affect

It's customary to distinguish two dimensions of the experience of pain: its sensory-discriminative dimension and its negative affective dimension. The negative affective aspect of pain is the *hurtfulness* or *felt badness* of pain. On an intentionalist view of pain, it's natural to suppose that the sensory-discriminative aspect of pain phenomenology is a matter of having a sensory representation of a certain kind of bodily disturbance. But how can the intentionalist account for the affective dimension of pain?

Some intentionalists have adopted a *cognitivist* account of pain-affect, according to which the negative affective quality of pain is a matter of its producing certain *cognitive* reactions, such as a desire that it should cease (Armstrong 1962, 1968; Tye 1995). A problem with the cognitivist account is that it seems to get matters backwards. It's not that pain feels bad because we desire that it should cease. Rather, we desire that it should cease because it feels bad.[4]

Another option for the intentionalist is to explain pain-affect in terms of the representation of *evaluative* properties (Helm 2002; Tye 2005a; Cutter and Tye 2011; Bain 2013). On the most natural way of developing this proposal, pain experience represents bodily disturbances as having two sorts of properties: "descriptive" properties, such as location and physiological characteristics, and "evaluative" properties, such as badness or harmfulness. We can then say that the descriptive content of pain accounts for its sensory-discriminative phenomenology, and the evaluative content of pain accounts for its affective phenomenology. Following Bain (2013), I shall call this view *evaluativism*.

A typical challenge for evaluativism is to give a plausible explanation of how we manage to represent evaluative properties. The challenge is especially pressing if one accepts an externalist "tracking" theory of intentionality. Aydede (2005b) puts the challenge forcefully:

> [Evaluative properties like badness] are simply not the kind of qualities that can be detected or tracked (in the technical information-theoretic sense). One reason for thinking this is ... there could be a molecule-by-molecule identical tissue damage which is not bad (not just experienced as bad, but just not bad – if we abstract away from the regular connotations of "damage" and think of it as composed of whatever physical features and their configurations constitute the damage). There doesn't seem to be any natural property of tissue damage simple and suitable enough to allow itself to be transduced.
>
> *(131)*

Cutter and Tye (2011) respond to this challenge, arguing that our internal states can, in some cases, causally depend on evaluative properties, and that a tracking theory of intentionality can therefore accommodate the representation of evaluative properties. Alternatively, the evaluativist could avoid Aydede's psychosemantic objection by giving forward-looking functional features a constitutive role in determining a state's evaluative content. Where a tracking theory explains content primarily in terms of a state's backward-looking functional role, we might instead hold that what makes it the case that a state assigns negative value to its object is the role that state plays in structuring the agent's motivations and priorities, generating avoidance behavior, and so forth.[5]

An important rival to the evaluativist account of pain-affect is the *imperativist* account (Klein 2007, 2015; Hall 2008; Martínez 2011). According to the imperativist, the intentional content of pain is akin to the content of a sentence in the imperative mood, e.g., "stop doing that!" In this way, the content of pain is very different from the contents of, say, visual experiences, which are naturally taken to have "indicative" contents – contents akin to those of sentences in the indicative mood, e.g., "there is a red and round object before me." On Klein's (2007) version of the view, the content of pain is a "negative imperative" of the form:

don't do action A.[6] On Hall's (2008) version: *Stop what you're doing with this body part!* On Martínez's (2011) version: *Don't have this bodily disturbance!* Imperativists typically endorse the intentionalist thesis that the phenomenal character of pain is determined by its content, though of course their view that pain's content is imperatival sets them apart from traditional intentionalist views of pain.

Imperativism comes in two forms: impure and pure. According to the impure version, pain has both imperative and indicative content (Hall 2008; Martínez 2011). It is natural for an impure imperativist to say, as Martínez (2011) does explicitly, that the indicative content accounts for the sensory-discriminative dimension of pain phenomenology and the imperative content accounts for the affective dimension. According to the pure version, pain *only* has imperative content (Klein 2007, 2015). A pure imperativist (assuming she's also an intentionalist) must account for all aspects of pain's phenomenology, affective and otherwise, in terms of its imperative content.

The pure version of imperativism faces several difficulties. First, pure imperativism arguably lacks the resources to account for qualitative differences between pains which don't seem to enjoin (or prohibit) different actions, e.g., a stinging pain vs. a throbbing pain in the wrist. The impure version can account for these phenomenal differences by claiming that the two experiences differ in indicative content. But how can the pure imperativist account for them?[7] The pure version of imperativism also seems to be at odds with pain phenomenology. The feeling of pain seems to have what we might call a "quality-placing phenomenology." When you pinch your forearm, for example, your experience seems to present you with a certain unpleasant quality pervading a small region of your forearm (cf. Pautz 2010: 364 n.). This quality-placing phenomenology would seem to demand at least some indicative content which attributes the qualities in question to the relevant bodily region, just as the quality-placing phenomenology of color experience would seem to demand some sort of indicative content for color experience, which attributes the relevant color qualities to items in one's environment.

There are other objections that apply to imperativism in both its pure and impure forms. For example, on the imperativist views of Klein and Hall, pains command us to perform, or refrain from performing, some *action*. But many pains don't seem to command or proscribe any action at all. For instance, what does my headache tell me to do? Or the brief sharp pain I feel in my side as I'm sitting silently in my chair? In these cases, it seems that there is no action that my pain is telling me to perform or refrain from performing.[8]

4 Conclusion

Over the last few decades, philosophy of mind has been largely concerned with a cluster of interrelated questions about the representational content and phenomenal character of experience: Do all experiences have representational content? In virtue of what does an experience have the content that it has? Does the phenomenal character of an experience supervene on its representational content? As we've seen, pain bears on each of these questions in interesting ways. Specifically, pain presents important challenges for certain popular answers to these questions, such as those given by intentionalist theories of phenomenal consciousness and reductive externalist theories of intentionality. Whether or not these challenges can be overcome, we shall be better positioned to answer the questions about representation and phenomenology that have dominated recent philosophy of mind once we come to a better philosophical understanding of pain.

Related topics

Chapter 3: Evaluativist accounts of pain's unpleasantness (Bain)
Chapter 4: Imperativism (Klein)
Chapter 5: Fault lines in familiar concepts of pain (Hill)

Acknowledgements

Thanks to Jennifer Corns and Adam Pautz for helpful feedback on an earlier draft of this chapter.

Notes

1 This gloss on the notion of experiential content will have to be qualified somewhat in Section 3.2, when we consider a view according to which certain experiences have *imperative* content. The imperative content of an experience is a specification of *what the experience commands the subject to do* rather than *the way the subject experiences things to be*. Until then, it will be convenient to ignore the possibility of imperative experiential content and to conceive of experiential content in the manner suggested above.
2 For a more detailed discussion of this proposal, see Hill's contribution to this volume: Chapter 5.
3 This is so even if we think that a peripheral disturbance only counts as a pain$_o$ if it is the object of an experience of pain (Tye 2005a). In that case, it would not be possible for there to be a pain$_o$ in the absence of an experience of pain, but it would be possible for there to be an experience of pain in the absence of a pain$_o$, e.g., in the case of phantom limb pain.
4 For further discussion, see Schroeder 2004: ch. 3, and Corns 2014.
5 For a more detailed discussion of the evaluativist view, see David Bain's contribution to this volume: Chapter 3.
6 Klein's (2015) account proposes instead a "protective imperative" of the form: *keep body part B from E (with priority P)!*
7 I owe this point to Adam Pautz (personal communication).
8 For a more detailed discussion of the imperativist view of pain, see Klein's contribution to this volume: Chapter 4.

References

Armstrong, D.M. (1962) *Bodily Sensations*. London: Routledge.
Armstrong, D.M. (1968) *A Materialist Theory of Mind*. London: Routledge.
Aydede, M. (ed.) (2005a) *Pain: New Essays on Its Nature and the Methodology of Its Study*. Cambridge, MA: MIT Press.
Aydede, M. (2005b) The main difficulty with pain: commentary on Tye. In M. Aydede (ed.), *Pain: New Essays on Its Nature and the Methodology of Its Study*. Cambridge, MA: MIT Press.
Bain, D. (2013) What makes pains unpleasant? *Philosophical Studies* 166 (suppl. 1): S69–S89.
Block, N. (2005) Bodily sensations as an obstacle for representationism. In M. Aydede (ed.), *Pain: New Essays on Its Nature and the Methodology of Its Study*. Cambridge, MA: MIT Press.
Byrne, A. (2001) Intentionalism defended. *Philosophical Review* 110(2): 199–240.
Chalmers, D. (2006) Perception and the fall from Eden. In T. Gendler and J. Hawthorne (eds.), *Perceptual Experience*. Oxford: Oxford University Press, pp. 49–125.
Corns, J. (2014) Unpleasantness, motivational oomph, and painfulness. *Mind & Language* 29(2): 238–254.
Cutter, B. and Tye, M. (2011) Tracking representationalism and the painfulness of pain. *Philosophical Issues* 21(1): 90–109.
Davidson, D. (1980) Mental events. In *Essays on Actions and Events*. Oxford: Oxford University Press, pp. 207–227.
Dretske, F. (1995) *Naturalizing the Mind*. Cambridge, MA: MIT Press.
Hall, R.J. (2008) If it itches, scratch! *Australasian Journal of Philosophy* 86(4): 525–535.
Hardin, C.L. (1988) *Color for Philosophers: Unweaving the Rainbow*. Indianapolis, IN: Hackett.

Harman, G. (1990) The intrinsic quality of experience. *Philosophical Perspectives* 4: 31–52.

Helm, B.W. (2002) Felt evaluations: a theory of pleasure and pain. *American Philosophical Quarterly* 39(1): 13–30.

Hill, C. (2009) *Consciousness*. Cambridge: Cambridge University Press.

Hill, C. (2012) Locating qualia: do they reside in the brain or in the body and the world? In C. Hill and G. Simone (eds.), *New Perspectives on Type Identity: The Mental and the Physical*. Cambridge: Cambridge University Press.

Klein, C. (2007) An imperative theory of pain. *Journal of Philosophy* 104(10): 517–532.

Klein, C. (2015) *What the Body Commands*. Cambridge, MA: MIT Press.

Lowe, E.J. (2000) *An Introduction to the Philosophy of Mind*. Cambridge: Cambridge University Press.

Lycan, W.G. (1996) *Consciousness and Experience*. Cambridge, MA: Bradford Books / MIT Press.

McGinn, C. (1982) *The Character of Mind*. Oxford: Oxford University Press.

McGinn, C. (1989) *Mental Content*. Oxford: Blackwell.

Martínez, M. (2011) Imperative content and the painfulness of pain. *Phenomenology and the Cognitive Sciences* 10(1): 67–90.

Pautz, A. (2010) Do theories of consciousness rest on a mistake? *Philosophical Issues* 20(1): 333–367.

Peacocke, C. (1983) *Sense and Content*. Oxford: Oxford University Press.

Pitcher, G. (1970) Pain perception. *Philosophical Review* 79: 368–393.

Pitcher, G. (1971) *A Theory of Perception*. Princeton: Princeton University Press.

Price, D. (1999) *Psychological Mechanisms of Pain and Analgesia*. Seattle: IASP Press.

Reid, T. (1997/1785) *An Inquiry into the Human Mind: On the Principles of Common Sense*. London: T. Cadell.

Schroeder, T. (2004) *Three Faces of Desire*. Oxford: Oxford University Press.

Searle, J. (1983) *Intentionality*. Cambridge: Cambridge University Press.

Searle, J. (1992) *Rediscovering the Mind*, Cambridge, MA: MIT Press.

Shoemaker, S. (2001) Introspection and phenomenal character. *Philosophical Topics* 28(2): 247–273.

Siegel, S. (2006) Subject and object in the contents of visual experience. *Philosophical Review* 115(3): 355–388.

Strawson, G. (1994) *Mental Reality*. Cambridge, MA: MIT Press.

Tye, M. (1992) Visual qualia and visual content. In T. Crane (ed.), *The Contents of Experience*. Cambridge: Cambridge University Press, pp. 158–176.

Tye, M. (1995) *Ten Problems of Consciousness: A Representational Theory of the Phenomenal Mind*. Cambridge, MA: MIT Press.

Tye, M. (2005a) Another look at representationalism about pain. In M. Aydede (ed.), *Pain: New Essays on Its Nature and the Methodology of Its Study*. Cambridge, MA: MIT Press.

Tye, M. (2005b) In defense of representationalism: Reply to commentaries. In M. Aydede (ed.), *Pain: New Essays on Its Nature and the Methodology of Its Study*. Cambridge, MA: MIT Press.

3

EVALUATIVIST ACCOUNTS OF PAIN'S UNPLEASANTNESS

David Bain

Evaluativism is best thought of as a way of enriching a perceptual view of pain to account for pain's unpleasantness or painfulness.[1]

Once it was common for philosophers to contrast pains with perceptual experiences (McGinn 1982; Rorty 1980). It was thought that perceptual experiences were *intentional* (or *content-bearing*, or *about* something), whereas pains were representationally blank. But today many of us reject this contrast. For us, your having a pain in your toe is a matter not of your sensing "pain-ly" or encountering a sense-datum, but of your having an interoceptive experience representing (accurately or inaccurately) that your toe is in a particular experience-independent condition, such as undergoing a certain "disturbance" or being damaged or in danger (Armstrong 1962; Tye 1995).[2] But even if such representational content makes an experience a pain, a further ingredient seems required to make the pain *unpleasant*. According to evaluativism, the further ingredient is the experience's possession of *evaluative* content: its representing the bodily condition as *bad* for the subject.

Below, I elaborate evaluativism, locate it among alternatives, and explain its attractions and challenges.

1 Locating evaluativism

One *could* use "evaluativism" broadly, for any view invoking evaluations to explain pain's unpleasantness or pain itself, whether these evaluations are experiences, beliefs, or desires, and whether what is evaluated are bodily conditions or experiences. But I'm using the term more narrowly for a view whose essentials are endorsed by Bennett Helm (2001, 2002), Brian Cutter and Michael Tye (Cutter and Tye 2011), and myself (Bain 2013):

Evaluativism

1   Your being in pain consists in your undergoing an interoceptive experience (the pain or pain experience) that represents a bodily condition of a certain sort.

2 Your pain being *unpleasant* consists in its additionally representing that condition as *bad* for you.

Notice the following. First, like most accounts of unpleasant pain, this is a *composite view*, invoking distinct ingredients to explain pain and its unpleasantness respectively. This structure makes room for pains that are not unpleasant (see Section 2.3). Suppose your pain yesterday was unpleasant and your otherwise identical pain today isn't (thanks to morphine, say). For evaluativists, this is a matter of the two pains representing the same kind of bodily condition, but only yesterday's representing it as *bad for you*.[3]

Second, evaluativism is a *first-order view*. It explains pains' unpleasantness in terms of states directed at the *extramental* world, not at other mental states. In particular, crucially, the badness that evaluativism says pains represent is the badness not of pains, but of certain bodily conditions.[4] As I'll put it, they represent *bodily* or *b-badness*.

Third, evaluativism is a *content view*. It says that a pain's being unpleasant consists in its having the right representational content. Contrast, for example, functionalist views that say a pain's unpleasantness consists in its causal role or mode of processing, where this is not taken to constitute the possession of content (Aydede 2014; Aydede and Fulkerson, submitted; see Section 3.2 below).

Fourth, evaluativism is a *cognitivist view*, in the sense that it not only explains pain's unpleasantness in terms of content, but says that pains have, partly in virtue of their unpleasantness, truth conditions. Contrast those *imperativist* views that explain pain's unpleasantness in terms of the receipt of body-issued, experiential commands, such as "Stop this bodily condition!" (Hall 2008; Klein 2007; Martínez 2011).[5, 6]

Finally, evaluativism is a *phenomenological view*, taking your pain's unpleasantness to constitute part of *what it is like* for you to undergo your pain. It might even be elaborated as a *feeling view*, in the sense of a view on which a pain's unpleasantness is not only phenomenal, but phenomenal *in a way that non-perceptual, central states such as beliefs and desires are not*. (For some reason, however, "feeling view" is usually reserved in the literature for views rejecting intentional explanations of the relevant feeling [Rachels 2000; Bramble 2013].)

Illustrating the preceding remarks, we might contrast evaluativism with two *desire views*: the first-order desire view (FOD) and – the orthodoxy – the second-order desire view (SOD). These respectively substitute for evaluativism's second claim – (2) above – something like the following:

FOD

3 Your pain being unpleasant consists in your having an experience-based intrinsic desire that *that bodily condition*, represented by the pain, not obtain (Jacobson in preparation; Aydede 2014; Aydede and Fulkerson, submitted).[7]

SOD

4 Your pain being unpleasant consists in your having an intrinsic desire that your *pain experience* not occur (Armstrong 1962; Pitcher 1970; Heathwood 2007; Brady 2015).

Both desire views differ from evaluativism. SOD, after all, is a second-order account. And, assuming that desires lack truth conditions *and* lack the kind of phenomenology that perceptual experiences have, neither SOD nor FOD is a cognitivist or feeling view.[8]

2 Motivating evaluativism

2.1 *Representationalism, affective intensity, and pain talk*

Why be an evaluativist? Brian Cutter and Michael Tye's answer focuses on the representationalist idea that an experience's phenomenal character consists in its representational content (Cutter and Tye 2011).[9] If representationalism is to be accepted, then a pain's unpleasantness – assuming its phenomenality – had better be explicable in terms of the pain's content. If evaluativism is right, it is.

But what reason is there to reach for evaluative contents specifically? Cutter and Tye are led to do so by a process of elimination. They worry that pain's unpleasantness undermines their representationalism, since their psychosemantics – their account of the determinants of perceptual content (Section 3.3) – allows for two pains to *differ* in unpleasantness while being *identical* in respect of descriptive contents: contents concerning, for instance, the shape, location, and type of disturbance represented. But representationalism and their psychosemantics survive, they argue, *provided* unpleasant pains also have non-descriptive, evaluative content, since their psychosemantics predicts the two pains will – for all their intentional overlap – differ in respect of how *bad for oneself* they represent the disturbances as being (Cutter and Tye 2011: 96, 98–101).

Another reason some think evaluative contents a promising candidate for explaining pain's unpleasantness is that, like unpleasantness, b-badness admits of degree. This allows us to explain differing intensities of pain's unpleasantness as follows. Just as a visual experience might represent one wall as *brighter* than it represents another, your interoceptive experience might represent one disturbance as *worse* for you than it represents another (Cutter and Tye 2011: 98, 104). Alternative explanations, evaluativists argue, are considerably less attractive (Cutter and Tye 2011: 103–105; Bain 2011).[10]

It is also occasionally hinted that evaluativism is supported by our tendency to report – when, say, our feet hurt – that things (or our feet, say) feel *bad*. But such utterances are not really probative, since they might alternatively be interpreted in ways not requiring evaluativism, for instance as saying that the feeling we're having is *itself* bad, or that our feet are in a state that is *causing* a bad feeling, or that we are having an experience that allows us to *infer* – without its *representing* – that our feet are in a bad state.

2.2 *Motivation and rationalization*

To appreciate another route to evaluativism, suppose you are standing in front of a boulder and *see* that it is wide. This visual experience, many think, is not itself motivational.[11] You will be moved to act only given further, motivational states of yours, such as a desire to walk around the boulder. Consider now another case: your hand is dangling in water that is hot enough to cause unpleasant pain, but not to trigger a reflex. Many think that, by contrast with your visual experience, this unpleasant pain *is* itself motivational, perhaps motivating you to lift your hand from the water, and doing so without the need for further motivational states such as a desire to not feel pain or damage your hand (this is compatible with your nevertheless not lifting your hand if – say – your pain is overridden by a stronger motivation, e.g., a desire to recover a wedding ring from the hot water). Now, according to some, what explains this contrast between your motivational pain and your inert visual experience is that the former alone has evaluative content (Helm 2002; Bain 2013).

The point is not just *that* unpleasant pains motivate, but *how* they do so. Rather than brutely causing movement, the idea goes, pains are motivating *reasons*, rationalizing action

(Helm 2002; Bain 2013, in preparation-a). Again, the way your pain explains your lifting your hand contrasts with the way the fullness of a volcano's magma chamber explains its eruption. Like belief–desire explanations of action, pain explanations are perspectival and normative. An explanation of your hand-lifting in terms of your pain allows me to put myself in your shoes and see from your perspective why your action *should* have seemed reasonable to you. In short, pains figure in rationalizations; and crucially, evaluativists argue, they do so courtesy of their evaluative content. In particular, they are motivating reasons by dint of representing *justifying reasons*: you are moved to lift your hand because your pain represents a *good reason* for doing so, namely your hand's bad state.

Other views arguably make less good sense of unpleasant pains as motivating reasons. Imperativism, for instance, models pains on commands. But a child might command you to stand without your having any inclination to do so (Bain 2011). And even were the command issued by a police officer, and you obeyed, what motivated and rationalized your standing would arguably not be the command per se, but further motivational states, such as a desire not to be arrested (Bain 2011, 2013, in preparation-a).[12]

Might a desire view prove a more potent rival than imperativism? Competing conceptions of desire complicate the answer. For instance, one view – an attempt to make sense of the rationalizing capacity of *desire* – is that desires are truth-apt, experience-like evaluative episodes: your wanting the beer, for instance, involves it striking you as good (Oddie 2005; Helm 2002). Now, on this conception, some desire views of pain risk *collapsing* into evaluativism. In particular, FOD's body-directed desires start to look a lot like evaluativism's body-directed evaluative experiences.[13]

Alternative conceptions of desire avert the threat of collapse. But some doubt that desires on these alternative conceptions can rationalize (Bain 2013). Moreover, even if they can, evaluativism arguably still makes better sense than desire views of pain's rationalizing role. For pains arguably constitute a distinctive category of motivation, intermediate between brute causes, on the one hand, and desires, on the other (Bain in preparation-a). While pains rationalize, they are nonetheless more basic than desires: more peripheral, less (in one sense) cognitive. They are, it might be said, reason-constituting *urges*, not instances of *your* wanting to act in this or that way, or to achieve this or that end, but rather ways in which *the world* (in particular, your own body) gives you reasons for action, reasons indeed for *desire*, rather as visual experiences are not *themselves* judgments, but ways in which the world gives you *reasons* for judgment (Evans 1982; McDowell 1994; O'Sullivan and Schroer 2012). This picture belongs with the idea that pain's unpleasantness is an experiential, phenomenal matter (Section 1). Like that idea, some will reject it. But evaluativists are not alone in finding it attractive.[14] And evaluativism is a compelling way of accommodating it.[15]

2.3 *Extending evaluativism*

Evaluativism arguably illuminates more than the intensity and rationalizing capacity of pain's unpleasantness.

There are, for instance, data that some construe as showing that beliefs evaluating bodily conditions can influence the unpleasantness of the pains those conditions cause. In one case, for instance, it is suggested that soldiers' beliefs that their wounds had saved them from an horrific battlefield made the pains those wounds caused less unpleasant (Hall 1989; Beecher 1959). If real, this phenomenon can be attractively explained by evaluativism as a case of cognitive penetration, involving our doxastic evaluations of bodily conditions having a top–down influence on our experiential evaluations of the same conditions.[16]

Evaluativism also illuminates pain asymbolia, a bizarre and rare disorder resulting from brain damage (Berthier et al. 1988). Asymbolics, when pinched and the like, *say* they feel pain. But, remarkably, they deny it is unpleasant and don't attempt to prevent or stop the stimuli. Call these anomalies their pain indifference. Less often reported is their general *threat* indifference: the ways in which they fail to respond even to bodily threats that are *not* causing pain, for instance threats that are issued verbally or presented only in *visual* experience. So what might explain both kinds of indifference? Colin Klein's answer is that asymbolics' brain damage makes them incapable of a basic kind of *care* about their own bodies (Klein 2015a). But while this would illuminate their threat indifference – they don't protect bodies they don't care about – how might it explain their pain indifference, in particular their pain's not being unpleasant? Evaluativism supplies an attractive answer (Bain 2014). Caring about *x* is plausibly a condition on representing threats to *x* as bad for you (Helm 2002). Hence it is argued that, just as you won't regard a threat to a vase as bad for you *if* you don't care about the vase, so too your interoceptive experience won't represent a condition of your body as bad for you – hence won't be unpleasant – if you don't care about your body.[17]

Evaluativism is also attractively adaptable. It can be tweaked to account for sensory unpleasantness *in general*, and sensory pleasure too. For instance, the latter might be taken to involve experiences representing certain circumstances as *good* for oneself. Consider, by contrast, an imperativist view on which an unpleasant pain in your foot is a command to *protect* your foot. It is unclear how this might be tweaked to account for other unpleasures, let alone pleasure.[18] Notice, finally, that standard accounts of emotions such as grief invoke evaluative states. Hence evaluativism about pain might be the key to capturing the intuitive kinship between sensory and emotional suffering.

3 Challenges

3.1 Bodily badness

One challenge for evaluativists is to say something sensible about the nature of b-badness.[19] If b-badness seems spooky, one worry goes, then those like Cutter and Tye who adopt evaluativism in order to avert the threat that pain's unpleasantness poses to naturalism have really only deferred the problem.

Cutter and Tye try to overcome the worry by explaining b-badness as an objective, natural property, explicable without reference to mental states. A bodily condition's badness for you, they claim, is its aptness to *harm* your body, in the sense of impeding its *proper functioning* in a Darwinian sense (Cutter and Tye 2011: 99–100). This account's naturalistic purity is attractive; but some may fear that harmfulness in this sense is insufficiently normative to sustain the sorts of arguments for evaluativism sketched in Section 2.2: that a state's b-badness for you defeasibly *justifies* your intrinsically desiring that state to end, for instance, or that representations of b-badness can themselves *rationalize* action.

We might alternatively construe b-badness as subjective. One subjectivist view identifies a bodily condition's being b-bad for you with its frustrating an intrinsic desire of yours. This, notice, is not FOD. Whereas FOD explains pain's unpleasantness in terms of a desire for an experientially represented bodily condition to cease, the current view explains it in terms of an experience representing the desire-frustrating-ness (if you will) of a bodily condition, albeit representing that property not *as such* but under the mode of presentation, *being bad for me* [Bain in preparation-b; see also Section 3.3 below]).[20]

A different subjectivism identifies a bodily condition's being b-bad for you with its causing – or being disposed to cause – unpleasant pains in you. Most evaluativists eschew such accounts, perhaps worried that explaining unpleasantness in terms of the representation of b-badness would be viciously circular if b-badness is in turn explained in terms of the production of unpleasantness experiences. It is worth noticing, however, that *some* philosophers are happy to explain the phenomenal character of an object's *looking red* in terms of the visual representation of redness, even while explaining redness in terms of an object's disposition to cause experiences with that character (McDowell 1994).

There are yet other approaches to b-badness, some modeled on metaethical accounts of moral badness. For instance, Helm holds a no-priority view of b-badness (Helm 2001)[21] and there is also room for a projectivist or error theory according to which b-badness is represented but never instantiated. But I shall not explore or add to these options here.

Another challenge for evaluativists, less often noticed, is to ensure their specifications of pain's neutral, pain-constituting content and its evaluative, unpleasantness-constituting content cohere. Some, for instance, take pain's neutral content to represent "bodily disturbances," a phrase some use to refer to *nociceptor activity* (Armstrong 1968: 315, 319). But it is implausible that nociceptor activity might be accurately represented as *bad* for you, at least on some accounts of b-badness. Sometimes, Cutter and Tye instead take pain's neutral content to represent "tissue damage" (Cutter and Tye 2011: 91–92). But there is a worry here too, for *your foot's being damaged* is not obviously distinct from *your foot's being in a state apt to harm you*, which content Cutter and Tye invoke in their account of pain's distinct *evaluative* content.[22] Sometimes, they seem inclined to say instead that pains represent only determinate kinds of damage: one representing a toe as *burned*, say, another a finger as *cut* (Cutter and Tye 2011: 92). But unless these two experiences represent the cut and burn as instances of damage, or at least of some common kind, it is unclear what representational commonality makes them both pains.

In short, while evaluativists (including me) often intend the phrase "bodily disturbances" only as a promissory note for an account of pain's neutral content, cashing that note may turn out to be a challenge.[23]

3.2 Evaluative content

Worries about b-badness go hand-in-hand with worries about its perceptual representation. Evaluativism's critics argue, for instance, that if Cutter and Tye's account of b-badness *and* their psychosemantics were both correct, then b-badness could not be perceptually represented (Aydede 2005).

On Cutter and Tye's psychosemantics, your current experience represents blue (say) just in case the following holds: in the circumstances in which the human visual system evolved, you undergo experiences of your current experience's type if and only if and *because* something blue is present. As we might put it, perceptual representation consists in experience types *tracking* properties in *ancestral circumstances*. Why think this rules out the interoceptive representation of b-badness as Cutter and Tye understand it? One reason is that the "because" in Cutter and Tye's psychosemantics seems to require, in order for b-badness to be perceptually represented, that it *cause* the tracking states; but Cutter and Tye think b-badness is an *extrinsic* property – the same cut to your hand might be *very* bad for you in a bacteria-rich environment but only *moderately* bad for you in a cleaner environment – which some think prevents it being causally efficacious.

As well as entertaining non-causal interpretations of the crucial "because," Cutter and Tye insist that extrinsic properties in general and b-badness in particular *can* cause (Cutter and Tye

2011: 101–102). To see this, begin by noticing that Cutter and Tye characterize the tracking states in the pain case *functionally*. One kind of tracking state, for instance, is what we might call *H-states*, states whose role is to produce a *high* degree of damage-avoidance behavior. Suppose, then, that you right now have a cut finger; that you are in ancestral (bacteria-rich) circumstances; and that you are in an H-state. Surely, Cutter and Tye argue, it is – thanks to natural selection – *because* conditions of your cut's intrinsic type cause *severe harm* in ancestral circumstances (that is, are *very bad* for humans in those circumstances) that they typically cause H-states in humans in those circumstances, hence that yours causes an H-state in you *now* (Cutter and Tye 2011: 100–101). Others, however, will question whether this shows that your current cut's aptness to harm you has caused your H-state. They will point out that the very same cut as caused an H-state in you now in ancestral circumstances would have caused the very same H-state in you *even in cleaner, non-ancestral circumstances*, circumstances in which the cut would *not* have been apt to severely harm you, that is (crucially) would not have been *very bad* for you. So it can seem to be the cut's intrinsic properties rather than its severe badness for you that causes the H-state. The debate continues.[24]

There is, notice, no obligation for other evaluativists to follow Cutter and Tye's lead in trying to explain pain's evaluative content within the strictures of their tracking psychosemantics. For one thing, other psychosemantics exist. One possibility, for instance, is a functionalist psychosemantics on which an experience's occupying the right functional role *constitutes* its possession of evaluative content. This appeal to functional role, notice, contrasts with Aydede and Fulkerson's (Section 1): it is an explanation of, not an alternative to, evaluative content.[25]

It must be admitted that other evaluativists, including me, have said little about what if any psychosemantics we have in mind. But three points assuage the worry that we are simply ignoring an obvious problem. First, it is quite unclear that *anyone* has, in respect of *any* perceptual contents, an acceptable reductive psychosemantics. Second, you need not be a dualist to think no reductive account can be given. Finally, beyond the pain case – regarding emotional experience, for instance, and vision too – the idea that experiences might enjoy so-called high-level contents, concerning (for instance) natural kinds, affordances, threats, or indeed values, is rather widespread. In crediting pains with evaluative content, it is not clear that evaluativists are saying anything more outré than what is often said in other cases.

3.3 The badness of unpleasantness

Recall that the badness that evaluativists think pain's unpleasantness *represents* is not the badness of pain or its unpleasantness (Section 1). Nevertheless, that unpleasant pain is bad, indeed *non-instrumentally* bad (bad independently of the badness of its consequences), can seem like common sense. And this, four critics have argued, poses a problem for evaluativism (Aydede and Fulkerson, submitted; Brady 2015; and Jacobson 2013).

Evaluativism takes your unpleasant pain to consist in your undergoing a representation that a body part of yours is in a state that is bad for you – yet this representational state, the critics argue, is not *itself* a state that it would be non-instrumentally bad to be in. After all, experiences rarely instantiate the properties they represent; a visual experience of a cube is not itself cuboid. So why think an experience representing badness-for-you is itself bad for you (non-instrumentally)? The critics often make this point in terms of *belief*. Suppose you believe you're terminally ill and that your being so is bad for you. If your belief is true, then of course your situation is indeed bad for you. But is your *believing* it is bad for you *additionally* bad for you (non-instrumentally)? Does it itself make your situation non-instrumentally *worse*? Surely not, they argue. And we should say the same about *any* representations that things are bad for you, including the interoceptive experiences with which evaluativists identify unpleasant pains. Call this the *normative objection*.[26]

The problem might be sidestepped by denying the non-instrumental badness of unpleasant pain, as some non-evaluativists do (Martínez 2015). But, evaluativists have not taken this route; and indeed I have recently argued that the badness of pain's unpleasant is *not* entirely a matter of its bad effects, such as anxiety and distraction (Bain in preparation-b).

Another response is to question whether the critics themselves can accommodate the badness of pain's unpleasantness. The critics tend to explain the badness of unpleasant pain in terms of some notion of desire-frustration. But three of them embrace something like FOD, which arguably compromises their explanation.[27] Suppose you have an unpleasant pain in your foot that you know to be caused not by a condition of the foot, but by a central neuropathy. FOD says your pain's unpleasantness consists in a foot-directed desire for the pain-represented state of damage (say) not to obtain. The problem is that in this case the desire is *not* frustrated, or even *believed* to be frustrated.

The critics might reply that you nonetheless *experience* desire-frustration. But what does this mean? Perhaps that your experience represents (illusorily) a state of affairs that, though you know it doesn't, *would* frustrate a desire of yours if it obtained. But it is unclear that this situation would be non-instrumentally bad for you. Perhaps, instead, the idea is that the property you experience a state of your foot as instantiating is *desire-frustrating-ness*, even if you do not experience it under that mode of presentation. But if, as seems plausible, the mode of presentation under which you represent it is *being bad for me*, this suggestion collapses into evaluativism, in particular the version that explains b-badness in terms of desire-frustration (Section 3.1; Bain in preparation-b).

Evaluativists can also respond to the normative objection more positively. One strategy is to explain your pain's badness in terms of your intrinsic desire for its unpleasantness not to obtain (Cutter and Tye 2014; Bain in preparation-b). This strategy should not be confused with instrumentalism or SOD. It does not explain the badness of pain's unpleasantness in terms of the badness of its consequences; and the idea is not that pain's unpleasantness consists in anti-*pain* desires, but that the *badness* of pain's unpleasantness consists in anti-*unpleasantness* desires. However, the strategy has consequences some find awkward. Suppose that, instead of having anti-unpleasantness desires, a person (call her Strangelove) intrinsically wants the *continuation* of her pains' unpleasantness. Except in respect of their practical inconsistency with her other desires, Strangelove's pro-unpleasantness desires are not rationally criticizable, for they are directed at nothing antecedently bad. Moreover, they render her pains' unpleasantness non-instrumentally *good* for her.

An alternative strategy avoids these consequences (Bain in preparation-b). It starts by disentangling what is being asked of evaluativists. Suppose the question is: "Why *think* that experientially representing that your body is in a condition that is bad for you is *itself* bad for you, given that *believing* it is bad for you is not?" Given that question, evaluativism itself is arguably a plausible answer. For it is plausible, evaluativists argue, that your pain's *felt* unpleasantness consists in your experientially representing – contrast *believing* – that your body is in a state that is bad for you. So, if we are right, it is plausible that if pain's unpleasantness is non-instrumentally bad for you, then experientially representing the badness-for-you of certain bodily states is *also* non-instrumentally bad for you. This would be question-begging if the case for evaluativism were based on the non-instrumental badness of such representations. But, as we have seen, it isn't.

If the question is instead, "Can evaluativism *explain* the non-instrumental badness of pain's unpleasantness?," evaluativists might reply that normative explanation comes to an end somewhere. FOD theorists, after all, invoke the badness of desire-frustration to explain pain's badness while tending not to say *what* is bad about desire-frustration. If such quietism is permissible, it should be available to evaluativists too.

Suppose, finally, the question is, "If the badness of an unpleasant pain consists in its content, why isn't a belief with the same content also bad?" In reply, evaluativists might note the parallel with the following question, sometimes put to representationalists: "If the phenomenal character of a visual experience that a red apple is before you consists in its content, why doesn't a belief with the same content have the same phenomenal character as the experience?" The parallel is illuminating because if you take pain's unpleasantness to be an aspect of how it *feels*, as some evaluativists do (Section 1), an answer to the latter question might also answer the former. Again, something more generally needed might also meet the normative objection: namely, an account of why the content of a perceptual experience constitutively contributes to a *feel* in a way in which the content of a belief does not. And even the barest sketch of what philosophers say on this front is suggestive in the present context.

For instance, some say that a visual experience of a red apple – unlike a belief that a red apple is before you – is an episode in which you do not merely *represent* but putatively *encounter* an apple and its redness, or are *acquainted* or in *contact* with it, or have the apple putatively *present* to you. Sometimes, these ideas are fleshed out via a broadly Kantian distinction between spontaneity and receptivity – between *thinking*, construed as a process you are in some sense in charge of, and *experiencing*, construed as a process in which the world instead *impresses* itself on your senses. Now, if the idea of the non-instrumental badness of *representing* that a situation is bad for you is uncompelling, evaluativists might well point out that we do not invoke just *any* representations; we invoke episodes in which you putatively *encounter* or have *impressed* on you the badness of your situation, episodes in which its badness is putatively *present* to you. The idea that episodes of *this* sort should themselves be bad for you is considerably more compelling. The metaphors need cashing, of course, but that is something philosophers of perception are working to do. In short, there is an alternative to answering the normative objection in terms of second-order desires.

A residual worry, concerning motivation, remains. Construing unpleasant pains as representations of the badness of bodily conditions, evaluativism arguably explains how pains motivate actions aimed at minimizing *those bodily conditions* (Section 2.2). But it does not explain what motivates behavior aimed at *pain itself*, such as the taking of painkillers. Even if evaluativists can explain what *justifies* taking painkillers, the worry goes, they cannot explain what *motivates* it. But replies are available (Bain in preparation-b). Evaluativists might argue, for instance, that whether or not anti-unpleasantness desires explain the badness of pain's unpleasantness, such desires exist and are what motivate our reaching for the aspirin. In short, the worry about motivation doesn't look fatal.

Related topics

Acknowledgements

This work was supported by the John Templeton Foundation.

Notes

1 "Unpleasantness" and "painfulness" aren't synonyms. Nausea is unpleasant but not painful. But "is painful," as applied to experiences, may yet mean "is an unpleasant pain."
2 See Chapters 9 (Price) and 2 (Cutter).
3 Helm (2002: nn. 2 and 28) may not intend a composite view.
4 Klein, by contrast, approves of a view on which a pain's unpleasantness consists in the evaluation of the *pain* (Klein 2015b: 185).
5 Imperativists tend to think contents (contrast sentences) have moods, e.g., indicative and imperative (Martínez 2011: 79–81). My formulation of cognitivism remains neutral on this. Cognitivism might also be put in terms of "direction of fit," but see Bain 2013: S84, for complications.
6 See also Chapter 4 (Klein). Notice that Klein (2015b) explains only pain, not its unpleasantness, in terms of commands.
7 In fact Aydede and Fulkerson invoke only "desire-like" states. Not everything I say about FOD, e.g., that it's not a feeling view, applies to their position.
8 Klein's account of pain's unpleasantness sometimes appears to invoke (second-order) judgements. If so, it is also not a feeling view (Klein 2015b: 186). Nelkin's oft-cited approach invokes (first-order) judgements, but it is an account of pain, not its unpleasantness (Nelkin 1994).
9 See also Chapter 2 (Cutter).
10 See Klein and Martínez, submitted, for reply.
11 This allows that *some* visual experiences are motivational, as for instance Siegel thinks those representing "mandates" are (Siegel 2014).
12 For reply, see Klein 2015b.
13 This conception is also problematic for SOD (Bain 2013: S79–S80).
14 Hall 2008: 530–532; Klein 2015b: 17, 128.
15 See Chapter 19 (Fulkerson and Cohen).
16 On cognitive penetration, see Stokes 2013 and Chapter 22 (Jacobson).
17 Against Klein's and my appeal to "care-lack," see de Vignemont 2015.
18 I assume this is one reason Klein's imperativism (invoking protective commands) is an account of pain, not its unpleasantness (Klein 2015b). Martínez's imperativism (which *is* an account of its unpleasantness) looks easier to extend; but see Cutter and Tye 2011: 105.
19 See also Chapter 27 (Massin).
20 Schroeder explains unpleasantness in terms of experiential representations *that one's intrinsic desires as a whole are on balance less well satisfied than expected* (Schroeder 2004: 97).
21 Aspects of Helm's story are redolent of both the desire-frustration account and the allegedly circular account just mentioned.
22 They might say damage is harm whereas b-badness is *aptness* to harm. But the resulting view would be unattractive: that your unpleasant pain represents a condition both as harming you and as apt to harm you.
23 Kindred challenges include assigning different bodily sensations (e.g., pain and itch) different neutral contents, and assigning different displeasures different *evaluative* contents *if* it is thought that their unpleasantness differs.
24 See also Chapter 2 (Cutter).
25 Cutter and Tye's functional characterizations of the tracking states may seem to approximate this approach.
26 It is also known as the messenger-shooting objection (Bain 2013; Jacobson 2013, in preparation).
27 The exception is Brady (2015).

References

Armstrong, D. (1962) *Bodily Sensations*. London: Routledge & Kegan Paul.
Armstrong, D. (1968) *A Materialist Theory of the Mind*. London: Routledge & Kegan Paul.

Aydede, M. (2005) The main difficulty with pain: commentary on Tye. In M. Aydede (ed.), *Pain: New Essays on Its Nature and the Methodology of Its Study*. Cambridge, MA: MIT Press.

Aydede, M. (2014) How to unify theories of sensory pleasure: an adverbialist proposal. *Review of Philosophy and Psychology* 5: 119–133.

Aydede, M. and Fulkerson, M. (Submitted) Reasons and theories of sensory affect. In D. Bain, M. Brady, and J. Corns (eds.), *The Nature of Pain*.

Bain, D. (2011) The imperative view of pain. *Journal of Consciousness Studies* 18: 164–185.

Bain, D. (2013) What makes pains unpleasant? *Philosophical Studies* 166 (suppl. 1): S69–S89.

Bain, D. (2014) Pains that don't hurt. *Australasian Journal of Philosophy* 92: 305–320.

Bain, D. (In preparation-a) Pain and action.

Bain, D. (In preparation-b) Why take painkillers?

Beecher, H.K. (1959) *Measurement of Subjective Responses*. Oxford: Oxford University Press.

Berthier, M., Starkstein, S., and Leiguarda, R. (1988) Asymbolia for pain: a sensory-limbic disconnection syndrome. *Annals of Neurology* 24(1): 41–49.

Brady, M. (2015) Feeling bad and seeing bad. *Dialectica* 69(3): 403–416.

Bramble, B. (2013) The distinctive feeling theory of pleasure. *Philosophical Studies* 162: 201–217.

Cutter, B. and Tye, M. (2011) Tracking representationalism and the painfulness of pain. *Philosophical Issues* 21: 90–109.

Cutter, B. and Tye, M. (2014) Pains and reasons: why it is rational to kill the messenger. *Philosophical Quarterly* 64(256): 423–433.

de Vignemont, F. (2015) Pain and bodily care: whose body matters? *Australasian Journal of Philosophy* 93(3): 542–560.

Evans, G. (1982) *Varieties of Reference*. Oxford: Oxford University Press.

Hall, R. (1989) Are pains necessarily unpleasant? *Philosophy and Phenomenological Research* 49: 643–659.

Hall, R. (2008) If it itches, scratch! *Australasian Journal of Philosophy* 86(4): 525–535.

Heathwood, C. (2007) The reduction of sensory pleasure to desire. *Philosophical Studies* 133: 23–44.

Helm, B. (2001) *Emotional Reason: Deliberation, Motivation, and the Nature of Value*. Cambridge: Cambridge University Press.

Helm, B. (2002) Felt evaluations: a theory of pleasure and pain. *American Philosophical Quarterly* 39(1): 13–40.

Jacobson, H. (2013) Killing the messenger: representationalism and the painfulness of pain. *Philosophical Quarterly* 63(252): 509–519.

Jacobson, H. (Submitted) Not just a messenger: towards a hybrid conative-representational theory of pain.

Klein, C. (2007) An imperative theory of pains. *Journal of Philosophy* 104(10), 517–532.

Klein, C. (2015a) What pain asymbolia really shows. *Mind* 124(494): 493–516.

Klein, C. (2015b) *What the Body Commands*. Cambridge, MA: MIT Press.

Klein, C. and Martínez, M. (Submitted) Imperativism and pain intensity. In D. Bain, M. Brady, and J. Corns (eds.), *The Nature of Pain*.

McDowell, J. (1994) *Mind and World*. Cambridge, MA: Harvard University Press.

McGinn, C. (1982) *The Character of Mind*, Oxford: Oxford University Press.

Martínez, M. (2011) Imperative content and the painfulness of pain. *Phenomenology and the Cognitive Sciences* 10: 67–90.

Martínez, M. (2015) Pains as reasons. *Philosophical Studies* 172: 2261–2274.

Nelkin, N. (1994) Reconsidering pain. *Philosophical Psychology* 7(3): 325–343.

O'Sullivan, B. and Schroer, R. (2012) Painful reasons: representationalism as a theory of pain. *Philosophical Quarterly* 62(249): 737–758.

Oddie, G. (2005) *Value, Reality, and Desire*. Oxford: Clarendon Press.

Pitcher, G. (1970) Pain perception. *Philosophical Review* 79(3): 368–393.

Rachels, S. (2000) Is unpleasantness intrinsic to unpleasant experiences? *Philosophical Studies* 99(2): 187–210.

Rorty, R. (1980) *Philosophy and the Mirror of Nature*. Oxford: Basil Blackwell.

Schroeder, T. (2004) *Three Faces of Desire*. Oxford: Oxford University Press.

Siegel, S. (2014) Affordances and the contents of perception. In B. Brogaard (ed.), *Does Perception Have Content?* New York: Oxford University Press.

Stokes, D. (2013) The cognitive penetrability of perception. *Philosophy Compass* 8(7): 646–663.

Tye, M. (1995) *Ten Problems of Consciousness*. Cambridge, MA: MIT Press.

4

IMPERATIVISM

Colin Klein

1 Imperativism

Pains differ from sensations in other modalities. Visual and auditory sensations are *indicative*: they tell you something about what the world is like. The sight of a gum tree or the sound of a magpie tell you, respectively, that there's a gum tree and a magpie nearby. Since they indicate, they could be false. You might have *misperceived* or *hallucinated*. Furthermore, the appropriate thing to do about what you see or hear depends on your expectations, your desires, and your goals. The sound of the magpie might motivate you to pursue, to flee, or to remain entirely indifferent. In part because of this, we often have to deliberate about the appropriate response to a particular sight or sound.

Not so with pain. Pains are remarkably uninformative: we often hurt without knowing what in the world has caused our pain. The idea of a pain hallucination strikes many as deeply odd – perhaps even a conceptual mistake (see Hardcastle, this volume, Chapter 1). The adaptive thing to do in response to particular pains is often quite inflexible and context *in*sensitive: the pain of a broken ankle weighs against walking, quite regardless of your other goals. That is why pains motivate you *directly*. That is, pains motivate without requiring further deliberation on your current plans and goals. The pain in my broken ankle gives me a reason not to walk. My goals and desires, at best, can *override* that motivation, but can't make it go away. It is hard to imagine being completely indifferent to pain.

Imperativism is a theory of pain crafted to make sense of these differences. It claims that ordinary bodily pains are *imperatives*, akin to ordinary-language imperatives like "Close the door!" So, for example, the pain of a broken ankle has a content that conveys something like that expressed by the ordinary-language imperative: "Keep from putting weight on your ankle!" This means, minimally, that pains have a content, and that content expresses a *command* to do certain things.

The parallels between pain and ordinary imperatives already explain some puzzling features of pain. Imperatives aren't truth-apt; the commands they express have *satisfaction-conditions* rather than truth conditions (Hamblin 1987). A command like "Close the door!" doesn't tell us anything about how the world *is*, and therefore cannot be true or false.[1] Imperatives also motivate directly, without requiring the addressee to deliberate about whether to satisfy them. If you understand the imperative, and you have accepted its source as authoritative, you're just motivated to act accordingly. That might be overridden, and you may deliberate on *how* you'll do it, but in general accepting a command as authoritative is sufficient to get you to act (Raz 1975; Klein 2015a).

Imperativism is more than just an analogy, however. In what follows, I explicate imperativism by discussing both the core commitments and a few variations on the position. I then discuss some of the arguments in favor of imperativism as well as a few of the problems it faces. I will conclude by elaborating some future directions for imperativism.

2 Why imperativism?

I will motivate imperativism in three ways. First, by shared features with ordinary linguistic imperatives. Second, by consideration of the biological role of pain. Third, by imperativism's philosophical advantages.

As noted in Section 1, pains share two important features with linguistic imperatives: they are (comparatively) uninformative, and they are directly motivating. Neither are obvious, and so both could use a bit of commentary.

First, there is a long tradition in the philosophical literature of assuming that pains *are* informative: about tissue damage or "disturbances" or some similar state of acute injury.[2] Some pains are indeed caused by actual tissue damage. Yet a focus on damage ignores the great variety of situations in which pains are adaptively evoked. Pains are also caused by *potential* damage, as when I press a needle to my skin just to the point of breaking the surface. Pains of *recuperation* are caused by the ongoing effects of past damage, which may outlast the damage itself. Indeed, the pains of recuperation probably form the bulk of the pains we feel: a single broken bone can cause pain for months. Finally, there are pains of *exertion:* as I bike long distances my thighs burn and ache. But I probably can't bike hard or long enough to injure myself.

The diversity of pains is, in turn, one of the reasons why they are uninformative. There is no obvious property that is both common to the states that cause pain and that can be specified in purely objective terms (though for an attempt, see Hill, this volume, Chapter 5). Instead, pains seem to be unified by the *action* that one ought to take with respect to them: something like *protecting* the body part that is in danger.

Second, pains have a strongly motivating phenomenology: there is something bizarre, as Hall (2008) notes, about the idea of someone being in pain but completely unmotivated by it. Of course, the motivational force of pain is not absolute: one might feel pain and have a stronger reason not to act. However, those stronger reasons *override* pain rather than eliminate it.

A second argument for imperativism comes from consideration of the *biological role* of pain. Biological entities must adapt to changing environments. *Homeostasis* is the name for the processes that implement that adaptation (Cannon 1932). Some homeostatic processes are entirely internal to the body: they don't require us to do anything in particular, and they occur without our awareness. Others require us to take some action to eliminate a threat to survival. If I am low on fluid, I need to take a drink to survive.

Behaviorally mediated homeostasis is usually associated with particular bodily sensations. Lack of fluid drives me to drink *by* making me thirsty. That thirst motivates me to take action that eliminates the threat to my body. Hunger moves me to eat, thirst moves me to drink, itches to scratch, and so on. In each case, the specific causes for my motivation – the underlying physiological states – are both obscure and irrelevant for taking adaptive action.

All homeostatic sensations are good candidates for an imperative treatment. Hunger says "Eat!" an itch says "Scratch here!" and so on. The underlying physiological state, no matter how complex, need give rise only to the appropriate imperative sensation in order to be addressed. Imperative sensations are thus both sufficient and efficient ways of maintaining homeostasis through appropriate action.

Pain plays a similar role in behavioral homeostasis. P.D. Wall (1979, 2000) emphasized the important role of pain in limiting motion so as to aid in recuperation. The congenitally insensitive to pain, for example, rarely succumb to acute injury. Rather, they succumb to the wear and tear of unhealed injuries that they fail to guard. Conversely, an imperative that directly leads you to favor damaged areas would promote bodily integrity by leading to rest and recuperation.

Several scientific treatments have also emphasized the similarities between the homeostatic sensations and pains. A.D. Craig (2003; Strigo and Craig, this volume, Chapter 8) dubs pain a "homeostatic emotion," while Derek Denton (2006) notes the role of pain as among the "primordial emotions." Both treatments emphasize not only the strongly motivational force of pains, but also the peripheral and central pathways shared among pains and other bodily sensations. Merker (2005) also emphasizes that homeostatic sensations are important, evolutionarily old, and play a different role in action selection than do the mechanisms involved in perception of the external world.

Third and finally, imperativism confers a number of philosophical advantages. None of these may be compelling on their own (indeed, some authors may disagree on whether some features are desirable), but on the whole they make imperativism more attractive.

The most notable of these is the compatibility between imperativism and *intentionalism*. Intentionalists claim that the phenomenal character of any experience supervenes on the intentional content of that experience (Byrne 2001). Intentionalism is attractive because it opens the prospect of naturalizing phenomenal states. Most intentionalist treatments have focused on *representational* content. Imperative content is another, equally valid, type of content available to ground phenomenology (Klein 2007).

Intentionalism is sometimes thought to falter on bodily sensations, precisely because of the differences between pains and normal exteroceptive sensations (Block 2005; Cutter, this volume, Chapter 2). In addition to the motivational force of pain, introspective reports about pain appear to have a distinct logic from those about representational sensations: the latter can be easily recast as reports about the world, while the former seem to be reports about a sensation (Aydede 2001, this volume, Chapter 18). Imperativism is crafted to make sense of the motivational differences between pains and other sensations. Further, the fact that imperatives have a different direction of fit from indicatives neatly explains the difference in introspective reports: reports about pains cannot be translated into reports about the world because pains tell you what to do, not how the world is (Klein 2015a: ch. 9).

In sum, imperativism says that pains have the particular, strongly motivating phenomenology that they do because the imperative content that constitutes pain is the best way for the body to handle threats to its physical integrity. A good theory of pain ought to capture both the phenomenological and biological features of pain and show how the latter illuminate the former. Imperativism does just that.

3 Varieties of imperativism

Imperativism is a relatively new position, with only a few defenders in print. As such, several of the possible regions in the logical space that I will outline remain unoccupied.

First, *pure* imperativists hold that pains are entirely exhausted by their imperative contents, while *hybrid* imperativists claim that pains are constituted by imperatives *and* some other state(s). In the literature, Klein (2007, 2015a) is the primary defender of pure imperativism, while Hall (2008) and Martínez (2010) both defend versions of hybrid imperativism. The typical extra ingredient for hybrid imperativism is a representational state. In Hall's account, for example, pains are composed of a representation of damage plus an imperative to deal with that damage (Hall 2008: 534).

The choice between pure and hybrid imperativism is a complex one. Pure imperativism offers a simple, unified account. Hybrid imperativism, by contrast, has a richer set of explanatory resources from which to draw. That can simplify the account, sometimes dramatically. Klein's (2015a) pure account requires half a chapter to explain pain location, whereas a hybrid imperativist can, with the representationalist, simply locate pains at the location of represented damage.

An interesting middle ground is represented by Martínez's more recent work (Martínez 2015, forthcoming). In this, pain expresses a command to see to a particular located bodily disturbance. While a formally pure account, this inherits many of the virtues of the hybrid story by baking the location and properties of the disturbance into the content of the imperative.

Second, imperativism can be *first-order* or *higher-order*. Most imperative treatments are first-order: that is, they treat the content of pains as an imperative concerning some actions to be performed or avoided. (I'll consider some of those possible contents shortly.)

First-order accounts fit well with the biologically based motivations for imperativism outlined in Section 2. There is a possible role for a higher-order account, however. Following Hare (1964), Klein distinguishes pain proper (sometimes called "physical pain") from *hurt* or *painfulness* or *suffering*, feelings that can quantify a variety of different sensations. Extant imperative theories concern pain proper. Klein suggests, however, that hurt might be considered a second-order imperative: a command to stop having some first-order sensation (Klein 2015a: ch. 14). This is largely independent of the argument for imperativism. In theory, one could be (say) a representationalist about pain and a second-order imperativist about hurt.

Third, *narrow* imperativists restrict their claims to pain alone, while *wide* imperativists include other sensations. Strictly speaking a wide imperativist could extend the thesis to all sensations (treating, e.g., visual sensations as commands to believe that such-and-such is the case). In practice, wide imperativism is typically restricted to other bodily sensations: pain, itch, hunger, thirst, dyspnea, and so on. Imperativism about all bodily sensations is attractive for the biologically based reasons outlined in Section 2. Narrow imperativism might become attractive, however, if one is drawn to second-order imperativism about hurt.

Fourth, imperativism can be *fully* or *partially* intentionalist. The former claims that the phenomenal properties of pain are entirely exhausted by their intentional content (imperative or otherwise), while the latter claims that some features require distinct treatment. As intentionalism is one of the attractive features of imperativism, current defenders are all full intentionalists. Partial intentionalism has been suggested mainly by those who are sympathetic to imperativism but who doubt its ability to fully account for some aspects of pain experience. Ganson and Bronner (2013), for example, suggest that the motivational force of pain can't be exhausted by content alone, and requires an additional functionalist treatment.

Fifth and finally, imperativists have proposed a variety of distinct commands expressed by pain. Early versions of imperativism held that pains are stop commands that *proscribe motion*. Hall (2008) focused on the immediate cessation of movement. Klein (2007, 2010) included proscriptions against future use of the affected body part as well: the pain of a broken ankle expressed the command "Don't use this ankle!" understood as applying both to the present and to one's future plans.

As Maura Tumulty (2009) pointed out, however, motion-proscription accounts struggle with pains in body parts over which one has no voluntary control or that don't "act" in a relevant sense – headaches, kidney pain, and the like. Klein's more recent account has abandoned motion proscription in favor of commands to *protect* a certain body part, in which case Tumulty's critique doesn't apply: one can still protect a body part over which one has no voluntary control (Klein 2015a, 2015b). Martínez, by contrast, proposes the *removal of a disturbance* (Martínez 2010, 2015) as the relevant command. Both are contextually flexible and so can handle a wide variety of pains. They do not coincide, however: taking morphine for a sprained ankle is a way of removing a disturbance in the ankle but not of protecting the ankle.

4 Issues with imperativism

Imperativism faces both empirical and philosophical challenges. I will canvass several. I will focus on some of the persisting challenges and the imperativist strategies for dealing with them. What follows is not intended to be comprehensive, but rather to show some of the outstanding issues and arguments around imperativism.

Some pains are associated with injuries for which there are obvious adaptive solutions: it's easy to see what you ought to do about a broken arm or a burn. Other pains are more puzzling. What could be commanded by a headache, or by kidney stones, or by pain in a phantom limb?

Problem cases for the imperativist can be divided into three rough classes. *Maladaptive* pains are ones where the command is clear – the agent is under no illusions about how to act – but the effect is unhelpful. Sciatica might cause you to favor your leg, even though that does nothing for the underlying pinched nerve. *Impossible* pains present commands that can't be satisfied: as you can't do anything with a phantom limb, you can't possibly do whatever the phantom pain commands. Finally, *cryptic* pains are ones where it is hard to even see what one could do in response. There is nothing under your control that solves the underlying problem that causes kidney stones, and so it is hard to see what such pains could command.

Maladaptive pains probably aren't a problem for the imperativist. All accounts of pain concede that even the pain *system* is prone to numerous mistakes.[3] The imperativist cashes that out in a straightforward way: maladaptive pains are just ones that command you to do something that does not contribute to survival. The other two categories are more pressing. Imperativism is only compelling if it is comprehensive, and these seem like counterexamples (Tumulty 2009; Bain 2011).

The devil is in the details. Kidney stones are hard to account for if the relevant imperative is to stop motion, but trivial if it is a protection imperative. Further, Klein (2010, 2012) has argued that unsatisfiable imperatives are still both semantically meaningful and motivating, which may explain why (for example) chronic pains are uniquely demoralizing.

A distinct sort of problem case comes from cases of pains that do not appear to motivate at all. Clean cases are controversial, but minimally include so-called "morphine pain" (Hall 1989) and pain asymbolia, a rare effect of damage to the brain region known as the insula (Grahek 2007). In these cases, patients report feeling pain, but by all accounts are completely unmoved by it.

As imperativism is intended to make pains intrinsically motivating, such cases are potentially devastating. They are hardest for pure imperativists to deal with. Hybrid imperativists can arguably avail themselves of the usual response: that non-motivating pains are one half of a double dissociation between the sensory and motivational aspects of pain (Hardcastle 1999; Grahek 2007).

Pure imperativism, by contrast, needs a principled story on which pains can sometimes fail to motivate. The most common story is that such pains represent a kind of breakdown of agency itself, leading to an alienation from pain experiences (Klein 2015b). This faces its own challenges, however (Bain 2014), and so the jury is still out.

Imperativists assume that there must be a clear distinction between indicatives and imperatives, and that this difference manifests in content. But if imperatives differ from indicatives only in (say) their illocutionary force (Searle 1969), then imperativism is not cleanly distinguishable from other theories. This might occur on a local level as well. Cutter and Tye (2011), for example, argue that the *force* of an imperative is an illocutionary matter, and thus imperativists cannot deal with the varieties of pain intensity in a fully intentionalist way. Here, some progress has been made. Klein (2015a) relates pain quality to particular details of protective actions, for example, while Klein and Martínez (forthcoming) develop a theory of pain intensity that links it to variations in imperative force. What is clear, however, is that the pure imperativist will probably need to posit a relatively complex content for pains, one with enough varying parameters to capture the variations present in everyday pains.

Conversely, some think that imperatives can be reduced to indicative statements with evaluative content. "Close the door!" might, on such accounts, be equivalent to statements like "You should close the door" or "Closing the door would be good." It is perhaps telling that one of the closest competing theories to imperativism, *evaluativism*, treats pains as expressing precisely such evaluative propositions (Helm 2002; Bain 2013, 2014, this volume, Chapter 3).

The issue is a complex one. On the philosophy of language side, the trend has been away from reductive accounts of imperatives.[4] What it does show, however, is the need for imperativists to develop a naturalistic theory of imperative content rather than rely on simple linguistic analogies.

Martínez (2010) made headway on this issue by appealing to Millikan's naturalistic theory of content. More recently, Martínez and Klein have developed a theory that relies on the Lewis–Skyrms signaling framework.[5] Within this framework, imperatives are simply those messages in the optimal scheme that correspond to a degenerate set of external states and a single resulting action. As noted above, both pain and the other homeostatic sensations have this structure: the same action can be the adaptive response to a variety of underlying states. The Lewis–Skyrms framework allows for a spectrum of messages between indicatives and imperatives, however, further complicating the matter. Whether this framework is sufficient, or whether some other approach might be preferable, remain open questions.

A final challenge to imperativism involves the extent to which pains motivate by giving *reasons* for action rather than simply pushing us around (Bain 2013, 2014; Fulkerson and Cohen, this volume, Chapter 19). Intuitively, it does seem that a broken ankle gives us a *reason* not to walk, rather than simply *causing* us not to do so. Imperativist responses mostly emphasize the degree to which ordinary imperatives are actually reason-conferring (Martínez, forthcoming; Klein 2015a). If a traffic cop says "Turn right!" you're not merely more inclined to turn right – that command actually gives you a *reason* to turn right.

For the analogy to hold, one must be able to treat the body as something like a practical authority.[6] The literature on command and authority in the political tradition stresses the extent to which commands can be reason-giving without deliberation on the content of the command (Hart 1982). Further, as Raz (1975) notes, legitimate commands also give second-order reasons to take the first-order reasons into account in our deliberations. This arguably captures a core theory of pain: a pain doesn't stop motivating us just because we know it is maladaptive (Klein 2015a). Conversely, Klein (2015b) argues that the breakdown of bodily authority is precisely how the pure imperativist ought to treat phenomena like pain asymbolia (though for a counter-argument, see de Vignemont 2015). Finally, lurking in the background may be a deeper disagreement between imperativists and others about whether reason-giving requires presenting some object *as* good or bad; imperativists must deny this stronger form of the so-called "guise of the good" thesis (Schroeder 2008).

5 Future directions

Many of the controversies listed above will, hopefully, generate further discussion. In this section I will instead focus on places where imperativists have had relatively *little* to say, but might fruitfully say more in the future.

First, there are a number of features of pain about which imperativists have had little to say. Pains are strongly *attention-grabbing*, for example, a feature they share with most of the more intense forms of bodily sensation. Here an imperativist treatment, while not offered, would seem to be in reach. Merker (2005), for example, notes that most of the bodily sensations would lead to death or serious disability if ignored for long, and so builds their ability to intrude into awareness into the heart of his theory of consciousness.

Similarly, imperativists have had little to say about the connection between pain and *learning*. Pain seems like the paradigmatic signal of disutility, and so one might think there must be a close connection between the two. The story may actually be more complex, though. It is clear, however, that not all stimuli which are aversive – that is, stimuli which reduce the frequency of behaviors associated with them – are pains. Conversely, not all pains are aversive. Research on pleasure now distinguishes the feeling of pleasure proper from *reward*; the latter need not even be conscious (Berridge 2009). A similar distinction might apply to pain and aversion.

Along the same lines, imperativism has had relatively little to say about the relationship between pain and pleasure,[7] or between pain and touch. The latter was traditionally connected to pain (Armstrong 1962), though modern theories have not emphasized that connection. Given the recent revival of interest in touch as a philosophical question (e.g., Fulkerson 2013), the relationship might be fruitfully explored. Finally, there is some obvious but complex relationship between physical pains and the *social* pains of rejection and jealousy (Corns 2015).

Imperativism also has potential consequences for ethics, particularly ethical theories that place weight on the badness of pain. One might wonder, for example, whether there is any deep ethical difference between types of pain – is the chronic pain of allodynia, for example, much worse than the sum of the pains from many small pinpricks?

Imperativists have suggested yes. Klein (2010, 2012) in particular has emphasized that chronic pains sometimes have the character of *unsatisfiable* imperatives, and that these can be uniquely demoralizing and discomfiting. Similarly, writers addressing the wrongs of torture have emphasized the way in which torture turns the body back against itself, making the victim at once cause and victim of their own commands (Scarry 1985; Sussman 2005). Sussman's treatment even makes reference to the "primitive language of bodily commands and pleasure" (Sussman 2005: 21), suggesting a fruitful avenue for further research.

6 Conclusion

Imperativism is a young theory. Yet it is also a theory worth taking seriously. It provides a clean link between the phenomenal feel and the biological role of pains. It is flexible enough to account for many problem cases, and might shed light on otherwise puzzling phenomena. There are gaps left to fill, and unanswered questions – but it also provides a powerful framework within which to expand and to explore these issues.

Related topics

Chapter 1: A brief and potted overview on the philosophical theories of pain (Hardcastle)
Chapter 2: Pain and representation (Cutter)
Chapter 3: Evaluativist accounts of pain's unpleasantness (Bain)
Chapter 5: Fault lines in familiar concepts of pain (Hill)
Chapter 8: A neurobiological view of pain as a homeostatic emotion (Strigo and Craig)
Chapter 18: Pain: perception or introspection? (Aydede)

Notes

1 At best, it can *presuppose* something false. For more on imperative presupposition, see Klein (2012).
2 Note that "disturbance" must ultimately refer to something that can be concretely specified, if pains are to be distinguished from other bodily sensations (especially itches). I doubt that this can be done; see Klein 2015a: ch. 3, §4, for an argument.
3 A point that goes back at least to Descartes' remarks on pain in Meditation 6. For an intriguing argument that Descartes was himself an imperativist, see Joe Gottlieb and Saja Parvizian, "Cartesian Imperativism" (draft ms).
4 The issue has a long and storied past. For useful discussions, see Hamblin (1987) and Parsons (2012). Vranas (2008), in addition to being valuable in its own right, contains an excellent bibliography focusing on attempts to construct imperative logics, the traditional ground upon which this question was fought.
5 In Martínez and Klein "Pain Signals are Predominantly Imperative" (draft ms). See Skyrms 2010 for the general framework. Huttegger (2007), expanding on remarks by Lewis (1969), provides the criteria for imperatives.
6 Contra Bain (2011), who assumes that imperativism must appeal to epistemic authority, and (plausibly) notes that epistemic authority would be insufficient to ground pain.
7 Though see Klein (2014) on masochism. Klein's treatment involves treating pleasure as the dual of *suffering* rather than of physical pain, however, and so in a different category altogether.

References

Armstrong, D. (1962) *Bodily Sensations*. New York: Routledge & Kegan Paul.
Aydede, M. (2001) Naturalism, introspection, and direct realism about pain. *Consciousness & Emotion* 2(1): 29–73.
Aydede, M. (ed.) (2005) *Pain: New Essays on Its Nature and the Methodology of Its Study*. Cambridge, MA: MIT Press.
Bain, D. (2011) The imperative view of pain. *Journal of Consciousness Studies* 18(9–10): 164–185.
Bain, D. (2013) What makes pains unpleasant? *Philosophical Studies* 166 (suppl. 1): S69–S89.
Bain, D. (2014) Pains that don't hurt. *Australasian Journal of Philosophy*, 92(2): 1–16.
Berridge, K.C. (2009) Wanting and liking: observations from the neuroscience and psychology laboratory. *Inquiry* 52(4): 378–398.
Block, N. (2005) Bodily sensations as an obstacle for representationism. In M. Aydede (ed.), *Pain: New Essays on Its Nature and the Methodology of Its Study*. Cambridge, MA: MIT Press, pp. 137–142.
Byrne, A. (2001) Intentionalism defended. *Philosophical Review* 110(2): 199–240.
Cannon, W.B. (1932) *The Wisdom of the Body*. New York: W.W. Norton & Co.

Corns, J. (2015) The social pain posit. *Australasian Journal of Philosophy* 93(3): 561–582.

Craig, A. (2003) A new view of pain as a homeostatic emotion. *Trends in Neurosciences* 26(6): 303–307.

Cutter, B. and Tye, M. (2011) Tracking representationalism and the painfulness of pain. *Philosophical Issues* 21(1): 90–109.

Denton, D. (2006) *The Primordial Emotions*. New York: Oxford University Press.

de Vignemont, F. (2015) Pain and bodily care: whose body matters? *Australasian Journal of Philosophy* 93(3): 542–560.

Fulkerson, M. (2013) *The First Sense: A Philosophical Study of Human Touch*. Cambridge, MA: MIT Press.

Ganson, T. and Bronner, B. (2013) Visual prominence and representationalism. *Philosophical Studies* 164(2): 405–418.

Grahek, N. (2007) *Feeling Pain and Being in Pain*, 2nd ed. Cambridge, MA: MIT Press.

Hall, R. (1989) Are pains necessarily unpleasant? *Philosophy and Phenomenological Research* 49(4): 643–659.

Hall, R. (2008) If it itches, scratch! *Australasian Journal of Philosophy* 86(4): 525–535.

Hamblin, C. (1987) *Imperatives*. Oxford: Basil Blackwell.

Hardcastle, V.G. (1999) *The Myth of Pain*. Cambridge, MA: MIT Press.

Hare, R.M. (1964) Symposium: pain and evil. *Proceedings of the Aristotelian Society, Supplementary Volumes* 38: 91–124.

Hart, H.L.A. (1982) *Essays on Bentham: Studies in Jurisprudence and Political Theory*. Oxford: Clarendon Press.

Helm, B. (2002) Felt evaluations: a theory of pleasure and pain. *American Philosophical Quarterly* 39(1): 13–30.

Huttegger, S.M. (2007) Evolutionary explanations of indicatives and imperatives. *Erkenntnis* 66(3): 409–436.

Klein, C. (2007) An imperative theory of pain. *Journal of Philosophy* 104(10): 517–532.

Klein, C. (2010) Response to Tumulty on pain and imperatives. *Journal of Philosophy* 107(10): 554–557.

Klein, C. (2012) Imperatives, phantom pains, and hallucination by presupposition. *Philosophical Psychology* 25(6): 917–928.

Klein, C. (2014) The penumbral theory of masochistic pleasure. *Review of Philosophy and Psychology* 5(1): 41–55.

Klein, C. (2015a) *What the Body Commands: The Imperative Theory of Pain*. Cambridge, MA: MIT Press.

Klein, C. (2015b) What pain asymbolia really shows. *Mind*, 124(494): 493–516.

Klein, C. and Martínez, M. (Forthcoming). Imperativism and pain intensity. In M. Brady (ed.), *The Nature of Pain: Hedonic Tone, Motivation, and Non-human Animals*. Oxford: Oxford University Press.

Lewis, D. (1969) *Convention: A Philosophical Study*. Cambridge, MA: Harvard University Press.

Martínez, M. (2010) Imperative content and the painfulness of pain. *Phenomenology and the Cognitive Sciences* 10: 67–90.

Martínez, M. (2015) Disgusting smells and imperativism. *Journal of Consciousness Studies* 22(5–6): 191–200.

Martínez, M. (Forthcoming). Pains as reasons. *Philosophical Studies*.

Merker, B. (2005) The liabilities of mobility: a selection pressure for the transition to consciousness in animal evolution. *Consciousness and Cognition* 14(1): 89–114.

Parsons, J. (2012) Cognitivism about imperatives. *Analysis* 72(1): 49–54.

Raz, J. (1975) Reasons for action, decisions and norms. *Mind* 84(336): 481–499.

Scarry, E. (1985) *The Body in Pain: The Making and Unmaking of the World*. New York: Oxford University Press.

Schroeder, M. (2008) How does the good appear to us? *Social Theory and Practice* 34(1): 119–130.

Searle, J.R. (1969) *Speech Acts: An Essay in the Philosophy of Language*. Cambridge: Cambridge University Press.

Skyrms, B. (2010) *Signals: Evolution, Learning, and Information*. New York: Oxford University Press.

Sussman, D. (2005) What's wrong with torture? *Philosophy & Public Affairs* 33(1): 1–33.

Tumulty, M. (2009) Pains, imperatives, and intentionalism. *Journal of Philosophy* 106(3): 161–166.

Vranas, P. (2008) New foundations for imperative logic I: Logical connectives, consistency, and quantifiers. *Noûs* 42(4): 529–572.

Wall, P. (1979) On the relation of injury to pain (The John J. Bonica Lecture). *Pain* 6(3): 253–264.

Wall, P. (2000) *Pain: The Science of Suffering*. New York: Columbia University Press.

5

FAULT LINES IN FAMILIAR CONCEPTS OF PAIN

Christopher S. Hill

This chapter is primarily concerned with three topics: conscious awareness of pain, the commonsense concept of pain, and the definition of pain that is recommended by the International Association for the Study of Pain. (The IASP defines pain as "an unpleasant sensory and emotional experience associated with actual or potential damage, or described in terms of such damage" (Mersky and Bogduk 1994: 210).)

I will begin by describing a theory of conscious awareness of pain that I will call the *bodily disturbance model*. According to this theory, awareness of pain is a type of perceptual state, and pain itself is a bodily disturbance that normally involves actual or potential damage. As we will see, this theory fits normal cases of awareness of pain reasonably well, and even some abnormal cases, such as situations in which morphine has been administered to a patient, and situations in which an agent is suffering from pain asymbolia. (Asymbolia patients say that they continue to experience pains, and in fact insist that their pains are often just as intense as they were before the damage occurred. But they show no aversion to their pains, and have no tendency to engage in palliative behavior; Grahek 2011.)

There are other phenomena, however, that the bodily disturbance model cannot easily accommodate. These principally include phantom limb pains, neuropathic pains, and certain aspects of second pain (e.g., its tendency to last longer than the aversive stimulus that gave rise to it). Phenomena of these kinds are better described by a second theory I will call the *central state model*. Roughly speaking, the central state model claims that pains are identical with the high-level perceptual states that represent bodily disturbances. In effect, then, instead of locating pains in peripheral regions of the body, it claims that they are grounded in activity in the brain. Its great virtue is that it can explain why we can be so strongly inclined to say that we are in pain in certain situations (such as those involving phantom limb pain) in which there is no bodily disturbance in the relevant location.

Because these models are incompatible, and because they both receive strong support from theoretical arguments and from empirical data as well, it is tempting to conclude that pain is involved in a paradox. The paradox can be resolved, however, by distinguishing between two kinds of pain – *peripheral pain* and *central state pain*. Instead of supposing that the two theories give conflicting accounts of a single phenomenon, we should suppose that they give correct accounts of different phenomena. The paradox arises only because common-sense psychology attempts to use a single concept of pain to keep track of different states. The same is true of recent scientific theories of pain, which tend to incorporate the definition proposed by the International Association for the Study of Pain (IASP) that I quoted above. It is possible to get by with a single concept when one is focusing on normal cases of pain, but normal cases are congeries of different components that have turned out to be dissociable. In order to keep more accurate track of these components, we should abandon the attempt to make do with a single concept of pain and commit to using an array of new concepts instead, including especially concepts for peripheral pain and central state pain.

1 The bodily disturbance model

The bodily disturbance model makes seven main claims:

1   In a normal case of awareness of pain, the sufferer is perceptually aware of a bodily disturbance of a certain sort.
2   More specifically, awareness of pain is awareness of a type of disturbance that generally involves actual or potential damage, and that is grounded principally in the activity of nociceptive neurons known as *C-fibers* and *Aδ-fibers*. (In the interests of brevity, I will refer to disturbances of this sort as *P-states*.)
3   Like other types of perceptual awareness, awareness of pain involves a perceptual experience that *represents* the object of awareness and also represents some of its properties. In this case, the experience represents a P-state as being a pain of a certain kind (piercing, burning, throbbing, etc.), as having a certain intensity, and as being located in a certain part of the body.
4   Represented properties of these three kinds constitute the *sensory phenomenology* of pain.
5   In a normal case, awareness of pain is accompanied by an affective/behavioral response. This response is a complex state that includes an attitude of aversion and dispositions to behave in ways that tend to reduce the intensity of the disturbance and may eliminate the disturbance altogether. (The affective and behavioral components of the response are of course separable, but I will treat them as a unit here.)
6   The three main components of a normal case that I have distinguished – the P-state, the perceptual experience that represents the P-state, and the affective/behavioral response – are bound intimately together by causal relations. Thus, the P-state causes the perceptual representation, and the perceptual representation causes the affective/behavioral response. (There are also causal pathways linking the P-state directly to the response.) Like all other causal relations, however, these relations are contingent. It is possible for each of the components to occur without the others.
7   Pains are P-states. The other components of normal cases are merely correlates of pains.

Variants of this model have been defended by Dretske (1995), Tye and Cutter (2011), and myself (Hill 2009, 2014). (See also Chapter 27, this volume.) In explaining the grounds for the model, I will focus on (1), (2), (4), and (7). There isn't sufficient space to discuss all of the components, and these four are the ones that are most in need of defense. Also, I will assume that the awareness of the sensory dimension of pain is primarily grounded in somatosensory cortex. There is good evidence for this (see, e.g., Hofbauer et al. 2001), though there is reason to believe that awareness of the sensory dimension involves other sites, including especially the insula, as well (Coghill et al. 1999; Ostrowsky et al. 2002).

Why should we suppose that awareness of pain is a form of perceptual awareness? This view receives strong support both from science and from introspection.

To begin with the relevant scientific considerations, it is well established that the somato-sensory mechanisms that support awareness of pain are very similar to the somatosensory mechanisms that support touch (awareness of pressure). The similarity involves the locations of these mechanisms, their structure, and the informational pathways linking them to peripheral phenomena (Basbaum and Jessell 2012; Gardner and Johnson 2012; Gardner and Johnson 2012). Now touch is widely regarded as a paradigmatic form of perceptual awareness. Hence, to the extent that awareness of pain resembles it, there are grounds for regarding awareness of pain as perceptual.

To be sure, awareness of pain differs from touch in that some of the neural structures that support it are polymodal. The peripheral neural structures that support touch respond only to pressure, but certain peripheral nociceptors are sensitive to extremes of pressure, to extremes of temperature, and also to some forms of chemical stimulation. Since these neurons have no one proprietary physical stimulus, it might be argued that they register a subject-dependent property, such as harm or damage, rather than an objective physical magnitude, and that this difference overturns the analogy with touch (Cevero 2012: 42). This line of thought has a certain appeal, but I don't think that it really establishes its conclusion. It could hardly be maintained that the neurons in question detect the highly generic property *damage*, because there are many kinds of bodily damage to which they are not sensitive (e.g., radiation damage). The claim would have to be that the neurons detect a disjunction of specific types of damage. But if we say that, we might as well say that they detect a disjunction of purely physical properties – a disjunction consisting of a specific range of pressures, a specific range of temperatures, and a specific range of chemicals. But anyway, the fact that a property is subject-dependent isn't a reason to deny that awareness of it is perceptual. There is good reason to think that the visual system measures heights and distances in body units (Warren 1984). These measures are of course subject-dependent.

There is also another important feature of awareness of pain that might be thought to preclude its being classified as perceptual: it is affected by the influence of top–down processing to a very substantial degree. Thus, awareness of pain seems to be modulated by a variety of high-level factors that include attention, emotion, expectation, and hypnotic suggestion (Bushnell et al. 2004; Rainville 2004; Price et al. 2007; Hofbauer et al. 2001; Chapter 32, this volume). At first sight this might seem to pose a challenge to the idea that awareness of pain is perceptual, but reflection shows that this is not the case. Even vision, the gold standard of the perceptual, involves large amounts of downward influence from a range of high-level factors: as is well known, such factors can control the allocation of attention, and attention can transform visual processing.

It appears, then, that there are strong analogies between awareness of pain and touch, and that these points of similarity are not outweighed by disanalogies.

This brings me to the *introspective* data that support thesis (1), the claim that awareness of pain is a form of perceptual awareness. I will mention data of three kinds. (I discuss others in Hill 2009.) First, introspection reveals that awareness of pain is associated with a phenomenology that parallels the phenomenology of vision, hearing, and touch in complexity and vividness. Other alleged types of phenomenology are much less robust. Second, introspection shows that attention can enhance the resolution of awareness of pain. We know from Marissa Carrasco's work that the same is true of vision – attention enhances the resolution of objects of visual awareness (Yeshuran and Carrasco 1998). Moreover, there is reason to think that this is also true of other paradigmatic forms of perceptual awareness, and reason to doubt that it is true of non-perceptual forms of awareness, such as introspective awareness of thoughts. (What would it mean to claim that attention enhances awareness of the fine-grained organization of thoughts, improving our grasp of their smaller parts?) Third, introspection shows that experiences of pain assign bodily locations to pains. The paradigmatic forms of perception also assign locations to their objects. To be sure, in the case of vision, hearing, and touch, the locations are positions in physical space rather than locations in the body, but that difference seems less important when one recalls that the relevant locations in physical space are largely egocentric, defined by relations to the subject's body.

I turn now to thesis (2), which claims that awareness of pain is directed on P-states. Why should we accept this view? One reason is provided by the first of the foregoing arguments for thesis (1). Awareness of pain is similar to awareness of pressure, and awareness of pressure is directed on occurrences in peripheral regions of the body. By analogy, then, awareness of pain is directed on occurrences in peripheral regions of the body. The obvious candidates are P-states. (Cf. Chapter 4, this volume.) There is also a second reason – one that is grounded in part in scientific fact and in part in assumptions about the nature of representation. As is well known, awareness of pain is supported by a number of somatotopic maps, including a highly detailed map in somatosensory cortex. Since awareness of pain is grounded in these maps, the objects of awareness must be whatever is represented by the relevant positions on the maps. But it is very plausible that positions on the maps represent P-states. This can be seen by reflecting on three considerations. First, positions on the maps encode information about P-states (in the sense that activity at a position is generally correlated with and indeed caused by a P-state at a particular bodily location). Second, it is plausible that activity at the positions on the maps has the *function* of encoding information about corresponding P-states, for the information that is encoded is information that the brain desperately needs if it is to respond to potentially harmful stimuli in appropriate ways. And third, it is plausible that perceptual representation occurs when perceptual states have the function of encoding information of a certain sort. (I am here opting for a Dretskean account of perceptual representation, but that is not essential; Dretske 1986.)

It is plausible, then, that an experience of pain is a perceptual state that represents a P-state. This is not to say that every experience of pain corresponds to a P-state. Like all forms of perceptual awareness, awareness of pain can give rise to illusions and hallucinations. This is what occurs in cases of neuropathy and cases of phantom limb pain. In a normal case, however, an experience that represents a P-state as occurring will always be accompanied by (and will in fact be caused by) an actual P-state.

This brings us to thesis (4), the claim that the phenomenology of pain is exhausted by *sensory* properties of three kinds – a specific qualitative character (e.g., burning pain), a specific intensity, and a specific location. I submit that introspection provides strong evidence that the phenomenology of pain includes properties of *at least* these three kinds. The question before us is whether it also includes other properties.

It is sometimes claimed that it does (Tye and Cutter 2011; Aydede and Fulkerson 2014). Thus, it is sometimes said that the sensory dimension of pain includes the quality that we refer to as *hurting*. I think, however, that this view is called into question by the testimony of people who have been given morphine or who have the disorder known as pain asymbolia. Testimony from subjects of these kinds shows that they experience their pains as having specific characters, specific intensities, and specific locations. They do not, however, experience them as hurting or noxious or bad.

To elaborate, instead of maintaining that the phenomenology of their pains has changed, these subjects seem to be affirming that the phenomenology has remained the same, but that they are no longer *bothered by* that phenomenology. *That phenomenology* has lost its power to command attention, and to cause aversion. Equally, it has lost its power to compel withdrawal and nursing behavior. The patients are able to view pain with detachment. Asymbolia patients are sometimes even amused by their pains, precisely because they recognize them as having all of the phenomenal properties by which they used to be distressed (Grahek 2011). It seems incongruous that the *same sensation* should now be insignificant.

How then should we think of the feature of pains that we refer to when we describe pains as hurting or noxious or bad? If it isn't a phenomenal feature of pains, what is it? I suggest that it is more in keeping with the relevant testimony to think of hurting or noxiousness as a causal power – specifically, the power to cause pain-affect or pain-specific aversion. In normal cases, P-states have this causal power, and so do representations of P-states. Their having the power depends on the integrity of the neural pathways linking nociceptive centers in the thalamus and in somatosensory cortex to the limbic system, which is the seat of pain-effect. When these pathways are compromised or interrupted, as occurs when opiates are administered and in asymbolia, the casual power is diminished or extinguished. But this has nothing to do with the phenomenology of pain itself.

To be sure, it may be that pain-affect has a phenomenology that adds to the total phenomenology of an experience of pain. If the testimony of asymbolia subjects is to be trusted, however, this phenomenology is independent of the phenomenology that is proprietary to pain. It is not an essential component of the phenomenology that guides us in identifying pains as such. By the same token, there is no obligation for a theory of pain to explain it. Explaining it is rather an obligation of theories of the emotions.

There are several reasons to accept thesis (7), which identifies pains with P-states. First, as we have just seen, awareness of pain is a form of perceptual awareness that is directed on P-states. This is an excellent reason for thinking that pains *are* P-states. Second, pains share many of the properties of P-states. For example, experiences of pain represent their objects as located in specific regions of the body. In normal cases, there are P-states in exactly the locations that experiences assign to pains. Moreover, pains and P-states seem to have the same causal powers. Both pains and P-states can cause automatic withdrawals from aversive stimuli; both can cause pain-affect (the form of aversion that normally accompanies awareness of pain); both can cause beliefs and other propositional attitudes that are directed on pains; and both can cause palliative or nursing behaviors, such as immobilizing an afflicted body part and pressing on the areas that immediately surround the site of an injury. Third, pains are correlated with P-states in normal cases: in normal cases, pains occur when and only when P-states occur. This correlation breaks down in many cases, such as phantom limb pain and neuropathic pain, but it is arguably possible to account for such cases by pleading hallucination and illusion. For example, it can be argued that in a case of phantom limb pain the sufferer is undergoing a hallucination, albeit a hallucination that causes the same kind of aversion and distress as a real pain. And fourth, people are willing to describe themselves as being in pain in cases in which the affective and behavioral phenomena that normally accompany awareness of pain are considerably attenuated, as happens when morphine or other opiates have been administered, and even when the normal affective and behavioral accompaniments have been eliminated altogether, as happens in cases of pain asymbolia. In other words, it appears that awareness of pain can exist even when a number of its liaisons are pared away, provided only that an appropriate perceptual experience and the corresponding P-state are intact. If this is right, then pains must either be perceptual experiences or P-states. Could they be perceptual experiences? No. If they were perceptual experiences, then we could only be aware of them by introspection. Being aware of them would be a matter of second-order awareness of a mental state. But as we have seen, awareness of pain is not like that. Awareness of pain is perceptual, not introspective. (Cf. Chapter 18, this volume.) Hence, pains must be P-states.

This completes the case for the bodily disturbance model. I will turn now to consider an objection to this line of thought.

2 The intensity objection

There are a number of reasons for thinking that the perceived intensities of pains are not very well correlated with levels of P-state activity. (See also Chapter 2, this volume.) They are correlated much more strongly with levels of activity in the dorsal horn of the spinal cord, a key site in the processing of nociceptive information, and correlated more strongly still with levels of nociceptive activity in the thalamus and cerebral cortex (Porro et al. 1998; Coghill et al. 1999). Accordingly, there is reason to think that intensities are identical with properties of states that occur at a much higher level of the nervous system than P-states – for example, properties of states of the dorsal horn (*D-states*, for short). But intensities are properties of pains. Hence, if intensities are properties of D-states, it is natural to think that pains are identical with D-states, as opposed to being identical with P-states. (I will continue to focus on this *D-state identity hypothesis* in the interests of simplicity. The corresponding identity hypotheses concerning states of the thalamus and cortex are similar, but require more detailed exposition. The reply to the D-state identity hypothesis that I offer below can be generalized so as to apply to these other identity hypotheses as well.)

This objection to the bodily disturbance model has been pressed forcefully by Adam Pautz in several papers (e.g., Pautz 2010 and 2014). Related objections have been raised by Price and Barrell (2012: 201, 203).

There are several reasons why the intensities of pains are more strongly correlated with D-states than with P-states. I will mention three. First, perceived intensities often reflect the history of nociceptive activity in a particular location, not just the current level of activity. This is *temporal summation* (see, e.g., Price 1999). Second, perceived intensities reflect *long-term sensitization* – a condition of hypersensitivity in dorsal horn regions that results from long-term stimulation (Basbaum and Jessell 2012). Third, as we noticed earlier, there is downward influence on nociceptive processing from higher-level states, such as attention, emotion, expectation, and hypnotic suggestion. Intensities attest to this influence. This is *higher-level modulation*.

In view of all this, it must be acknowledged that there is a strong case for identifying perceived intensities with properties of D-states. By the same token, there is a strong case for thinking that the somatosensory representations that support awareness of pain have components or aspects that stand for such properties. Let us grant that this is true. But should we also grant that pains *are* the states that possess these properties? That is, should we grant that pains are D-states? The case for this additional claim is much weaker. Indeed, it can be shown to rest on a false principle. Thus, the argument clearly presupposes the following *state/property principle*:

> (SPP) If a representational state R represents a property P as instantiated, and P is in fact instantiated by X, then R attributes P to X.

This principle holds across a wide spectrum of cases, but we quickly run into problems if we try to apply it across the board. To see this, recall Treisman's results concerning illusory conjunctions (Treisman and Schmidt 1982). She found that when attention to specific objects is attenuated, due to its being spread across a wide array, visual representations can misattribute properties in the array, assigning them to the wrong objects. It follows that (SPP) is mistaken. By the same token, even though we are granting that perceived intensities are properties of D-states, there is no compelling reason for going on to conclude that pains are D-states.

Further, there is an alternative to the claim that pains are D-states that can be seen on reflection to be much more plausible. This is the view that pains are P-states, but that the somatosensory representations that support awareness of pain systematically misrepresent P-states by attributing properties of D-states to them. This can also be put by saying that awareness of pain involves a systematic illusion. Some of the properties of pains – and in particular, their locations – are perceived accurately, at least in normal cases, but intensities are not, because the mechanisms that support awareness of pain are unable to discriminate between levels of activity in peripheral regions and levels of activity in the dorsal horn.

Why should we suppose that it is the locations of pains that are perceived accurately rather than their intensities? I will give one reason. (There are others.) As is well known, the somatotopic maps that support awareness of pains are integrated with visual and motor maps of bodily regions. Thus, when we experience pain at a site in the body, visual attention is drawn to that site, and motor programs that target the site swing into action, directing appropriate withdrawal and palliative behaviors. It's hard to see how the experienced locations of pains could be *universally* illusory when these locations coincide with the locations on other maps that are essential parts of the organism's response to pain.

If there is an illusion, then, it is much more likely that the illusion involves perceived intensities rather than perceived locations. But is there a plausible story as to why the nociceptive mechanisms should generate this illusion? I think so. The neural pathways carrying information about properties of P-states are the same as the pathways carrying information about the properties of D-states. Accordingly, the nociceptive mechanisms in somatosensory cortex are unable to distinguish between the former properties and the latter properties. Now as we have just seen, the mechanisms that are responsible for processing information about locations are integrated with other mechanisms associated with vision and behavior, so they are in effect parts of a system that can *triangulate* on the locations of P-states. But it appears that no such teamwork is possible for the mechanisms that process information about intensities. Accordingly, they cannot discriminate between the levels of activity of P-states and the levels of the corresponding D-states. Moreover, since D-states occur farther up the processing hierarchy, information about their levels of activity screens off information about the levels of P-states. Accordingly, there is a much closer correlation between cortical representations and the levels of D-states than between the representations and the levels of P-states. But this is a reason for supposing that the representations stand for the levels of D-states.

3 The central state model

I have been at pains to develop a strong case for the bodily disturbance model because the alternative model is supported by a simple argument that can seem to be absolutely irresistible. Unless the case for the bodily disturbance model is developed carefully, it can seem to be negligible in comparison.

The main claims of the central state model are as follows:

1   Experiences of pain are perceptual states that represent P-states.
2   Pains are identical with these perceptual states.

3   Hence, pains can occur even when there are no corresponding P-states.
4   In cases of this sort, the somatosensory system represents P-states as occurring, but these are misrepresentations, on a par with the illusions and hallucinations associated with the visual system.
5   Perceptual states of the sort in question cause pain-affect. Hence, experiences of pain are almost always accompanied by states of aversion, even when they are not accompanied by P-states.
6   Awareness of pain is a form of introspective awareness.

The argument for the model is simple: it is that cases of neuropathic pain and phantom limb pain are definitely cases of *pain*. It would be very confusing to describe them as cases in which agents are subject to illusions or hallucinations of pain. Yes, they may involve illusions or hallucinations concerning P-states. This is explicitly acknowledged by the model. But it would clearly create serious communications problems for a doctor to attempt to console a patient by telling him that his *pain* is a hallucination, on a par with Macbeth's dagger. Any such claim would be dismissed by the patient as absurd – unless it was accompanied by a full presentation of the bodily disturbance theory, and perhaps also a suggestion that a linguistic reform was due. Whatever its deficiencies may be in other respects (for example, its account of awareness of pain seems quite unsatisfactory; consider the earlier arguments that awareness of pain is perceptual), the central state model accommodates facts of this sort beautifully. On the other hand, the bodily disturbance model can make no sense of them.

There is another way to put this point. Folk psychology makes no allowance for an appearance/reality distinction with respect to pain. That is, according to folk psychology, if it seems to one that one is in pain, then one really is in pain; and if one really is in pain, then it seems to one that one is in pain. The central state model accommodates this feature of the folk picture of pain by identifying pain with a perceptual experience. There is an appearance/reality distinction with respect to objects of perceptual experience, such as daggers, but there is no appearance/reality distinction with respect to perceptual experiences themselves. Although folk psychology will allow you to say that you seem to be seeing a dagger, but perhaps aren't really seeing one, it won't allow you to say that you seem to seem to be seeing a dagger, but perhaps don't really seem to be seeing one.

The definition of pain that is offered by the IASP seems to coincide in this respect with the picture that is embedded in folk psychology. As we saw, the definition represents pain as an unpleasant *experience*. In claiming that pain is an experience, it is in effect denying that pain is governed by an appearance/reality distinction. (For further discussion, see Chapter 31, this volume.) Scientific thought joins folk wisdom in holding that in the case of pain, what you (seem to) see is what you get.

If we were to seek an explanation for the absence of an appearance/reality distinction in the case of pain, we would probably conclude that it has to do with the fact that pain bothers us, often quite terribly. That fact is responsible for much of our interest in pain, and therefore, for much of our willingness to apply the concept of pain. Now the perceptual states that represent P-states can cause deep aversion, of the sort characteristic of awareness of pain, whether or not they are actually accompanied by P-states. That is, it is these perceptual states that most directly control our emotional response to pain. In view of this, it is not surprising that we are disposed to apply the concept whenever the perceptual states occur.

4 A paradox and its resolution

As we observed earlier, it is possible to build a strong case for the bodily disturbance model of pain, which identifies pains with bodily states. But also, as we have just now been noticing, it is possible to build a strong case for the opposing central state model, which identifies pain with mental states. Since the models conflict, they cannot both be correct. This is the paradox of pain.

I hope I have said enough above to show that we cannot respond to the paradox by just dismissing one of the two theories. They both capture very important aspects of the folk and scientific pictures of pain. We should try to preserve them both, insofar as possible. If we can agree on this, I think we can also agree on the sources of the paradox, and also on how it should be resolved. One of the sources is the fact that awareness of pain has a number of distinct aspects or components that are always present in normal cases, and that are in fact causally connected under normal background conditions, but that are nonetheless dissociable. The other source is the fact that both folk psychology and cognitive science try to keep track of these dissociable components by a single concept. This works well enough in normal cases, but serious problems emerge when normal causal relations are suspended. When the various normal companions part company, two or more concepts are needed to draw the necessary distinctions. What we should do, then, in order to resolve the paradox, is to replace the single concept of pain that is offered us by folk psychology, and the single concept that is offered us by ISAP, with a bevy of new ones. It would be a good start to introduce a concept of *peripheral pain* to stand for P-states, and a concept of *central state pain* to stand for the perceptual states that represent P-states.

All of this is good news for the philosopher who wishes to give a representationalist account of the phenomenology of pain. (For discussion see Chapter 2, this volume.) In effect, the lines of thought of the present chapter show that resistance to the bodily disturbance theory, while partly grounded in important facts, largely derives from a conceptual confusion. It arises because we erroneously attempt to use a single concept to keep track of phenomena that are different and indeed dissociable. Once this is appreciated, it is easy to see that the bodily disturbance theory provides a correct account of the sensory awareness that is involved in the overall experience of pain. The theory errs only insofar as it claims to explain all of the dimensions of pain. It follows that the bodily disturbance theory is available for use by anyone who is trying to account for the phenomenology of pain. More particularly, it is available to the representationalist. Indeed, it is a natural bedfellow of representationalism, since it implies that the sensory awareness that is involved in pain constitutively involves perceptual representations. Accordingly, the representationalist is entitled to all of the tools he or she employs in explaining the phenomenologies associated with the standard perceptual modalities in explaining the phenomenology of pain.

Related topics

Chapter 2: Pain and representation (Cutter)
Chapter 4: Imperativism (Klein)
Chapter 18: Pain: perception or introspection? (Aydede)
Chapter 27: Bad by nature: an axiological theory of pain (Massin)
Chapter 31: An introduction to the IASP's definition of pain (Wright)
Chapter 32: Philosophy and "placebo" analgesia (Moerman)

References

Aydede, M. and Fulkerson, M. (2014) Affect: representationalists' headache. *Philosophical Studies* 170: 175–198.

Basbaum, A.I. and Jessell, T.M. (2012) Pain. In E.R. Kandel, J.H. Schwartz, T.M. Jessell, S.A. Siegelbaum, and A.J. Hudspeth (eds.), *Principles of Neural Science*, 5th ed. New York: McGraw Hill, pp. 530–555.

Bushnell, M.C., Villemure, C., and Duncan, G.H. (2004) Psychophysical and neurophysiological studies of pain modulation by attention. In D.D. Price and M.C. Bushnell (eds.), *Psychological Methods of Pain Control: Basic Science and Clinical Perspectives*. Seattle: IASP Press, pp. 99–116.

Cevero, F. (2012) *Understanding Pain*. Cambridge, MA: MIT Press.

Coghill, R.C., Sang, C.N., Maisog, J.M., and Iadarola, M.J. (1999) Pain intensity processing within the human brain: a bilateral distributed mechanism. *Journal of Neurophysiology* 82(4): 1934–1943.

Dretske, F. (1986) Misrepresentation. In R. Bogdan (ed.), *Belief: Form, Content, and Function*. Oxford: Oxford University Press, pp. 597–610.

Dretske, F. (1995) *Naturalizing the Mind*. Cambridge: MIT Press.

Gardner, E.P. (2012) Touch. In E.R. Kandel, J.H. Schwartz, T.M. Jessell, S.A. Siegelbaum, and A.J. Hudspeth (eds.), *Principles of Neural Science*, 5th ed. New York: McGraw Hill, pp. 498–529.

Gardner, E.P. and Johnson, K.O. (2012). The somatosensory system: receptors and central pathways. In E.R. Kandel, J.H. Schwartz, T.M. Jessell, S.A. Siegelbaum, and A.J. Hudspeth (eds.), *Principles of Neural Science*, 5th ed. New York: McGraw Hill, pp. 475–497.

Grahek, N. (2011) *Feeling Pain and Being in Pain*, 2nd ed. pbk. Cambridge, MA: MIT Press.

Hill, C.S. (2009) *Consciousness*. Cambridge: Cambridge University Press.

Hill, C.S. (2014) *Meaning, Mind, and Knowledge*. Oxford: Oxford University Press.

Hofbauer, R.K., Rainville, P., Duncan, G.H., and Bushnell, M.C. (2001) Somatosensory representation of the sensory dimension of pain. *Journal of Neurophysiology* 85: 402–411.

Mersky, H. and Bogduk, N. (1994) *Classification of Chronic Pain*, 2nd ed. Seattle: ISAP Press.

Ostrowsky, K., Magnin, M., Ryvlin, P., Isnard, J., Guenot, M., and Mauguiére, F. (2002) Representation of pain and somatic sensation in the human insula: a study of responses to direct electrical cortical stimulation. *Cerebral Cortex* 12: 376–385.

Pautz, A. (2010) Do theories of consciousness rest on a mistake? *Philosophical Issues* 20: 333–367.

Pautz, A. (2014) The real trouble for phenomenal externalists. In R. Brown (ed.), *Consciousness Inside and Out: Phenomenology, Neuroscience, and the Nature of Experience*. Dordrecht: Springer, pp. 237–298.

Porro, C.A., Cettolo, V., Francescato, M.P., and Baraldi, P. (1998) Temporal and intensity coding of pain in human cortex. *Journal of Neurophysiology* 80(6): 3312–3320.

Price, D.D. (1999) *Psychological Mechanisms of Pain and Analgesia*. Seattle: IASP Press.

Price, D.D. and Barrell, J.J. (2012) *Inner Experience and Neuroscience: Merging Both Perspectives*. Cambridge, MA: MIT Press.

Price, D.D., Craggs, J., Verne, G.N., Perlstein, W.M., and Robinson, M.E. (2007) Placebo analgesia is accompanied by large reductions in pain-related brain activity in Irritable Bowel Syndrome patients. *Pain* 127: 63–72.

Rainville, P. (2004) Pain and emotions. In D.D. Price and M.C. Bushnell (eds.), *Psychological Methods of Pain Control: Basic Science and Clinical Perspectives*. Seattle: IASP Press, pp. 117–141.

Treisman, A. and Schmidt, H. (1982) Illusory conjunctions in the perception of objects. *Cognitive Psychology* 14: 107–141.

Tye, M. (2000) *Consciousness, Color and Content*. Cambridge: MIT Press.

Tye, M. and Cutter, B. (2011) Tracking intentionalism and the painfulness of pain. *Philosophical Issues* 21: 90–109.

Warren, W.H. (1984) Perceiving affordances: Visual guidance of stair climbing. *Journal of Experimental Psychology: Human Perception and Performance* 10(5): 683–703.

Yeshuran, Y. and Carrasco, M. (1998) Attention improves or impairs visual performance by enhancing spatial resolution. *Nature* 396: 72–75.

PART I-II

Modeling pain in neuroscience

6

ADVANCES IN THE NEUROSCIENCE OF PAIN

Vania Apkarian

> The substance of the mind must therefore be material, since it is affected by the impact of material weapons.
>
> *Lucretius (100–50 BCE),* On the Nature of the Universe

Over the last twenty years or so there has been a veritable revolution in the science of pain. Many of these discoveries have direct implications as to processes involved in perception and/or consciousness, and thus impact philosophical discussions on the topic. This chapter covers recent advances in our understanding of brain mechanisms involved in nociception and acute and chronic pain. It expounds on the state of our knowledge regarding the differentiation between conscious pain perception and subconscious nociception; and on neural circuitry underlying both acute pain and mechanisms that reorganize the brain through learning processes that engage emotion/addiction related circuitry, to carve the chronic brain state.

1 Introduction

As a neuroscientist who has dedicated a lifetime to uncovering brain mechanisms of pain, both in animal and human studies, using technologies that span cellular electrophysiology to whole-brain functional imaging in humans, I do not question the link between neurons and perception. Establishing grounding rules regarding this relationship guides this research enterprise. Different philosophers continue to argue regarding the extent to which consciousness can or is being explained; while some purport that neuroscientific advances have already all but solved the problem, others insist the question is too hard: "how could mere matter be conscious?" (Fodor 2007). Scientists have the luxury of circumventing these arguments by posing testable questions with which one can establish relationships, hoping to eventually reveal mechanisms and even laws, between neurons and consciousness or perception. It remains unclear whether this approach will be sufficient in the long run; however, the advances made in the last decades have been plentifully fruitful and demonstrate that there is more work to be done; quoting Fodor again: "there is plenty of tunnel at the end of the light," especially regarding the neuroscience of perception. Welcome news for those who revel in exploring long, dark tunnels.

73

The last fifteen to twenty years have all but revolutionized our understanding of brain mechanisms of pain. These advances now point to a vast circuitry that hitherto was not suspected to be involved in pain, imposing new conditionals regarding subjectivity, incommunicability, free will, multiple realizability, and attention/salience, and even forcing us to revisit the definition of pain itself. The subject is briefly reviewed below.

It is first appropriate to review necessary definitions to clarify the topic in review. From a physiological/psychological viewpoint and in relation to the neuroscience of the sense of pain, pain is defined as the conscious perception associated with tissue damage or potential tissue damage. (Cf. philosophical positions presented in Chapters 1–5, 17, and 18 in this volume.) This subjective perception has florid behavioral correlates that can be observed in animals as well, thus providing the opportunity to study mechanisms associated with pain-like behaviors in species other than humans. (Cf. Chapter 15, this volume.) Sherrington coined the terms nociception/nociceptive referring to neural elements that respond to tissue injuries and which may give rise to pain. Importantly, nociceptive activity may or may not result in pain perception. The rest of this chapter expands on new concepts regarding (1) the distinction between pain and nociception, (2) modern psychophysical rules for pain, (3) brain circuitry transforming nociception into pain, and (4) brain circuitry transforming acute pain into chronic pain.

2 Conscious pain, subconscious nociception, and blindness to pain

Since the work of Beecher in the 1950s, there has been the realization that pain and nociception do not necessarily correspond to each other. Baliki and I recently proposed the more extreme position that pain and nociception should be considered distinct processes and must be studied separately (Baliki and Apkarian 2015). Additionally, we argued that the functional role of nociception remains to be scientifically elucidated. We proposed that nociception is in fact by and large the machinery that usually and continuously and *subconsciously* protects the body from being injured. In contrast, acute conscious perception of pain signals *the failure* to protect tissue from injuries or from potential injuries, and as such it is coupled with negative affect. Note our definition for pain is essentially the opposite of the more common definition where pain is linked with protecting tissue from impending or further injury. We instead relegate this function specifically to subconscious nociception.

The strongest argument for a continuous injury-protecting mechanism, nociception, is the fact that most organisms, for most of their lifetimes, live free of injuries and free of experiencing pain even though our environments, including modern urban sprawls, are highly noxious. My body weight is around 64 kilograms. How many minutes can you lift me without reporting pain? Perhaps five to ten minutes, certainly not much longer than thirty minutes. But, your nociceptors innervating your own soles carry your own weight – approximately equivalent to mine – for a lifetime, yet you never feel this weight and it is not painful. Similarly, individual afferent nociceptor thresholds and supra-threshold response curves are very similar across rodents, humans, and presumably even elephants, and moreover they remain constant across a lifetime. However, the body weight that your soles are carrying increases by about ten times from childhood to adulthood, and varies across species. Therefore, the rate of afferent nociceptor activity impinging on the brain cannot be linearly related to pain. This concept in turn implies an active central thresholding process, which fine-tunes the shift between subconscious nociception-related behavior and conscious pain. Given that even simple motor movements, like flexion and extension or walking are all potentially noxious outside of the natural behavioral boundaries, we conclude that for most of life and across species the experience of pain is actually blind to most noxious stimuli.

If the subconscious nociceptive system can properly protect the organism most of the time from injuries, why have a conscious pain at all? One reason is the opportunity that conscious perceptions provide regarding making choices across multiple possibilities, and the second is the need to bind the environmental situational multisensory details with each other and form higher-order learned memory traces that provide venues for future planning as well as opportunities for more complex experiences. As Tse states: "... the only time most of our actions require a conscious feeling of willing will be cases where the action involves a deci-sion point that cannot be preprogrammed ..." (Tse 2013: 176). Taking Tse's position to heart, the implication is that nociceptive subconscious decisions are mostly "exogenously controlled and closed-ended" and thus fundamental to the integrity of the organism. In fact, in our perspective article (Baliki and Apkarian 2015), we present the evidence that lack of nociceptors (for example in congenital insensitivity to pain) compromises life, as such indi-viduals usually cannot survive past puberty due to the massive tissue damages they incur on themselves. On the other hand, subjects who do not have the conscious qualia of pain but normal nociception (for example patient "H.M.") can lead a normal life (although most likely with a somewhat diminished quality of experiences).

3 Pain psychophysics obeys mathematical rules

Psychophysics from its inception in the nineteenth century has attempted to demonstrate that at least parts of human subjective experience/perception can be captured quantitatively and described with simple mathematical models. Beginning with the work of E.H. Weber and culminating with S.S. Stevens' law of magnitude perception (power functions that define sensory stimulus intensity transformation to perceived magnitudes), statistical properties of pain have been quantified and modeled using simple equations (Stevens 1957; Weber 1978; Price 1988). Currently, statistics of pain are quantified with questionnaire-based tools (for example, the McGill Pain Questionnaire), and these have become the main instruments with which the efficacy of pain therapies is studied in clinical trials (Hansson and Haanpaa 2007).

As pain fluctuates slowly, due to slow transmission from the periphery to the brain, subjects can readily and continuously rate how much pain they are experiencing, for example by varying the expanse of thumb to pointing finger separation (Apkarian et al. 2001; Davis et al. 2002). Subjects can be instructed to rate the intensity of specific properties of their pain, such as sharpness, burning, etc. If one plots the temperature applied to the skin relative to the reported pain intensity ratings, then one can derive a differential equation relating the temperature to perceived pain intensity (Cecchi et al. 2012). This mathematical formula-tion, where the equation is determined for individual subjects using a few parameters, captures thousands of values of pain reports highly accurately (70–90-percent accuracy), and with almost the same accuracy predicts the same subject's ratings of pain stimuli that the subject had not experienced before, and generalizes across subjects. This discovery should surprise, and shock, at least the philosopher and even pain clinicians and scientists who for decades have been instructed to accept the personalized, subjective incommunicability of pain. One is forced to conclude that the subjectivity of pain follows, at least for specific stimuli and under specific lab conditions, objective mathematically deterministic rules, rules of which the participants themselves do not have any conscious knowledge.

A second similar study complements the above observations (Jepma et al. 2014). This study shows that the habituation and sensitization effects (changes in perceived pain intensity over many minutes due to the same or different tissues receiving repeated stimulation) can be captured by a simple mathematical model, which accurately predicts the group-average reported pain, independently of the stimulus intensity (Jepma et al. 2014). Thus, multiple properties of experimental pain show objectively determinable rules.

In 1978, D. Dennett argued, based on the neuroscience of the period and due to the subjectivity of pain, and in contrast to visual perception, that it cannot be captured in computational models (Dennett 1978). The passage of time seems to have demonstrated the opposite. We now have elegant mathematical models for intensity of pain but none for vision. Therefore, at least some properties of pain, in the lab setting, are precise and predictable, and follow strict mathematical rules.

4 Neural elements of nociception and acute pain

The fundamental cellular and molecular elements of the machinery that underlie nociceptive processing are solidly established (Melzack and Wall 1999). There is extensive evidence for the existence of a specific neural substrate engaged in pain-related information processing. Nociceptive free nerve endings (nerve endings that signal tissue-injury-related energies) innervate almost all tissue outside of the brain and transduce through a variety of receptors acidity, high temperatures, heat, cold, and potentially or starkly painful mechanical stimuli to the central nervous system (CNS). A long list of receptors is now uncovered with specializations that encode injury-related energies.

There is a wonderful continuity across species regarding transduction mechanisms signaling nociceptive energies. Similarly, small myelinated afferents and non-myelinated C-fibers are observed across at least the mammalian species and their spinal circuitry also seems highly preserved between species, and the same presynaptic, postsynaptic, and excitatory/inhibitory neurotransmitters and associated peptides are observed in the spinal cord circuitry across species. Multiple ascending pathways from the spinal cord to the brainstem and thalamus convey nociceptive information cephalad. Descending modulatory pathways from the cortex to the brainstem and then down to the spinal cord also constitute an essential system that seems crucial in modulating the gain of spinal cord nociceptive information transmission cephalad. Thus the concept of a sensory system (transduction, transmission, and representation) as initially illustrated by Descartes specifically for pain (see Figure 6.1) has been solidly established; for more details see Melzack and Wall 1999).

5 Cortical encoding of acute pain, in contrast to vision

A multiplicity of pathways transmit innocuous and nociceptive information to the cortex. The spinothalamic pathway is the projection most studied (Hodge and Apkarian 1990). It is the homolog to the optic tract in vision. Both pathways transmit peripheral information (nociceptive vs. visual), from first-order information processing (spinal cord vs. retina), to specific thalamic relay regions to the cortex (somatosensory regions vs. visual cortex). Therefore, it is informative to directly compare the informational content between the two pathways.

The optic tract is composed of about 1.0–1.7 million axons, and this count does not differ between cat, monkey, and human tissues (Sanchez et al. 1986). On the other hand, the spinothalamic pathway contains 12,000–20,000 axons, in cat and monkey tissue (Apkarian and Hodge 1989; Klop et al. 2004), and no more than 70 percent of these axons convey nociceptive information. Thus, the visual channel transmits a hundred times more

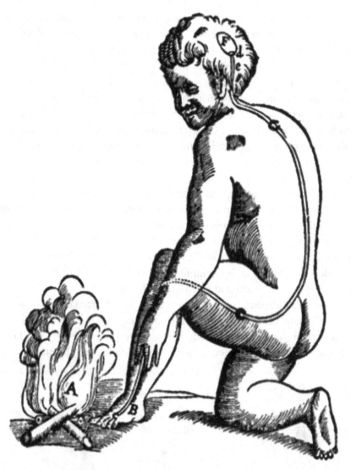

Figure 6.1 Descartes' depiction in 1644 of pain perception. Even though his description of the components illustrated is no longer viable in modern neuroscience, the drawing amply exemplifies the fundamental concepts that underlie a sensory system. A stimulus A being transduced to a signal at B, then transmitted (through afferents and spinal pathways), and finally encoded or represented at F is completely in accordance with nociceptive afferents giving rise to pain perception. Moreover, its equivalent can readily be extrapolated to other sensory modalities from this concept.

data to the thalamus than the nociceptive channel. This discrepancy further balloons at the cortical level. The human brain is composed of about 80 billion neurons, 20 billion of which constitute the neocortex, and around one third of cortical tissue is dedicated to visual information processing. In contrast, very few nociceptive cortical neurons have been found. In fact this effort has yet to find a single cortical column dedicated to the representation of nociceptive information (in the visual cortex every neuron shows visual responsiveness). Anatomically it is clear that thalamic nociceptive pathways project to multiple cortical targets (Gingold et al. 1991; Dum et al. 2009; Craig 2014), including the primary and secondary somatosensory cortex, posterior insula, and anterior cingulate, and in each of these areas a handful of nociceptive-responsive neurons are found always embedded within regions where tactile innocuous responses are dominantly represented (Kenshalo and Isensee 1983; Sikes and Vogt 1992; Peyron et al. 2002; Chen et al. 2009).

Thus, there is a stark computational difference between vision and pain. In the case of vision thalamic inputs are boosted by about 5,000 times in the cortex, while the nociceptive signal is scattered and intermingled across diverse brain regions.

The paucity of nociceptive neurons in the cortex had for decades forced questioning whether the cortex is involved in pain experience. Human brain imaging over the last twenty years overturned the discussion. There is now a highly replicable set of cortical regions consistently activated for acute painful stimuli across many different labs and in hundreds of studies (see Figure 6.2 and Chapter 7, this volume). Here it should be emphasized that putting the electrophysiology and human neuroimaging studies together, one has to assert that none of the regions seen activated with neuroimaging can be said to represent a nociceptive-specific cortical tissue. Therefore, unlike vision where a hierarchical construct seems to transform inputs to visual perception (details of which remain unclear), pain must depend on non-specific brain regions cooperating, during enhanced nociceptive inputs, to give rise to the emergent conscious percept of pain.

Since the nineteenth century there has been accumulating evidence that the cortical mantle performs sophisticated integration and feature extraction across sensory modalities. This view in modern neuroscience is exemplified by our penchant to report brain activity for a given task or perception by Cartesian coordinates (location x, y, z, in Figure 6.2 associated with pain or not) in a standardized human brain atlas. The Cartesian view dictates that if we can separately manipulate the different attributes of pain then we should identify specializations of different cortical territories regarding the additive properties of pain. For example, by analogy to cortical visual regions where color, motion, faces, or objects are associated with

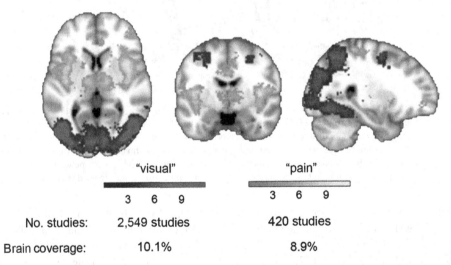

	"visual"	"pain"
No. studies:	2,549 studies	420 studies
Brain coverage:	10.1%	8.9%

Figure 6.2 Brain regions associated with the terms "visual" (blue; see online, www.routledge.com/ 9781138823181) and "pain" (yellow) based on a meta-analysis of papers collected from PubMed. The number of studies associated with "visual" was 2,549 while for "pain" the number of identified studies was 420 (mainly studies of acute pain). Confidence of association is indicated by z-values ranging from 2.3 to 14 (color brightness). The two terms engage equivalent and almost completely distinct brain tissue (10.1 percent for visual, 8.9 percent for pain). The yellow map is commonly referred to as the "pain matrix." There is a fundamental difference between the two maps. Within the regions in blue, there is very high-quality electrophysiological evidence that almost every neuron responds to some type of visual stimuli. In contrast, none of the regions in blue exhibit tissue specifically dedicated to nociceptive information processing.

distinct brain-regional activity, for pain too we should uncover regions engaged in emotion, attention, and motor preparation, and the relative activity of each of these regions would then uncover the specific properties of the painful condition the subject is in. Alternatively or additionally, we could also test for brain regions specialized in mechanical, thermal, and chemical pains; or even for burning or throbbing or stabbing pains. Although some such claims have been made (Moulton et al. 2012), they have generally not been replicated or advanced to a convincing level of evidence. Where does this leave us as to the role of the cortex in pain? One simple alternative is the idea that interaction across disparate cortical circuits is necessary for pain; and in fact recent studies show that combining signals from across many brain regions (Wager et al. 2013), or calculating local patterns of activity (Liang et al. 2013), one can extract a signal that correlates to either a painful stimulus or to the experience of pain itself. The more general issue being discussed here relates to mechanisms that transform sensory inputs to conscious perception, regarding which long lists of potential mechanisms are advanced. Unfortunately, in the realm of nociception being transformed to conscious pain there are no convincing scientific data or palatable theories of underlying mechanisms.

6 Pain as emotion or sensation

Plato, Aristotle, Galen, and Darwin excluded pain from other sensory modalities and instead classified it with emotions. Avicenna (or Ibn Sīnā), the eleventh century Arab-Persian philosopher-physician, is credited with being the first to suggest pain as a specific skin sense, an idea more concretely reformulated by Descartes (Figure 6.1; see Finger 2001; Perl 2011). Perhaps surprisingly the issue remains unsettled even though the official definition of pain (almost universally accepted) advanced by the International Association for the Study of Pain states that pain is "an unpleasant sensory and emotional experience," asserting that pain sensation and pain emotion together constitute pain and that one component cannot, or can only very seldom and under very special conditions, be experienced without the other. (For discussion see Chapter 31, this volume.) Neuroscience is still ambivalent as to where and how to define the emotions, see (Phan et al. 2002), and thus linking nociceptive inputs with emotional attributes also remains incomplete and imprecise.

The classical concept divides the spinothalamic pathway into a medial and a lateral component, and assigns emotional evaluation to the medial spinothalamic pathway and sensory discrimination to the lateral pathway (Hodge and Apkarian 1990). This subdivision is consistent with the anatomy of thalamocortical projections. The medial pathway terminates in medial thalamic nuclei, which project to prefrontal and cingulate cortex, and these regions are best connected to sub-cortical limbic structures that are necessarily involved in the emotions, while the lateral spinothalamic projections gain access to somatosensory cortices and to the insula. Given this construct and human-brain-imaging technology, differentially manipulating painful stimuli to enhance emotional and sensory aspects should then segregate respectively specialized brain regions. This was in fact the approach used by Bushnell and colleagues who manipulated thermal-pain perception properties by hypnosis, suggestively enhanced the emotional salience of the stimulus, and observed increased brain activity in the anterior cingulate. The authors thus concluded that pain-affect is encoded in the anterior cingulate but not in the somatosensory cortex (Rainville et al. 1997). The study is complicated due to the use of hypnosis, where the experimenter has no idea what is being manipulated. A complementary study reported that when electrical recordings are done from neurons in anterior cingulate in patients undergoing neurosurgical procedures (precious and rare data), nociceptive neurons can be identified (eleven of sixty-eight tested) but electrical stimulation at these sites did not evoke the experience of pain (Hutchison et al. 1999), and in a later report further results indicated the region is more responsive to novelty, salience, and emotional demands (Davis et al. 2005; for a more recent discussion, see Wager et al. 2016). The other cortical region regularly espoused to be involved in encoding affective properties of pain is the insula. The region is the most commonly and reproducibly activated cortical structure for acute pain (Apkarian et al. 2005): the posterior insula is shown to receive spinothalamic-thalamocortical projections (Dum et al. 2009), and nociceptive-responsive neurons are described in the posterior insula in human neurosurgical procedures (Peyron et al. 2002; Mazzola et al. 2009). Still, direct evidence that any region in the insula is specialized in preferentially encoding emotional aspects of pain is lacking. Instead there is evidence that large lesions of the insula do not impair (and may even enhance) pain perception (Starr et al. 2009).

The lateral spinothalamic tract projects to primary and secondary somatosensory cortex, posterior insula, and motor regions. Different researchers continue to insist that any one of these cortical targets is essential for conveying sensory discriminative aspects of pain, although again the evidence remains minimal, and large lesions of the regions minimally compromise pain (Greenspan et al. 1999; Starr et al. 2009; see recent discussion regarding posterior insula in Davis et al. 2015).

Thus, overall evidence for cortical regional specificity for sensory discrimination or the negative emotional experience of pain remains unconvincing, and the same can be said for all other perceptual dimensions co-occurring with pain.

7 Pain as salience

The other defining property of pain is its close association with attention. There is ample brain-imaging evidence that distraction decreases perceived intensity for painful stimuli and such conditions are accompanied by decreased brain activity across most brain regions activated for acute pain (Bushnell et al. 2006, 2013). Earlier human-brain-imaging studies debated whether anterior cingulate activity reflects attention to or the emotion of pain. More recent studies have shown that painful or non-painful visual or auditory, but similarly salient, stimuli seem to activate almost all of the brain regions commonly observed for pain (Iannetti and Mouraux 2010). The latter observation questions the extent to which brain activity commonly seen for acute pain can be decomposed to its constituent properties.

The science of human-brain imaging for acute pain is treated here in rough strokes. The literature is vast and many elegant studies are not covered. My emphasis is the fact that the current literature remains correlative. Additionally, the brain-imaging literature for acute pain is heavily dominated by efforts to isolate regional activity (treating each brain voxel as an independent variable), and for the most part ignoring the interactive properties of the brain, that is, the brain as an integrated network. Pattern analysis studies are the first to begin to address the integrative properties of the brain as a network in pain (Liang et al. 2013; Wager et al. 2013; Chapter 7, this volume); much more remains to be done in this direction.

8 Chronic pain

Pain that persists following the initial inciting event and past the natural healing process after the injury is defined as chronic pain. (For further discussion on chronic pain, see also Chapter 10, this volume.) Chronic back pain, osteoarthritis joint pain, and headaches are the most common examples. In many cases the patients suffer from the condition for the rest of their lives, severely limiting their daily abilities, disrupting sleep, decreasing cognitive performance, and overall negatively impacting on quality of life. Chronic pain is now ranked as the most common disability condition in the US and seventh most common worldwide (Murray and Lopez 2013). Unlike acute pain, where variants of opiates or aspirin rapidly and significantly diminish the pain, treatment options for chronic pain are far more limited. Therapies, pharmacological or otherwise, show limited efficacy and none are scientifically validated. Until the advent of animal models mimicking chronic pain-like behaviors, clinicians commonly blamed the patient for the condition (unobservable subjectivity is easy to reject especially when pitted against health-care costs or resources; "you say you have pain, I do not believe you"), and many simply denied even the existence of chronic pain conditions. Fortunately, once human-brain-imaging technology became available and applied to the chronic pain patients, neuroscience started documenting brain anatomical and physiological abnormalities, and brain risk factors for chronic pain, compelling the scientific and medical communities to accept the concept that chronic pain is a pathological disease state (Tracey and Bushnell 2009).

Almost twenty years ago, at a time when my lab had already been engaged in human-brain-imaging studies for more than five years, I made the conscious decision that we needed to turn away from brain imaging of acute pain in healthy subjects, and develop methodologies to study chronic pain patients' brain properties. Twenty years hence we still continue on this path. The effort has provided important concepts regarding the human pain condition, many of which are now validated by different scientists and for a diversity of clinical pain conditions, and has begun to demystify chronic pain and lead to reverse translational studies where animal models study circuits identified in the human condition.

The main concept of studies, across animals and humans, regarding chronic pain is the general demonstration that as soon as painful conditions persist for more than some minutes in the peripheral nervous system (PNS), the CNS exhibits reorganization (changes in synaptic sensitivity, often accompanied with anatomical deformations, and even neuronal death) (Basbaum et al. 2009). The scale of this reorganization dictates whether it may be reversible or not, and the human evidence shows that the interaction between the injury and brain properties, especially regarding regions involved in emotions, is the primary conditional dictating whether the inciting event would give rise to chronic pain or to recovery back to health (Baliki and Apkarian 2015).

9 Animal models, and peripheral and spinal cord reorganization

A very large and growing literature documents peripheral and spinal cord reorganization following various injuries to the skin, to afferent fibers, and to the peripheral nervous system (Melzack and Wall 1999). In general, such studies indicate changes in stimulus–response properties of afferent fibers following peripheral injuries, with many specific changes unique to the types of injury incurred. The simplest example is a mild skin inflammation, such as sunburn. Within the territory of the injured skin, nociceptive afferents increase their response sensitivity. Behaviorally this translates into stimuli like light touch or warm water or mildly painful heat all feeling more painful. That is, taking a warm shower after sunburn becomes painful. In addition, tissue just adjacent to the injury develops increased sensitivity to light touch, where touch starts feeling painful, while other stimulus modalities remain unperturbed. The change in perception for the injured tissue is commonly referred to as peripheral sensitization because these effects are mediated by the change in properties of afferents innervating the tissue. On the other hand, the mechanical sensitivity seen outside of the injured tissue is mediated at the level of the first synapse in the spinal cord, and is thus defined as central (meaning spinal cord) sensitization. For the sunburn example, touching the skin outside of the burn feels painful due to spinal-cord-mediated synaptic activity. Even in the absence of any medication use, inflammatory injuries like the sunburn will dissipate in a few days with the tissue healing and all abnormal sensations reversed. Besides the reversible peripheral and central reorganization, another novelty of the inflamed tissue is that a large portion of the enhanced pain experience in such conditions is mediated by myelinated afferents that in healthy tissue only signal touch-related experiences. Thus, following injury the specificity of afferents involved in pain is perturbed and shows a complex relationship with type and duration of injury (Woolf et al. 2006b). When the injury involves neural tissue, usually nerve bundles, then associated behavior is dubbed neuropathic pain, and commonly animal models of such injuries tend to result in pain-like behaviors that can last for months or for a lifetime. Such injuries also show both peripheral and central sensitization, with many distinct properties from that seen following inflammatory injuries, and there is a very large literature on the specific receptor and channel property changes in the PNS as well as spinal cord circuitry reorganization, including descending modulatory control changes, all of which essentially exaggerate the signal transmitted to the brain (Woolf et al. 2006a).

10 Malleability of the cortex with chronic pain

As soon as one peers into the brain of chronic pain patients one observes abnormalities in its chemistry, anatomy, and physiology (in comparison to healthy subjects) (Apkarian et al. 2005, 2009, 2011; first demonstrated by Flor et al. 1995). These observations afford multiple implications. The evidence suggests that in a way similar to the reorganization observed in the periphery and the spinal cord, higher brain and especially cortical circuits also undergo reorganization with persistent pain. Moreover, we are confronted with the fact that at the cortex chronic pain is not simply the increased activity of acute pain (e.g., more activity in regions shown in Figure 6.2), but rather distinct chronic pain conditions exhibit different brain regional activity and different patterns of cortical anatomical reorganization. It remains unclear, however, whether the cortical plasticity is consequent or causal to the spinal cord central sensitization. A trivial explanation that also cannot be ruled out would be that these are simply a reflection of long-term cortical reorganization as a result of suffering and coping with the condition, including the effects of medication consumption, behavior modifications, lack of sleep, limited mobility, etc.

Studying patients longitudinally over three years, from initial onset of back pain to either recovery to health or transitioning to chronic pain indicates that chronification of pain is itself accompanied with brain anatomical and functional reorganization (Baliki et al. 2012).

11 Predictability of chronic pain

Clinically it is a common observation that, although a very large number of subjects suffer from similar injuries, a very small proportion of them actually develop chronic pain. Thus the tissue injury properties are not sufficient for the emergence of chronic pain. The longitudinal study also demonstrated that anatomical and physiological brain properties can predict who will develop chronic pain (Baliki et al. 2012; Mansour et al. 2013). Both brain anatomical and physiological properties were highly accurately predictive (80–100 percent). The predictive circuitry involved the emotion- and addiction-related limbic brain, suggesting that chronic pain can be conceptualized as the brain becoming addicted to the nociceptive barrage it is receiving (Baliki and Apkarian 2015).

12 Memory and chronic pain

Neonates show full-blown behavioral signs of pain: they withdraw from pinprick, and cry when pinched. Acute pain (and nociception), together with food, drink, and pleasure, are all primary reinforcers. That is, these sensory–behavioral repertoires provide elementary innate experiences upon which more complex associations are built, giving rise to more complex perceptions and behaviors. It has classically been assumed that chronic pain is simply the amplification of the nociceptive barrage. However, the longitudinal study as well as anatomical studies, and rodent-model studies now hint that hippocampal properties are also critically involved in the development of chronic pain, and hippocampal information processing itself is necessary and disrupted after neuropathic injury or with the development of chronic pain (Mutso et al. 2012, 2013; Apkarian et al. 2015). The important implication here is the idea that hippocampus-mediated learning mechanisms are involved in the development of chronic pain, and not the persistence of an innate sensation.

13 Concluding remarks

This review avoided discussing molecular details and minimized specifics of brain circuits, and instead emphasized more general concepts. The primary notion conveyed is the separation, both mechanistically and functionally, of nociception, acute pain, and chronic pain. Brain tissue dedicated to pain perception, especially for acute pain, remains contentious. Yet our ability to accurately model the intensity of perceived pain challenges long-standing discourse regarding its subjectivity. The topic of chronic pain is also reviewed minimally, emphasizing novel concepts. The field is in flux and important new advances have occurred very recently. Fundamental progress regarding chronic pain is driven by observations regarding brain properties in humans developing or suffering from chronic pain. These studies now place the brain circuitry involved in emotions, learning, and addiction squarely in the midst of processes causally linked to chronic pain. Yet, the specifics of the interaction between peripheral and spinal cord processes that accompany chronic pain and the brain emotional circuits remain almost wholly unknown. Clinically the science of pain has still not delivered tangible benefits – for example, efficient preventions or cures – but the future does look promising.

Related topics

Chapter 1: A brief and potted overview on the philosophical theories of pain (Hardcastle)
Chapter 2: Pain and representation (Cutter)
Chapter 3: Evaluativist accounts of pain's unpleasantness (Bain)
Chapter 4: Imperativism (Klein)
Chapter 5: Fault lines in familiar concepts of pain (Hill)
Chapter 7: Neuromatrix theory of pain (Wager and Roy)
Chapter 10: Pathophysiological mechanisms of chronic pain (Thacker and Moseley)
Chapter 17: Pain and consciousness (Pereplyotchik)

References

Apkarian, A.V. and Hodge, C.J. (1989) Primate spinothalamic pathways I: A quantitative study of the cells of origin of the spinothalamic pathway. *Journal of Comparative Neurology* 288: 447–473.

Apkarian, A.V., Krauss, B.R., Fredrickson, B.E., and Szeverenyi, N.M. (2001) Imaging the pain of low back pain: functional magnetic resonance imaging in combination with monitoring subjective pain perception allows the study of clinical pain states. *Neuroscience Letters* 299: 57–60.

Apkarian, A.V., Bushnell, M.C., Treede, R.D., and Zubieta, J.K. (2005). Human brain mechanisms of pain perception and regulation in health and disease. *European Journal of Pain* (London, UK) 9: 463–484.

Apkarian, A.V., Baliki, M.N., and Geha, P.Y. (2009) Towards a theory of chronic pain. *Progress in Neurobiology* 87: 81–97.

Apkarian, A.V., Hashmi, J.A., and Baliki, M.N. (2011) Pain and the brain: specificity and plasticity of the brain in clinical chronic pain. *Pain* 152(3 suppl.): S49–S64.

Apkarian, A.V., Mutso, A.A., Centeno, M.V., Kan, L., Wu, M., Levinstein, M., Banisadr, G., Gobeske, K.T., and Miller, R.J., Radulovic, J., Hen, R., and Kessler, J.A. (2015) Role of adult hippocampal neurogenesis in persistent pain. *Pain* 157(2): 418–428.

Baliki, M.N. and Apkarian, A.V. (2015) Nociception, pain, negative moods, and behavior selection. *Neuron* 87: 474–491.

Baliki, M.N., Petre, B., Torbey, S., Herrmann, K.M., Huang, L., Schnitzer, T.J., Fields, H.L., and Apkarian, A.V. (2012) Corticostriatal functional connectivity predicts transition to chronic back pain. *Nature Neuroscience* 15: 1117–1119.

Basbaum, A.I., Bautista, D.M., Scherrer, G., and Julius, D. (2009) Cellular and molecular mechanisms of pain. *Cell* 139: 267–284.

Bushnell, M.C., Apkarian, A.V., McMahon, S.B., and Koltzenburg, M. (2006) Representation of pain in the brain. In C.J. Woolf, M.W. Salter, S.B. McMahon, and M. Koltzenburg (eds.), *Wall and Melzack's Textbook of Pain*, 5th ed. London: Elsevier, pp. 107–124.

Bushnell, M.C., Čeko, M., and Low, L.A. (2013) Cognitive and emotional control of pain and its disruption in chronic pain. *Nature Reviews Neuroscience* 14: 502–511.

Cecchi, G.A., Huang, L., Hashmi, J.A., Baliki, M., Centeno, M.V., Rish, I., and Apkarian, A.V. (2012) Predictive dynamics of human pain perception. *PLoS Computational Biology* 8: e1002719.

Chen, L.M., Friedman, R.M., and Roe, A.W. (2009) Area-specific representation of mechanical nociceptive stimuli within SI cortex of squirrel monkeys. *Pain* 141: 258–268.

Craig, A.D. (2014) Topographically organized projection to posterior insular cortex from the posterior portion of the ventral medial nucleus in the long-tailed macaque monkey. *Journal of Comparative Neurology* 522: 36–63.

Davis, K.D., Pope, G.E., Crawley, A.P., and Mikulis, D.J. (2002) Neural correlates of prickle sensation: a percept-related fMRI study. *Nature Neuroscience* 5: 1121–1122.

Davis, K.D., Taylor, K.S., Hutchison, W.D., Dostrovsky, J.O., McAndrews, M.P., Richter, E.O., and Lozano, A.M. (2005) Human anterior cingulate cortex neurons encode cognitive and emotional demands. *Journal of Neuroscience* 25: 8402–8406.

Davis, K.D., Bushnell, M.C., Iannetti, G.D., St. Lawrence, K., and Coghill, R. (2015) Evidence against pain specificity in the dorsal posterior insula. *F1000Research* 4: 362.

Dennett, D.C. (1978) Why you can't make a computer that feels pain. *Synthese* 38: 415.

Dum, R.P., Levinthal, D.J., and Strick, P.L. (2009) The spinothalamic system targets motor and sensory areas in the cerebral cortex of monkeys. *Journal of Neuroscience* 29: 14223–14235.

Finger, S. (2001) *Origins of Neuroscience: A History of Explorations into Brain Function*. London: Oxford University Press.

Flor, H., Elbert, T., Knecht, S., Wienbruch, C., Pantev, C., Birbaumer, N., Larbig, W., and Taub, E. (1995) Phantom-limb pain as a perceptual correlate of cortical reorganization following arm amputation. *Nature* 375: 482–484.

Fodor, J. (2007) Headaches have themselves. *London Review of Books* 29(10): 9–10.

Gingold, S.I., Greenspan, J.D., and Apkarian, A.V. (1991) Anatomic evidence of nociceptive inputs to primary somatosensory cortex: relationship between spinothalamic terminals and thalamocortical cells in squirrel monkeys. *Journal of Comparative Neurology* 308: 467–490.

Greenspan, J.D., Lee, R.R., and Lenz, F.A. (1999) Pain sensitivity alterations as a function of lesion location in the parasylvian cortex. *Pain* 81: 273–282.

Hansson, P. and Haanpaa, M. (2007) Diagnostic work-up of neuropathic pain: computing, using questionnaires or examining the patient? *European Journal of Pain* (London, UK) 11: 367–369.

Hodge, C.J. Jr. and Apkarian, A.V. (1990) The spinothalamic tract. *Critical Reviews in Neurobiology* 5: 363–397.

Hutchison, W.D., Davis, K.D., Lozano, A.M., Tasker, R.R., and Dostrovsky, J.O. (1999) Pain-related neurons in the human cingulate cortex. *Nature Neuroscience* 2: 403–405.

Iannetti, G.D. and Mouraux, A. (2010) From the neuromatrix to the pain matrix (and back). *Experimental Brain Research* 205: 1–12.

Jepma, M., Jones, M., and Wager, T.D. (2014) The dynamics of pain: evidence for simultaneous site-specific habituation and site-nonspecific sensitization in thermal pain. *Journal of Pain* 15: 734–746.

Kenshalo, D.R. Jr. and Isensee, O. (1983) Responses of primate SI cortical neurons to noxious stimuli. *Journal of Neurophysiology* 50: 1479–1496.

Klop, E.M., Mouton, L.J., and Holstege, G. (2004) How many spinothalamic tract cells are there? A retrograde tracing study in cat. *Neuroscience Letters* 360: 121–124.

Liang, M., Mouraux, A., Hu, L., and Iannetti, G.D. (2013) Primary sensory cortices contain distinguishable spatial patterns of activity for each sense. *Nature Communications* 4: 1979.

Mansour, A.R., Baliki, M.N., Huang, L., Torbey, S., Herrmann, K.M., Schnitzer, T.J., and Apkarian, A.V. (2013) Brain white matter structural properties predict transition to chronic pain. *Pain* 154: 2160–2168.

Mazzola, L., Isnard, J., Peyron, R., Guenot, M., and Mauguiere, F. (2009) Somatotopic organization of pain responses to direct electrical stimulation of the human insular cortex. *Pain* 146: 99–104.

Melzack, R. and Wall, P.D. (1999) *Textbook of Pain*, 4th ed. London: Churchill Livingston.

Moulton, E.A., Pendse, G., Becerra, L.R., and Borsook, D. (2012) BOLD responses in somatosensory cortices better reflect heat sensation than pain. *Journal of Neuroscience* 32: 6024–6031.

Murray, C.J. and Lopez, A.D. (2013) Measuring the global burden of disease. *New England Journal of Medicine* 369: 448–457.

Mutso, A.A., Radzicki, D., Baliki, M.N., Huang, L., Banisadr, G., Centeno, M.V., Radulovic, J., Martina, M., Miller, R.J., and Apkarian, A.V. (2012) Abnormalities in hippocampal functioning with persistent pain. *Journal of Neuroscience* 32: 5747–5756.

Mutso, A.A., Petre, B., Huang, L., Baliki, M.N., Torbey, S., Herrmann, K., Schnitzer, T.J., and Apkarian, A.V. (2013) Reorganization of hippocampal functional connectivity with transition to chronic back pain. *Journal of Neurophysiology* 111(5): 1065–1076.

Perl, E.R. (2011) Pain mechanisms: a commentary on concepts and issues. *Progress in Neurobiology* 94: 20–38.

Peyron, R., Frot, M., Schneider, F., Garcia-Larrea, L., Mertens, P., Barral, F.G., Sindou, M., Laurent, B., and Mauguiere, F. (2002) Role of operculoinsular cortices in human pain processing: converging evidence from PET, fMRI, dipole modeling, and intracerebral recordings of evoked potentials. *Neuroimage* 17: 1336–1346.

Phan, K.L., Wager, T., Taylor, S.F., and Liberzon, I. (2002) Functional neuroanatomy of emotion: a meta-analysis of emotion activation studies in PET and fMRI. *Neuroimage* 16: 331–348.

Price, D.D. (1988) *Psychological and Neural Mechanims of Pain*. New York: Raven Press.

Rainville, P., Duncan, G.H., Price, D.D., Carrier, B., and Bushnell, M.C. (1997) Pain affect encoded in human anterior cingulate but not somatosensory cortex. *Science* 277: 968–971.

Sanchez, R.M., Dunkelberger, G.R., and Quigley, H.A. (1986) The number and diameter distribution of axons in the monkey optic nerve. *IOVS: Investigative Ophthalmology & Visual Science* 27: 1342–1350.

Sikes, R.W. and Vogt, B.A. (1992) Nociceptive neurons in area 24 of rabbit cingulate cortex. *Journal of Neurophysiology* 68: 1720–1732.

Starr, C.J., Sawaki, L., Wittenberg, G.F., Burdette, J.H., Oshiro, Y., Quevedo, A.S., and Coghill, R.C. (2009) Roles of the insular cortex in the modulation of pain: insights from brain lesions. *Journal of Neuroscience*, 29: 2684–2694.

Stevens, S.S. (1957) On the psychophysical law. *Psychological Review* 64: 153–181.

Tracey, I. and Bushnell, M.C. (2009) How neuroimaging studies have challenged us to rethink: is chronic pain a disease? *Journal of Pain* 10: 1113–1120.

Tse, P.U. (2013) *The Neural Basis of Free Will: Criterial Causation*. London: MIT Press.

Wager, T.D., Atlas, L.Y., Lindquist, M.A., Roy, M., Woo, C.W., and Kross, E. (2013) An fMRI-based neurologic signature of physical pain. *New England Journal of Medicine* 368: 1388–1397.

Wager, T.D., Atlas, L.Y., Botvinick, M.M., Chang, L.J., Coghill, R.C., Davis, K.D., Iannetti, G.D., Poldrack, R.A., Shackman, A.J., and Yarkoni, T. (2016) Pain in the ACC? *Proceedings of the National Academy of Sciences of the United States of America* 113(18): E2474–E2475.

Weber, E.H. (1978) *The Sense of Touch*, trans. H.E. Ross and D.J. Murray. London: Academic Press.

Woolf, C.J., Salter, M.W., McMahon, S.B., and Koltzenburg, M. (eds.) (2006a) *Wall and Melzack's Textbook of Pain*, 5th ed. London: Elsevier.

Woolf, C.J., Salter, M.W., McMahon, S.B., and Koltzenburg, M. (2006b) Plasticity and pain: role of the dorsal horn. In C.J. Woolf, M.W. Salter, S.B. McMahon, and M. Koltzenburg (eds.), *Wall and Melzack's Textbook of Pain*, 5th ed. London: Elsevier, pp. 91–105.

7

NEUROMATRIX THEORY OF PAIN

Mathieu Roy and Tor D. Wager

1 Pain, nociception, neurosignatures, and the body–self neuromatrix

Pain is generally subjectively perceived as a direct, intense, and unitary experience. However, despite this apparent simplicity, a comprehensive scientific explanation of the central nervous system (CNS) processes that generate the subjective experience of pain still remains elusive. Indeed, although two centuries of systematic neurophysiological studies have succeeded in mapping out many of the pathways and relays through which information about potentially harmful stimuli are conveyed from the periphery to the brain (Perl 2007), we still lack a clear understanding of the cerebral processes that convert these raw sensory signals into the subjective experience we feel as pain. Indeed, pain refers to the subjective "emotional and sensory experience associated with actual or potential tissue damage, or described in terms of such damage" (IASP 2014; see also Chapter 31, this volume). Therefore, by definition, pain implies consciousness. (Cf. Chapter 17, this volume.) By contrast, the term "nociception" is reserved to designate the "neural processes of encoding noxious stimuli" (IASP 2014), which may not be necessarily associated with either consciousness or pain. From that perspective, the question of how the brain generates the subjective experience of pain can be seen as the quintessential mind–body problem of how subjective experience arises from matter.

One simplistic way to solve the problem would be to simply deem it out of neuroscience's reach: Neuroscience can explain nociception, but not pain. Indeed, pain as a subjective experience cannot be ontologically reduced to neuronal activity: there isn't any pattern of neuronal activity that could possibly *be* pain (Searle 2007). Still, it is reasonable to think that pain is caused by the CNS. In other words, although pain cannot be *ontologically* reduced to any one state of neuronal activity, it may be *causally* reduced to neuronal activity. One possibility could be that all pain is caused by nociception. However, an emerging consensus is that nociception doesn't have a 1:1 relationship with pain, and that it is thus possible to have pain without nociception, and nociception without pain. Indeed, pain behaviors in animals and pain reports in humans can be influenced by brain processes that do not appear to be related to changes in nociception (Johansen and Fields 2004; Navratilova and Porreca 2014). Thus, there is likely another layer of neuroscientific phenomena between pain and nociception that may explain how brain activity causes pain, above and beyond (and perhaps in the absence of) nociception.

The kinds of neural processes that comprise this "intermediate layer" were first imagined by Ronald Melzack almost twenty years ago (Melzack 1999). Indeed, Melzack was puzzled by the fact that the pain experienced by patients with phantom limbs presented all the qualities of "normal" pain, despite the obvious absence of peripheral and/or spinal nociceptive activity (Baron and Maier 1995; Birbaumer et al. 1997). He concluded that the pain therefore had to be caused by the same cerebral processes that are responsible for normal pain perception. Melzack proposed that the experience of pain was generated by the flow of activity within a widespread network of convergent/divergent loops between the thalamus, cortex, and limbic system. He thought that the general function of this network, which he called the "body–self neuromatrix," was to produce a unified representation of the body and of the self. Moreover, he suggested that the various bodily states generated by the neuromatrix each had a particular "neurosignature," i.e., a characteristic pattern of neuronal activity stemming from the interaction between environmental inputs and the pre-existing state of the neuromatrix. According to Melzack, there is therefore no "pain center" in the brain, but rather a general-purpose body–self neuromatrix capable of representing a wide array of bodily states, of which pain is just one particular exemplar. Whereas Melzack's terminology had a profound impact on subsequent brain-imaging studies of pain, his ideas have been largely misinterpreted and the core hypothesis of his neuromatrix theory of pain – that pain is generated by a specific pattern of activity within a general-purpose system – still remains to be tested using modern neuroimaging techniques.

2 From neuron to voxels: a brief history of brain imaging of pain

Before the advent of functional brain imaging in the 1980s, physiologists had already mapped out several ascending pathways conveying nociceptive signals from the dorsal horn of the spinal cord up to the brainstem, thalamus, and a number of cortical and sub-cortical sites. The presence of neurons with nociceptive properties (sensitivity to potentially tissue-damaging high-intensity stimuli) was also beginning to be reported in a number of cortical and subcortical structures including the hippocampus, thalamus, amygdala, anterior cingulate, insula (Ins), and primary somatosensory cortex (Kenshalo et al. 2000; Millan 1999; Vogt and Sikes 2000). However, the techniques at their disposal generally only allowed examination of one local recording site in one brain region at a time. Typically, experiments would target a brain region and systematically test the response profiles of hundreds of neurons, isolated individually, in search of neurons that gradually increased their firing rate as a function of stimulus intensity (wide dynamic range neurons), or that only responded to high-intensity stimulation (nociceptive-specific neurons; Kenshalo et al. 2000). This approach became increasingly cumbersome as the targeted areas became larger and contained fewer and more dispersed nociceptive neurons (e.g., 9/125 tested neurons in the anterior cingulate cortex, ACC: Hutchison et al. 1999). Additionally, it remained unclear how nociceptive stimulus encoding in isolated cells relates to pain experience. In other domains, a growing set of studies focusing on population coding was suggesting that perceptual and motor processes are an emergent property of the overall pattern of activity in populations of neurons, rather than activity in any single neuron (Georgopoulos et al. 1986). Thus, it was (and is) uncertain how activity in nociceptive neurons is related to subjective pain perception.

With the advent of functional brain imaging in the late 1980s, researchers began to have the tools to image how the entire brain responded to noxious stimuli. The first technique to be used was positron emission tomography (PET), which was soon replaced by functional magnetic resonance imaging (fMRI). Both techniques use indirect measures of neuronal activity – cerebral blood flow for PET and blood oxygenation for fMRI – to measure brain activity in small parcels of the brain called voxels. In a typical fMRI experiment, each voxel has a volume of approximately 8–64 cubic millimeters. A typical 3-millimeter × 3-millimeter × 3-millimeter voxel (27 cubic millimeters) contains on the order of 5.5 million neurons (Logothetis 2008). Using these techniques, several studies found that high-intensity noxious stimuli (thermal, electrical, mechanical, or chemical) systematically produced more activity than low-intensity innocuous stimuli in a set of regions that included the thalamus, ACC, Ins, primary and secondary somatosensory cortices (S1 and S2) and prefrontal cortices (PFC) (Apkarian et al. 2005). Inspired by Melzack's methodology, researchers soon started to refer to this collection of regions as the "pain matrix" (Ingvar 1999; Jones 1998).

While many researchers mainly employed the term as shorthand for the regions generally activated by pain, the concept of the pain matrix quickly began to implicitly designate the brain's "pain center" (Ingvar 1999). More specifically, it was thought that each part of the pain matrix mapped onto different aspects or qualities of pain (e.g.: localization, intensity, unpleasantness, motivation, etc.), and that their combined activation is what creates the full experience of pain. In other terms, it was thought that it was the global pattern of activation across all of the pain matrix's regions that created pain, and not activity in any of its sub-regions taken independently. Based on prior neurophysiological evidence suggesting a parsing of the spinothalamic tract into a lateral/sensory system and a medial/emotional system, it was suggested that S1 and S2 subserved the sensory dimension of pain, while the Ins and ACC were responsible for pain's unpleasantness (Price 2000). Finally, the prefrontal cortex was thought to be involved in "secondary" cognitive and emotional reactions to pain, such as rumination, anxiety, and anger, which depend on higher-order appraisals of the meaning of the pain for the individual (Price 2000, Chapter 9, this volume). While this general architecture agrees relatively well with neurophysiological evidence (Millan 1999) and lesion data (Danziger 2006; Ploner et al. 1999), there is no evidence that any of the regions, or combination of regions, of the pain matrix is specific to pain. Indeed, several brain-imaging studies have shown that most, if not all, structures of the pain matrix are sensitive to different kinds of salient events that are not necessarily painful (Yarkoni et al. 2011; Chapter 6, this volume).

3 From voxels to pain: reverse inference and the problem of pain specificity

Debates around pain's specificity are as old as research on pain physiology itself (Perl 2007). Unlike the other senses that process a specific type of physical stimulus, like vision and light or audition and air waves, pain can be generated by a variety of somatosensory inputs (thermal, mechanical, chemical). It was therefore proposed that pain may be simply caused by the vigorous activation of nervous pathways normally concerned with somato- and viscero-sensation. However, based on observations that hemisections of the spinal cord produced a double-dissociation between pain and tactile sensation, it was also argued that pain may very well be a specific sense distinct from normal somatosensation. Up to this day, this opposition between specificity and intensity theories of pain still fuels debates regarding how the CNS generates pain. Needless to say, the question of pain specificity also drove important con-troversies regarding the interpretation of brain-imaging data. At the core of these controversies lies the problem of reverse inference, i.e., the conclusion that a certain experience (e.g., pain) has been elicited based on the presence of activity in regions shown to be activated by that same experience (e.g., pain-matrix regions) in previous studies, even if these regions may also be involved in a variety of other experiences or processes (e.g., attention, negative affect, conflict, etc.).

One example of reverse inference is the use of activity in the pain matrix to infer effects of non-pharmacological interventions on "pain processing" (Bushnell et al. 2013). Typically, brain modulation by conditions including hypnosis (Rainville et al. 1997), placebo/expectations (Wager et al. 2004), emotion (Roy et al. 2009), distraction (Tracey et al. 2002), and others, was used to corroborate effects on pain reports and infer meaningful changes in pain mechanisms. Moreover, some of these studies also found increased activity in brain neuro-chemical systems (Wager et al. 2007) and regions involved in descending pain modulatory systems, such as the rAAC (rostral ACC) or PAG (periaqueductal gray) (Tracey et al. 2002; Wager et al. 2004), which was interpreted as evidence that these interventions may alter spinal nociceptive processes. While it is perfectly plausible that non-pharmacological interventions influence activity in the same pain-processing regions that respond to noxious inputs, these results also tended to be interpreted by the greater scientific community as a proof that these interventions did not just induce biases in pain reports, but were really having an effect on subjective pain perception. Unfortunately, for decreased activity in pain-matrix regions to provide evidence that these interventions were really effective in decreasing pain requires that pain-matrix activity be specific to pain-processing, an interpretation that is not supported by analyses of imaging data across many types of tasks (Yarkoni et al. 2011).

Another example of reverse inference without evidence for specificity came from studies in social neuroscience examining the cerebral substrates of social rejection and pain empathy. When these studies were published, the concept of the pain matrix as a specific set of pain-processing regions had become insidiously entrenched in the minds of the greater cognitive neuroscience community. Therefore, it seemed natural to conclude that activity in pain-matrix regions (ACC, Ins, etc.) could be interpreted as proof that "pain systems" were involved when individuals experience social rejection (Eisenberger and Lieberman 2004) or observe others in pain (Singer et al. 2004). Again, the problem with these otherwise plausible conclusions is that other explanations, which do not rely on the shared involvement of pain systems, are equally valid. Indeed, because each of the structures of the pain matrix are involved in many processes other than pain, it is impossible to conclusively infer the presence of pain from activity in any of these regions (Poldrack 2006). In a strong critique of the pain matrix's alleged specificity, Iannetti and Mouraux (2010) proposed that regions of the pain matrix could be simply responsive to salient events in general. Indeed, they noted that intense or unexpected visual and auditory stimuli also strongly activated the thalamus, ACC, and Ins. Moreover, they found that in addition to activity in general salience-processing regions, intense non-painful tactile stimuli also activated S1, rendering their global pattern activity undistinguishable from the pattern associated with painful stimuli. On the basis of these findings, Iannetti and Mouraux concluded that activity in pain-matrix regions is not specific to pain, and could be better accounted for by a more general salience-processing interpretation.

However, this leaves intact the question of the cerebral substrates of pain: how can the experience of pain, which we feel as distinct from other salient events (e.g., receiving an unexpected reward), be caused by non-specific activity in a general salience-processing system? Our view is that it cannot. As originally suggested by Melzack, one possibility could be that the pain matrix constitutes a general-purpose architecture (i.e., the body–self neuromatrix) whose billions of neurons represent many states – and that pain constitutes a specific state (i.e., a neurosignature) or collection of states of the system. Indeed, nociceptive projections to the brain appear to converge in relatively well-defined subparts of pain-matrix regions, making the existence of such distinctive pain neurosignatures quite likely. For example, spinothalamic tract (STT) projections have been shown to target specific subparts of the posterior granular insular cortex (Ig; 41 percent of all projections), parietal operculum (S2; 29 percent of all projections), and cingulate cortex (24 percent of all projections) (Dum et al. 2009).

Interestingly, the relatively small insular (Ig) and parieto-opercular (S2) regions that receive most of STT projections appear to be relatively specific to nociceptive input. Indeed, they have been shown to respond to noxious heat, but not to innocuous warmth, cold, brushing, or proprioceptive inputs (Mazzola et al. 2012a). Moreover, they appear to be critical for the sensory-discriminative aspects of pain: their lesion results in a selective contralateral loss of temperature and pain sensation (Garcia-Larrea et al. 2010). Finally, these are the only two known cortical regions capable of generating painful sensations when stimulated (Mazzola et al. 2012b), suggesting that they may very well stand at the interface of nociceptive processing and pain perception. Still, neither of these two structures seems to be necessary or sufficient for pain. Indeed, a large proportion (more than 60 percent) of patients with operculo-insular lesions will develop central pain in proportion with their thermo-algesic deficits (Garcia-Larrea et al. 2010), suggesting that these patients' pain must be generated by neuronal activity outside of these two operculo-insular regions. Moreover, nociceptive sensations, such as "burning," "pricking," or "throbbing" sensations are not painful per se, because they are not necessarily accompanied by the negative affect that characterizes pain; it is only when they are interpreted as potentially tissue damaging and associated with negative affect that the overall experience can be labeled as "pain" (IASP 2014). Consequently, lesion of the cingulate and prefrontal structures responsible for pain unpleasantness, or of the white matter tracts connecting these regions to the operculo-insular region, can cause an intriguing dissociation between pain sensation and affect whereby nociceptive sensations are no longer perceived as unpleasant. Interestingly, this condition has been called "pain asymbolia" by the neurologists who first described it to signify that pain had lost its meaning (Danziger 2006). Thus, although the operculo-insular region appears to be very important for the processing of ascending nociceptive inputs, it does not have a 1:1 relationship with the subjective experience of pain.

4 From voxels to signatures: identifying the cerebral representation of pain

Unlike other sensations, pain always implies some evaluation of the meaning of the raw nociceptive sensation in order for the experience to have all the properties of pain, i.e., an emotional and sensory experience associated with actual or potential tissue damage. Consequently, pain cannot be simply generated by the passive reception of ascending nociceptive inputs to the brain; it has to emerge from the concerted activity of large-scale networks of neurons spanning sensory, emotional, and cognitive-evaluative regions of the brain (Melzack 1999; Tononi and Koch 2015). Moreover, as originally proposed by Melzack (1999), it is highly unlikely that any of the processes binding together the different aspects of pain are per se pain-specific. Indeed, it could be argued that most, if not all, of our conscious subjective experiences are the result of combined sensory, emotional, and cognitive processes (Tononi and Koch 2015). It is therefore not surprising that previous attempts to link pain to a specific macroscopic network of pain-processing structures have failed (Iannetti and Mouraux 2010).

However, as mentioned previously, it remains possible that fine-grained patterns of activity within a more general-purpose system may be relatively specific to pain. Unfortunately, the traditional fMRI analyses used in prior brain-imaging studies of pain typically examine each of the brain's voxels independently one from another, thereby ignoring the important information that may potentially lie in distributed patterns of neuronal activity and connections among regions. It is only with the recent development of multivariate pattern analyses (MVPA) that researchers were endowed with analytic tools capable of assessing the predictive power of distributed patterns of fMRI activity (Haxby et al. 2014). In a typical MVPA analysis, machine-learning algorithms are used to train multivariate classifiers – patterns of predictive weights distributed over hundreds to thousands of voxels – that aim to predict a certain outcome of interest (e.g., distinguish the presence of a face vs. an object). The predictive accuracy of these trained classifiers is then tested in a separate holdout validation set using cross-validation procedures. The resulting classifiers are therefore optimally tuned for making predictions for new, unseen data points. Using this principle, a wealth of applications are now being developed that allow researchers to "mind-read" or "decode" perceptions, intentions, and actions from patterns of brain activity (Haxby et al. 2014).

Inspired by these studies, we recently developed and tested a pain-predictive pattern that we have called the "neurologic pain signature" (NPS) (Wager et al. 2013). The NPS was originally trained to predict the subjective pain ratings associated with four levels of thermal stimulation, from innocuous warmth to highly painful heat. It is therefore designed to track the pain that arises from changes in temperature. As expected, NPS predictions were extremely accurate, with an average prediction error of 0.96 (plus or minus 0.33) on a 9-point visual analogue scale. Unsurprisingly, the NPS pattern of pain-predictive weights comprised positive weights in regions of the pain matrix such as the ACC, Ins, S2, and thalamus, and negative weights in default mode structures frequently deactivated by pain, such as the ventromedial prefrontal cortex (vmPFC) and precuneus (see Figure 7.1). However, contrary to earlier conceptions of the pain matrix, it wasn't the overall macroscopic pattern of regions of the signature that predicted pain, but rather the fine-grained pattern of weights within each structure.

We then examined how the NPS behaved across various independent data sets. We began by testing the NPS sensitivity to six predetermined levels of thermal stimuli, ranging from innocuous warmth to painful heat (44.3, 45.3, 46.3, 47.3, 48.3, and 49.3° C; stimuli were administered on the left forearm with a 3-centimeter × 3-centimeter contact thermode). Interestingly, the signature response proved to be much more sensitive to variations in temperatures above versus below pain threshold, suggesting that it is partly specific to temperatures in the noxious range. The signature was then used to test the idea that psychological interventions aiming at reducing perceived pain exert their effects by decreasing the pattern of brain activity underlying "normal," stimulus-driven, pain perception. More specifically, we examined the cerebral mechanisms underlying the effects of instructions to imagine thermal stimuli as more or less painful than they really are (Woo et al. 2015). Surprisingly, the NPS didn't track the changes in perceived pain associated with these instructions, although it was highly sensitive to equivalent changes in pain that were driven by changes in temperature. By contrast with temperature, self-regulation of pain exerted most of its effects through the Nac (nucleus accumbens) and vmPFC. While these two structures are not typically part of the pain matrix, they are crucial for self-related motivational processes (Roy et al. 2014), and would therefore perfectly fit Melzack's description of structures of the body–self neuromatrix. Interestingly, the connectivity between these two structures has been shown to be highly predictive of the development of chronic pain, suggesting that they may serve important

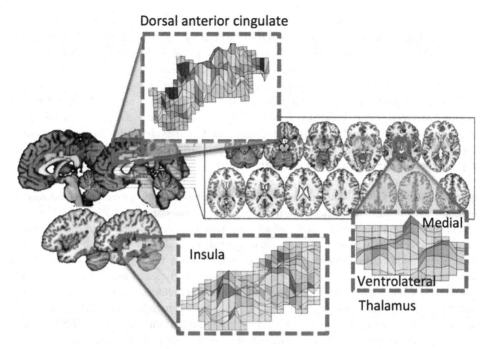

Figure 7.1 The neurologic pain signature map, consisting of voxels in which activity reliably predicted pain. Warm/cold colors (see online, www.routledge.com/9781138823181) indicate positive/ negative weights.
Source: Zaki et al. (2014).

cognitive and emotional aspects of pain that aren't bound to nociceptive stimulus intensity (see also Chapter 10, this volume).

We also used the signature to test the hypothesis that physical and social pains share a common cerebral representation. As mentioned previously, this hypothesis was mainly based on observations that social rejection activates the same brain regions as those involved in the physical experience of pain. More specifically, a prior study conducted within our laboratory had shown that looking at pictures of an ex-romantic partner who had rejected one activated the thalamus, Ins, ACC, S2, and dpIns (dorso-posterior insula) (Kross et al. 2011). Based on the relative pain-specificity of the operculo-insular region (see above), we had initially concluded that these results indicated that rejection may literally share a common somatosensory representation with physical pain. However, when we re-examined these results with the NPS, we came to a different conclusion. Indeed, the NPS didn't respond to social rejection, even when we only considered the patterns of activity within the operculo-insular region (Wager et al. 2013). Therefore, despite the apparent similarity in the large-scale networks of structures activated by pain and social rejection, the two phenomena differ at the level of the fine-grain patterns of activity within each of these commonly activated structures. In Melzack's terms, this would mean that both social rejection and physical pain are represented within the same body–self neuromatrix, but that they have distinct neurosignatures.

To follow-up on this idea, we also developed a signature that could reliably distinguish looking at pictures of ex-partners versus friends (Woo et al. 2015). Indeed, one possible explanation for the NPS's lack of sensitivity to social rejection could have been that social rejection is simply more difficult to identify from patterns of brain activity. By developing a signature that was sensitive to rejection, but insensitive to physical pain (painful heat), we demonstrated that the two experiences were "separately modifiable," i.e., that they are represented by distinct patterns of brain activity. These findings also suggested that the NPS isn't sensitive to all sorts of salient stimuli (Iannetti and Mouraux 2010), such as pictures of ex-partners, but is rather specific to physical pain. Finally, in a strong test of the shared representation hypothesis, we systematically searched the brain for a potential "shared representation" between physical and social pain – areas in which the patterns that encode pain and social rejection are similar (Woo et al. 2015). We found evidence for shared representations in parts of the striatum, temporoparietal junction, fusiform and parahippocampal gyrii, and posterior and retrosplenial cingulate cortices, suggesting the existence of shared processes. However, none of these shared processes were localized within any of the pain-matrix regions, suggesting that what is shared may be representations of negative affect and related mnemonic associations rather than activation of primary pain systems.

Finally, we examined the extent to which pain is represented similarly across individuals. Indeed, the NPS is amongst the first neural signatures capable of predicting a subjective experience in new individuals or new studies. One reason for this high inter-individual consistency in signature patterns may be that the seemingly dispersed nociceptive projections to the brain are also highly anatomically consistent across individuals (Dum et al. 2009). This again fits perfectly well with Melzack's idea of a partly genetically determined body–self neuromatrix. That being said, we should also expect important inter-individual differences in pain's representation due to gross inter-individual differences in brain anatomy and/or unique developmental histories. In order to test that hypothesis, we trained within-subject "idiographic" signatures, and tested the degree to which these idiographic signatures improved predictions made by the NPS across a set of seven different studies (Lindquist et al. 2015). Given an infinite amount of training data (e.g., hundreds of hours of imaging in the same subject), idiographic signatures should in principle always procure the optimal predictions. However, because we had limited training data (e.g., less than 1 hour of data per subject), predictions based solely on idiographic signatures were often imprecise. We therefore found that an optimized combination (weighted average) of idiographic signatures and of our group-based NPS always procured better predictions than idiographic signatures alone. Indeed, when idiographic signatures are found to be imprecise, a stronger weighting of the NPS can provide a fail-safe against poor predictions. Conversely, when idiographic signatures are found to be more precise, their contribution to the combined prediction can be increased so as to provide more flexibility to group-based NPS predictions. Altogether, these results support the idea that individual and contextual variations in the cerebral representation of pain exist, but that they are also constrained by the conserved neuroanatomical architecture of the nociceptive system.

A palette of signatures for a family of pains

Because pain subjectively feels like a very direct and unique experience, we are compelled to try to find an objective pattern of brain activity that would have a perfect, one-on-one, correspondence with pain, i.e., to find "pain" in the brain. However, unlike objective phenomena that exist regardless of the presence of an observer to witness them (i.e., natural kinds), subjective phenomena like pain cannot exist without a subject to experience them (Barrett 2009; Searle 2007; see also Chapters 16, 18, 20, and 21 for more advanced discussions on this topic). This is well recognized by IASP's definition of pain, which states that as long as an experience is described as pain, it should be recognized as pain (IASP 2014). In other terms, we are in pain as soon as we think that we are in pain. From that perspective, pain would therefore result from the act of categorizing an unpleasant, and potentially harmful, bodily sensation as an instance of "pain." However, this doesn't mean that nociceptive processes are irrelevant for understanding pain. Indeed, it is widely accepted that nociceptive sensations (e.g., burning, pricking, etc.) preferentially signal potential injury, like the alarm of a smoke detector may signal the presence of smoke. However, they do not, by themselves, constitute the experience of pain.

Indeed, pain rather seems to result from the combination of three core ingredients: (1) a bodily sensation, (2) negative affect, and (3) the appraisal – conscious or unconscious – that the experience indicates a potential injury. Therefore, various experiences that comprise these three basic ingredients in different proportions, or in slightly different kinds, could all be categorized as different instances of "pain": the pain of a bee sting, the pain of a frostbite, the pain of a stomach ache, the pain of sore muscles, etc. However, as for most of our categories, it seems almost impossible to find a set of necessary and sufficient properties that perfectly define "pain" (see the note attached to the IASP definition of pain; IASP 2014). Rather, "pain" should be conceived as a collection of exemplars that share a "family resemblance" (Wittgenstein 2001/1953). It follows that some members of the pain "family," like a stomach ache, may actually share more characteristics with closely related non-members of the family, like hunger, than with more distant members of the family, like the pain of a bee sting. In other words, it is possible that the category "pain" doesn't perfectly carve nature at its joints.

If this is correct, then it would be virtually impossible to derive a signature that would be highly sensitive to all types of pain, and at the same time highly selective to pain. In order to reflect pain's diversity, we could rather need a palette of signatures that would allow characterizing each type of pain with respect to other types of pain or pain-related phenomena, such as thermal pain, hunger, social rejection, etc. We have just begun to lay some of the methodological foundations for this vast program of research, which was initially envisioned by Melzack almost twenty years ago. However, it was just with the development of multivariate pattern analyses that we acquired the ability to decode the cerebral representation of pain, and to begin addressing Melzack's initial question: how can the brain generate the experience of pain in the absence of nociception (Woo et al., submitted)? As intuited by Melzack, the answer to that question may force us to imagine another, more representational layer of neuroscientific explanation, measurable in terms of signature patterns of distributed brain activity. Although it is too soon to say where this paradigm shift is taking us, we hope that it will enlighten our comprehension of the role of the brain in normal and pathological chronic pain syndromes, and ultimately enhance assessment and treatment.

Related topics

References

Apkarian, A.V., Bushnell, M.C., Treede, R. D., and Zubieta, J.K. (2005) Human brain mechanisms of pain perception and regulation in health and disease. *European Journal of Pain* 9: 463–484.

Baron, R. and Maier, C. (1995) Phantom limb pain: Are cutaneous nociceptors and spinothalamic neurons involved in the signaling and maintenance of spontaneous and touch-evoked pain? A case report. *Pain* 60: 223–228.

Barrett, L.F. (2009) The future of psychology: connecting mind to brain. *Perspectives on Psychological Science* 4: 326–339.

Birbaumer, N., Lutzenberger, W., Montoya, P., Larbig, W., Unertl, K., Topfner, S., Grodd, W., Taub, E., and Flor, H. (1997) Effects of regional anesthesia on phantom limb pain are mirrored in changes in cortical reorganization. *Journal of Neuroscience* 17: 5503–5508.

Bushnell, M.C., Čeko, M., and Low, L.A. (2013) Cognitive and emotional control of pain and its disruption in chronic pain. *Nature Reviews Neuroscience* 14: 502–511.

Danziger, N. (2006) Neurological basis of the emotional dimension of pain [In French]. *Revue Neurologique* (Paris) 162: 395–399.

Dum, R.P., Levinthal, D.J., and Strick, P.L. (2009) The spinothalamic system targets motor and sensory areas in the cerebral cortex of monkeys. *Journal of Neuroscience* 29: 14223–14235.

Eisenberger, N.I. and Lieberman, M.D. (2004) Why rejection hurts: a common neural alarm system for physical and social pain. *Trends in Cognitive Sciences* 8: 294–300.

Garcia-Larrea, L., Perchet, C., Creac'h, C., Convers, P., Peyron, R., Laurent, B., Mauguiere, F., and Magnin, M. (2010) Operculo-insular pain (parasylvian pain): a distinct central pain syndrome. *Brain* 133: 2528–2539.

Georgopoulos, A.P., Schwartz, A.B., and Kettner, R.E. (1986) Neuronal population coding of movement direction. *Science* 233: 1416–1419.

Haxby, J.V., Connolly, A.C., and Guntupalli, J.S. (2014) Decoding neural representational spaces using multivariate pattern analysis. *Annual Revue of Neuroscience* 37: 435–456.

Hutchison, W.D., Davis, K.D., Lozano, A.M., Tasker, R.R., and Dostrovsky, J.O. (1999) Pain-related neurons in the human cingulate cortex. *Nature Neuroscience* 2: 403–405.

Iannetti, G.D. and Mouraux, A. (2010) From the neuromatrix to the pain matrix (and back). *Experimental Brain Research* 205: 1–12.

IASP (International Association for the Study of Pain) (2014) *IASP Taxonomy.* IASP. Updated 2014. <http://www.iasp-pain.org/Taxonomy>, accessed 18 April 2016.

Ingvar, M. (1999) Pain and functional imaging. *Philosophical Transactions of the Royal Society B: Biological Sciences* 354: 1347–1358.

Johansen, J.P. and Fields, H.L. (2004) Glutamatergic activation of anterior cingulate cortex produces an aversive teaching signal. *Nature Neuroscience* 7: 398–403.

Jones, A. (1998) The pain matrix and neuropathic pain. *Brain* 121 (pt. 5): 783–784.

Kenshalo, D.R., Iwata, K., Sholas, M. and Thomas, D.A. (2000) Response properties and organization of nociceptive neurons in area 1 of monkey primary somatosensory cortex. *Journal of Neurophysiology* 84: 719–729.

Kross, E., Berman, M.G., Mischel, W., Smith, E.E., and Wager, T.D. (2011) Social rejection shares somatosensory representations with physical pain. *Proceedings of the National Academy of Sciences of the United States of America* 108: 6270–6275.

Lindquist, M.A., Krishnan, A., Lopez-sola, M., Jepma, M., Woo, C.W., Koban, L., Roy, M., Atlas, L. Y., Schmidt, L., Chang, L.J., Reynolds Losin, E. A., Eisenbarth, H., Ashar, Y. K., Delk, E., and Wager, T. D. (2015) Group-regularized individual prediction: theory and application to pain. *Neuroimage.* doi:10.1016/j.neuroimage.2015.10.074.

Logothetis, N.K. (2008) What we can do and what we cannot do with fMRI. *Nature* 453: 869–878.

Mazzola, L., Faillenot, I., Barral, F.G., Mauguiere, F., and Peyron, R. (2012a) Spatial segregation of somato-sensory and pain activations in the human operculo-insular cortex. *Neuroimage* 60: 409–418.

Mazzola, L., Isnard, J., Peyron, R., and Mauguiere, F. (2012b) Stimulation of the human cortex and the experience of pain: Wilder Penfield's observations revisited. *Brain* 135: 631–640.

Melzack, R. (1999) From the gate to the neuromatrix. *Pain* 6 (Suppl): S121–S126.

Millan, M.J. (1999) The induction of pain: an integrative review. *Progress in Neurobiology* 57: 1–164.

Navratilova, E. and Porreca, F. (2014) Reward and motivation in pain and pain relief. *Natural Neuroscience* 17: 1304–1312.

Perl, E.R. (2007) Ideas about pain, a historical view. *Nature Reviews Neuroscience* 8: 71–80.

Ploner, M., Freund, H.J., and Schnitzler, A. (1999) Pain affect without pain sensation in a patient with a postcentral lesion. *Pain* 81: 211–214.

Poldrack, R.A. (2006) Can cognitive processes be inferred from neuroimaging data? *Trends in Cognitive Sciences* 10: 59–63.

Price, D.D. (2000) Psychological and neural mechanisms of the affective dimension of pain. *Science* 288: 1769–1772.

Rainville, P., Duncan, G.H., Price, D.D., Carrier, B., and Bushnell, M.C. (1997) Pain affect encoded in human anterior cingulate but not somatosensory cortex. *Science* 277: 968–971.

Roy, M., Piché, M., Chen, J.I., Peretz, I., and Rainville, P. (2009) Cerebral and spinal modulation of pain by emotions. *Proceedings of the National Academy of Sciences of the United States of America* 106: 20900–20905.

Roy, M., Shohamy, D., Daw, N., Jepma, M., Wimmer, G.E., and Wager, T.D. (2014) Representation of aversive prediction errors in the human periaqueductal gray. *Nature Neuroscience* 17: 1607–1612.

Searle, J.R. (2007) Dualism revisited. *Journal of Physiology – Paris* 101: 169–178.

Singer, T., Seymour, B., O'Doherty, J., Kaube, H., Dolan, R.J., and Frith, C.D. (2004) Empathy for pain involves the affective but not sensory components of pain. *Science* 303: 1157–1162.

Tononi, G. and Koch, C. (2015) Consciousness: here, there and everywhere? *Philosophical Transactions of the Royal Society B: Biological Sciences* 370(1668). doi:10.1098/rstb.2014.0167.

Tracey, I., Ploghaus, A., Gati, J. S., Clare, S., Smith, S., Menon, R.S. and Matthews, P.M. (2002) Imaging attentional modulation of pain in the periaqueductal gray in humans. *Journal of Neuroscience* 22: 2748–2752.

Vogt, B.A. and Sikes, R.W. (2000) The medial pain system, cingulate cortex, and parallel processing of nociceptive information. *Progress in Brain Research* 122: 223–235.

Wager, T.D., Rilling, J.K., Smith, E.E., Sokolik, A., Casey, K.L., Davidson, R.J., Kosslyn, S.M., Rose, R. M., and Cohen, J.D. (2004) Placebo-induced changes in fMRI in the anticipation and experience of pain. *Science* 303: 1162–1167.

Wager, T.D., Scott, D.J., and Zubieta, J.K. (2007) Placebo effects on human mu-opioid activity during pain. *Proceedings of the National Academy of Sciences of the United States of America* 104: 11056–11061.

Wager, T.D., Atlas, L.Y., Lindquist, M.A., Roy, M., Woo, C. W., and Kross, E. (2013) An fMRI-based neurologic signature of physical pain. *New England Journal of Medicine* 368: 1388–1397.

Wittgenstein, L. (2001/1953) *Philosophical Investigations*, trans. G.E.M. Anscombe, ed. G.E.M. Anscombe and R. Rhees. Oxford: Blackwell.

Woo, C.W., Roy, M., Buhle, J.T., and Wager, T.D. (2015) Distinct brain systems mediate the effects of nociceptive input and self-regulation on pain. *PLoS Biology* 13: e1002036.

Woo, C.W., Schmidt, L., Krishnan, A., Jepma, M., Roy, M., Lindquist, M., Atlas, L., and Wager, T. (Submitted) Quantifying cerebral contributions to pain beyond nociception.

Yarkoni, T., Poldrack, R.A., Nichols, T.E., Van Essen, D.C., and Wager, T. D. (2011) Large-scale automated synthesis of human functional neuroimaging data. *Nature Methods* 8: 665–670.

Zaki, J., Wager, T.D., Singer, T., Keysers, C., and Gazzola, V. (2014) The anatomy of suffering: understanding the relationship between nociceptive and empathic pain. *Trends in Cognitive Sciences* 20(4): 249–259.

8

A NEUROBIOLOGICAL VIEW OF PAIN AS A HOMEOSTATIC EMOTION

Irina A. Strigo and Arthur D. ("Bud") Craig

1 Introduction

Our view of pain is grounded in functional neuroanatomy. The brain in our bodies is mysterious, but not mystical; it substantializes our phenomenal minds and engenders our feelings, thoughts, and urges, yet its pathways and activity are comprehensible. It is evolutionarily and reproducibly well-organized, and it guides behaviors that maintain the health and well-being of each individual and support the cooperative advancement of our species.

Mental appraisal of pain underlies suffering, but pain begins as an affective bodily feeling that signals an urgent need, like itch or hunger. All feelings from the body have a characteristic hedonic affect and are conjoined with autonomic activity and behavioral motivation that are aimed to restore homeostatic balance. Homeostasis is the process that dynamically maintains an optimal balance in the living body across all conditions at all times through neural, endocrinological, and behavioral functions. As explained below, we regard our bodily feelings as components of *homeostatic emotions* (for discussion and references, see Craig 2015a; see also Chapter 4, this volume).

We discuss first the functional and anatomical characteristics of the neural elements that substantialize bodily feelings and why the architecture of these substrates supports the concept that pain is a homeostatic emotion. Next, we briefly outline how homeostatic processing can explain our experience of feelings. Last, we present new evidence that illustrates how these ideas advance our understanding of pain clinically.[1]

2 The ascending homeostatic sensory pathway

In cats and macaque monkeys, sensory cells thought traditionally to mediate feelings of pain were found intermixed with neurons selectively responsive to stimuli that produce various affective feelings from the body, including cool, itch, muscle ache, and sensual touch. Altogether, these neurons constitute a representation of the physiological condition of the body, which we refer to as *interoception*, thus expanding the term to include skin along with muscle, viscera, and bone. Interoceptive activity is necessary first of all for homeostasis. The neural effector (or agent; see below) of homeostasis is the autonomic nervous system (ANS).

The thermal, mechanical, and chemical conditions of every tissue of the body are reported by small-diameter (Aδ and C) sensory fibers. These have slow conduction velocities and low firing rates, which is energy efficient because most are continuously active. They include functionally specific thermoreceptors, osmoreceptors, and metaboreceptors. Noxious stimuli that cause pain, such as pinch, strong heat or cold, and chemical irritants, activate *nociceptors*, which can be selective or polymodal. Notably, their thresholds vary broadly, and nearly all are sensitive to a major immunological modulator (interleukin-1β).

Small-diameter sensory fibers are fundamentally distinct from large-diameter sensory fibers, which innervate mechanoreceptors (skin) and proprioceptors (muscles/joints) and have fast conduction velocities and high firing rates. The small-diameter and large-diameter fibers have small and large cell bodies, respectively, with distinct embryological origins. Large-diameter fibers develop first and enter the spinal cord to contact large dorsal horn neurons, which connect to ventral horn motor neurons that drive skeletal muscle. Small-diameter fibers enter second, just in time to meet small neurons that migrate up to the superficial dorsal horn from the lateral horn, which is the origin of autonomic neurons (which drive smooth muscle). The migrating small neurons are synchronized with and facilitated by a structural rotation of the entire dorsal horn, which simultaneously moves the large neurons to the deep dorsal horn. These two embryological families are guided through this remarkable sequence by two ancient and distinct gene regulatory networks in all vertebrates.

Small-diameter fibers from all tissues terminate on *lamina I* neurons along the outer edge of the superficial dorsal horn. Consistent with their autonomic origin, lamina I neurons convey the interoceptive signals of small-diameter sensory fibers exclusively to the spinal autonomic cell columns and the brainstem homeostatic integration sites. The former contain autonomic output neurons, the latter pre-autonomic neurons with descending connections to the output neurons. This hierarchical sensorimotor homeostatic architecture is capped by bidirectional interconnections with the hypothalamus, the main homeostatic integration region of the forebrain, which sends descending terminations to exactly the same brainstem and spinal regions, including lamina I.

Thus, lamina I neurons provide the anatomical continuation of the homeostatic sensory (interoceptive) small-diameter fibers. Their functional properties confirm this role. Several classes of modality-selective lamina I neurons are differentiated by numerous characteristics. Each class consists of a morphologically identifiable type of neuron that receives input selectively from a particular subset of small-diameter sensory fibers. These functionally and genetically distinct classes constitute discrete sensory channels that, upon integration in the forebrain, engender distinct feelings from the body, such as cool, warm, itch, affective (sensual) touch, muscle ache, and so on. Each class is a virtual "labeled line" (Craig 2003; Ma 2010), which makes sense energetically.

Two classes of lamina I neuron engender pain: *nociceptive-specific* (NS) cells that respond only to noxious pinch and/or noxious heat, and *polymodal nociceptive* (HPC) cells that respond only to noxious *heat*, *pinch*, and noxious *cold*. The NS neurons are predominantly sensitive to myelinated Aδ fibers, display almost no ongoing activity, and have cigar-shaped cell bodies; the HPC neurons respond mainly to unmyelinated C-fibers, have slow ongoing activity, and are multipolar cells. These two classes correspond unequivocally with first (pricking) pain and second (burning) pain sensations, respectively, based on quantitative analyses using patterned stimuli that selectively elicit these clinically and psychophysically distinguished sensations.

Each class has subtypes, some with characteristics that are anomalous for "pain" cells. Two NS subtypes respond only to noxious heat or only to noxious pinch, but another responds to a subset of Aδ-fibers that encodes sharpness, whether painful or not. The most common type of HPC "burning pain" neuron responds to noxious cold, consistent with our burning cold sensation, yet responds also to cool temperatures (below 75° F [= 24° C]) that are normally not called painful (just as many polymodal C-nociceptors do). Such temperatures do cause increasing discomfort or unpleasantness (which corresponds with thermoregulatory behavioral motivation), and they can cause damage because, if maintained for hours, they ultimately produce hypothermia and tissue necrosis (e.g., "trench foot" in the First World War). Such temperatures do not normally cause pain because HPC cell actions in the forebrain are normally inhibited by cool-sensitive lamina I (COOL) neurons (which have ongoing activity and respond to temperatures below normal skin temperature, 90° F [= 32° C], but plateau at noxious cold temperatures, lower than 59° F [= 15° C]), to which HPC cell activity increases); thus, such temperatures do elicit burning pain if peripheral cool-sensitive Aδ-fibers are blocked or if lamina I COOL cells are inhibited by simultaneously applying cool and warm stimuli (in the "thermal grill illusion"). In other words, HPC cells generate "burning pain" if their activity exceeds COOL cell activity; otherwise, in a comfortable ambient environment (above 75° F [= 24° C]), their activity continuously follows the low ongoing activity of polymodal C-fibers, which can also signal metabolic homeostatic needs.

The clearest example of lamina I neurons subserving homeostasis is the HPC subtype that selectively conveys the activity of small-diameter sensory fibers from muscle. These fibers cause sensations of burning or cramping pain when strongly activated, yet many respond proportionately to metabolites that uniquely signal muscular work, or energy usage, while others respond to mild vascular distension and signal blood flow. Such lamina I neurons provide essential sensory feedback that continuously modulates homeostatic (cardio-respiratory) networks in the brainstem; those that project to the forebrain may in addition underlie the sentient feeling of being alive (see below). Respiration rate is similarly modulated by breathing air at cool temperatures, which only lamina I neurons report. Lamina I neurons can also respond to cytokines, steroids, and other modulators, consistent with the role of the ANS in immune and neuroendocrine mechanisms.

The small-diameter sensory fibers and lamina I neurons constitute a homeostatic sensory system that complements the sympathetic motor output of the ANS. Small-diameter sensory fibers in cranial nerves (e.g., vagus) that terminate in a specialized region of the lower brainstem (the nucleus of the solitary tract, NTS) similarly drive parasympathetic autonomic outputs.[2] Together, lamina I and NTS neurons that project to the forebrain represent homeostatic sensory input from the entire body. The ascending sensory neurons that generate affective bodily feelings of pain are elements of this homeostatic sensory pathway and, in at least some cases, are neurons that continuously convey homeostatic sensory signals.[3]

3 Homeostatic sensory projections to the primate forebrain

A key finding was that in anthropoid primates the discrete lamina I interoceptive sensory channels are conveyed directly to the forebrain (Craig 2004a, 2014, 2015a). This phylogenetically novel, anatomically distinct homeostatic sensory pathway surmounts the ancient mammalian brainstem homeostatic system, and it parallels a direct NTS forebrain projection also found only in primates. The forebrain targets of this pathway are most highly developed in humans. Convergent clinical, physiological and functional imaging evidence indicates that it underlies all affective feelings from the body, including pricking pain and burning pain, along with cool, warm, itch, muscle ache, affective (sensual) touch, and vasomotor flush, as well as taste, hunger, thirst, "air hunger," bowel or bladder distension, and so on. Thus, pain and all other affective feelings from the body are generated by the ascending projections of interoceptive neurons that extend the long-missing central sensory component of the ANS to the forebrain.

Importantly, this projection has three cortical targets (see Figure 8.1). A well-organized (high-resolution, topographic, modality-selective) pathway conveys lamina I and NTS inter-oceptive information to a discrete field in the dorsal posterior insular cortex (*interoceptive cortex*), with a corollary projection to a subregion of primary sensorimotor cortex (*area 3a*). A smaller pathway conveys interoceptive activity to the *cingulate* (motor) *cortex* (Dum et al. 2009; Craig 2014, 2015a).[4] The forebrain substrates of this pathway are much larger and more complex in humans than in monkeys. The hypermetric evolutionary growth of anterior insular cortex endowed humans with the benefits of far greater interoceptive integration (see below; Bauernfeind et al. 2013).[5]

A second key finding came in a functional imaging experiment on thermal sensation (Craig et al. 2000). It showed that the intensity of an innocuous cool stimulus is linearly correlated exclusively with cortical activation in the dorsal posterior insula. That finding matched the evidence in monkeys and suggested that the primary nociceptive cortical areas for first and second pain in humans are similarly located in the dorsal posterior insula. That result is now strongly supported by consonant evidence (see Craig 2014, 2015a), including electrical stimulation in awake humans (Mazzola et al. 2012), graded nociceptive laser-evoked potential recordings, functional imaging activation during various types of painful stimulation including direct correlation with human pain reports (e.g., Segerdahl et al. 2015), demonstrations of congruent topographical organization, and clinical deficits due to restricted infarcts.

Notably, about half of all imaging studies of cutaneous pain reported activation in the primary somatosensory cortex (S1, or area 3b); however, the focus was often clearly at the bottom of the central sulcus, which is area 3a (e.g., Chen et al. 2002). The corollary inter-oceptive projection to area 3a might have a role in pain sensation (Vierck et al. 2013), but it is more likely involved in cortical modulation of nocifensive ("viscerosomatic") reflexes because this region receives vestibular, visceral, and (predominantly) dense proprioceptive input and is a major source of descending motor control signals to the spinal cord. Reports of pain activation in the second somatosensory cortex (S2) are confounded by the mis-identification of dorsal posterior insula as S2 in early anatomical studies, which unfortunately persists in human brain atlases (see Craig 2014). It is noteworthy that most imaging studies of muscle and visceral pain (e.g., rectal, stomach, or esophageal distension) found strong activation in the insular and cingulate cortices but *not* in the somatosensory cortices. Finally, the cingulate cortex is activated in all imaging studies of pain. Several studies associate this activation with unpleasantness, or the affective motivation of pain, which fits with the evidence that this is homeostatic/emotional motor cortex described below (Rainville et al. 1997; Craig 2015a).

4 Interoceptive integration in the insula underlies all subjective feelings

The functional imaging experiment that identified thermosensory cortex further revealed that subjective thermosensory feelings are correlated with successive processing in the bilateral middle insula and the right anterior insula (Craig et al. 2000). Subsequent imaging data for all bodily feelings, including pain, affective touch, and taste, documented the same posterior–middle–anterior progression of insular cortical activity (Wiech et al. 2014). This pattern also

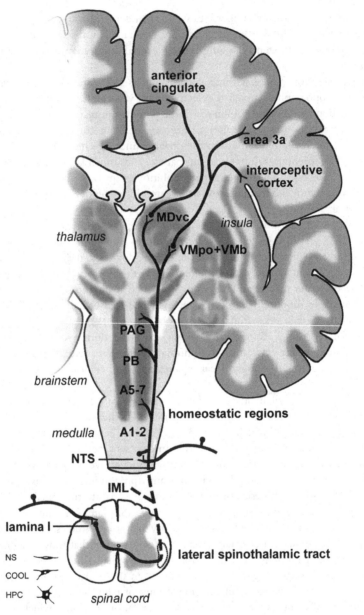

Figure 8.1 The ascending homeostatic sensory pathway in anthropoid primates. A1–2, 5–7, noradrenergic cell groups in the brainstem; area 3a, subregion of primary sensorimotor cortex in the fundus of the central sulcus; COOL, thermoreceptive-specific lamina I neurons responsive to cooling; HPC, polymodal nociceptive lamina I neuron responsive to *h*eat, *p*inch, and *c*old; IML, inter-*medio*lateral cell column (contains sympathetic motor output neurons); MDvc, ventral caudal part of the medial dorsal nucleus of the thalamus; NS, nociceptive-specific lamina I neuron; NTS, nucleus of the solitary tract; PAG, *peria*queductal *g*ray (homeostatic motor region in the brainstem); PB, *para*brachial nucleus (homeostatic sensory region in the brainstem); VMb, the *bas*al part of the *v*entral *m*edial nucleus in the thalamus (relays NTS activity to the interoceptive cortex); VMpo, the *p*osterior part of the *v*entral *m*edial nucleus in the thalamus (relays lamina I activity to the interoceptive cortex).

Source: Craig (2015a: figure 1).

fits clinical lesion evidence, functional connectivity analyses, and the integration gradient in other frontal cortices (Ongur and Price 2000; see Craig 2002, 2009, 2014, 2015a). The subjective feeling of pain is most closely associated with activation of the right anterior insular cortex.

In fact, the anterior insula and the anterior cingulate cortices are conjointly and uniquely activated in humans during all feelings and all emotions (Craig 2009; Lindquist and Barrett 2012). Most clinical evidence suggests that the anterior insula is in fact crucial for experiencing feelings; insular damage disrupts subjective feelings in patients with restricted infarcts, with fronto-temporal dementia, or with depersonalization disorder.[6]

These convergent findings support the idea that subjective awareness of the emotional state of the material self is based on neural integration of the body's physiological state, consistent with embodiment theories of emotion and psychological evidence (Barrett et al. 2004, see below, section 7). Key evidence was provided by several demonstrations of unique overlap between neural activation during subjective interoceptive feelings and emotional feelings in the anterior insula. Thus, we experience emotional feelings as if they were feelings from the body based on integration in the anterior insular cortex (Craig 2015a). Accordingly, the condition of the body affects our feelings and motivations continuously, and vice versa. For example, pain is more unpleasant and interoceptive circuitry more active when one feels acutely sad or clinically depressed, as described below (Ushinsky et al. 2013).

5 A sensorimotor architecture for emotion in the cortex

Like the classic sensorimotor system, the homeostatic/emotional system has identifiable sensory and motor components at each hierarchical level of the nervous system. The complementary components include: in the spinal cord, lamina I, and the autonomic columns; in the brainstem, PB (parabrachial nucleus) and PAG (periaqueductal gray); and, in the forebrain, the insular and cingulate cortices. The insular and cingulate regions both belong to the "limbic system" that earlier neuroscientists characterized, using lesions and electrical stimulation, as brain regions that are important both for overt emotional behaviors and for descending control of cardiorespiratory and visceral activity via the ANS. Modern evidence provides firm support for the idea that the insula serves as *limbic sensory cortex* and the cingulate (and medial prefrontal cortex) as *limbic motor cortex* (introduced in Craig 2002; see Heimer and van Hoesen 2006).

The insular and cingulate cortices interact strongly with each other and with other limbic forebrain regions (e.g., hypothalamus, amygdala, ventral striatum). In all mammals, the insular cortex receives ascending homeostatic sensory input via PB and has descending projections to PB and lamina I; functionally, it associates adaptive integration of olfactory, gustatory and viscerosensory activity with memory and homeostatic/emotional behavior, primarily ingestion (see Craig 2015a). The cingulate motor cortical area in all mammals is a major source of descending motoric projections to PAG and the spinal cord; functionally, it drives both autonomic activity and homeostatic/emotional behavior, including pain-related conditioned behavior (Johansen et al. 2001). This homeostatic sensorimotor perspective fits also with the global organization of frontal cortex into a sensory and a motor network (Ongur and Price 2000).

The anterior insular and anterior cingulate cortices bilaterally are the most commonly activated sites across all functional imaging studies and underlie the most common functional (EEG) microstate. They function as a core control network that links and coordinates activity across the entire forebrain, acting as a "predictive coding" system (Seth and Critchley 2013) that supports fluid intelligence (Duncan et al. 2012; see Craig 2009, 2015a). Notably, the insular and cingulate cortices are abnormal in an array of mental disorders, such as depression (Goodkind et al. 2015; see below).

In our view, subjective feelings engendered in the anterior insula and behavioral motivations (or, agency) engendered in the anterior cingulate together form the fundamental neuroanatomical basis for all human emotions. Closely related emotional feelings have overlapping but distinct activity foci in the anterior insula and differential activity in the cingulate and medial prefrontal cortex (see Craig 2015a). (A multivoxel meta-analysis for pain shows this differential pattern with additional sites; Wager et al. 2013 and Chapter 7, this volume, for discussion). This perspective fits with the view that an emotion in humans consists of a feeling and a motivation with direct autonomic sequelae (Rolls 1999). It fits also with modern evidence indicating that emotions guide all of our decisions and behaviors (Montague et al. 2006). From an evolutionary perspective, emotions are not simply episodic; rather they are continuously ongoing, and all of our behaviors are emotional behaviors, regardless of whether they occur with or without subjectively experienced feelings (Wegner 2003). Emotional behaviors evolved as energy-efficient means of producing goal-directed actions that fulfill social needs (Darwin 1965/1882) based on the same neural substrates that underlie homeostatic emotional behaviors.

6 Pain is a homeostatic emotion

Pain in humans consists of a feeling and a motivation that reflects an adverse condition in the body which the homeostatic spinal and brainstem mechanisms cannot rectify automatically and which urgently demands a behavioral response. The concept that pain and all affective feelings from the body constitute *homeostatic emotions* is compelled by the termination pattern of the homeostatic sensory pathway identified in primates and by how that dovetails with the functional neuroanatomical architecture described above; further, it explains why pain and all affectively charged feelings from the body have both strong autonomic sequelae and overwhelming behavioral urgency.

Thermosensory activity provides a good example of a homeostatic emotion. We normally think of temperature sensation as a discriminative cutaneous sensory capacity. However, with each thermal sensation we feel an obligatory hedonic affect (pleasantness or unpleasantness, unless neutral). For instance, in winter we put on or remove a glove based on a feeling of thermal discomfort or comfort in our hand. That affective feeling occurs along with a behavioral thermoregulatory motivation that guides an energy-efficient response to an interoceptive sensory condition which the homeostatic system cannot rectify automatically. It underscores the fundamental significance of temperature sensation for homeostasis *because* its valence depends directly on the body's thermoregulatory needs (Cabanac et al. 1972; Mower 1976; Strigo et al. 2000). For example, the cool glass of water that feels wonderful if you are overheated feels gnawingly unpleasant if you are chilled. Conversely, if you are "chilled to the bone," then a hot shower feels wonderful, even if it is prickly and stinging; however, that hot water would be called painful if you had a normal core temperature or were overheated. These affective feelings accompany behavioral motivations that are driven by the homeostatic needs of the body, and in humans the combination is a homeostatic emotion. Consonant with this view, our imaging studies of temperature sensation revealed that subjective thermosensory feelings are associated with the anterior insular cortex, while an intensifying thermal stimulus (which is arousing) additionally activates the cingulate cortex (Craig et al. 2000; Hua et al. 2005). Imaging and psychological evidence support the same concept for pain (Craig et al. 1996; Rainville et al. 1997); it "hurts" because it is *urgently* unpleasant, yet if other motivations are more urgent it just doesn't hurt as much, though it is usually still unpleasant.

7 A theoretical model for the generation of feelings

These considerations led to a model that offers plausible neurobiological explanations for how feelings are generated in our brains, what feelings represent, and how we experience our feelings (Craig 2009, 2015a). In this model, progressive interoceptive integration with all neural activity culminates in a complete representation of homeostatic salience as vivid feelings that are continuously changing in the immediate moment ("now"). The brain constructs feelings to represent the overall energy budget of any neural activity pattern, in order to facilitate choices that guide behavior in the most energy-efficient manner. Being able to "feel" every thought, perception, motivation, intention, or potential behavior provides a powerful common currency. The efficient utilization of energy is a crucial evolutionary arbiter, and the human brain consumes about 25 percent of the body's entire energy budget. Optimal energy utilization in highly social primates required interoceptive integration of activity in both the body and the brain in order to achieve homeostatic valuation of both actual and potential (or, fictive) energy utilization.

In this model, feelings from the body emerge from interoceptive integration in the middle insula with several types of activity. Integration with hedonically valenced activity from the ventral striatum of the reward behavioral system supplies the crucial appetitive and aversive incentives that underpin the affective pleasantness or unpleasantness of feelings from the body. Most important, interoceptive sensory activity is integrated with homeostatic motor activity that drives autonomic outputs to the body. The ongoing metaboreceptive and vasoreceptive activity essentially provides a high-fidelity sensory feedback image to the homeostatic motor system, in effect enabling this agent to sense what it's doing in the living body – to "feel" its own actions – at high resolution, in real time, with synchronous, rhythmic autonomic bursts driving immediate sensory responses from the body that pulsate with every breath, every heartbeat, and every emotion. In the model, this integration produces the feeling of being alive – "I feel that I am" – that constitutes the fundamental basis for the concept of *homeostatic sentience*. It enables the generation of vivid feelings from the body for any sensory event based on homeostatic motor outputs triggered by hereditary and learned emotional associations that are encoded at every level of the sensorimotor hierarchy. Inputs caused by "other" sensory signals are differentiated because those were not caused directly by the outputs of the homeostatic motor agent itself.

Integration in the anterior insula includes a moment-to-moment global representation of homeostatic salience that supports emotional awareness across time with a cinemascopic representation of the sentient self. This construct has remarkable emergent characteristics, and it offers sensible explanations for a variety of psychological constructs (the perceptual moment), philosophical concepts (subjective awareness), and clinical syndromes (anxiety, depression). While other authors assert a global network theory of pain or consciousness, rapidly accumulating studies support the localization of human emotional awareness to the anterior insular cortex (Smith et al. 2015; Tamietto et al. 2015; Warnaby et al. 2016; cf. Chapter 17, this volume).

Finally, this model includes the idea that a bivalent, opponent-regulated emotional control system is manifested in the bicameral vertebrate brain, with energy expenditure, negative affect, avoidance behavior, and sympathetic activity operationalized in the right forebrain and energy nourishment, positive affect, approach behavior, and parasympathetic activity in the left forebrain (see Craig 2009, 2015a). This asymmetry is demonstrated by ethological studies, clinical evidence, physiological results, and psychophysiological findings. Convincing neuroanatomical evidence in humans was recently obtained (Tomer et al. 2014). Two recent quantitative meta-analyses of functional imaging studies of emotional tasks revealed consonant asymmetric activation in the amygdala, anterior insular cortex, and cingulate cortex: during positive emotional conditions, strong activation occurred almost exclusively on the left side, while activation on the right side occurred exclusively during negative emotional conditions (Stevens and Hamann 2012; Duerden et al. 2013). Activation was observed on both sides during negative conditions, which is certainly consistent with the survival value of generating rapid escape behaviors with both hemispheres. Bilateral activation, or only left activation, during negative events can also be interpreted as evidence of coordinate opponent regulation.

8 Emotional pain in clinical patients

People that are depressed express how they feel by saying they live "in pain." This was eloquently described by Emily Dickinson as "I felt a funeral in my brain" and by William Styrone, who wrote that "the gray drizzle of horror induced by depression takes on the quality of physical pain." Below we provide evidence that the pain one feels when one is depressed can best be explained by viewing pain as a homeostatic emotion.

A key finding was that depressed individuals report feelings of unpleasantness in response to thermal stimuli that healthy individuals do not perceive as unpleasant. In the first study, we administered brief stimuli that ranged from warm to painfully hot on the left forearm of fifteen patients diagnosed with major depressive disorder (MDD), who at the time were not taking prescribed medications, and fifteen matched healthy comparison (HC) subjects. We asked the participants to rate the quality of each stimulus using three separate validated visual analog scales, one for intensity ("how strong was the stimulus?"), one for pain ("how painful was the stimulus?"), and one for unpleasantness ("how bothersome was the stimulus?"). We found that the relationship between the discriminative sensory scales and unpleasantness was strikingly different for MDD patients. They rated warm stimuli as quite unpleasant, even at temperatures they did not report as painful; for the HC participants, the same warm stimuli were neither unpleasant nor painful. The leftward shift in the unpleasantness ratings of MDD patients was profound, in that their unpleasantness rating of a normally non-painful stimulus was as high as the unpleasantness rating of a clearly painful heat stimulus for HCs. Statistical analyses showed that the temperatures at which MDD participants began to report unpleasantness were: (1) significantly lower than those of HCs, and (2) significantly lower than temperatures at which MDDs began to report pain (Strigo et al. 2008a).

We call this phenomenon *emotional allodynia*, because stimuli that are normally *not* unpleasant produce an unpleasant feeling in the MDD subjects. (Clinical "allodynia" means unpleasant light touch.) Their affective feeling of unpleasantness is uncoupled from their sensory discrimination of intensity or pain, in stark contrast to HCs, who begin to report unpleasantness at pain threshold (Strigo et al. 2008a, 2008b, 2013). This is distinct from hyperalgesia or sensitization, which mean enhanced pain sensation, because, even though MDD subjects can have lower heat pain thresholds than HCs, they report normal intensity and unpleasantness at normally painful higher temperatures.

We further found that neither attentional nor mood mechanisms altered emotional allodynia. Diverting attention away from the temperature stimulus reduced all intensity ratings (both painful and non-painful) for HCs, but for MDD subjects it reduced only the intensity ratings of the warm stimuli that were not rated unpleasant (Strigo et al. 2008b). In other words, the MDD subjects displayed emotional allodynia irrespective of whether they paid attention to the warm stimuli or not. In another psychophysical study, we used mood induction procedures to compare the effects of acute states of sadness and happiness in a group of twenty-one individuals diagnosed with current MDD and a matched comparison group of twenty-one HC subjects. We found the same pattern of significantly lower temperatures that produced unpleasantness in individuals with MDD despite the fact that they reported similar levels of sad or happy mood as the HCs did (Ushinsky et al. 2013). In other words, the temperatures at which the MDD subjects reported unpleasantness were not changed by the acute mood; they were abnormally reduced in both sad and happy moods. By contrast, in the HCs, we observed that the temperatures that were unpleasant were lower in a sad than in a happy mood, as others have found (see Ushinsky et al. 2013). These findings thus support the notion that emotional allodynia in MDD is not simply a reflection of the lower baseline affect or increased self-focus found in this disorder. Rather, these findings imply that emotional allodynia is a stable characteristic of major depression, that is, a measurable manifestation of emotional dysfunction that is fundamentally inherent to this disorder.

Several lines of evidence suggest that emotional allodynia is homeostatically driven. The most relevant is the phenomenon of thermal *alliesthesia*, whereby a thermal stimulus can be hedonically pleasant or unpleasant depending on the core body temperature, as described above (Cabanac et al. 1972). Considering that the core temperatures of depressed individuals tend towards hyperthermia (Rausch et al. 2003), warm stimuli would naturally be homeostatically aversive; warm stimuli applied to a body that is already too warm potentially threaten to increase the deviation from thermoregulatory neutrality. This mechanism could underlie the phenomenon of emotional allodynia that we have observed, in accordance with our view of pain as a homeostatic emotion. Homeostatic sensory integration is pivotal for thermoregulation (Craig 2003) and for emotional dysfunction in MDD.

9 Abnormal activation in the anterior insula in depression

The homeostatic sensory pathway and the insular and cingulate cortices are involved in the interactions between emotion and homeostasis. Our initial brain-imaging experiments showed that MDD subjects display hyperactivation in the bilateral anterior insula and dorsal cingulate during anticipation of pain. Considering that individuals with MDD rated warm temperatures as significantly more unpleasant than HC subjects, the abnormally increased activation in the cortical projection targets of the homeostatic sensory pathway could be directly related to the observed emotional allodynia in MDD (Strigo et al. 2008a). Further support for this possibility was provided by a meta-analysis of functional activation during negative emotional processing in MDD patients, in which we found that the focus of activation was shifted almost 10 millimeters from the location observed in HC subjects, so that it overlapped abnormally with the foci of acute pain and somatosensory processing in HCs (Mutschler et al. 2012). When we specifically examined the relation between warmth-related activation in a group of MDD subjects and the magnitude of emotional allodynia using a statistical model, we found that emotional allodynia was *inversely* related to warmth-related activation in the *left* anterior insula (Strigo and Craig 2016), consistent with the asymmetry described above. Functional connectivity analyses showed strong interactions between the left anterior insula and the right insula, dorsal cingulate, and right posterolateral thalamus, all of which are activated by the homeostatic sensory pathway. Finally, we also found that emotional allodynia is greater in individuals with reduced heart-rate variability, a common symptom of MDD that suggests an autonomic imbalance and reduced parasympathetic tone (Kemp et al. 2014). Dysfunctional homeostatic sensory integration in the limbic sensory and motor cortical regions that tightly link emotional and autonomic processing can parsimoniously explain these observations.

10 Emotional asymmetry, depression, and pain

An imbalance between the left and right hemispheres has been described in depressed patients (Hecht 2010), whereby the right hemisphere is hyperactive and the left hypoactive, in direct correspondence with depression severity (Grimm et al. 2008). Accordingly, therapeutically effective vagus nerve stimulation (VNS) in treatment-resistant depressed patients decreased activity on the right and increased activity on the left (Conway et al. 2013), while patients with the greatest activity in the right anterior insula were non-responders to VNS (Conway et al. 2012) and to antidepressant medications (Bruder et al. 2008). Similarly, transcranial magnetic stimulation has antidepressant effects if applied over the left frontal cortex (Lefaucheur et al. 2014); the more effective sites had EEG activity that correlated positively with left and negatively with right anterior insular activity, while at less-effective sites the opposite pattern was observed (Fox et al. 2012). Likewise, reduced right insula activation was associated with antidepressant response to ketamine (Carlson et al. 2013).

We have found that depressive symptom severity in MDD patients is predicted by the activation in the right dorsal anterior insula during anticipation of painful heat stimuli (Strigo et al. 2013). Furthermore, activity in the right dorsal anterior insula correlates with a measure of activity in the ascending lamina I pathway (Strigo et al. 2013). The right dorsal anterior insula is an important component of the forebrain network that controls attention, and so together these findings suggest that attention in MDD subjects is linked more to the neural processing of interoception and feelings from the body than to cognitive networks, which is consistent with the increased internal focus in this disorder (Sliz and Hayley 2012) and with the likely role of the right anterior insular cortex in emotional allodynia described above.

Related topics

Notes

1 Specialized terms are in parentheses.
2 The sacral parasympathetic system is not discussed here.
3 In contrast, large-diameter sensory fibers terminate on deep dorsal horn neurons that project to ventral horn motor neurons and to central motoric regions (cerebellum, tectum, motor thalamus). Such neurons respond to cutaneous mechanoreceptors and tonically active muscle proprioreceptors (Bannatyne et al. 2006); they are modulated by descending (rubro-spinal and cortico-spinal) signals that control skeletal muscle movements. Deep dorsal horn neurons are musculotopically, not somatotopically, organized (Schouenborg et al. 1995), consistent with their role in motoric integration.

Some deep dorsal horn neurons are activated by myelinated nociceptors from skin, muscle, or viscera, in particular a subtype with fast-conducting fibers and receptors in the outer epidermis that are adapted for external noxious stimuli (Lawson 2002). These neurons generate nocifensive reflexes (e.g., withdrawal, guarding) that serve a homeostatic function (Cannon 1932), and they constitute a vital ("viscerosomatic") coupling between small-diameter and large-diameter functions. Conversely, other deep dorsal horn neurons convey mechanoreceptive activity to the autonomic cell columns.

Deep dorsal horn neurons that receive multisynaptic C-fiber nociceptive input and display intensity-related ("wide dynamic range") discharge (as do many motor neurons) are said by certain authors to signal pain (Price 2013). However, because they are modality ambiguous and cannot differentiate touch from pressure or pinch from noxious heat, a central pattern detector must be imputed, which doesn't make sense developmentally (see Craig 2003, 2015a). Our recordings demonstrated that such cells in monkeys cannot explain the temporal summation of second pain following repeated brief-contact heat stimuli or the ice-like burning pain of the thermal grill illusion, whereas lamina I HPC neurons explain these phenomena quantitatively (Craig 2004b, 2015a).

4 The insula is a cortical "island" buried within the lateral sulcus, or Sylvian fissure. It is a well-developed, operculated fifth lobe only in the brains of species that have this pathway, the anthropoid primates. The three adjacent inward folds of cortex that process direct interoceptive inputs also exist only in these species. This morphology minimizes the distance between these continuously interacting sites, thereby supporting the central goal of homeostasis, energy efficiency.

5 The identification of distinct interoceptive forebrain areas in primates validated the neural distinctness of regions that process small-diameter fiber activity and serve smooth muscle control, which are separate from regions that process large-diameter fiber activity and serve skeletal muscle control. Since it made sense to call the former interoceptive, we suggested calling the latter *exteroceptive*. But, that led to mis-understandings (Lawson 2002; Price 2013; cf. also Price, Chapter 9, this volume). From the perspective of autonomic output, W.B. Cannon (1932) had suggested the similar terms "interofective" and "exterofective" to no avail. The *visceral* and *somatic* categories used by early neuroanatomists capture only some of these differences. It seems likely that ongoing work differentiating the corresponding embryologic gene regulatory networks noted above will eventually provide definitive nomenclature.

6 Contradictory evidence was reported in two patients whose insular cortex was "completely" destroyed bilaterally, but in both cases dorsal anterior insular cortex can be seen in the published images (see Craig 2015a). Nearly all recent clinical and imaging studies affirm that the insula is crucial for subjective emotional awareness (Smith et al. 2015; Tamietto et al. 2015; Warnaby et al. 2016).

References

Bannatyne, B.A., Edgley, S.A., Hammar, I., Jankowska, E., and Maxwell, D.J. (2006) Differential projections of excitatory and inhibitory dorsal horn interneurons relaying information from group II muscle afferents in the cat spinal cord. *Journal Neuroscience* 26: 2871–2880.

Barrett, L.F., Quigley, K.S., Bliss-Moreau, E., and Aronson, K.R. (2004) Interoceptive sensitivity and self-reports of emotional experience. *Journal of Personality and Social Psychology* 87; 684–697.

Bauernfeind, A.L., De Sousa, A.A., Avasthi, T., Dobson, S.D., Raghanti, M.A., Lewandowski, A.H., Zilles, K., Semendeferi, K., Allman, J.M., Craig, A.D., Hof, P.R., and Sherwood, C.C. (2013) A volumetric comparison of the insular cortex and its subregions in primates. *Journal of Human Evolution* 64: 263–279.

Bruder, G.E., Sedoruk, J.P., Stewart, J.W., Mcgrath, P.J., Quitkin, F.M., and Tenke, C.E. (2008) Electroencephalographic alpha measures predict therapeutic response to a selective serotonin reuptake inhibitor antidepressant: pre- and post-treatment findings. *Biological Psychiatry* 63: 1171–1177.

Cabanac, M., Massonnet, B., and Belaiche, R. (1972) Preferred skin temperature as a function of internal and mean skin temperature. *Journal of Applied Physiology* 33: 699–703.

Cannon, W.B. (1932) *The Wisdom of the Body*. New York: W.W. Norton. Repr. Birmingham, AL: Classics of Medicine Library, 1989.

Carlson, P.J., Diazgranados, N., Nugent, A.C., Ibrahim, L., Luckenbaugh, D.A., Brutsche, N., Herscovitch, P., Manji, H.K., Zarate, C.A. Jr., and Drevets, W.C. (2013) Neural correlates of rapid antidepressant response to ketamine in treatment-resistant unipolar depression: a preliminary positron emission tomography study. *Biological Psychiatry* 73: 1213–1221.

Chen, J.I., Ha, B., Bushnell, M.C., Pike, B., and Duncan, G.H. (2002) Differentiating noxious- and innocuous-related activation of human somatosensory cortices using temporal analysis of fMRI. *Journal of Neurophysiology* 88: 464–474.

Conway, C.R., Chibnall, J.T., Gangwani, S., Mintun, M.A., Price, J.L., Hershey, T., Giuffra, L.A., Bucholz, R.D., Christensen, J.J., and Sheline, Y.I. (2012) Pretreatment cerebral metabolic activity correlates with antidepressant efficacy of vagus nerve stimulation in treatment-resistant major depression: a potential marker for response? *Journal of Affective Disorders* 139: 283–290.

Conway, C.R., Chibnall, J.T., Gebara, M.A., Price, J.L., Snyder, A.Z., Mintun, M.A., Craig, A.D., Cornell, M.E., Perantie, D.C., Giuffra, L.A., Bucholz, R.D., and Sheline, Y. (2013) Association of cerebral metabolic activity changes with vagus nerve stimulation antidepressant response in treatment-resistant depression. *Brain Stimulation* 6: 788–797.

Craig, A.D. (2002) How do you feel? Interoception: The sense of the physiological condition of the body. *Nature Reviews Neuroscience* 3: 655–666.

Craig, A.D. (2003) Pain mechanisms: labeled lines versus convergence in central processing. *Annual Review of Neuroscience* 26: 1–30.

Craig, A.D. (2004a). Distribution of trigeminothalamic and spinothalamic lamina I terminations in the macaque monkey. *Journal of Comparative Neurology* 477: 119–148.

Craig, A.D. (2004b) Lamina I, but not lamina V, spinothalamic neurons exhibit responses that correspond with burning pain. *Journal of Neurophysiology* 92: 2604–2609.

Craig, A.D. (2009) How do you feel – now? The anterior insula and human awareness. *Nature Reviews Neuroscience* 10: 59–70.

Craig, A.D. (2014) Topographically organized projection to posterior insular cortex from the posterior portion of the ventral medial nucleus in the long-tailed macaque monkey. *Journal of Comparative Neurology* 522: 36–63.

Craig, A.D. (2015a) *How Do You Feel?: An Interoceptive Moment with Your Neurobiological Self*. Princeton: Princeton University Press.

Craig, A.D. (2015b) Referee report for: The dorsal posterior insula is not an island in pain but subserves a fundamental role – Response to: "Evidence against pain specificity in the dorsal posterior insula" by Davis *et al*. F1000Research, 4, 1207.

Craig, A.D., Reiman, E.M., Evans, A., and Bushnell, M.C. (1996) Functional imaging of an illusion of pain. *Nature* 384: 258–260.

Craig, A.D., Chen, K., Bandy, D., and Reiman, E.M. (2000) Thermosensory activation of insular cortex. *Nature Neuroscience* 3: 184–190.

Darwin, C. (1965/1882) *The Expression of the Emotions in Man and Animals*. Chicago: University of Chicago Press.

Duerden, E.G., Arsalidou, M., Lee, M., and Taylor, M.J. (2013) Lateralization of affective processing in the insula. *Neuroimage* 78: 159–175.

Dum, R.P., Levinthal, D.J., and Strick, P.L. (2009) The spinothalamic system targets motor and sensory areas in the cerebral cortex of monkeys. *Journal of Neuroscience* 29: 14223–14235.

Duncan, J., Schramm, M., Thompson, R., and Dumontheil I. (2012) Task rules, working memory, and fluid intelligence. *Psychon Bull Rev* 19: 864–870.

Fox, M.D., Buckner, R.L., White, M.P., Greicius, M.D., and Pascual-Leone, A. (2012) Efficacy of transcranial magnetic stimulation targets for depression is related to intrinsic functional connectivity with the subgenual cingulate. *Biological Psychiatry* 72: 595–603.

Goodkind, M., Eickhoff, S.B., Oathes, D.J., Jiang, Y., Chang, A., Jones-Hagata, L.B., Ortega, B.N., Zaiko, Y.V., Roach, E.L., Korgaonkar, M.S., Grieve, S.M., Galatzer-Levy, I., Fox, P.T., and Etkin, A. (2015) Identification of a common neurobiological substrate for mental illness. *JAMA Psychiatry* 72: 305–315.

Grimm, S., Beck, J., Schuepbach, D., Hell, D., Boesiger, P., Bermpohl, F., Niehaus, L., Boeker, H., and Northoff, G. (2008) Imbalance between left and right dorsolateral prefrontal cortex in major depression is linked to negative emotional judgment: an fMRI study in severe major depressive disorder. *Biological Psychiatry* 63: 369–376.

Hecht, D. (2010) Depression and the hyperactive right-hemisphere. *Neuroscience Research* 68: 77–87.

Heimer, L., and Van Hoesen, G.W. (2006) The limbic lobe andits output channels: implications for emotional functions and adaptive behavior. *Neuroscience and Biobehavioral Reviews* 30: 126–147.

Hua, L.H., Strigo, I.A., Baxter, L.C., Johnson, S.C., Craig, A.D. (2005) Anteroposterior somatotopy of innocuous cooling activation focus in human dorsal posterior insular cortex. *American Journal of Physiology – Regulatory, Integrative and Comparative Physiology* 289: R319–R325.

Johansen, J.P., Fields, H.L., and Manning, B.H. (2001) The affective component of pain in rodents: direct evidence for a contribution of the anterior cingulate cortex. *Proceedings of the National Academy of Sciences of the United States of America* 98: 8077–8082.

Kemp, A.H., Quintana, D.S., Quinn, C.R., Hopkinson, P., and Harris, A.W. (2014) Major depressive disorder with melancholia displays robust alterations in resting state heart rate and its variability: implications for future morbidity and mortality. *Frontiers of Psychology* 5: 1387.

Lawson, S.N. (2002) Phenotype and function of somatic primary afferent nociceptive neurones with C-, Adelta- or Aalpha/beta-fibres. *Experimental Physiology* 87: 239–244.

Lefaucheur, J.P., Andre-Obadia, N., Antal, A., Ayache, S.S., Baeken, C., Benninger, D.H., Cantello, R. M., Cincotta, M., de Carvalho, M., De Ridder, D., Devanne, H., Di Lazzaro, V., Filipović, S.R., Hummel, F.C., Jääskeläinen, S.K., Kimiskidis, V.K., Koch, G., Langguth, B., Nyffeler, T., Oliviero, A., Padberg, F., Poulet, E., Rossi, S., Rossini, P.M., Rothwell, J.C., Schönfeldt-Lecuona, C., Siebner, H. R., Slotema, C.W., Stagg, C.J., Valls-Sole, J., Ziemann, U., Paulus, W., and Garcia-Larrea, L. (2014) Evidence-based guidelines on the therapeutic use of repetitive transcranial magnetic stimulation (rTMS). *Clinical Neurophysiology* 125: 2150–2206.

Lindquist, K.A. and Barrett, L.F. (2012) A functional architecture of the human brain: emerging insights from the science of emotion. *Trends in Cognitive Sciences* 16: 533–540.

Ma, Q. (2010) Labeled lines meet and talk: Population coding of somatic sensations. *Journal of Clinical Investigation* 120: 3773–3778.

Mazzola, L., Isnard, J., Peyron, R., and Mauguiere, F. (2012) Stimulation of the human cortex and the experience of pain: Wilder Penfield's observations revisited. *Brain* 135: 631–640.

Montague, P.R., King-Casas, B., and Cohen, J.D. (2006) Imaging valuation models in human choice. *Annual Review of Neuroscience* 29: 417–448.

Mower, G.D. (1976) Perceived intensity of peripheral thermal stimuli is independent of internal body temperature. *Journal of Comparative and Physiological Psychology* 90: 1152.

Mutschler, I., Ball, T., Wankerl, J., and Strigo, I.A. (2012) Pain and emotion in the insular cortex: evidence for functional reorganization in major depression. *Neuroscience Letters* 520: 204–209.

Ongur, D. and Price, J.L. (2000) The organization of networks within the orbital and medial prefrontal cortex of rats, monkeys and humans. *Cerebral Cortex* 10: 206–219.

Price, D.D. (2013) Dorsal horn neuronal responses and quantitative sensory testing help explain normal and abnormal pain. *Pain* 154: 1161–1162.

Rainville, P., Duncan, G.H., Price, D.D., Carrier, B., and Bushnell, M.C. (1997) Pain affect encoded in human anterior cingulate but not somatosensory cortex. *Science* 277: 968–971.

Rausch, J.L., Johnson, M.E., Corley, K.M., Hobby, H.M., Shendarkar, N., Fei, Y., Ganapathy, V., and Leibach, F.H. (2003) Depressed patients have higher body temperature: 5-HT transporter long promoter region effects. *Neuropsychobiology* 47: 120–127.

Rolls, E.T. (1999) *The Brain and Emotion*. Oxford: Oxford University Press.

Schouenborg, J., Weng, H.R., Kalliomaki, J., and Holmberg, H. (1995) A survey of spinal dorsal horn neurones encoding the spatial organization of withdrawal reflexes in the rat. *Experimental Brain Research* 106: 19–27.

Segerdahl, A.R., Mezue, M., Okell, T.W., Farrar, J.T., and Tracey, I. (2015) The dorsal posterior insula subserves a fundamental role in human pain. *Nature Neuroscience* 18: 499–500.

Seth, A.K. and Critchley, H.D. (2013) Extending predictive processing to the body: emotion as interoceptive inference. *Behavioral and Brain Sciences* 36: 227–228.

Sliz, D. and Hayley, S. (2012) Major depressive disorder and alterations in insular cortical activity: a review of current functional magnetic imaging research. *Frontiers in Human Neuroscience* 6: 323.

Smith, R., Braden, B.B., Chen, K., Ponce, F.A., Lane, R.D., and Baxter, L.C. (2015) The neural basis of attaining conscious awareness of sad mood. *Brain Imaging and Behavior* 9: 574–587.

Stevens, J.S. and Hamann, S. (2012) Sex differences in brain activation to emotional stimuli: a meta-analysis of neuroimaging studies. *Neuropsychologia* 50: 1578–1593.

Strigo, I.A., Carli, F., and Bushnell, M.C. (2000) Effect of ambient temperature on human pain and temperature perception. *Anesthesiology* 92: 699–707.

Strigo, L.A and Craig, A.D (2016) Why depression hurts: initial evidence for neural correlates of emotional allodynia. *Neuropsychopharmacology* 41: 455-630.

Strigo, I.A., Simmons, A.N., Matthews, S.C., Craig, A.D., and Paulus, M.P. (2008a) Increased affective bias revealed using experimental graded heat stimuli in young depressed adults: evidence of "emotional allodynia". *Psychosomatic Medicine* 70: 338–344.

Strigo, I.A., Simmons, A.N., Matthews, S.C., Craig, A.D., and Paulus, M.P. (2008b) Association of major depressive disorder with altered functional brain response during anticipation and processing of heat pain. *Archives of General Psychiatry* 65: 1275–1284.

Strigo, I.A., Matthews, S.C., and Simmons, A.N. (2013) Decreased frontal regulation during pain anticipation in unmedicated subjects with major depressive disorder. *Translational Psychiatry* 3: e239.

Tamietto, M., Cauda, F., Celeghin, A., Diano, M., Costa, T., Cossa, F.M., Sacco, K., Duca, S., Geminiani, G.C., and de Gelder, B. (2015) Once you feel it, you see it: insula and sensory-motor contribution to visual awareness for fearful bodies in parietal neglect. *Cortex* 62: 56–72.

Tomer, R., Slagter, H.A., Christian, B.T., Fox, A.S., King, C.R., Murali, D., Gluck, M.A., and Davidson, R.J. (2014) Love to win or hate to lose? Asymmetry of dopamine D2 receptor binding predicts sensitivity to reward versus punishment. *Journal of Cognitive Neuroscience* 26: 1039–1048.

Ushinsky, A., Reinhardt, L.E., Simmons, A.N., and Strigo, I.A., (2013) Further evidence of emotional allodynia in unmedicated young adults with major depressive disorder. *PLoS One* 8: e80507.

Vierck, C.J., Whitsel, B.L., Favorov, O.V., Brown, A.W., and Tommerdahl, M. (2013) Role of primary somatosensory cortex in the coding of pain. *Pain* 154: 334–344.

Wager, T.D., Atlas, L.Y., Lindquist, M.A., Roy, M., Woo, C.-W., and Kross, E. (2013) An fMRI-based neurologic signature of physical pain. *New England Journal of Medicine* 368: 1388–1397.

Warnaby, C.E., Seretny, M., Mhuircheartaigh, R.N., Rogers, R., Jbabdi, S., Sleigh, J., and Tracey, I. (2016) Anesthesia-induced suppression of human dorsal anterior insula responsivity at loss of volitional behavioral response. *Anesthesiology* 124(4): 766–778.

Wegner, D.M. (2003) *The Illusion of Conscious Will*. Cambridge, MA: MIT Press..

Wiech, K., Jbabdi, S., Lin, C.S., Andersson, J., and Tracey, I. (2014) Differential structural and resting state connectivity between insular subdivisions and other pain-related brain regions. *Pain* 155: 2047–2055.

9

A VIEW OF PAIN BASED ON SENSATIONS, MEANINGS, AND EMOTIONS

Donald D. Price

Views about what constitute the fundamental dimensions and functions of pain are remarkably different. Until the late 1960s pain was mainly seen as a specific neuronal system that functioned like other sensory systems (Melzack and Wall 1983): pain sensation intensity and duration were considered to be determined only by the intensity and duration of the peripheral stimulus, much like other exteroceptive systems directed toward the external environment (tactile, visual, auditory). Wall's (1979) functional account of pain departed radically from this classical view and claimed that pain was more like a need state such as hunger and thirst and functioned as a homeostatic mechanism involved in recuperation and healing. More recently, this homeostatic view has been expanded to consider pain a basic feeling or emotion that serves an interoceptive function, one that provides a representation of the physiological condition of the body (Craig 2003; see also Chapter 8, this volume). A major problem with homeostatic and interoceptive views of pain is that they seem to entirely leave out considerable evidence that demonstrates that many types of pain have distinct sensory qualities and provide highly sensitive information about stimulus location, stimulus intensity, and intensity differences (Price et al. 2003). This chapter provides an inclusive view of pain as serving interoceptive and exteroceptive functions and as having sensory and affective dimensions. This account integrates an experiential perspective with results of studies of experimental and clinical pain.

1 Defining pain through a perspective of direct experience

A definition of pain agreed upon by the International Association for the Study of Pain's (IASP's) taxonomy committee is as follows: "*Pain is an unpleasant sensory and emotional experience associated with actual or potential tissue damage, or described in terms of such damage*" (Mersky and Bogduk 1994). This definition is unique in that it was the first to explicitly recognize that the phenomenon of pain is an *experience*, yet one that comprises both sensory and affective dimensions. It is a bit confusing because it is ambiguous as to whether the *association with actual or potential tissue damage* is from the perspective of the person who has the pain or from an external observer (Price 1999). The definition could be construed to imply that if an observer (e.g., health-care professional) cannot establish an association between a self-reported experience of pain and tissue damage, then the experience may not be considered painful (for further discussion on the IASP definition, see Chapter 31, this volume). An association between unpleasant sensation and tissue injury or even the potential for tissue injury is neither necessary nor sufficient for pain. It may not even be a common factor in pain from the perspective of those who have it. Does someone with a stomach ache associate the sensation with actual or potential tissue damage? Similarly, some patients with pain from nerve injury experience repeated gentle stroking of the hand as "burning," "aching," or "throbbing" but do not really associate the burning sensations with actual or potential tissue damage (Melzack and Torgerson 1971; Price 1999).

There seem to be common factors within the experiences of very different types of pain, as reviewed elsewhere (Melzack and Wall 1983; Price 1999). Based on common factors, an alternative definition of pain closely resembles the widely accepted IASP definition yet mitigates the problems inherent in the latter: *Pain is a somatic or visceral experience that is comprised of (1) unique sensory qualities that are like those which occur during tissue-damaging stimulation, (2) a closely related meaning of intrusion and/or threat, and (3) an associated feeling of unpleasantness and/or other immediate negative emotion(s)* (based on a revision of Price 1999). Each of these factors is necessary and taken together jointly sufficient for pain. It was derived using considerations of patients' and healthy volunteers' direct experiences of considerably different types of pain and on numerous studies of the experience of pain (Price 1999).

2 Unique sensory qualities of pain

Sensory qualities of pain are unique and distinct from other body sensations (Melzack and Torgerson 1971; Merskey and Nicholas 1994). For example, unlike sensations of other modalities, pain often spreads in area as it becomes more intense, even when the stimulus itself is not spreading. It can be highly localized (e.g., a pin prick) or very diffuse and poorly localized. Yet the sensory qualities of pain contain a common meaning of intrusion or threat to the body. This is clearly evident when pain patients endorse sensory descriptive words on the McGill Pain Questionnaire (MPQ) (Melzack 1975; Melzack and Torgerson 1971; Melzack and Wall 1983). The vast majority of sensory descriptors on the MPQ refer to a rudimentary meaning of intrusion and/or threat to body tissues. For example, words such as "pinching," "pressing," or "crushing" connote constrictive pressure to tissues, and words such as "pricking," "boring," or "stabbing" connote intense punctuate pressure or penetration of tissues. "Burning," "scalding," and "searing" connote destructive thermal stimulation. These words seem at least partly metaphorical – patients often describe pain *as if* their skin is being stabbed or burned. The intrusive, disturbing, and threatening qualities relate to the meaning that something is happening to or within the body in such as way as to evoke harm. Pain always involves a meaning of *threat or intrusion of the self* that is directed toward one's body, well-being, sense of psychological stability, or all of these components (Price et al. 1987). However, this meaning is not necessarily that of an association with tissue damage, as implied by the IASP pain definition.

3 Exteroceptive and interoceptive functions of sensory qualities of pain

Pain sometimes has an exteroceptive function, extracting information about events in the environment in order to execute behaviors that protect the organism from external threats (Price et al. 2003). When the skin of mammals comes into contact with external objects that can cause tissue damage, specialized nociceptors are activated, ultimately leading to the initiation of escape and avoidance behaviors providing for self-protection. This is analogous to visual or auditory receptors which signal events in the external environment. Hence, extero-ceptors, as defined by Sherrington (1906), can lead to escape and avoidance. In contrast, interoceptors are activated when deep tissues are injured or there is a state of dysfunction or disease within them. Unlike exteroceptor-initiated pain, interoceptive functions of pain are accompanied by homeostatic behaviors such as quiescence and guarding of injured body regions and autonomic responses that promote recuperation and healing (Wall 1979). Thus, one can envision two biological functions of pain: escape/avoidance of external threats, and protection of injured or dysfunctional tissues that disrupt homeostasis. Both functions serve to protect the integrity of the body. (Cf. Chapters 5 and 8, this volume.) The sensory qualities of exteroceptive- and interoceptive-initiated pain are distinct, perhaps helping to account for the two types of general behaviors. Interoceptive pains referred to deep tissues are often felt as aching, throbbing, and spatially vague or diffuse. Exteroceptive pains more likely are referred to superficial tissues and felt as punctuate, piercing, or pricking. Despite these general differences, the sense of intrusion/threat applies to both interoception and exteroception.

If the sensory qualities themselves contain part of the meaning of intrusion/threat, one might question whether pain-like sensory qualities and the sense of intrusion/threat are identical factors. They are not identical, because the meanings of intrusion and threat can be based on more than just the sensory qualities of pain. Pain always occurs within a psychosocial and physical context and is influenced by several contextual factors. For example, a backache is likely to be experienced as less intrusive and threatening when someone is sitting in their living room as compared to when they are trying to work. Parallel influences from contextual and psychosocial factors abound in pain experience (see Figure 9.1). Thus, although pain-like sensory qualities may contain part of the sense of intrusion or

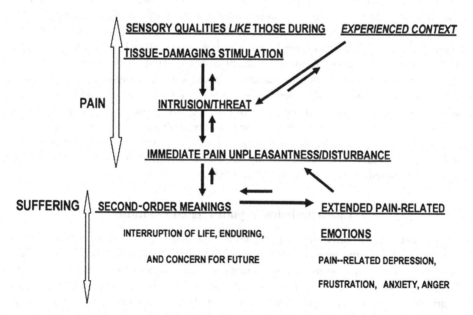

Figure 9.1 A schematic used to illustrate interactions between the basic meanings and dimensions of pain and pain-related suffering. Direct positive effects are denoted by large arrows and smaller effects in the reverse direction are denoted by small arrows. Note that serial and parallel effects occur for contextual and sensory factors. See text for descriptions and explanations of these concepts.

threat, this meaning can be strongly combined with contextual factors. (See Chapters 11 and 12, this volume.)

4 Immediate pain-related emotional feelings

Experienced threat/intrusion determines whether or not an experience is labeled as physically painful. For example, an experiment showed that when laser stimuli were applied at intensities near pain threshold, instructions that induced a high degree of threat resulted in a much greater likelihood of labeling the experience as pain as compared to instructions that induced a low degree of threat (Wiech et al. 2010). In other words, when all other variables, such as stimulus intensity, were held constant, labeling the experience as painful or non-painful was dependent on the extent of experienced threat. These results provide direct support for the new definition of pain proposed above.

Finally, the meaning of intrusion/threat is not only closely related to the feeling of unpleasantness or disturbance, but it can sometimes be accompanied by other negative emotion(s). The inclusion of this alternative, "*other immediate negative emotion(s),*" helps to mitigate a problem with the IASP definition that uses only one word "unpleasantness" to denote the emotional component of pain (Melzack and Wall 1983). The revised definition also accommodates the observation that in addition to immediate feelings of unpleasantness or disturbance, pain can be linked to suffering or extended emotional feelings, such as pain-related depression, anxiety, or anger (Wade et al. 1996; Harkins et al. 1989). However, pain can occur without suffering and therefore suffering is not necessary for pain. The meaning of intrusion/threat reflects a physical *meaning* of pain that is a part of the sensory experience. The emotional feeling of unpleasantness or disturbance reflects the felt sense of that physical meaning often in relation to its physical and psychosocial context. A major reason that emotional feelings during pain are shaped by context is that they are often accompanied by a desire to reduce or terminate the pain combined with a level of expectation that it can or will be reduced, as is evident in several studies of both experimental and clinical pain (Price et al. 1987; Price 1999, 2000; Rainville et al. 2005; Wiech et al. 2010). Desires and expectations are integrally related to one's situation. Meanings of intrusion/threat, feelings of unpleasantness/disturbance, and sometimes extended emotions (i.e., suffering) are separate though often closely related. Pain-related emotional feelings are often most important to us, especially when pain persists over time. Unique sensory qualities, a sense of intrusion/threat, and immediate pain-related emotional feelings are each necessary and taken together sufficient for pain, consistent with a long held consensus that pain contains sensory, evaluative, and emotional dimensions (Melzack and Wall 1983).

5 Characteristics of pain-related emotions

The stage of immediate unpleasantness of pain is about the meaning of pain as it relates to what is taking place in the present and is sustained by what Damasio (1999) refers to as "core consciousness." Core consciousness can be thought of as the moment-by-moment awareness of the state of the body and self and the perceptual aspects of what is taking place in the present. The link between immediate pain unpleasantness and core consciousness is evident when one directly experiences the distress, intrusion, and threat that occur in the present (see again Figure 9.1). To put it simply, whenever we experience the immediate unpleasantness/ disturbance of pain we are aware of that feeling. That awareness is sustained by brain structures involved in the regulation of consciousness (Damasio 1999; cf. Chapter 17, this volume).

6 Multisensory contributions to immediate pain unpleasantness

Certainly the sensory qualities of pain dispose us to experience them as threatening, intrusive, disturbing, and unpleasant under most circumstances. Thus, similar to nausea or intense thirst, painful sensations are usually closely linked to the immediate threat and intrusiveness and hence unpleasantness/disturbance of pain. However, this immediate response sometimes includes additional sensory components that are part of a more integrated experience. Consider a hypothetical example of being suddenly stung by an insect such as a bee. This negative experience is accompanied by abrupt visual, auditory, and somatic attention to the bee. The stinging sensation is only part of what is threatening. Seeing and hearing the bee at the same time only makes the experience more threatening and fearful. The stinging sensation, the arousal, and the feelings of one's own autonomic and motor responses all culminate in an experience of sudden intense threat, intrusion, and fear. Memory of past consequences of bee stings can also add to this experience. One can easily appreciate that a bee sting would be even more emotionally disturbing if one remembered their previous allergic reaction to a sting.

This example illustrates that emotional feelings that are a part of pain experience are based on meanings derived from the integration of different sense modalities and from the contexts in which they occur. Some contextual factors, including psychosocial interactions, can lead to the association of pain sensations with present or near-future consequences as a result of someone's immediate situation. The affective dimension of pain is integrally related to the evaluative dimension of pain and is not separate from it. (See Chapter 3, this volume.) Meanings and evaluations are *integral components* of the emotional dimension of pain. They trigger somatic and visceral responses in neural pathways that project to brain areas involved in emotions and emotional feelings (e.g., insular cortex) (Damasio 1999; Price 1999, 2000; see also Chapter 8, this volume).

7 How do pain sensation and immediate pain unpleasantness/ disturbance interact?

Given the three-factor definition of pain, functional hypotheses pertaining to how these pain-related factors interact can be tested in studies that use psychophysical scaling methods. Numerous studies support the view that the sensory and immediate affective dimensions of pain are separate and unique, even though they are often closely associated (Price 2000). Two related experiments clearly illustrate this view and help establish the direction of causation between the sensory and affective dimensions (Rainville et al. 1999). Both experiments were part of a hypnosis study in which pain was induced in subjects by immersing their left hands in a moderately painful water bath heated to 47° C (about 5 on a 10-point scale). In the first experiment, hypnotic suggestions were alternately given to enhance or decrease pain unpleasantness without changing pain sensation intensity. In the second, the hypnotic suggestions were targeted specifically toward enhancing or decreasing pain sensation intensity and nothing whatsoever was stated about pain unpleasantness. Pain unpleasantness but not pain sensation intensity ratings were changed in the directions suggested in the first experiment, a result that unsurprisingly followed the hypnotic suggestion. However, both pain sensation intensity and pain unpleasantness ratings changed in parallel in the second experiment despite the fact that the suggestions were about pain sensation intensity and did not mention pain unpleasantness at all. In other words, pain unpleasantness decreased and increased passively as a consequence of alternations between reduced and increased pain sensation intensity. This study helps to establish that pain sensation is more of an immediate cause of pain unpleasantness than is the latter a cause of pain sensation. Thus, there is a sequential or serial relationship between the sensation of pain and its associated unpleasantness, as shown in Figure 9.1. For this reason and others, hypnotic or placebo suggestions that are targeted toward pain sensations reduce unpleasantness as an additional consequence (e.g., second experiment of Rainville et al. 1999). Other experiments and studies of pain patients also support a sequential relationship between pain sensation intensity and the immediate emotional dimension of pain (Wade et al. 1996; Price et al. 1987). At the same time, Rainville et al.'s first experiment showing selective effects on unpleasantness also suggests parallel influences on pain unpleasantness. If pain unpleasantness can be selectively diminished without changing pain sensation intensity, the latter cannot be the exclusive cause of pain-related unpleasantness. In clinical contexts, parallel influences appear quite frequently because patients' emotional responses are often not just about the pain, but also about the physical and social implications of having the pain. These kinds of influences can be illustrated by a study in which different types of pain patients were studied, including patients with cancer pain and women who were in labor (Price et al. 1987). This study hypothesized that the ratio of unpleasantness ratings to pain sensation intensity ratings would be higher in cancer patients whose pain is likely to be associated with a serious threat to health or life in comparison to labor-pain patients whose pain is very intense but likely to be less threatening. Labor-pain patients and cancer-pain patients used visual analogue scales (VAS) to rate their levels of pain sensation intensity and degree of unpleasantness that occurred at different times during their clinical condition. Cancer-pain patients were distinguished by the fact that their VAS unpleasantness ratings were higher than their VAS sensory ratings, whereas the reverse was true for labor-pain patients.

The combination of these results indicates that someone's goals (e.g., having baby/avoiding pain), desires, and expectations about outcomes can strongly influence unpleasant feelings associated with different clinical pain conditions. The influence of these factors is most apparent when divergent psychological orientations exist *within* a clinical pain condition. Thus, the emotional dimension of cancer pain was enhanced by meanings that extended beyond that provided by the sensory qualities, including thoughts and images about the tumor location and the implication that having this pain is a result of cancer. In contrast, labor pain had an immediate implication for some patients that a baby is being born. The positive emotional consequences of this implication may offset to some degree the unpleasantness of labor pain. This interpretation is further supported by the much greater degree of labor-pain unpleasantness among women who mainly focused on avoiding pain (an avoidance goal) as compared to those who focused on the birth of the baby (an approach goal). Unpleasantness ratings of the latter were approximately half those of the former (Price et al. 1987). Part of what constitutes pain disturbance and unpleasantness is the *immediate implication* of the pain condition. Results obtained in studies of experimental and clinical pain demonstrate that evaluative factors can selectively and sometimes powerfully modify the immediate emotional dimension of pain.

8 Suffering: extended pain-related emotions based on reflection/ rumination

Both empirical studies of experiential factors in pain and consideration of the experience of pain itself indicate that there can be two stages of pain-related feelings distinguished by the time frame over which cognitive appraisals are directed (Wade et al. 1996; Price 2000). These stages and their interrelationships are illustrated schematically in Figure 9.1. The first, discussed already, is the *immediate unpleasant or disturbing feelings* that are often closely linked with the intensity of the painful sensation and its accompanying arousal. The next stage is more complex, and is based on more elaborate reflection related to that which one remembers or imagines. These involve meanings directed toward the longer-term implications of having pain. These meanings are related to perception of how pain has or will interfere with different aspects of living, the experienced difficulty of enduring the pain over time, and concern for future consequences of having pain (Figure 9.1). Persistent pain can be experienced as a serious threat to one's freedom, significance of life, and ultimately self-esteem. Whereas the *immediate unpleasantness and disturbance* is based on the present, secondary pain-related emotions have been hypothesized as being based on consideration of the past and future. It is important to note that this consideration can take place immediately after injury and pain onset (e.g., a broken arm or leg after a fall), though often it is based on the persistence of pain over time. Thus, just as one may be immediately fearful, distressed, or annoyed during the immediate intrusion and disturbance of pain, one can also feel anxious or depressed about long-term implications of persistent pain. Pain is often experienced not only as an immediate threat to the body, comfort, or activity, but also to one's well-being and life in general. It is, then, the meanings of how pain influences life activities and future that fuel much of the *secondary* stage of pain-related emotions (i.e., suffering).

This stage of pain-related emotions has been tested by administering VAS for each of five pain-related negative emotions – depression, anxiety, frustration, anger, and fear – and for three meanings that are likely to be main contributors to these emotions: interruption of life activities, difficulty of enduring, and concern for future consequences (Wade et al. 1996). It was critical for the patients to rate the magnitudes of these emotions and meanings in relationship to their chronic pain. Thus, a question about anxiety, for example, was framed in the following way: "In relationship to your pain, how anxious have you felt over the past week?" The combined ratings of these five emotions in combination with ratings of interruption, difficulty of enduring, and concern for future have been hypothesized as representing a psychological stage that is unique and separate from that of immediate pain unpleasantness. The quantitative evidence for this secondary stage of pain-related emotions consists of two types of studies: (1) studies testing pathways between the psychological stages of pain and suffering; (2) studies testing selective effects of personality traits and demographic factors on this stage of pain-related emotions (i.e., suffering). The first uses a form of "path analysis" to test the functional interactions between the stages of pain (e.g., Wade et al. 1996; Lackner et al. 2005). The second establishes the stage of pain-related emotions to be unique and separate from immediate pain emotions because it demonstrates a selective effect of personality trait or psychosocial factor on the secondary emotions related to pain (e.g., Harkins et al. 1989; Wade et al. 1996). In combination, these two types of results support the existence of two stages of pain-related emotions even though there may not be a sharp distinction between them. I also think they can be verified by noticing one's direct experience of pain unpleasantness and pain-related extended emotions (i.e., first-person observations). The reasoning behind testing relationships between these stages is similar to that which has been used to demonstrate pain unpleasantness to be unique and separate from pain sensation intensity, as when some types of hypnotic suggestions alter the unpleasantness of pain without changing the strength of the pain sensation. The selective effects on extended emotions related to pain have largely confirmed the causal relationships between early stages of pain and the later stage of suffering, as well as the extrinsic effects of environmental, personality, and demographic factors. Suffering is probably more commonly conceptualized as an effect of pain rather than part of the pain itself. Neuroticism, a trait involving high levels and expression of negative emotions, selectively enhances extended emotions related to pain and age selectively reduces them, with less intense effects on the immediate unpleasantness and/or disturbance of pain. Finally, later states of more complex emotions (anxiety, depression) can feed back on and either enhance or diminish pain unpleasantness (Figure 9.1; see also Chapter 8, 11, and 12, this volume).

9 Neural processing of pain: types of nociceptive neurons and ascending pathways

The sequential-parallel model of sensory intensity–unpleasantness/disturbance–suffering is supported by several studies using large samples of pain patients (Lackner et al. 2005; Wade et al. 1996). This model is related to ascending pathways and brain circuits, as well as mechanisms by which pain can be modified. Ideally, the neuroscience of pain-related ascending pathways and brain circuitry should further explain psychological models of pain. A framework that draws upon direct human experience can guide the neuroscience of pain, reflecting an integration of a science of inner experience and science based on "external" observations.

The principal ascending pathways for pain originate in specialized receptors in body tissues, called nociceptors. These receptors are specialized to respond to the stimulation of tissues that either causes damage or would cause damage if it were maintained for a sufficient length of time. Nociceptors are connected to primary afferent neuron axons that synapse onto neurons of the dorsal gray matter of the spinal cord shown at the bottom right in Figure 9.2. Wide dynamic range (WDR) neurons respond differentially over a wide range of skin stimulation extending from very gentle to noxious levels (tissue damaging). Nociceptive-specific (NS) neurons respond mainly to levels of stimulation that would be painful, although their thresholds are often below pain threshold. There are different classes of primary nociceptive afferent neurons that supply different types of tissues, such as skin, muscle, joints, and viscera. Spinal cord neurons that receive primary nociceptive neuron input are at the origin of ascending pathways to the brain, and they have different roles in pain. A major somatosensory pathway is that of the spinothalamic tract that originates mainly in the spinal cord dorsal horn and projects to an area in the back of the thalamus, termed VPL (ventro-posterior-lateral) and other thalamic areas (Figure 9.2). VPL, in turn, projects to the somatosensory cortices (S1 and S2). Other thalamic areas project to limbic cortical areas. Both pathways to the somatosensory cortices and insular cortex (elongated dashed ovals of Figure 9.2, denoting anterior and posterior insula) play roles in sensory qualities and intensity of pain as well as feelings of unpleasantness or disturbance by reason of *both* serial and parallel connections to brain areas involved in emotions. Other spinal cord pathways project to the medulla, midbrain, and hypothalamus involved in autonomic nervous system responses and arousal (related to the reticular activating system). There is also an ascending pathway that targets a small area at the base of each temporal lobe, termed the amygdala, involved in fear and anger. This pathway projects to brain areas involved in emotions that can be quickly initiated (e.g., fear). This path to the amygdala may be more selectively involved in emotional aspects of pain and behaviors that are rapidly expressed. Pain-related cortical regions are functionally interconnected in reciprocal directions (Figure 9.2). Central projections of ascending pathways and the strength of functional connections between their targets form cortical and sub-cortical networks that provide the neural causes and correlates of unique types of pains. Some of these functional connections change dynamically and often reverse themselves during conditions such as placebo analgesia for example (Craggs et al. 2007; cf. Chapter 32, this volume).

Based largely on their central connections, *all of these pathways*, including somatosensory cortices, are very likely to contribute to the emotional dimension of pain. Thus, there are serial pathways (A→B→C) that connect somatosensory cortices (S1, S2) to limbic areas involved in emotions (e.g., insula, ACC) and there are parallel ascending pathways that more

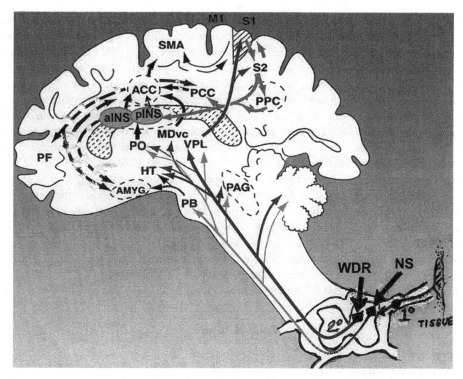

Figure 9.2 Schematic of ascending pathways, sub-cortical structures, and cerebral cortical structures involved in processing pain. ACC, anterior cingulate cortex; aINS, anterior insula; AMYG, amygdala; HT, hypothalamus; MDvc, ventrocaudal part of the medial dorsal nucleus; M1, primary motor cortex; NS, nociceptive-specific dorsal horn neuron; PAG, periaqueductal gray; PB, parabrachial nucleus of the dorsolateral pons; PCC, posterior cingulate cortex; PF, prefrontal cortex; pINS, posterior insula; PO, pain-related areas of the posterior thalamus; PPC, posterior parietal complex; S1 and S2, first and second somatosensory cortical areas; SMA, supplementary motor area; Stage 1, tissue stimulation; stage 2: spinal cord reception and projection; VPL, ventroposterior lateral nucleus; WDR, wide dynamic range dorsal horn neuron.

Source: Updated from data reviewed in Price (1999, 2000).

selectively influence the affective dimensions of pain such as pathways to the reticular formation, amygdala, and hypothalamus. Both serial and parallel pathways are consistent with psychophysical studies by Rainville et al. (1999) described earlier. Both unique sensory responses in combination with arousal and autonomic activation contribute to the overall experience of pain, especially its immediate unpleasantness. Some pain-related emotions such as fear may sometimes occur automatically as a result of direct input to the amygdala (Damasio 1999; Price 1999). Integration of inputs from multiple senses (e.g., bee sting) and higher-order evaluative functions associated with activity in frontal cortical areas contribute to secondary pain-related emotions known as suffering.

10 Pain-related neurons involved in exteroceptive, interoceptive, sensory, and affective functions

Spinal cord WDR and NS neurons are at the origin of multiple ascending pathways discussed above and serve different aspects of sensory and affective dimensions of pain. As just discussed, brain structures are serially connected in some of these pathways (e.g., spinal dorsal horn – thalamus – S2/S2 cortex) and connected in parallel in others (e.g., spinothalamic tract is in parallel with the spinoreticular pathway as shown in Figure 9.2). WDR and NS neurons are also likely to serve both exteroception and interoception. Both classes of neurons serve exteroception because they progressively increase their impulse frequency over a broad range of nociceptive stimulus intensity and can detect very small changes in stimulus intensity (e.g., 0.2° C for WDR and greater than 0.2° C for NS), even before tissue damage occurs. Both classes are somatotopically organized into a body map at all levels of the central nervous system. Thus, they provide exquisitely precise information about stimulus intensity and location at the surface of the body and are therefore exteroceptive. Many of the same WDR and NS neurons also serve interoception because they also receive synaptic input from several types of deep tissues involved in homeostasis (i.e., muscles, joints, blood vessels, viscera). Convergence of input from both skin and deep tissues on individual sensory projection neurons of the dorsal horn forms the basis of referred pain as has been established over the last fifty years (Janig 2009). This view of pain as serving both exteroceptive and interoceptive functions and as having sensory and affective dimensions contrasts with views of pain as serving only a single function or dimension or even those that propose only one or two major pathways for pain (Craig 2003; Chapter 8, this volume; Wall 1979).

Related topics

Chapter 3: Evaluativist accounts of pain's unpleasantness (Bain)
Chapter 4: Imperativism (Klein)
Chapter 8: A neurobiological view of pain as a homeostatic emotion (Strigo and Craig)
Chapter 11: Psychological models of pain (Williams)
Chapter 12: Biopsychosocial models of pain (Hadjistavropoulos)
Chapter 17: Pain and consciousness (Pereplyotchik)
Chapter 31: An introduction to the IASP's definition of pain (Wright)
Chapter 32: Philosophy and "placebo" analgesia (Moerman)

Further reading

Donald D. Price and James J. Barrell, *Inner Experience and Neuroscience: Merging Both Perspectives* (Cambridge, MA: MIT Press, 2012), is a thought-provoking treatise on how to integrate the science of human experience with the natural sciences, similar to the overall perspective of this chapter. This approach is very applicable to the study of pain. Max Velmans' *Understanding Consciousness*, 2nd ed. (London and New York: Routledge, 2009) provides a philosophical underpinning of the main ideas in Price and Barrell.

References

Craggs, J.G., Price, D.D., Verne, N., Perlstein, W.M., and Robinson, M.E. (2007) Functional interactions within brain areas serving cognitive-affective processing during pain and placebo conditions. *Neuroimage* 38(4): 720–729.
Craig, A.D. (2003) A new view of pain as a homeostatic emotion. *Trends in Neurosciences* 6: 303–307.
Damasio, A. (1999) *The Feeling of What Happens.* New York: Avon Books.
Harkins, S.W., Price, D.D., and Braith, J. (1989) Effects of extraversion and neuroticism on experimental pain, clinical pain, and illness behavior. *Pain* 36: 209–218.
Janig, W. (2009) Autonomic nervous system and pain. In A.I. Basbaum and M.C. Bushnell (eds.), *Science of Pain.* Amsterdam: Elsevier, pp. 194–226.

Lackner, J.M., Jaccard, J., and Blanchard, E.B. (2005) Testing the sequential model of pain processing in Irritable Bowel Syndrome: a structural equation modeling analysis. *European Journal of Pain* (London, UK) 9: 207–218.

Melzack, R. (1975) The McGill Pain Questionnaire: major properties and scoring methods. *Pain* 1: 277–299.

Melzack, R. and Torgerson, W.S. (1971) On the language of pain. *Anesthesiology* 34: 50–59.

Melzack, R. and Wall, P.D. (1983) *The Challenge of Pain*. New York: Basic Books.

Mersky, H. and Bogduk, N. (1994) *Classification of Chronic Pain*, 2nd ed. Seattle: IASP Press.

Price, D.D. (1999) *Psychological and Neural Mechanisms of Pain and Analgesia*. Seattle: IASP Press.

Price, D.D. (2000) Psychological and neural mechanisms of the affective dimension of pain. *Science* 288: 1769–1772.

Price, D.D., Harkins, S.W., and Baker, C. (1987) Sensory-affective relationships among different types of clinical and experimental pain. *Pain* 28: 291–299.

Price, D.D., Greenspan, J.D., and Dubner, R. (2003) Neurons involved in the exteroceptive function of pain. *Pain* 106: 215–219.

Rainville, P., Benoit, C., Hofbauer, R.K., Duncan, G.H., and Bushnell, M.C. (1999) Dissociation of sensory and affective dimensions of pain using hypnotic modulation. *Pain* 82(2): 159–171.

Rainville, P., Bao, Q.V., and Chrétien, P. (2005) Pain-related emotions modulate experimental pain perception and autonomic responses. *Pain* 118(3): 306–318.

Sherrington, C.S. (1906) *The Integrative Action of the Nervous System*. London: Constable.

Wade, J.B., Dougherty, L.M., Archer, L.M., and Price, D.D. (1996) Assessing the stages of pain processing: a multivariate approach. *Pain* 68: 157–168.

Wall, P.D. (1979) On the relation of injury to pain (The first John J. Bonica Lecture). *Pain* 6: 253–264.

Wiech, K., Lin, C., Broderson, H.H., Bingel, U., Ploner, M., and Tracey, I. (2010) Anterior insula transforms information about salience into perceptual decisions about pain. *Journal of Neuroscience* 30(48): 16324–16331.

10

PATHOPHYSIOLOGICAL MECHANISMS OF CHRONIC PAIN

Mick Thacker and Lorimer Moseley

"Chronic pain" (also referred to as persistent pain) is a term usually applied to pain that persists past normal healing time and often lacks the acute warning function of physiological nociception, although many authors apply the term pragmatically to pain that lasts or recurs for more than three to six months (Treede et al. 2015; see also Chapter 6, this volume). Unfortunately chronic pain is a common occurrence that affects an estimated 20 percent of the world's population (Breivik et al. 2006; Goldberg and McGee 2011; Hart et al. 2014) and accounts for 15 to 20 percent of the total visits to physicians (Treede et al. 2015). Adequate treatment of chronic pain is a basic human right according to the World Health Organization, who further recommend that the management of chronic pain be a global health priority (Bond et al. 2006).

This account focuses on the pathophysiological mechanisms responsible for chronic pain. These mechanisms are largely "neuroplastic" in nature. Neuroplasticity is defined "as a change to the nervous system as a result of age and/or experience" (Shaw and McEachern 2000). Here we focus on how the experience of noxious inputs may lead to neuroplastic changes that are thought responsible for the development and maintenance of chronic pain.

The pathophysiological (neuroplastic) mechanisms of chronic pain may be split fairly neatly into two main groups: the first underpinned by functional plasticity, involving biochemical alterations within and between neurons and other cell types; and the second, structural plasticity, involving anatomical changes within the system. A detailed discussion of these neuroplastic mechanisms with a focus on the central nervous system (CNS) forms the basis of the main body of this chapter, following a brief overview of the somatosensory system which is included in order to help the reader better understand how changes in function and/or alterations in structure are responsible for chronic pain.

1 Neuroplastic mechanisms of the central nervous system

1.1 The somatosensory system

Classical neuroanatomical approaches to pain revealed pathways that begin in the periphery and end in the brain and it became standard to outline the somatosensory nociceptive system in this way. (Cf. discussions in Chapters 6, 7, and 8, this volume.) While we adhere to this approach here for convenience, we hope that the account reveals the limitations of this way of thinking to the reader.

1.2 Nociceptors

Nociceptors are normally small-diameter sensory neurons involved in the transduction (the conversion of external stimuli into electrochemical messages) and transmission (the relay of these electrochemical messages from receptor terminals – normally centrally – to the CNS) of damaging or potentially damaging stimuli (McMahon and Priestly 2005; Carlton 2014; Gold 2013; Ringkamp et al. 2013). Electrical transmission is rapid while chemical signaling transmission occurs over longer time frames (Gold 2013). Both functions are initiated following the activation of receptors on the receptive terminal of nociceptors. These terminals innervate specific target tissues including skin, muscle, tendons, ligaments, blood vessels, and nerves themselves. The constellation of receptors expressed on the membrane of nociceptors determines the stimuli to which they respond with three main categories of receptor described: chemical, thermal, and mechanical stimuli.

While transduction is dependent on the properties of specialized receptors, electrical transmission via action potentials is largely dependent on the interaction of several types of ion channels and the relative distribution of several specific ions (see Habib et al. 2015; Hoeijmakers et al. 2015). Ion channels and in particular voltage-gated sodium channels have formed the mainstay of research into nociceptive transmission (Cummins et al. 2007). Alterations in structure and density of these and other channels are associated with significant changes in the behavioral characteristics of neurons, including nociceptors (Hoeijmakers et al. 2015). These changes have been associated with heightened sensitivity to peripheral stimuli so that touch for example may elicit a pain experience and spontaneous firing of afferent fibers independent of external stimuli where pains may be experienced suddenly and for no obvious reason (Ringkamp et al. 2013; Habib et al. 2015; Hoeijmakers et al. 2015).

1.3 Dorsal horn

Nociceptors terminate in the dorsal horn (sensory horn) of the spinal cord. The cord is highly arranged, consisting of several distinct layers (correctly called Rexed laminae I–XI). Primary afferent fibers show a marked preference for specific lamina, e.g., C-fibers terminate in the outer (more peripheral) laminae I and II (classically called substantia gelatinosa Rolandi) while larger myelinated fibers penetrate deeper within the horn, e.g., Aδ synapse preferentially (but not exclusively) in lamina V. Within each lamina, the primary afferent fibers synapse with spinal cord neurons that extend throughout the cord and, potentially supraspinally, to nuclei within the brain. In addition, fibers may make contact with local interneurons that communicate intraspinally between sites within the same level or immediately adjacent levels of the cord (see Todd and Koerber 2013 for an exhaustive review).

The anatomy and physiology of the dorsal horn neurons, also referred to as "second order neurons," "transmission neurons," or "projection neurons" have received much attention (see Todd and Koerber 2013 for review). Two main types of cell have been described: *nociceptive-specific* (NS) neurons which are limited almost exclusively to laminae I and II and therefore receive only inputs from C-fibers; and *wide dynamic range* (WDR) neurons found in deeper laminae, including lamina V, where they receive inputs from Aδ and other large myelinated fibers and also inputs from superficial laminae via spinal interneurons.

Primary afferents may also make functional connections with descending neurons that traverse the cord from many areas of the brain including the cortex, midbrain, and brainstem. Thus the cord acts as a "selective hub" where sensory information is initially processed and modulated; peripheral inputs are not merely transmitted centrally.

1.4 Ascending pathways

While the spinothalamic is best known as the main nociceptive pathway, noxious inputs ascend via several spinal cord tracts (Heinricher and Fields 2013; Baccei and Fitzgerald 2013; Dostrovesky and Craig 2013). These pathways have been broadly grouped into medial (spino-reticular) and lateral systems (spino-mesencephalic) (Heinricher and Fields 2013; Dostrovesky and Craig 2013). There is much debate about the degree of specificity within these tracts with two opposing groups, the "line labelists" who insist specific "sensations" ascend in specific tracts (e.g., Chapter 8, this volume) and "multimodalists" who suggest that, while specialized for certain afferent inputs (e.g., Tracey and Mantyh 2007), the pathways have the residual ability to transmit several modalities of sensory afferent inputs.

1.5 Brain

The projections from the spinal cord terminate in many disseminated nuclei within the brain (see Tracey and Mantyh 2007; Apkarian et al. 2013b for reviews). Attempts to understand the complexity of the neuroanatomical/physiological organization as it relates to nociception and pain perception have led to several models; perhaps the most widely accepted of these is the neuromatrix model first proposed by Ron Melzack and discussed in detail by Roy and Wager in Chapter 7 of this volume.

2 Functional plasticity

2.1 Central sensitization

The ongoing pain of many clinical syndromes, e.g., low-back pain, fibromyalgia, chronic headaches, no longer serves any known protective function and may therefore be considered maladaptive. Central sensitization has provided a mechanistic explanation for many of the temporal, spatial, and threshold changes in pain sensibility in chronic clinical pain and is implicated in all the etiological groups above (Bruehl 2010; Kehlet et al. 2006; Mantyh et al. 2002; Mantyh et al. 2002; Scholz and Woolf 2007; Woolf and Costigan 1996).

Central sensitization (see Ji and Woolf 2001; Latremoliere and Woolf 2009; Sandkühler 2000, 2009, 2013; Woolf 2011; Woolf and Salter 2000 for extensive reviews) affords novel inputs the ability to activate nociceptive pathways; for example, large myelinated fibers, Aβ neurons, normally associated with touch, produce allodynic responses. It also produces hypersensitivity in non-inflamed tissue by changing the sensory response elicited by normal inputs, and increases sensitivity long after the initiating cause may have disappeared and when no peripheral pathology may be present. Because central sensitization results from changes in the properties of neurons in the CNS, the pain is no longer coupled to the presence, intensity, or duration of particular peripheral stimuli. Instead, central sensitization represents an abnormal state of responsiveness or increased gain of the nociceptive system (see above reviews). The pain experience is effectively generated by changes within the CNS that then alter how it responds to sensory inputs, rather than reflecting the presence of peripheral noxious stimuli. Central sensitization therefore represents a major functional shift in the somatosensory system from high-threshold nociception to low-threshold sensory hypersensitivity.

"Sensitization" is an umbrella term used to refer to a group of processes that may be reduced to a general schema of events (Ji et al. 2003; Sandkühler 2000; Woolf 1996). This simplified schema is dependent on interactions between primary messengers, normally neurotransmitters (most notably glutamate, but may also involve growth factors, cytokines and chemokines [see section below]) acting on specific receptors on the postsynaptic membrane (particularly the glutamate receptors AMPA (α-amino-3-hydroxy-5-methyl-4-isoxazolepropionic acid) and NMDA (*N*-Methyl-D-aspartate). The first part of these processes is characterized by an increase in synaptic efficiency so that the same stimulus level produces enhanced effects in terms of both intensity and duration, e.g., noxious stimuli will be felt as stronger and last longer than before. These receptor interactions drive a plethora of intracellular mechanisms, normally governed by the release of intracellular calcium stores and enzyme activation.

The activation of intracellular signaling systems or secondary messenger systems (generally enzymes) acts to increase intracellular metabolism, resulting in greater activation and sensitivity of the cell to ongoing inputs or responses to novel inputs (see Ji and Woolf 2001; Ji et al. 2003; Latremoliere and Woolf 2009). There is huge interaction and overlap in secondary messenger functions; some act specifically on individual intracellular organelles, while others translocate (move) throughout the cell, altering cell metabolism at several sites (Ji and Woolf 2001; Ji et al. 2003; Latremoliere and Woolf 2009). Several secondary messengers act directly upon the nucleus by crossing the nuclear envelope (the membrane that separates the nucleus from the rest of the cell). Secondary messengers that cross the envelope become known as "tertiary messengers," as here their main role is to influence the cell's production of amino acids and ultimately functional protein synthesis via controlling effects on the expression of messenger RNA (Woolf and Costigan 1999). These alterations of protein synthesis have functional consequences as they form the receptors or neurotransmitters involved in noxious processing – therefore increasing their number increases the likelihood that pain will be experienced.

Five individual mechanisms have been implicated in central sensitization, namely wind-up; long-term potentiation (LTP); classical central sensitization (CCS); late-onset transcription-dependent central sensitization; and neuroimmune/neurogenic inflammation. The first four mechanisms essentially operate via all or parts of the general schema outlined above. Each mechanism has unique temporal and spatial characteristics that set them apart. What follows is a rather brief and highly simplified summary of the key features of each of these five mechanisms.

Wind-up is a progressive increase in the magnitude of C-fiber-evoked responses of spinal dorsal horn neurons produced by low-frequency, repetitive stimulation. Spatially it is homosynaptic, occurring only at the active synapse, and is short-lasting in duration, demonstrating extinction within around ninety seconds following cessation of the evoking stimulus. Activation of these fibers elicits slow synaptic potentials lasting several-hundred milliseconds in dorsal horn projection neurons. Wind-up results from the summation of these slow synaptic potentials at relatively low afferent input frequencies. This produces a cumulative depolarization that leads to removal of the voltage-dependent Mg^{2+} channel blockade in NMDA receptors. By increasing glutamate sensitivity, this progressively increases the action potential response to each stimulus in a train of inputs. This produces a pain experience that is disproportionate to the stimulus experienced, e.g., light touch on the skin leads to pain.

LTP (see Ji and Woolf 2001; Ji et al. 2003; Sandkühler 2000, 2007, 2009; Scholz and Woolf 2007; Woolf 1996; Woolf and Salter 2000) is a long-lasting strengthening of the response of a postsynaptic nerve cell to stimulation across the synapse that occurs with repeated stimulation. LTP is a form of long-term synaptic plasticity lasting for an extended period of time (tens of minutes to hours *in vitro* and hours to days and months, or even years, *in vivo*). Two distinct phases of LTP have been described; early- and late-phase LTP. Early-phase LTP is independent of *de novo* (novel) protein synthesis, i.e., it involves existing neurotransmitters and receptors, and lasts for up to two to three hours. Late-phase LTP involves protein synthesis and lasts longer than three hours, up to the lifespan of an animal/person, and may be accompanied by structural changes at synapses and involve increased number/new neurotransmitters and receptors.

LTP, like wind-up, is spatially homosynaptic, affecting only those synapses where activity has directly occurred. Both phases of LTP involve a plethora of transmitters and receptors and the reader is referred to the extensive literature above for detail. The action of glutamate on NMDA and subsequent release of intracellular messengers critically underpin the impact of nociceptive inputs on the dorsal horn neurons. However, some components of LTP are known to be independent of NMDA pathways, suggesting critical role/s for other neurotransmitter–receptor complexes (see references above). Together these transmitter–receptor interactions allow more positively charged ions into the cell which in turn activate intracellular signaling mechanisms, leading to a lowering in the firing threshold of the dorsal horn neurons.

These processes allow low-threshold inputs to activate the cell (allodynia) and amplify the response to high-threshold inputs (hyperalgesia) so that stimuli that are not expected to produce pain do and those that are expected to, produce more than expected; both produce a more painful experience.

Key secondary messenger molecules in dorsal horn cells include protein kinases, phospholipases, and MAPkinases (again see references above). Protein kinases have established roles in the modulation of synaptic functional plasticity. Enhancing responsiveness to further stimuli, phospholipases are linked to receptor trafficking and MAPkinases to alterations in amino acid synthesis. This results in a great number of receptors embedded in the membrane of the nociceptive neurons, effectively meaning that incoming stimuli have enhanced effects so that inputs produce greater effects, i.e., amplification in nociceptive pathways.

It is important to note that these changes are not isolated to the spinal cord. Luo et al. (2014) review both *in vitro* and *vivo* evidence for pain-related LTP and reported similar processes at the level of the cord and thalamus, as well as the anterior cingulate, insular cortices, and the amygdala – suggesting an impact on not only sensory processing but all mood and affect.

CCS (see Ji and Woolf 2001; Ji et al. 2003; Sandkühler 2000, 2007, 2009; Scholz and Woolf 2007; Woolf 1996; Woolf and Salter 2000) refers to a prolonged synaptic plasticity after a noxious stimulus. Activity in nociceptors, caused either experimentally or clinically, evokes a period of facilitated transmission in dorsal horn neurons, the dorsal horn is in a charged-like state where inputs more easily evoke a response. This augments responses in the conditioning nociceptor pathway (homosynaptic potentiation, as in wind-up or LTP) and recruits novel inputs from non-stimulated afferents (heterosynaptic potentiation). This activity-dependent form of central sensitization is the consequence of activation of multiple intracellular signaling pathways, most importantly tertiary messengers, in dorsal horn neurons due to glutamate neurotransmission and neuromodulators (these increase the action of neurotransmitters thereby increasing neuronal activity), such as substance P and brain-derived neurothrophic factor (BDNF), and again involves NMDA receptors, other glutamate, and non-glutamate receptors (see above references for full details). The induced intracellular signaling cascades lead to significant effects on the cell's nucleus, leading to a multitude of biochemical consequences including increased cellular production and trafficking of receptor proteins. This in turn increases the number of functional receptors present at the synapse, leading to an increased responsiveness to the initiating and/or other neurotransmitters essentially establishing a self-sustaining chemical couple. This effect is amplified by several molecules synthesized and released by the postsynaptic cell that act as retrograde (go in the opposite direction) messengers from the postsynaptic back on to the presynaptic terminus, with the effect of further increasing the release of presynaptic neurotransmitters. These processes may become self-sustaining, i.e., a feedback loop, negating the need for ongoing peripheral inputs and leading to spontaneous non-evoked experiences of pain. CCS may last from several hours to days, weeks, months, years, up to a lifetime for some particularly following neuropathic injury (Ji and Woolf 2001).

CCS, unlike wind-up and LTP, is not limited to the synapses which initiated the neuro-chemical response; rather it alters both local and remote receptor complexes, making them more likely to be activated. This has several important effects including the unsilencing of normally "silent" synapses to form functional synapses, functionally apparent as increases in the receptive fields of the postsynaptic neurons.

Late-onset transcription-dependent central sensitization, simply put, is the result of the action of tertiary messengers altering the expression of amino acids and functional proteins synthesized by neurons, and overlaps greatly with CCS so that these two mechanisms are likely to be coexistent (see Costigan and Woolf 2002; Ji and Woolf 2001; Woolf and Costigan 1999; von Hehn et al. 2012).

Many see these four mechanisms as a continuation that begins with wind-up and ends in CCS, but this is slightly too oversimplified, as the stimulus parameters required are different for each mechanism in terms of the firing frequency of nociceptors; i.e., LTP is dependent on nociceptors firing at high frequencies, whereas CCS is dependent on the same fibers firing at low frequencies (see above references for detail). However, it is certainly possible that the four processes may coexist in the same individual. These mechanisms not only coexist with one another but also with other mechanisms of central sensitization, such as neuroimmune interactions at various sites throughout the neuroaxis.

2.2 Neuroimmune interactions

Traditional approaches to pain failed to recognize any role for the immune system in the generation and/or maintenance of pain. Several groups helped establish neuroimmune interactions as key generators of ongoing pain (Arruda et al. 1998; DeLeo et al. 2004; Sorkin and Doom 2000; Sommer and Kress 2004; Thacker et al. 2007). Most of these groups employed neuropathic (involving direct nerve injury) models to demonstrate the role of the immune system in the generation of pain. Ongoing pain associated with injury to neurons was thought to be due entirely to injury-induced reactions within the neurons themselves, but a more complex picture emerged to reveal processes that involve the phenotypic alteration of cells normally associated with the immune system, including macrophages, microglia, and other glial cells (Beggs and Salter 2013; Clark and Malcangio 2012, 2014; Clark et al. 2013; Old et al. 2015; Thacker et al. 2009; Salter and Beggs 2014; Scholz and Woolf 2007; Tsuda et al. 2013).

These processes have now been confirmed as nociceptive, capable of acting directly on dorsal horn neurons to produce ongoing afferent input to the somatosensory nervous system, and are dependent on interactions between neuronal and glial cells activated by molecular products including neurotransmitters, cytokines, and chemokines (Schäfers and Sorkin 2008; Thacker et al. 2007). Work focused on the dorsal horn where microglia and astrocytes form functional synapses with the pre- and postsynaptic neurons in structures known as "tripartite" and "quadripartite" synapses (see Papa et al. 2014 for a detailed review of the anatomy and pathophysiology). In addition, there is a reciprocal expression of receptors to key chemical messengers on the respective cells in these synapses in both the spinal dorsal horn and higher centers, suggesting communication between neuronal and non-neuronal cells is part of normal physiological processing (Papa et al. 2014). These chemical interactions provide a potential site for maladaptive plasticity following nociception, as discussed below.

The most widely studied of these cells is the spinal microglia. Following injury to a peripheral nerve, these cells respond rapidly with a series of cellular and molecular changes (see Beggs and Salter 2013; Clark and Malcangio 2012, 2014; Clark et al. 2013; Old et al. 2015; Thacker et al. 2009; Salter and Beggs 2014; Scholz and Woolf 2007; Tsuda et al. 2013). Microglia enlarge abnormally and up-regulate (increase production of) and increase their expression of various genes resulting in the *de novo* expression of cytokines (including chemokines), growth factors and cell-surface receptor complexes (see references above) under the influence of activity-dependent intracellular signaling molecules. The most important of these cell-surface molecules are purinergic receptors that respond preferentially to ATP (adenosine triphosphate). ATP is released within the dorsal horn following nociceptor activity and acts directly on the microglia causing them to increase their production of the same and/or other novel signaling molecules. The induced molecules may have both autocrine (acting on the same cell) and/or paracrine (acting on other cells) actions including direct stimulatory effects on adjacent neurons. The exact molecular pathways underpinning the release and trafficking of purinergic receptors is highly complex and not entirely resolved, but is a multiconvergent cascade involving classical intracellular signaling molecules similar to those seen in the sensitization of neurons (see Beggs and Salter 2013; Salter and Beggs 2014; Tsuda et al. 2013).

A basic schema involves the injury-induced release of chemokines from injured neurons and adjacent astrocytes and the microglia themselves. These act on pre-existing toll-like receptors, expressed on resident astrocytes and microglia, which in turn causes activation of intracellular signaling pathways in these cells, altering their phenotype, so they express and translocate purine receptor functional proteins (Tsuda et al. 2013). The receptor proteins are embedded into the cellular membrane via the action of intracellular enzymes. The main result of activation of purine receptors is the release of BDNF, a known algogen (Clark et al. 2015). BDNF not only has direct excitatory effects, i.e., increases nociception, but decreases the inhibitory pathways particularly in the outer laminae of the dorsal horn, with the resultant effect that inhibition of nociception is adversely affected, leading to a greater pain experience (Tsuda et al. 2013).

While these mechanisms have been established from experiments in the dorsal horn of rodents, some studies of neuroimmune interactions have been reported in the brains of human pain sufferers. Banati (2002) demonstrated increased microglial activity within the thalamus of a small group of individuals with chronic pain following neuropathic injury using PET (positron emission tomography) scanning. Of particular note was that some of the participants had suffered nerve injury several years before scanning, suggesting that the effect either persisted for long periods or may be an ongoing consequence of being in pain. Unfortunately, due to the specificity of the ligand available at this time, these findings have to be questioned on methodological grounds.

Loggia et al. (2015) combined PET–MRI (positron emission tomography–magnetic resonance imaging) with a recently developed microglial specific TSPO (18-kD translocator protein) receptor radioligand. This pioneering study revealed that ligand uptake values were significantly higher in patients than controls in multiple brain regions, including the thalamus and the putative somatosensory representations of the lumbar spine and leg. Interestingly, the increased ligand binding was negatively correlated with clinical pain and circulating levels of the proinflammatory cytokines, suggesting that TSPO expression exerts pain-protective/anti-inflammatory effects in humans, i.e., is analgesic. This suggests that these changes may be considered adaptive as opposed to maladaptive, suggesting that microglia may play different roles at different sites within the neuroaxis, or that their function alters in a temporal fashion: first being pro-nociceptive/inflammatory and at later time points becoming anti-nociceptive/anti-inflammatory.

Thus, Loggia et al.'s study confirms that microglia are active within the human nervous system in an ongoing pain state. This has important consequences for pharmacological management of pain as glial activation is known to occur in response to opioid compounds as well. Opioid-induced glial activation has potentially negative effects for the use of opioid analgesia and enhances opioid tolerance, dependence, reward, and respiratory depression (see Hutchinson et al. 2011 for an exhaustive review of mechanisms and supporting data).

While less is known about the role of astrocytes in nociceptive regulation, there is mounting evidence concerning their involvement in maintaining chronic pain (Gao et al. 2009). In particular, the signaling molecule c-Jun N-terminal kinase (JNK) is activated in spinal astrocytes in neuropathic pain conditions in rodents (Gao et al. 2009). This activation is thought necessary for the maintenance of neuropathic pain because spinal infusion of JNK inhibitors reverses mechanical allodynia. It is envisaged that a more extensive investigation of astrocytes in humans will identify more detail about their role in nociceptive signaling.

3 Supraspinal functional plasticity

3.1 Vagal afferent system

Although most of the mechanisms above are associated with nerve injury, immune cells are also activated in response to infection, inflammation, or trauma to non-neuronal tissues (Grace et al. 2014). A key component of cellular immunity is the release of proinflammatory cytokines (Grace et al. 2014; Thayer and Sternberg 2009, 2010). These proinflammatory cytokines signal to the CNS in a unique immune-privileged manner (this refers to the fact that these chemicals cross into the brain easily) involving the vagus nerve. It appears that "vagal afferents" express receptors to circulatory and tissue-released cytokines following injury which in turn leads to the release of neurotransmitters and cytokines supraspinally at their terminus in the solitary nucleus (Grace et al. 2014; Thayer and Sternberg 2009, 2010). Here they activate toll-like receptors (Grace et al. 2014; Thayer and Sternberg 2009, 2010) expressed on non-neuronal cells in processes similar to those described above that lead to increased nociception. The effect is a spread of neuronal–glial-cell interactions throughout the brain and spinal cord, which produces a constellation of signs and symptoms including altered sensory perceptions, such as allodynia and hyperalgesia, and expansion of receptive fields.

These neuroimmune interactions also lead to the characteristic behaviors often referred to as "the sickness response," including general malaise, tiredness, and loss of clarity of thought, all of which are also reported by patients with ongoing pain states including fibromyalgia and low-back pain (Grace et al. 2014; Thayer and Sternberg 2009, 2010).

3.2 Supraspinal functional neuroplasticity revealed by neuroimaging

Functional magnetic resonance imaging (fMRI) and related neuroimaging techniques may be used to demonstrate both structural and functional alterations in blood flow as a surrogate of neuronal activity. Techniques such as VBM (voxel-based morphometry) and cortical thickness analysis reveal structural changes (discussed below) while methods such as BOLD (blood oxygen level-dependent) imaging and ASL (arterial spin labeling) reveal functional alterations in blood flow. Although structural and functional alterations may be interdependent to some degree, i.e., there is a presumed reduction in blood flow where there is a "loss" of neural tissue, the methods should not be confused. In addition to fMRI, EEG (electroencephalography, a non-invasive measure of electrical activity in the brain) and magnetoencephalography (MEG, a non-invasive measure of magnetic induced flux across the brain) have been used to demonstrate alterations in neuronal function in chronic pain. The physics underpinning, and the assumptions made for, these techniques are beyond the scope of this account; each has individual merit and limitations (see Davis 2003).

Many classic studies demonstrate that cortical reorganization is associated with persistent pain, both increases and decreases in cortical activation in ongoing pain states have been reported; for example, phantom limb pain using MEG has been associated with an increase in representation within S1 (Flor et al. 1995) and similar findings have been reproduced for persistent low-back pain (Flor et al. 1997). This is in contrast to studies on those suffering Complex Regional Pain Syndrome 1 (CRPS-1) which demonstrated decreases in the cortical representation in S1 using MEG (Pleger et al. 2005). One difficulty is that we still do not know whether these changes are a response to, or causative for, pain. Nevertheless, treatment approaches aimed at enhancing and correcting sensorimotor input have been shown to result in pain relief in patients with CRPS-1 (Pleger et al. 2005 and Moseley et al. 2008) and amputees (Lotze et al. 1999). See Lotze and Moseley (2015) for an in-depth review of these fascinating treatment approaches. These analgesic effects are often accompanied by an apparent "normalization" of the supraspinal representation suggesting that these methods are able to positively impact on altered brain function associated with chronic pain (see Moseley and Flor 2012 for greater detail). While most of this work has focused on the sensory cortex, similar findings have been demonstrated in the same conditions in several other supraspinal sites including the motor cortex, brainstem, and cerebellum (see Lotze and Moseley 2007, 2015 for extensive reviews).

These changes in neuronal function remain poorly understood in terms of cellular response and health, mechanisms ranging from alterations in cellular phenotype to outright cell death are postulated (Lotze and Moseley 2007, 2015).

Detailed discussion of the vast literature now available based on studies of chronic pain utilizing fMRI are beyond the scope of this account; they may however be summarized (after Martucci and Mackey 2016) as:

- No single region within the human CNS is responsible for chronic pain; altered function (and structure, see below) occurs across all regions of the neuroaxis including spinal cord, brainstem, midbrain, and cortices with different patterns of altered activity varying both within and across studies of the same and different pain states (Apkarian et al. 2013a; Davis 2004; Davis et al. 2003, 2011; Di Pietro et al. 2013a, 2013b; Martucci and Mackey 2016; Mouraux et al. 2011; Tracey and Mantyh 2007).
- Resting-state fMRI has revealed multiregional alterations in brain function within various resting-state networks, including salience, executive control, and default-mode networks,

across different pain states (Apkarian et al. 2013b; Baliki et al. 2008, 2011a, 2014; Howard et al. 2012; Jiang et al. 2016).

- Multivariate pattern analysis methodologies (MVPAMs) are new and powerful machine-learning paradigms that allow for a whole-brain approach to identifying altered brain function (and structure) in chronic pain. MVPAMs may ultimately help to develop brain-based objective biomarkers of pain (O'Muircheartaigh 2015; Ung et al. 2014; Chapter 7, this volume).

4 Structural plasticity

Structural plasticity refers to an alteration to the normal anatomy and includes changes across all levels of the neuroaxis and involves processes ranging from the microscopic, e.g., synaptic reconfiguration, to the macroscopic, such as fMRI-revealed supraspinal volume loss. The two most widely studied areas of the nervous system that undergo structural reorganization associated with chronic pain are the dorsal horn and the brain.

Dorsal horn reorganization involves several processes, but the most widely recognized (but contested, see Sandkühler 2015) involves excitotoxicity whereby the release of excitatory neurotransmitters (particularly glutamate and associated excitatory amino acids) leads to the selective neuronal death of both local inhibitory interneurons and descending inhibitory neurons within the spinal cord, with the resultant effect of reducing the efficacy of both local inhibitory and descending inhibitory connections with negative consequences for endogenous pain relief.

Another pathologically driven structural alteration is dorsal horn sprouting (Woolf et al. 1992). Due to the selective loss of small-fiber afferents in the superficial layers of the spinal dorsal horn following nerve injury, large myelinated fibers, normally confined to the deeper laminae, "sprout" onto the vacant nociceptive specific neurons providing a structural model to underpin large-fiber-induced allodynia. The methods used to establish this sprouting have since been widely criticized (see Sandkühler 2015 for a complete review), with the suggestion that these are pre-existing silent connections as opposed to injury-induced sprouting (Costigan et al. 2009; Sandkühler 2015).

Supraspinal structural plasticity has become one of the hottest topics in pain neuroscience (Martucci and Mackey 2016). Functional imaging has revealed a plethora of structural changes associated with ongoing pain although the specific mechanisms are still poorly understood (Coppieters et al. 2016; Martucci and Mackey 2016). Several conditions typified by ongoing pain have revealed structural neuroplasticity that is thought to be closely allied to alterations in the level of neuronal activity (Coppieters et al. 2016; Davis 2003; Martucci and Mackey 2016).

The literature reports almost exclusively on anatomical sites that are associated with the so-called "pain matrix." Experiments are often driven by prior hypotheses about the sites that are expected to demonstrate change in these pain states. (For further discussion, see Chapter 7.) More detailed analysis of the changes reveals that a constellation of "non-matrix" anatomical sites also demonstrates structural plasticity in ongoing pain states (Davis 2011).

Vania Apkarian and co-workers have been at the forefront of structural MRI studies in chronic pain, with a particular focus on chronic low-back pain (CBP) (Baliki et al. 2011a, 2011b, 2012; Baliki and Apkarian 2007). They compared brain morphology of patients with CBP to matched control subjects and initially demonstrated a modest decrease in gray matter volume in the subjects with CBP compared with control subjects (Baliki and Apkarian 2007). However, when these volumes were compared again, correcting for age, gender, and duration of pain, the resultant gray matter volume was equivalent to the loss of neocortical gray matter volume associated with ten to twenty years of normal ageing (Baliki and Apkarian 2007). This seemingly staggering finding has to be carefully interpreted, as we have no clue whether these changes precede the onset of pain or are the result of the ongoing pain. They may be an adaptive mechanism to reduce the representation of the spine within the cortex in an attempt to reduce the impact of sensory inputs.

The results from Apkarian's group have demonstrated that CBP is associated with decreased gray matter density of the bilateral DLPFC (dorsolateral prefrontal cortex), anterior thalamus, brainstem, and somatosensory cortex, and increased gray matter bilaterally in the basal ganglia and left thalamus (Baliki et al. 2011a, 2011b, 2012; Baliki and Apkarian 2007).

Baliki et al. (2012) used structural MRI to compare global, local, and architectural changes in gray matter properties in patients suffering from CBP (chronic back pain), CRPS (complex regional pain syndrome), and knee osteoarthritis, compared with healthy controls. They found unique anatomical "brain signatures" for each pain condition. The CBP group only showed altered whole-brain gray matter volume; regional gray matter density was distinct for each group. There was a general pattern of gray matter density loss across the brains of the patient group, compared with controls. Using a custom analysis method they were able to demonstrate an exponential increase for structural brain reorganization with pain chronicity.

Geha and co-workers (Geha et al. 2008) investigated gray matter morphometry and white matter anisotropy (a measure of connectivity between brain regions) in CRPS patients with persistent pain and matched controls. The patient group exhibited a disrupted relationship between white matter anisotropy and whole-brain gray matter volume. While regional atrophy related to pain intensity and duration, the strength of connectivity between specific atrophied regions was closely correlated to anxiety, suggesting that not all alterations are linked specifically to pain. These abnormalities encompass regions involved in emotional, autonomic, and pain perception, implying that they play a critical role in the global clinical picture of CRPS (see also Bailey et al. 2013 and Di Pietro 2013a, 2013b for additional reviews).

Reports of gray matter changes in fibromyalgia are highly contradictory (see Jorge and Amaro 2012 and Gracely and Ambrose 2011 for a detailed review), varying according to functional differences among subjects and techniques, unsurprisingly due to the heterogeneous nature of the condition. A summary of gray matter atrophy in fibromyalgia demonstrates alterations within DLPFC, medial frontal cortex, left mid-insular cortex, left rostral and left mid-anterior cingulate cortex, thalamus, mid-posterior cingulate cortex, parahippocampal gyrus, supplementary motor area, and temporal cortex (Jorge and Amaro 2012).

Robinson et al. (2011) suggest that the results of imaging in fibromyalgia are, however, consistent. They found that fibromyalgia patients have a significantly lower global volume of gray matter than controls and 3.3 times greater age-associated decline in gray matter than controls. This suggests that the longer one suffers fibromyalgia, the greater the gray matter loss. These results seem to support the theory of premature ageing of brain nuclei as a cause for fibromyalgia but caution is indicated, as they may be consequential as opposed to causative. Conversely, increases in gray matter volumes have also been reported in fibromyalgia.

5 Conclusion

Specific alterations in the CNS may result in an experience of pain in the absence of either peripheral pathology or noxious stimuli, and the target/challenge for treatment in these situations must be the CNS, not the periphery. We hope that this rather simplified account reflects the quality and depth of work undertaken by many neuroscientists all over the world and may in some small part move those still attached to the C-fiber as a source of pain to seek different and more plausible constructs in order to attempt to understand what is unfortunately a huge worldwide problem.

Related topics

Chapter 6: Advances in the neuroscience of pain (Apkarian)
Chapter 7: Neuromatrix theory of pain (Roy and Wager)
Chapter 8: A neurobiological view of pain as a homeostatic emotion (Strigo and Craig)

References

Apkarian, A.V., Baliki, M.N., Farmer, M.A. (2013a) Predicting transition to chronic pain. *Current Opinion in Neurology* 26(4): 360–367.

Apkarian, A.V., Bushnell, M.C., and Schweinhardt, P. (2013b) Representation of pain in the brain. In S.B. McMahon, M. Koltzenburg, I. Tracey, and D.C. Turk (eds.), *Wall and Melzack's Textbook of Pain*, 6th ed. London: Elsevier.

Arruda, J.L., Colburn, R.W., Rickman, A.J., Rutkowski, M.D., and DeLeo, J.A. (1998) Increase of interleukin-6 mRNA in the spinal cord following peripheral nerve injury in the rat: potential role of IL-6 in neuropathic pain. *Brain Research: Molecular Brain Research* 62(4): 228–235.

Baccei, M.L. and Fitzgerald, M. (2013) Development of pain pathways and mechanism. In S.B. McMahon, M. Koltzenburg, I. Tracey, and D.C. Turk (eds.), *Wall and Melzack's Textbook of Pain*, 6th ed. London: Elsevier.

Bailey, J., Nelson, S., Lewis, J., and McCabe, C.S. (2013) Imaging and clinical evidence of sensorimotor problems in CRPS: utilizing novel treatment approaches. *Journal of Neuroimmune Pharmacology* 8(3): 564–575.

Baliki, M.N. and Apkarian, A.V. (2007) Neurological effects of chronic pain. *Journal of Pain and Palliative Care Pharmacotherapy* 21(1): 59–61.

Baliki, M.N., Geha, P.Y., Apkarian, A.V., and Chialvo, D.R. (2008) Beyond feeling: chronic pain hurts the brain, disrupting the default-mode network dynamics. *Journal of Neuroscience* 28(6): 1398–1403.

Baliki, M.N., Schnitzer, T.J., Bauer, W.R., and Apkarian, A.V. (2011a) Brain morphological signatures for chronic pain. *PLoS One* 6(10): e26010.

Baliki, M.N., Baria, A.T., and Apkarian, A.V. (2011b) The cortical rhythms of chronic back pain. *Journal of Neuroscience*, 31(39): 13981–13990.

Baliki, M.N., Petre, B., Torbey, S., Herrmann, K.M., Huang, L., Schnitzer, T.J., Fields, H.L., and Apkarian, A.V. (2012) Corticostriatal functional connectivity predicts transition to chronic back pain. *Nature Neuroscience* 15(8):1117–1119.

Baliki, M.N., Mansour, A.R., Baria, A.T., and Apkarian, A.V. (2014) Functional reorganization of the default mode network across chronic pain conditions. *PLoS One* 9(9): e106133.

Banati, R.B. (2002) Brain plasticity and microglia: is transsynaptic glial activation in the thalamus after limb denervation linked to cortical plasticity and central sensitisation? *Journal of Physiology* (Paris) 96(3–4): 289–299.

Beggs, S. and Salter, M.W. (2013) The known knowns of microglia-neuronal signalling in neuropathic pain. *Neuroscience Letters* 557 (pt. A): 37–42.

Bond, M., Breivik, H., Jensen, T.S., Scholten, W., Soyannwo, O., and Treede, R.D. (2006) Pain associated with neurological disorders. In J.A. Aarli, T. Dua, A. Janca, and A. Muscetta (eds), *Neurological Disorders: Public Health Challenges*. Geneva: WHO Press.

Breivik, H., Collett, B., Ventafridda, V., Cohen, R., and Gallacher, D. (2006) Survey of chronic pain in Europe: prevalence, impact on daily life, and treatment. *European Journal of Pain* (London, UK) 10(4): 287–333.

Bruehl, S. (2010) An update on the pathophysiology of complex regional pain syndrome. *Anesthesiology* 113(3): 713–725.

Carlton, S.M. (2014) Nociceptive primary afferents: they have a mind of their own. *Journal of Physiology* 592(16): 3403–3411.

Clark, A.K. and Malcangio, M. (2012) Microglial signalling mechanisms: Cathepsin S and Fractalkine. *Experimental Neurology* 234(2): 283–292.

Clark, A.K. and Malcangio, M. (2014) Fractalkine/CX3CR1 signalling during neuropathic pain. *Frontiers in Cellular Neuroscience* 7(8): 121.

Clark, A.K., Old, E.A., and Malcangio, M. (2013) Neuropathic pain and cytokines: current perspectives. *Journal of Pain Research* 21(6): 803–814.

Clark, A.K., Gruber-Schoffnegger, D., Drdla-Schutting, R., Gerhold, K.J., Malcangio, M., and Sand-kühler, J. (2015) Selective activation of microglia facilitates synaptic strength. *Journal of Neuroscience* 35(11): 4552–4570.

Coppieters, I., Meeus, M., Kregel, J., Caeyenberghs, K., De Pauw, R., Goubert, D., and Cagnie, B. (2016) Relations between brain alterations and clinical pain measures in chronic musculoskeletal pain: a systematic review. *Journal of Pain* 17(9): 946–962.

Costigan, M. and Woolf, C.J. (2002) No DREAM, no pain: closing the spinal gate. *Cell* 108(3): 297–300.

Costigan, M., Scholz, J., and Woolf, C.J. (2009) Neuropathic pain: a maladaptive response of the nervous system to damage. *Annual Review of Neuroscience* 32: 1–32.

Cummins, T.R., Sheets, P.L., and Waxman, S.G. (2007) The roles of sodium channels in nociception: implications for mechanisms of pain. *Pain* 131(3): 243–257.

Davis, K.D. (2003) Neurophysiological and anatomical considerations in functional imaging of pain. *Pain* 105(1–2): 1–3.

Davis, K.D. (2004) Neuroimaging of pain. *Supplements to Clinical Neurophysiology* 57: 72–77.

Davis, K.D. (2011) Neuroimaging of pain: what does it tell us? *Current Opinion in Supportive and Palliative Care* 5(2): 116–121.

DeLeo, J.A., Tanga, F.Y., and Tawfik, V.L. (2004) Neuroimmune activation and neuroinflammation in chronic pain and opioid tolerance/hyperalgesia. *Neuroscientist* 10(1): 40–52.

Di Pietro, F., McAuley, J.H., Parkitny, L., Lotze, M., Wand, B.M., Moseley, G.L., and Stanton, T.R. (2013a) Primary somatosensory cortex function in complex regional pain syndrome: a systematic review and meta-analysis. *Journal of Pain* 14(10): 1001–1018.

Di Pietro, F., McAuley, J.H., Parkitny, L., Lotze, M., Wand, B.M., Moseley, G.L., and Stanton, T.R. (2013b) Primary motor cortex function in complex regional pain syndrome: a systematic review and meta-analysis. *Journal of Pain* 14(11): 1270–1288.

Dostrovsky, J.O. and Craig, A.D. (2013) Ascending projection systems. In S.B. McMahon, M. Koltzenburg, I. Tracey, and D.C. Turk (eds.), *Wall and Melzack's Textbook of Pain*, 6th ed. London: Elsevier.

Flor, H., Elbert, T., Knecht, S., Wienbruch, C., Pantev, C., Birbaumer, N., Larbig, W., and Taub, E. (1995) Phantom-limb pain as a perceptual correlate of cortical reorganization following arm amputation. *Nature* 375(6531): 482–484.

Flor, H., Braun, C., Elbert, T., and Birbaumer, N. (1997) Extensive reorganization of primary somatosensory cortex in chronic back pain patients. *Neuroscience Letters* 224(1): 5–8.

Gao, Y.J., Zhang, L., Samad, O.A., Suter, M.R., Yasuhiko, K., Xu, Z.Z., Park, J.Y., Lind, A.L., Ma, Q., and Ji, R.R. (2009) JNK-induced MCP-1 production in spinal cord astrocytes contributes to central sensitization and neuropathic pain. *Journal of Neuroscience* 29(13): 4096–4108.

Geha, P.Y., Baliki, M.N., Harden, R.N., Bauer, W.R., Parrish, T.B., and Apkarian, A.V. (2008) The brain in chronic CRPS pain: abnormal gray-white matter interactions in emotional and autonomic regions. *Neuron* 60(4): 570–581.

Gold, M.S. (2013) Molecular biology of sensory transduction. In S.B. McMahon, M. Koltzenburg, I. Tracey, and D.C. Turk (eds.), *Wall and Melzack's Textbook of Pain*, 6th ed. London: Elsevier.

Goldberg, D.S. and McGee, S.J. (2011) Pain as a global public health priority. *BMC Public Health* 6(11): 770.

Grace, P.M., Hutchinson, M.R., Maier, S.F., and Watkins, L.R. (2014) Pathological pain and the neuroimmune interface. *Nature Reviews Immunology* 14(4): 217–231.

Gracely, R.H. and Ambrose, K.R. (2011) Neuroimaging of fibromyalgia. *Best Practice & Research: Clinical Rheumatology* 25(2): 271–284.

Habib, A.M., Wood, J.N., and Cox, J.J. (2015) Sodium channels and pain. *Handbook of Experimental Pharmacology* 227: 39–56.

Hart, O.R., Uden, R.M., McMullan, J.E., Ritchie, M.S., Williams, T.D., and Smith, B.H. (2014) A study of National Health Service management of chronic osteoarthritis and low back pain. *Primary Health Care Research & Development* 27: 1–10.

Heinricher, M.M. and Fields, H.L. (2013) Central nervous systems mechanisms of pain modulation. In S.B. McMahon, M. Koltzenburg, I. Tracey, and D.C. Turk (eds.), *Wall and Melzack's Textbook of Pain*, 6th ed. London: Elsevier.

Hoeijmakers, J.G., Faber, C.G., Merkies, I.S., and Waxman, S.G. (2015) Painful peripheral neuropathy and sodium channel mutations. *Neuroscience Letters* 596: 51–59.

Howard, M.A., Sanders, D., Krause, K., O'Muircheartaigh, J., Fotopoulou, A., Zelaya, F., Thacker, M., Massat, N., Huggins, J.P., Vennart, W., Choy, E., Daniels, M., and Williams, S.C. (2012) Alterations in resting-state regional cerebral blood flow demonstrate ongoing pain in osteoarthritis: an arterial spin-labeled magnetic resonance imaging study. *Arthritis & Rheumatology* 64(12): 3936–3946.

Hutchinson, M.R., Shavit, Y., Grace, P.M., Rice, K.C., Maier, S.F., and Watkins, L.R. (2011) Exploring the neuroimmunopharmacology of opioids: an integrative review of mechanisms of central immune signaling and their implications for opioid analgesia. *Pharmacological Reviews* 63(3): 772–810.

Ji, R.R. and Woolf, C.J. (2001) Neuronal plasticity and signal transduction in nociceptive neurons: implications for the initiation and maintenance of pathological pain. *Neurobiology of Disease* 8(1): 1–10.

Ji, R.R., Kohno, T., Moore, K.A., and Woolf, C.J. (2003) Central sensitization and LTP: do pain and memory share similar mechanisms? *Trends in Neurosciences* 26(12): 696–705.

Jiang, Y., Oathes, D., Hush, J., Darnall, B., Charvat, M., Mackey, S., and Etkin, A. (2016) Perturbed connectivity of the amygdala and its subregions with the central executive and default mode networks in chronic pain. *Pain*. 157(9): 1970–1978.

Jorge, L.L. and Amaro, E. Jr. (2012) Brain imaging in fibromyalgia. *Current Pain and Headache Reports* 16(5): 388–398.

Kehlet, H., Jensen, T.S., and Woolf, C.J. (2006) Persistent postsurgical pain: risk factors and prevention. *Lancet* 367(9522): 1618–1625.

Latremoliere, A. and Woolf, C.J. (2009) Central sensitization: a generator of pain hypersensitivity by central neural plasticity. *Journal of Pain* 10(9): 895–926.

Loggia, M.L., Chonde, D.B., Akeju, O., Arabasz, G., Catana, C., Edwards, R.R., Hill, E., Hsu, S., Izquierdo-Garcia, D., Ji, R.R., Riley, M., Wasan, A.D., Zürcher, N.R., Albrecht, D.S., Vangel, M.G., Rosen, B.R., Napadow, V., and Hooker, J,M. (2015) Evidence for brain glial activation in chronic pain patients. *Brain* 138 (pt. 3): 604–615.

Lotze, M. and Moseley, G.L. (2007) Role of distorted body image in pain. *Current Rheumatology Reports* 9(6): 488–496.

Lotze, M. and Moseley, G.L. (2015) Theoretical considerations for chronic pain rehabilitation. *Physical Therapy* 95(9):1316–1320.

Lotze, M., Laubis-Herrmann, U., Topka, H., Erb, M., and Grodd, W. (1999) Reorganization in the primary motor cortex after spinal cord injury – a functional magnetic resonance (fMRI) study. *Restorative Neurology and Neuroscience* 14(2–3): 183–187.

Luo, C., Kuner, T., and Kuner, R. (2014) Synaptic plasticity in pathological pain. *Trends in Neurosciences* 37(6): 343–355.

McMahon, S.B. and Priestly, J.V. (2005) Nociceptor plasticity. In S. Hunt and M. Koltzenburg (eds.), *The Neurobiology of Pain*. Oxford: Oxford University Press.

Mantyh, P.W. (2002) A mechanism based understanding of cancer pain. *Pain* 96(1–2): 1–2.

Mantyh, P.W., Clohisy, D.R., Koltzenburg, M., and Hunt, S.P. (2002) Molecular mechanisms of cancer pain. *Nature Reviews Cancer* 2(3): 201–209.

Martucci, K.T. and Mackey, S.C. (2016) Imaging pain. *Anesthesiology Clinics* 34(2): 255–269.

Moseley, G.L. and Flor, H. (2012) Targeting cortical representations in the treatment of chronic pain: a review. *Neurorehabilitation & Neural Repair* 26(6): 646–652.

Moseley, G.L., Parsons, T.J., and Spence, C. (2008) Visual distortion of a limb modulates the pain and swelling evoked by movement. *Current Biology* 18(22): 1047–1048.

Mouraux, A., Diukova, A., Lee, M.C., Wise, R.G., and Iannetti, G.D. (2011) A multisensory investigation of the functional significance of the "pain matrix." *Neuroimage* 54(3): 2237–2249.

Old, E.A., Clark, A.K., and Malcangio, M. (2015) The role of glia in the spinal cord in neuropathic and inflammatory pain. *Handbook of Experimental Pharmacology* 227: 145–170.

O'Muircheartaigh, J., Marquand, A., Hodkinson, D.J., Krause, K., Khawaja, N., Renton, T.F., Huggins, J.P., Vennart, W., Williams, S.C., and Howard, M.A. (2015) Multivariate decoding of cerebral blood flow measures in a clinical model of on-going postsurgical pain. *Human Brain Mapping* 36(2): 633–642.

Papa, M., De Luca, C., Petta, F., Alberghina, L., Cirillo, G. (2014) Astrocyte-neuron interplay in maladaptive plasticity. *Neuroscience and Biobehavioral Reviews* 42: 35–54.

Pleger, B., Tegenthoff, M., Ragert, P., Förster, A.F., Dinse, H.R., Schwenkreis, P., Nicolas, V., and Maier, C. (2005) Sensorimotor retuning [corrected] in complex regional pain syndrome parallels pain reduction. *Annals of Neurology* 57(3): 425–429.

Ringkamp, M., Raja, S.N., Campbell, J.N., and Meyer, R.A. (2013) Peripheral mechanisms of cutaneous nociception. In S.B. McMahon, M. Koltzenburg, I. Tracey, and D.C. Turk (eds.), *Wall and Melzack's Textbook of Pain*, 6th ed. London: Elsevier.

Robinson, M.E., Craggs, J.G., Price, D.D., Perlstein, W.M., and Staud, R. (2011) Gray matter volumes of pain-related brain areas are decreased in fibromyalgia syndrome. *Journal of Pain* 12(4): 436–443.

Salter, M.W. and Beggs, S. (2014) Sublime microglia: expanding roles for the guardians of the CNS. *Cell* 158(1): 15–24.

Sandkühler, J. (2000) Learning and memory in pain pathways. *Pain* 88(2): 113–118.

Sandkühler, J. (2007) Understanding LTP in pain pathways. *Molecular Pain* 3(3): 9.

Sandkühler, J. (2009) Models and mechanisms of hyperalgesia and allodynia. *Physiological Reviews* 89(2): 707–758.

Sandkühler, J. (2013) Spinal cord plasticity and pain. In S.B. McMahon, M. Koltzenburg, I. Tracey, and D.C. Turk (eds.), *Wall and Melzack's Textbook of Pain*, 6th ed. London: Elsevier.

Sandkühler, J. (2015) Translating synaptic plasticity into sensation. *Brain* 138 (pt. 9): 2463–2464.

Schäfers, M. and Sorkin, L. (2008) Effect of cytokines on neuronal excitability. *Neuroscience Letters* 437(3): 188–193.

Scholz, J. and Woolf, C.J. (2007) The neuropathic pain triad: neurons, immune cells and glia. *Nature Neuroscience* 10(11): 1361–1368.

Shaw, C.A. and McEachern, J.C. (2000) Is there a general theory of neuroplasticity? In C.A. Shaw and J. C. McEarhern (eds.), *Towards a General Theory of Neuroplasticity*. London: Taylor & Francis.

Sommer, C. and Kress, M. (2004) Recent findings on how proinflammatory cytokines cause pain: peripheral mechanisms in inflammatory and neuropathic hyperalgesia. *Neuroscience Letters* 361(1–3): 184–187.

Sorkin, L.S., and Doom, C.M. (2000) Epineurial application of TNF elicits an acute mechanical hyperalgesia in the awake rat. *Journal of the Peripheral Nervous System* 5(2): 96–100.

Thacker, M.A., Clark, A.K., Marchand, F., and McMahon, S.B. (2007) Pathophysiology of peripheral neuropathic pain: immune cells and molecules. *Anesthesia & Analgesia* 105(3): 838–847.

Thacker, M.A., Clark, A.K., Bishop, T., Grist, J., Yip, P.K., Moon, L.D., Thompson, S.W., Marchand, F., and McMahon, S.B. (2009) CCL2 is a key mediator of microglia activation in neuropathic pain states. *European Journal of Pain* (London, UK) 13(3): 263–272.

Thayer, J.F. and Sternberg, E.M. (2009) Neural concomitants of immunity – focus on the vagus nerve. *Neuroimage* 47(3): 908–910.

Thayer, J.F. and Sternberg, E.M. (2010) Neural aspects of immunomodulation: focus on the vagus nerve. *Brain, Behavior, and Immunity.* 24(8): 1223–1228.

Todd, A.J. and Koerber, H.R. (2013) Neuroanatomical substrates of spinal nociception. In S.B. McMahon, M. Koltzenburg, I. Tracey, and D.C. Turk (eds.), *Wall and Melzack's Textbook of Pain*, 6th ed. London: Elsevier.

Tracey, I. and Mantyh, P.W. (2007) The cerebral signature for pain perception and its modulation. *Neuron* 55(3): 377–391.

Treede, R.D., Rief, W., Barke, A., Aziz, Q., Bennett, M.I., Benoliel, R., Cohen, M., Evers, S., Finnerup, N.B., First, M.B., Giamberardino, M.A., Kaasa, S., Kosek, E., Lavand'homme, P., Nicholas, M., Perrot, S., Scholz, J., Schug, S., Smith, B.H., Svensson, P., Vlaeyen, J.W., and Wang, S.J. (2015) A classification of chronic pain for ICD-11. *Pain* 156(6): 1003–1007.

Tsuda, M., Beggs, S., Salter, M.W., and Inoue, K. (2013) Microglia and intractable chronic pain. *Glia* 61(1): 55–61.

Ung, H., Brown, J.E., Johnson, K.A., Younger, J., Hush, J., and Mackey, S. (2014) Multivariate classification of structural MRI data detects chronic low back pain. *Cerebral Cortex* 24(4): 1037–1044.

von Hehn, C.A., Baron, R., and Woolf, C.J. (2012) Deconstructing the neuropathic pain phenotype to reveal neural mechanisms. *Neuron* 73(4): 638–652.

Woolf, C.J. (1996) Wind up and central sensitization are not equivalent. *Pain* 66(2–3): 105–108.

Woolf, C.J. (2011) Central sensitization: implications for the diagnosis and treatment of pain. *Pain* 152(3) (suppl.): S2–S15.

Woolf, C.J. and Costigan, M. (1999) Transcriptional and posttranslational plasticity and the generation of inflammatory pain. *Proceedings of the National Academy of Sciences of the United States of America* 96(14): 7723–7730.

Woolf, C.J. and Salter, M.W. (2000) Neuronal plasticity: increasing the gain in pain. *Science* 288(5472): 1765–1769.

Woolf, C.J., Shortland, P., and Coggeshall, R.E. (1992) Peripheral nerve injury triggers central sprouting of myelinated afferents. *Nature* 355(6355): 75–78.

PART I-III

Modeling pain in psychology

11

PSYCHOLOGICAL MODELS OF PAIN

Amanda C. de C. Williams

This chapter describes the definition and understanding of pain, for which some neurophysiological background is provided; the predominant psychotherapeutic models, their integration and the evidence base; and a brief note on philosophical contribution to psychological model development. It introduces important models that are further developed in other chapters within this section.

1 Definition of pain

"An unpleasant sensory and emotional experience associated with actual or potential tissue damage, or described in terms of such damage." (Merskey and Bogduk 1994).

This definition of pain is discussed in much more detail in Chapter 31 of this volume, but remains an important starting point for any consideration of the psychology of pain. It represented a significant advance on earlier definitions that referred primarily to sensation or perception (Auvray et al. 2010), and only to emotional components, if at all, as part of a response. Here emotion is identified as integral to the experience, as envisaged in the paradigm-changing gate-control model of pain (Melzack and Wall 1965; described below in Section 2, "Neurophysiology of Pain").

A note accompanying the definition gave equal importance to sensory and emotional components, acknowledged the unreliable relationship between pain and tissue damage, and recognized pain experience in those who lack language, human and non-human. But cognitive, social, and behavioral dimensions are missing, despite evidence for them in various animals (Langford et al. 2010; Low 2013; Mogil 2015; Sneddon 2011); the primacy given to verbal report overshadows reliable behavioral signs (Williams 2002; Hadjistavropoulos et al. 2011); and pain in the absence of tissue damage or disease is assigned to undefined "psychological reasons." The last statement reintroduces a psychosomatic model that is neither required nor helpful: known pain processes explain the generation and modulation of pain within the nervous system without lesion or pathology. Adding an undefined psychosomatic basis for pain reintroduces dualistic processes into an integrated understanding of pain. Patrick Wall (1994), one of the authors of the gate-control theory, proposed in characteristically robust terms three reasons why pain cannot be satisfactorily explained by reference to observable pathology:

First, I find it unwise arrogance to believe that our present techniques of diagnosis are capable of detecting all relevant forms of peripheral pathology. Second, we are now beginning to realise ... that a peripheral event may trigger long lasting changes in the spinal cord and brain ... This means that overt peripheral pathology is capable of initiating a cascade of changes which may persist in the central nervous system long after peripheral pathology has disappeared. Third, we are now beginning to discover that sensory systems are not dedicated and hard wired but are normally held in a stable state by elaborate dynamic control mechanisms. The rules of the physiology of these control mechanisms allow them to be pushed outside their normal working range in which state they will oscillate or fire continuously.

(4)

Many pains, from mild and momentary to severe and prolonged, originate from an identifiable cause, often external. Pain is a warning of actual or impending injury, and after injury a constant or repeated reminder to take care of the injury. These processes are essential for survival, since they maximize chances of healing and recovery (Williams 2002, 2016; Walters 1994). Injuries that become infected or infested, broken bones which further disintegrate through continued use, repeated encounters with noxious plants or animals that are not remembered and avoided: all lower chances of survival. So it is reasonable to look for causes of injury when pain is felt. What is unreasonable is to deny pain when no such cause can be found, and yet such statements are ubiquitous in medical texts and teaching, design of medical services, and decisions made about patients and their treatment (Donaldson 2009: 32–39). Psychiatry and psychology have speculatively filled the apparent gap in explanation with concepts such as "hysteria" or faulty pre-pain personality (Pilowsky and Spence 1975), now formulated as psychosomatic pain in clinical and empirical work, despite the dearth of theory or evidence (Williams and Johnson 2011; Crombez et al. 2009; Merskey 2009; see Chapter 13, this volume). Both in medical and in common-sense or lay understanding of pain, people with pain but no corresponding physical signs may be suspected of imagining, exaggerating, or fabricating it, and of malingering or seeking benefits without being entitled through genuine illness or disability (Eccleston et al. 1997; Patients' Association 2010; Williams 2002).

2 Neurophysiology of pain: the basis for psychological models

The gate-control theory (Melzack and Wall 1965) proposed an integration at the first synapse in the dorsal horn of the spinal cord of fast- and slow-conducted input from peripheral nerve endings and input descending from the brain and representing central control over peripheral input: "The model suggests that psychological factors such as past experience, attention and emotion influence pain response and perception by acting on the gate control system" (Melzack and Wall 1965: 978). Initially, this control was conceptualized as inhibitory but the proliferation of pain research which resulted from their model found far more excitatory than inhibitory mechanisms. Not only could these mechanisms amplify pain, but changes from the dorsal horn of the spinal cord onwards could produce afferent signals in the pain system from peripheral stimulation – such as light touch, or mild warmth – not normally associated with pain experience.

Research inspired by the gate-control model focused on the periphery and on processing at the spinal cord level, often using restrained animals with acute pain and evoked pain responses. It was challenging to translate to humans with chronic pain, manifest distress, and spontaneous behaviors. The development of brain-imaging techniques allowed some insight into the processing of pain in the brain, subject to the shortcomings of models available for interpretation (Tracey and Bushnell 2009). This established correlation between processing in particular networks and subjective pain rating (Coghill et al. 2003), and the prominence of emotional processing even of expected experimental stimuli in people with chronic pain (Baliki et al. 2006). In brief, the signature of pain in the brain (Tracey and Bushnell 2009) bore out the definition as a sensory and emotional experience, with impact on cognitive and emotional function even in non-human animals (Low 2013).

It is useful to distinguish between the immediate pain experienced when tissue is damaged, and that prompts rapid escape, from the persistence of pain during healing. An evolutionary understanding is helpful but almost entirely neglected in the field of pain (Williams, 2016). Evident even in invertebrates with a fairly simple nervous system (Walters 1994), nociception is generally unmodulated and the response is often reflexive. From that point, the inflammatory response and other systemic changes increase the sensitivity of the area around the injury, prompting wound care and adjustments to movement (such as guarding or limping) and reduction of usual activities to minimize disturbance during healing (Walters 1994; Woolf 2010). The wounded animal – best described in mammals – conserves resources, losing interest in eating, exploration, and pursuing social and sexual contact, while resting and sleeping more (Wall 1979; Williams 2016). In normal recovery, as healing proceeds and pain recedes, the individual becomes more active and loses the hypersensitivity and the changes to movement and activity that are also behavioral signs of pain.

In chronic pain, by contrast, the behavioral changes persist, as does pain. The injury (such as from trauma or surgery), if any, has healed; there may be ongoing disease such as rheumatoid arthritis or endometriosis, but the relationship of pain to pathology is very variable; or there may be neither injury nor pathology detected but the pain starts and continues without identifiable cause. One further possibility is neuropathic pain, when nerve tissue is damaged and multiple changes within the nervous system, peripheral, central, or both, generate pain on the slightest stimulus or spontaneously (Woolf 2010). It is chronic pain in particular that is often judged in medical or lay settings to lack a biological basis, and that has provided fertile ground for psychological models of pain. (Cf. Chapter 10, this volume.)

The psychological models described and discussed here are the behavioral model, the cognitive and combined cognitive-behavioral models, and Third Wave models (see also Chapters 12 and 33). All are implicitly or explicitly compared with what is often referred to as the "medical model," an oversimplified and concrete account of pain as described above, that recognizes tissue damage or pathology as the basis of pain, and the complaint of pain in the absence of identifiable tissue damage as suspect: as discussed above, this fails to integrate the contribution of the brain to the experience of pain.

3 The behavioral model

The foundation of psychology in chronic pain lies in the operant behavioral model developed by Fordyce (1976; Main et al. 2014), drawing on clinical experience in one of the earliest multidisciplinary pain clinics. If there was no longer a peripheral driver of pain (on the basis of medical assessment), his model focused on behaviors that indicated pain, verbal and non-verbal, from limping, guarding, or sighing to taking analgesics, soliciting social support, and seeking medical help. Fordyce explicitly rejected assumptions of covert psychological motivation as the explanation for pain, and took a neutral and compassionate stance towards chronic pain patients. Rest, attention, medication, but also recognition of progress were commonly used reinforcers.

Fordyce emphasized the distinction between "respondent pain," where behavior was a response to onset or exacerbation of pain, often acute-on-chronic pain (that is, acute exacerbation of chronic pain), and "operant pain" where the timing and frequency of behavior in relation to its consequences appeared to confirm that those consequences controlled the behavior. A common example of respondent knee pain would be evidenced by limping when under particular strain; of operant knee pain, of limping only when sympathetic others were present. Pain behaviors were addressed because they were accessible (Fordyce et al. 1968), not through any presumption of cause. Fordyce was careful to engage with the wider context of the patient's life, to share the model with the patient, and to involve the patient's family members, workmates, or employers in behavioral change. Alongside the reduction of pain behaviors, he stressed the importance of increasing well behaviors, again using operant methods, based on the patient's choice of leisure and other activities.

In experimental settings, where the pain has little or no threat value, and social relationships are constrained by design, it is possible to manipulate some pain-related behaviors, particularly verbal ones, by systematic positive or negative reinforcement: the model predicts behaviors well. In clinical settings many other variables apply and it is difficult to isolate or observe behavioral contingencies. Despite this, and the objections of Fordyce and colleagues (Fordyce et al. 1968), behavioral explanations were adopted in psychiatric practice and often subsumed in adverse moral judgements of patients. Rewarding behavioral consequences, such as attention, sympathy, and relief from unwanted duties, were assumed to govern behavior, rather than observed, and were therefore reversed in order to change the behavior. While this is not a failure of the model itself, it was clear that contingencies alone could not adequately explain behavior in chronic pain, in clinical settings or in the patients' own environments. Just as in the conceptualization of anxiety in the broader field of psychology, behavioral theories gave way to cognitive theory.

4 Cognitive and cognitive-behavioral models

In contrast to the behavioral model, there is no original authoritative statement of principles or practice for the cognitive model, nor has one emerged with time. Cognitive models were (like behavioral models) extrapolated from mainstream psychology, but piecemeal and predominantly from treatment studies rather than from experimental study of normal behavior. Early models drew heavily on cognitive processes of attention control, and on treatment for stress (Turk et al. 1983); subsequently, information-processing theories in mainstream psychology directed attention to beliefs and predictions (not least about behavioral choices and their consequences), and to the beliefs about pain and the ways of coping with which they were associated (Turk and Okifuji 2002).

Other than by self-report, there was little access to cognitive processes in clinical settings: tests for implicit cognitive processes used in experimental settings were impractical. Studies of people with pain focused on a variety of cognitive processes by self-report: control and self-efficacy; coping (Turk et al. 1983; Keefe et al. 1992). In clinical settings, behavior such as avoiding use of a painful although functioning limb, or turning every conversation to the hopeless situation of having chronic pain, remained the target for clinical intervention, now indirectly by addressing cognitive content (such as beliefs about pain) and processes (such as pessimistic thinking about pain). Many treatment trials (Morley and Williams 2006) refer to a book by Turk and colleagues (1983) in which the cognitive-behavioral model is briefly summarized:

> Behavioral change is a reflection of the intimate interrelationships among the patient's cognitive structures (schemata, beliefs), cognitive processes (automatic thoughts, internal dialogue, images), interpersonal behaviors, and resulting intrapersonal and interpersonal consequences.
>
> *(5)*

Above all, the individual's interpretation of his or her situation and of the world around, and its implications for mood, particularly depression, underpinned the targeting in treatment of the beliefs of the person with pain. Some even used cognitive concepts to explain all behavioral phenomena (Ciccone and Grzesiak 1984). In clinical settings, the language of "distorted" cognitions, "excessive" disability was widely used, as if correct adjustment to pain could be specified and shaped by changing patients' beliefs. This was not borne out by cognitive interventions (Turner and Jensen 1993), or by experimental tests of cognitive strategies such as distraction and use of imagery (Fernandez and Turk 1989), both of which bodies of work showed at best weak effects, despite patients' accounts of frequent use of the strategies. The use of the term "coping" for the strategies people used to try to sustain a reasonable lifestyle despite pain was generally unhelpful. The notion that strategies could in themselves be adaptive or maladaptive without reference to context was widespread, although some asked questions such as "Coping with what?" (Keefe et al. 1992).

A highly influential model that arose from the integration of cognitive and behavioral models was the "fear–avoidance" cycle of Vlaeyen and colleagues (1995; Vlaeyen and Linton 2000), most recently critically reformulated (Crombez et al. 2012) in the light of evidence and theory. The original version remains the foundation of psychological understanding of pain in pain medicine. It postulated that the individual in pain *either* had little fear and therefore confronted the pain and found that it did not prevent activity, nor did activity worsen the pain or the original injury (if any), *or* s/he was fearful, with catastrophic interpretation of pain as implying serious damage or disease, therefore rested and avoided activity, so becoming more disabled by disuse and depression. These in turn produced more pain with less and less activity. Despite its testability, very few attempts were made to challenge or to assemble evidence for the model; its strength lay in its roots in established work on phobia and in its apparent fit with patients seen in the clinic. It was rapidly adopted as an explanatory framework, and disuse and depression, in particular, became targets of treatment in their own right, as did catastrophic thinking (appraising everything pain-related in a very negative way), consistent with cognitive targets of therapy.

As with the cognitive component of pain, there is no coherent theory of emotion, and much work originates in pragmatic clinical settings. While Vlaeyen's model focused on fear, often used as if synonymous with anxiety (or catastrophizing, despite some important differences), people with chronic pain often seemed depressed, although because of the prevalence of theories of psychogenic pain they were not always willing to discuss it with doctors (Eccleston et al. 1997; see Chapter 13, this volume). Standard diagnostic criteria and questionnaires risked overestimating depression by attributing physical symptoms, such as sleep disturbance, to mood alone (Pincus and Williams 1999). At the same time, pessimism and hopelessness in patients undermined attempts to treat them, so were important to identify. Importing pathological constructs such as phobia and major depression from mainstream mental health has, in general, been unhelpful, and efforts to build a normal psychology of pain are welcomed (Eccleston 2011).

5 The Third Wave

The "Third Wave" is a collective term for diverse treatments arising from what is claimed as a common philosophy, but is hard to represent as such other than by its recognition of suffering as part of life rather than something that can be avoided or vanquished. The treatments may be provided together or separately. The most prominent in the field of pain – and based far more in clinical settings and directed towards treatment, rather than in experimental settings exploring the nature of pain psychology – are Acceptance and Commitment Therapy (ACT: Hayes 2004) and Mindfulness (McCracken and Vowles 2014). The roots of ACT are in the behavioral theory of language, recognizing the shortcomings of attempting to teach the "right" cognitive strategies and coping approaches (McCracken 2009), and building on some elements of cognitive-behavioral therapy while rejecting others, particularly implicit and explicit tenets of cognitive therapy that involve controlling thought content. In particular, unwelcome thoughts are accepted as thoughts, and recognized as possibly mistaken and therefore to be observed but not necessarily followed. The extent of difference from cognitive and behavioral therapy is disputed (Hofmann and Asmundson 2008). There is a focus on accepting pain (rather than trying to avoid it or fight it), disengaging and disinvesting in thoughts and emotions associated with pain, and acting according to personal values (McCracken 2009), the individual discovering for him or herself what works best. This may seem to require a wise homunculus who controls actions and responses, but this is rarely addressed. It is also an individualist philosophy – a contrast to some Eastern philosophies to which it refers. Although acceptance of pain emerged as a heuristic construct (Eccleston and McCracken 2003) that was relatively easy to share with patients and those around them (although sometimes mistaken for defeated resignation in the face of pain), current theory emphasizes psychological flexibility rather than acceptance (McCracken and Morley 2014). Unfortunately, psychological flexibility, defined as the capacity to persist in or change behavior in relation to thoughts and feelings, in relation to the situation, and in relation to personal goals and values (McCracken and Morley 2014), has so far resisted quantification, and its component parts are assessed by rather transparent self-report.

Mindfulness was first used in chronic pain in the 1980s (Kabat-Zinn 1982) but not again (in the research literature) until it was well-established in mainstream psychology (Teasdale et al. 2000). Contributions to its development have come from academic settings, including neuroscience (Zeidan et al. 2012), and from Buddhist philosophy and practice (Burch and Penman 2013; Carson et al. 2005). Mindfulness emphasizes being in the present, rather than in regrets over the past or anxieties about the future, and fully in the present, encompassing awareness using all senses and recognizing the many experiences other than pain. Daily meditation is for some practitioners an essential element to cultivate mindfulness, and it is encouraged in patients in mindfulness-based treatments for pain (Burch and Penman 2013).

6 Problems with evidence

Much of the presumed support for each of the models above consists of reports of efficacy of the practice in clinical settings in improving pain, mood, and disability. However, meta-analyses of cognitive-behavioral and behavioral therapy have yielded successively smaller effects with each update (Williams et al. 2012; Morley et al. 2013), while early meta-analyses of ACT trials look promising (Veehof et al. 2011). The apparently diminishing effects occur for a complex combination of reasons, many methodological but some related to health-care systems in which trials are run. More and bigger compound trials are unlikely to provide a definitive estimate of efficacy (Morley et al. 2013), nor is treatment efficacy a demonstration that treatment outcome is attributable to the specific techniques of treatment rather than to the non-specific effects of contact with therapeutic services and personnel (Wampold 2005). Assertions that one treatment type might suit one kind of patient better than another, and that each will be the best for someone, may be wishful thinking and have no theoretical basis. Attempts to type patients at entry to treatment have been superficial and unlikely to succeed (Morley and Williams 2006). On the other hand, trials of single methods of treatment with selected patients, such as behavioral exposure to feared activities (Vlaeyen et al. 2012), or mindfulness methods for modulation of pain (Zeidan et al. 2012) show impressive results of a clinically relevant magnitude, and suggest that we are not realizing the potential of psychological methods. The field seems to be in stasis, with diverse research groups pursuing patient selection, treatment refinement, or treatment delivery.

Even if we were to design a more potent intervention, difficulties remain in conceptualization and measurement of outcome. Constructs which were reasonably well founded in the field of psychological disorders are adopted and adapted in pain, particularly in clinical settings, in ways which do disservice to the theories and to patients: the reformulation of some behavioral methods to incorporate moral values, as described above, is a strong example. Further, psychologists' weakness for believing that any quality or experience can be measured by self-report on a questionnaire that presumes a simple linear, measurable underlying construct, by no means true (Michell 2009), made for a proliferation of measures which, whatever their claimed domain, often overlapped considerably in content and produced unsurprising correlations interpreted as association of the two domains, such as (lack of) confidence in activity and disability. There is little evidence that people can accurately report their thinking or emotional processes, or their behavior, and yet the assumption underpins most clinical (Morley and Williams 2006) and many experimental studies. Any face-to-face assessment, such as of pain, is a social event (Schiavenato and Craig 2010), not a "read-out" of a stable internal state. Self-report is a behavior, and like any behavior, may serve a function, consciously or not, for the individual in pain in that particular context (Williams 2002): self-presentation as needy, or brave, or deserving of some specific consideration or exception. (Cf. Chapters 20 and 21, this volume.)

While the neuroscience and experimental psychology fields have contributed substantially to our understanding (Bushnell et al. 2013; Legrain et al. 2009), much human research is essentially trivial, involving pain inflicted briefly and unthreateningly on healthy and willing participants, volunteer or paid. This usually has little to tell us about clinical pain that is threatening, unpredictable, unwanted, and unrewarded (Eccleston and Crombez 1999; Moore et al. 2013; Wiech et al. 2010). Research on people with problematic pain produces far more complex and less newsworthy results than, for instance, an assertion such as that social rejection and physical pain (both minor and in healthy volunteers) are essentially similar (Eisenberger et al. 2003). At first the area lacked any theory, but coherent frameworks have been built around findings, in this case using evolutionary understanding (Chester et al. 2012) in which all emotions trace their roots to pain (Walters 1994), and a neural systems model. Nevertheless, Iannetti et al. (2013) demonstrated serious weaknesses in the thesis: problems of logical error (reverse inference) and loose interpretation of neuroimaging evidence (see also Chapter 7, this volume).

7 Philosophical observations on pain

Philosophical and religious understandings of pain are represented in clinical discourses and practices. Dualism has dogged the study and understanding of pain, and persists in language, concepts, and the therapeutic options and their delivery to people with pain (Kleinman et al. 1992: 10).

Philosophical discussions of pain often invoke evidence on whether non-human animals feel pain (Dawkins 2015; Rose 2002: ch. 15), or whether humans feel pain without full consciousness. It is important to note that pain is evident in behavior and brain processing of unconscious patients (Arif-Rahu and Grap 2010; Schnakers et al. 2012), and that arguments about the completeness and functioning of the nervous system were used to deny – and so fail to treat – pain in infants and in people with cognitive impairment (such as dementia), despite behavioral evidence to the contrary (Hadjistavropoulos et al. 2011; Fitzgerald and McIntosh 1989; Rodkey and Pillai Riddell 2013). Craig (1997) argues persuasively that pain has been poorly understood in many writings on consciousness, and concepts of consciousness misleadingly used in pain studies (see also Chapter 17, this volume).

8 Conclusions

Despite the predominance of clinical concerns in driving research on pain, treatment failure is common and availability of psychological methods alone or integrated with other treatment fall so far short of need (Breivik et al. 2006; Von Korff 2013) that there is no possibility of adequate provision for all those whose lives are affected by chronic pain. Understanding of pain needs to change in both lay and health-care fields. Psychology of pain has largely developed without adequate reference to somatic experience (Eccleston 2016), to biological underpinnings, or to the social nature of humans, and has sought solutions before defining the problems. There is not yet any truly integrated bio-psycho-social model: most models which claim that title are predominantly psychological (see also Chapter 12, this volume). Arguably, to integrate with the biological and the social, psychology needs to adopt a framework, such as that provided by evolutionary theory, that relates behaviors common in pain across animals to its original functions, and to possible mismatches of those functions with the current environment (Williams 2016).

Related topics:

Chapter 6: Advances in the neuroscience of pain (Apkarian)
Chapter 7: Neuromatrix theory of pain (Roy and Wager)
Chapter 10: Pathophysiological mechanisms of chronic pain (Thacker and Moseley)
Chapter 12: Biopsychosocial models of pain (Hadjistavropoulos)
Chapter 13: Psychogenic pain: old and new (Sullivan)
Chapter 14: Pain, voluntary action, and the sense of agency (Beck and Haggard)
Chapter 15: The lives of others: pain in non-human animals (Droege)
Chapter 17: Pain and consciousness (Pereplyotchik)
Chapter 20: Pain and incorrigibility (Langland-Hassan)
Chapter 21: Can I see your pain? An evaluative model of pain perception (de Vignemont)
Chapter 31: An introduction to the IASP's definition of pain (Wright)
Chapter 33: Pain management (Berryman, Catley, and Moseley)

References

Arif-Rahu, M. and Grap, M.J. (2010) Facial expression and pain in the critically ill non-communicative patient: State of science review. *Intensive Critical Care Nursing* 26(6): 343–352.

Auvray, M., Myin, E., and Spence, C. (2010) The sensory-discriminative and affective-motivational aspects of pain. *Neuroscience and Biobehavioral Reviews* 34: 214–223.

Baliki, M.N., Chialvo, D.R., Geha, P.Y., Levy, R.M., Harden, R.N., Parrish, T.B., and Apkarian, A.V. (2006) Chronic pain and the emotional brain: specific brain activity associated with spontaneous fluctuations of intensity of chronic back pain. *Journal of Neuroscience* 26: 12165–12173.

Breivik, H., Collett, B., Ventafridda, V., Cohen, R., and Gallacher, D. (2006) Survey of chronic pain in Europe: prevalence, impact on daily life and treatment. *European Journal of Pain* (London, UK) 10: 287–333.

Burch, V. and Penman, D. (2013) *Mindfulness for Health: A Practical Guide to Relieving Pain, Reducing Stress and Restoring Wellbeing.* London: Piatkus.

Bushnell, M.C., Čeko, M., and Low, L.A. (2013) Cognitive and emotional control of pain and its disruption in chronic pain. *Nature Neuroscience Reviews* 14: 502–511.

Carson, J.W., Keefe, F.J., Lynch, T.R., Carson, K.M., Goli, V., Fras, A.M., and Thorp, S.R. (2005) Loving-kindness meditation for chronic low back pain: results from a pilot trial. *Journal of Holistic Nursing* 23(3): 287–304.

Chester, D.S., Pond, R.S., Richman, S.B., and DeWall, C.N. (2012) The optimal calibration hypothesis: how life history modulates the brain's social pain network. *Frontiers in Evolutionary Neuroscience* 4: art. 10.

Ciccone, D.S. and Grzesiak, R.C. (1984) Cognitive dimensions of chronic pain. *Social Science and Medicine* 19: 1339–1345.

Coghill, R.C., McHaffie, J.G., and Yen, Y.-F. (2003) Neural correlates of interindividual differences in the subjective experience of pain. *Proceedings of the National Academy of Sciences* 100: 8538–8542.

Craig, K.D. (1997) Implications of concepts of consciousness for understanding pain behavior and the definition of pain. *Pain Research and Management* 2(2): 111–117.

Crombez, G., Beirens, K., Van Damme, S., Eccleston, C., and Fontaine, J. (2009) The unbearable lightness of somatization: a systematic review of the concept of somatization in empirical studies of pain. *Pain* 145: 31–35.

Crombez, G., Eccleston, C., Van Damme, S., Vlaeyen, J.W.S., and Karoly, P. (2012) The fear avoidance model of chronic pain: the next generation. *Clinical Journal of Pain* 28: 475–483.

Dawkins, M. (2015) Animal welfare and the paradox of animal consciousness. *Advances in the Study of Behavior* 47: 5–37.

Donaldson, L. (2009) *150 Years of the Annual Report of the Chief Medical Officer: On the State of Public Health 2008.* London: Department of Health.

Eccleston, C. (2011) A normal psychology of chronic pain. *Psychologist* 26: 422–425.

Eccleston, C. (2016) *Embodied: the psychology of physical sensation.* Oxford: Oxford University Press.

Eccleston, C. and Crombez, G. (1999) Pain demands attention: a cognitive–affective model of the interruptive function of pain. *Psychological Bulletin* 125(3): 356.

Eccleston, C. and McCracken, L.M. (2003) Coping or acceptance: what to do about chronic pain? *Pain* 105: 197–204.

Eccleston, C., Williams, A., and Stainton Rogers, W. (1997) Patients and professionals understandings of the causes of chronic pain: blame, responsibility and identity protection. *Social Science and Medicine* 45: 699–709.

Eisenberger, N.I., Lieberman, M.D., and Williams, K.D. (2003) Does rejection hurt? An fMRI study of social exclusion. *Science* 302: 290–292.

Fernandez, E. and Turk, D.C. (1989) The utility of cognitive coping strategies for altering pain perception: a meta-analysis. *Pain* 38: 123–135.

Fitzgerald, M. and McIntosh, N. (1989) Pain and analgesia in the newborn. *Archives of Disease in Childhood* 64: 441–443.

Fordyce, W.E. (1976) *Behavioral Methods for Chronic Pain and Illness.* St. Louis, MO: C.V. Mosby & Co.

Fordyce, W.E., Fowler, R.S., Lehmann, J.F., DeLateur, and B.J. (1968) Some implications of learning on problems of chronic pain *Journal of Chronic Diseases* 21: 179–190.

Hadjistavropoulos, T., Breau, L., and Craig, K.D. (2011) Pain assessment in adults and children with limited ability to communicate. In D.C. Turk and R. Melzack (eds.) *Handbook of Pain Assessment*, 3rd ed. New York: Guilford Press.

Hayes, S.C. (2004) Acceptance and commitment therapy, relational frame theory, and the Third Wave of behavioral and cognitive therapies. *Behavioral Therapy* 35: 639–665.

Hofmann, S.G. and Asmundson, G.J.G. (2008) Acceptance and mindfulness-based therapy: new wave or old hat? *Clinical Psychology Review* 8: 1–16.

Iannetti, G.D., Salomons, T.V., Moayedi, M., Mouraux, M., and Davis, K.D. (2013) Beyond metaphor: contrasting mechanisms of social and physical pain. *Trends in Cognitive Sciences* 17(8): 371–378.

Kabat-Zinn, J. (1982) An outpatient program in behavioral medicine for chronic pain patients based on the practice of mindfulness meditation: theoretical considerations and preliminary results *General Hospital Psychiatry* 4(1) 43–47.

Keefe, F.J., Salley, A.N., and Lefebvre, J.C. (1992) Coping with pain: conceptual concerns and future directions. *Pain* 51: 131–134.

Kleinman, A., Brodwin, P.E., Good, B.J., and Good, M-J. Del V. (1992) Pain as human experience: an introduction. In M.J. Del V. Good, P.E. Brodwin, B.J. Good, and A. Kleinman (eds.), *Pain as Human Experience: An Anthropological Perspective.* Berkeley: University of California Press.

Langford, D.J., Tuttle, A.H., Brown, K., Deschenes, S., Fischer, D.B., Mutso, A., Root, K.C., Sotocinal, S.G., Stern, M.A., Mogil, J.S., and Sternberg, W.F. (2010) Social approach to pain in laboratory mice. *Social Neuroscience* 5(2): 163–170.

Legrain, V., Van Damme, S., Eccleston, C., Davis, K.D., Seminowicz, D.A., and Crombez, G. (2009) A neurocognitive model of attention to pain: behavioral and neuroimaging evidence. *Pain* 144: 230–232.

Low, L.A. (2013) The impact of pain upon cognition: what have rodent studies told us? *Pain* 154: 2603–2605.

McCracken, L.M. (2009) *Contextual Cognitive-Behavioral Therapy for Chronic Pain.* Seattle: IASP Press.

McCracken, L. and Morley, S.J. (2014) The psychological flexibility model: a basis for integration and progress in psychological approaches to chronic pain management. *Journal of Pain* 15(3): 221–234.

McCracken, L.M. and Vowles, K.E. (2014) Acceptance and commitment therapy and mindfulness for chronic pain: model, process, and progress. *American Psychologist* 69(2): 178–187.

Main, C.J., Keefe, F.J., Jensen, M.P., Vlaeyen, J.W.S., and Vowles, K.E. (eds.) (2014) *Fordyce's Behavioral Methods for Chronic Pain and Illness: Republished with Invited Commentaries.* Philadelphia: Lippincott Williams & Wilkins.

Melzack, R. and Wall, P.D. (1965) Pain mechanisms: a new theory. *Science* 150(3699): 971–979.

Merskey, H. (2009) Somatization: or another God that failed. *Pain* 145: 4–5.

Merskey, H. and Bogduk, N. (eds.) (1994) *Classification of Chronic Pain*, 2nd ed. Seattle: IASP Press. [Definitions available at the IASP website, <http://www.iasp-pain.org/Taxonomy#Pain>.]

Michell, J. (2009) The psychometricians' fallacy: too clever by half. *British Journal of Mathematical and Statistical Psychology* 62: 41–55

Mogil, J.S. (2015) Social modulation of and by pain in humans and rodents. *Pain* 156(4) (suppl. 1): S35–S41.

Moore, D.J., Keogh, E., and Eccleston, C. (2013) The effect of threat on attentional interruption by pain. *Pain* 154: 82–88.

Morley, S. and Williams, A.C. de C. (2006) Editorial: RCTs of psychological treatments for chronic pain: progress and challenges. *Pain* 121: 171–172.

Morley, S., Williams, A., and Eccleston, C. (2013) Examining the evidence of psychological treatments for chronic pain: time for a paradigm shift? *Pain* 154: 1929–1931.

Patients' Association (2010) *Public Attitudes to Pain.* Harrow: Patients' Association.

Pilowsky, I. and Spence, N.D. (1975) Patterns of illness behavior in patients with intractable pain. *Journal of Psychosomatic Research* 19: 279–285.

Pincus, T. and Williams, A. (1999) Models and measurements of depression in chronic pain. *Journal of Psychosomatic Research* 47: 211–219.

Rodkey, E.N. and Pillai Riddell, R. (2013) The infancy of infant pain research: the experimental origins of infant pain denial. *Journal of Pain* 14: 338–350.

Rose, J.D. (2002) The neurobehavioral nature of fishes and the question of awareness and pain. *Reviews in Fisheries Science* 10(1): 1–38

Schiavenato, M. and Craig, K.D. (2010) Pain assessment as a social transaction: beyond the "gold standard." *Clinical Journal of Pain* 26(8): 667–676.

Schnakers, C., Chatelle, C., Demertzi, A., Majerus, S., and Laureys, S. (2012) What about pain in disorders of consciousness? *AAPS Journal* 14: 437–444.

Sneddon, L.U. (2011) Pain perception in fish. *Journal of Consciousness Studies* 18(9–10): 209–229

Teasdale, J.D., Segal, Z.V., Williams, J.M.G., Ridgeway, V.A., Soulsby, J.M., and Lau, M.A. (2000) Prevention of relapse/recurrence in major depression by mindfulness-based cognitive therapy. *Journal of Consulting and Clinical Psychology* 68: 615–623.

Tracey, I. and Bushnell, M.C. (2009) How neuroimaging studies have challenged us to rethink: is chronic pain a disease? *Journal of Pain* 10(11): 1113–1120.

Turk, D.C. and Okifuji, A. (2002) Psychological factors in chronic pain: evolution and revolution. *Journal of Consulting and Clinical Psychology* 70: 678–690.

Turk, D.C., Meichenbaum, D., and Genest, M. (1983) *Pain and Behavioral Medicine: A Cognitive-Behavioral Perspective*. New York: Guilford Press.

Turner, J.A. and Jensen, M.P. (1993) Efficacy of cognitive therapy for chronic low back pain. *Pain* 52: 169–177.

Veehof, M.M., Oskam, M.-J., Schreurs, K.M.G., and Bohlmeijer, E.T. (2011) Acceptance-based interventions for the treatment of chronic pain: a systematic review and meta-analysis. *Pain* 152: 533–542.

Vlaeyen, J.W.S. and Linton, S.J. (2000) Fear-avoidance and its consequences in chronic musculoskeletal pain: a state of the art. *Pain* 85: 317–332.

Vlaeyen, J.W.S., Kole-Snijders, A.M.J., Boeren, R.G.B., and van Eek, H. (1995) Fear of movement/(re)injury in chronic low back pain and its relation to behavioral performance. *Pain* 62: 363–372.

Vlaeyen, J.W.S., Morley, S., Linton, S., Boersma, K., and de Jong, J. (2012) *Pain-Related Fear: Exposure-Based Treatment of Chronic Pain*. Seattle: IASP Press.

Von Korff, M. (2013) Healthcare for chronic pain: overuse, underuse, and treatment needs. *Medical Care* 51(10): 857–858.

Wall, P.D. (1979) On the relation of injury to pain. *Pain* 6: 253–264.

Wall, P.D. (1994) Introduction to P.D. Wall and R. Melzack (eds.), *Textbook of Pain*, 3rd ed. Edinburgh: Churchill Livingstone.

Walters, E.T. (1994) Injury-related behavior and neuronal plasticity: an evolutionary perspective on sensitization, hyperalgesia and analgesia. *International Review of Neurobiology* 36: 325–427.

Wampold, B.E. (2005) Establishing specificity in psychotherapy scientifically: design and evidence issues. *Clinical Psychology Science and Practice* 12: 194–197.

Wiech, K., Lin, C.S., Brodersen, K.H., Bingel, U., Ploner, M., and Tracey, I. (2010) Anterior insula integrates information about salience into perceptual decisions about pain. *Journal of Neuroscience* 30(48): 16324–16331.

Williams, A.C. de C. (2002) Facial expression of pain: an evolutionary account. *Behavioral and Brain Sciences* 25: 439–488.

Williams, A.C. de C. (2016) What can evolutionary theory tell us about chronic pain? *Pain* 157(4): 788–790.

Williams, A.C. de C. and Johnson, M. (2011) Persistent pain: not a medically unexplained symptom. *British Journal of General Practice* 61(591): 638–639.

Williams, A.C. de C., Eccleston, C., and Morley, S. (2012) Psychological therapies for the management of chronic pain (excluding headache) in adults. *Cochrane Database of Systematic Reviews*, no. 11: CD007407.

Woolf, C.J. (2010) What is this thing called pain? *Journal of Clinical Investigation* 120(11): 3742–3744.

Zeidan, F., Grant, J.A., Brown, C.A., McHaffie, J.G., and Coghill, R.C. (2012) Mindfulness meditation-related pain relief: evidence for unique brain mechanisms in the regulation of pain. *Neuroscience Letters* 520: 165–173.

12

BIOPSYCHOSOCIAL MODELS OF PAIN

Thomas Hadjistavropoulos

The definition of pain that has been adopted by the International Association for the Study of Pain (IASP) recognizes its complexity. According to IASP, pain is "an unpleasant sensory and emotional experience associated with actual or potential tissue damage, or described in terms of such damage" (Merskey and Bogduk 1994). The definition (see Chapter 31 of this volume for more details) underscores both the subjectivity of pain and its emotional elements. As such, it is consistent with the idea that pain represents a complex psychological phenomenon that cannot be objectively measured nor directly observed. In contrast to IASP's modern conceptualization of pain, earlier influential views, such as the specificity theory of pain (see Melzack 1973 for a review), construed pain as having a direct one-to-one correspondence with tissue damage: the greater the tissue damage, the greater the pain. Despite increases in our understanding of the complexity of pain physiology, biocentric conceptualizations of a one-to-one correspondence between pain and tissue damage remained influential and continue to exert their influence today despite compelling evidence that the experience of pain is determined by a multitude of factors, only one of which is tissue damage (see Chapter 6, this volume, for more details).

1 The gate-control theory of pain

Melzack (1973) highlighted many compelling examples demonstrating an absence of a one-to-one correspondence between pain and tissue damage and such examples were considered in the development of the gate-control theory of pain, which represents the most evidence-based comprehensive conceptualization of the experience (Mendell 2014). For instance, it had been observed that, during the Second World War, wounded soldiers in combat hospitals did not complain of much pain and did not require as much analgesia as one would expect (Beecher 1959). In contrast, civilians with similar injuries were in severe pain and pleading for analgesia. In interpreting the findings of his study, Beecher highlighted that the meaning of the situation had played a role in the pain experience. In the case of soldiers, the injury meant that they would escape alive from the battlefield. For civilians, however, injuries could have severe economic and other negative consequences.

Thinking leading to the gate-control theory was also influenced by anthropological work (e.g., Kosambi 1967; Melzack and Chapman 1973) that documented rituals practiced in various cultures and involve substantial tissue damage (e.g., steel hooks attached to strong ropes and shoved under the skin and muscles in order to allow the celebrant to be suspended from the hooks) with little or no evidence of pain. Moreover, anecdotally, it is easy to think of day to day examples such as being hit in the context of play, as opposed to an assault situation, not being perceived as painful.

The gate-control theory was the first theory to recognize the role of psychological influences in the pain experience. It provided an explanatory mechanism of how ascending peripheral physiological fibers and systems (i.e., transmitting stimulation from the body and the tissues to the spinal cord and, eventually, the brain) and descending input from the brain interact together to determine the nature and extent of the pain experience. The central ideas of the gate-control theory are well supported by research although recent investigations have led to improved descriptions of some of the physiological mechanisms involved in the pain experience (see Mendell 2014) and to recognition that pain can also occur even in the absence of external stimulation through brain mechanisms (Melzack 2001; see also Chapter 5, this volume, for discussion). The original gate-control theory idea that brain activity, reflecting processes such as attention and thoughts, can affect pain experiences is well supported by neuroscience research involving fMRI (functional magnetic resonance imaging) as well as other methodologies (see Hadjistavropoulos et al. 2011; also see Chapter 9, this volume) and provides the basis for the integration of social and psychological parameters in theoretical frameworks related to pain and most notably in biopsychosocial models.

2 Biopsychosocial models

The biopsychosocial model of health and illness, as originally proposed by Engel (1977), reflected dissatisfaction with the biomedical conceptualization of health which construed illness as an entity independent of social, psychological and behavioral influences (Day et al. 2012). In its most general form the biopsychosocial model of health and illness specifies that health and associated quality of life are determined by an interplay of biological (e.g., transmission of ascending inputs from damaged tissue to the brain), social (e.g., social support and cultural factors) and psychological parameters (e.g., catastrophic thoughts about the potential consequences of pain or optimism that the pain problem can be overcome). As a general example, one could consider a problem such as obesity. Genetic/biological factors affect metabolic rates that play a role in weight determination. Cultural factors may affect the extent to which an individual values a certain body weight (e.g., thinness) and may cause that individual to strive (or not) toward that ideal. Social support can also contribute to dieting success. Psychological factors could play a key role as well. For example, an individual may be more likely to overeat and less likely to exercise when he or she is feeling depressed or has lower self-esteem.

The general biopsychosocial conceptualization of pain represents a specific application of a broader conceptualization of disease and illness. This conceptualization is empirically supported. Certainly, biological factors, such as tissue damage, play a role in the pain experience. Social elements also affect this experience. For example, in a series of studies it has been demonstrated that exposure to pain-intolerant models (e.g., experimental confederates instructed to simulate intolerance for experimental pain stimuli by reporting relatively high pain intensities in response to such stimuli) leads participants to report a greater degree of pain (e.g., Craig and Weiss 1971; Craig 1986). Moreover, mothers of young children taught to interact with children in a pain-promoting way, led children to report more pain (e.g., Chambers et al. 2002) and the amount of social support that an individual receives affects responses to pain and related outcomes (Burckhardt 1985; Faucett and Levine 1991; Murphy et al. 1988; Turner and Noh 1988). Finally, psychological factors are predominant. For example, beliefs and attitudes about pain affect the experience, with those who catastrophize about pain being more likely to experience poorer outcomes (Hadjistavropoulos et al. 2011; Sullivan and Stanish 2003). The role of social/psychological factors in the pain experience has also been demonstrated through fMRI research. Coan et al. (2006), for example, studied women who were subjected to electric shock while holding the experimenter's hand, their spouse's hand, or no hand at all. Participants communicated reduced pain unpleasantness when holding their spouse's hand as compared to the other experimental conditions. Consistent with the reports of reduced pain unpleasantness during the spousal hand-holding condition, fMRI results showed a simultaneous pervasive attenuation of activation in the neural systems supporting behavioral and emotional threat responses.

Although studies are supportive of the broad ideas of the biopsychosocial model, the model's general nature makes it very difficult, if not impossible, to test it in its entirety. That is, finding one instance in which the model applies does not necessarily imply that the model applies in all instances (i.e., finding one white cat cannot lead us to conclude that all cats are white). Given this difficulty with the breadth of the general biopsychosocial model, a variety of more specific biopsychosocial models have been developed. These models focus on specific aspects of functioning such as the impact of catastrophic thinking and excessive activity avoidance on the experience and functioning of the individual with pain.

2.1 The Fear Avoidance Model of Pain

An example of a prominent biopsychosocial model is the Fear Avoidance Model of Pain (Vlaeyen and Linton 2000). Upon confrontation with persistent pain, there are two main pathways that a patient could follow. The first is an adaptive pathway. That is, the individual who does not consider the pain experience to be excessively threatening, will react to pain in adaptive ways seeking appropriate rehabilitation and beneficial physical activity. This approach would increase the probability of a positive outcome. On the other hand, a patient who has catastrophic thoughts about the consequences of pain and injury will show high levels of fear of pain and may become excessively avoidant of activity, including beneficial activity such as physiotherapy. Such excessive activity avoidance could contribute to stiffness and deconditioning prolonging chronicity and leading to unfavorable outcomes. Support for aspects of this model exists. For example, fear of pain has been shown to correlate with pain intensity and disability (Crombez et al. 2012; Ditre et al. 2013): fear appears to predict performance on some movement-related tasks, although the findings are mixed (Crombez et al. 1999) and catastrophizing relates to negative outcomes such as increased disability (Quartana et al. 2009). However, the relationship between fear of pain and future disability may not always be mediated by avoidance. In fact, supportive evidence for the Fear Avoidance Model is mostly cross-sectional, not all studies are supportive (e.g., Swinkels-Meewisse et al. 2006), and there may be other pathways leading to excessive avoidance (unrelated to fear) such as recommendations from family and health professionals (Pincus et al. 2010).

2.2 The Communal Model of Pain Catastrophizing

A second example of a model elaborating on a specific aspect of the broader biopsychosocial formulation of pain, is the Communal Model of Pain Catastrophizing (Sullivan et al. 2001b). The Communal Model, like most others, recognizes the importance of physiology in the pain experience. In also recognizing the potential impact of psychological variables and social variables, it focuses specifically on the role of catastrophic thinking (i.e., a psychological variable) about pain in interpersonal contexts. This model postulates that, within an interpersonal context, catastrophizing is a coping strategy utilized to elicit support from others. People who tend to catastrophize may, for example, present with excessive displays of pain in the hope of eliciting better support and pain management within a social/interpersonal context. Unfortunately, social reinforcement of exaggerated illness behavior can serve to sustain it, thus minimizing optimal adjustment to pain. Literature support for the model exists. For example, associations between catastrophizing and intensity of pain behavior have been found (Sullivan et al. 2004; Goubert et al. 2009). That said, there remain central tenets of the model that require more support such as the notion that people who catastrophize display increased pain behavior *in order to garner support from others.*

2.3 The Communications Model of Pain

In contrast to the Fear Avoidance Model and the Communal Model of Pain Catastrophizing that focus on a specific subset of social/psychological variables, the Communications Model of Pain (CMP; e.g., Hadjistavropoulos et al. 2011; Hadjistavropoulos and Craig 2002; Prkachin and Craig 1995) is much broader and describes a wide variety of pain phenomena. The CMP (see Figure 12.1) is based on an earlier A→B→C formulation by Rosenthal (1982) wherein the internal experience of pain (A) is determined by biological, sociocultural and

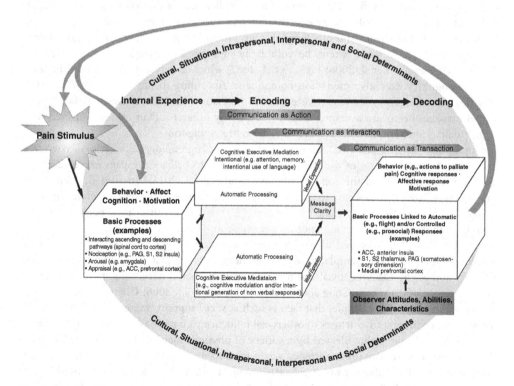

Figure 12.1 The Communications Model of Pain. ACC, anterior cingulated cortex; S1, somatosensory area; S2, second somatosensory area; PAG, periaqueductal gray.
Source: Hadjistavropoulos et al. (2011)

psychological parameters and is encoded in expressive behavior (B) that can then be decoded by observers (C) who then have the capacity of palliating, ignoring or even worsening the pain experience. As Figure 12.1 shows, the ABC sequence is situated in a broad context of socio-cultural, interpersonal, situational and intrapersonal parameters which can affect the experience at any stage (i.e., A, B or C).

The internal experience (A) is represented in the figure by a large solid. The model describes the affective, behavioral, cognitive and motivational manifestations of pain (shown at the top side of the solid) as well as the basic processes that are activated during the pain experience (represented on the side of the solid). It is important to emphasize, from the definition of pain, that affect (emotion) is a necessary component of pain but there can also be additional psychological/cognitive and behavioral components in the pain response. To summarize, pain is characterized by emotions such as fear (e.g., Hale and Hadjistavropoulos 1997), cognitive responses (Sullivan et al. 2005; Sullivan et al. 2001a), behavioral reactions (e.g., facial expressions, paralinguistic vocalizations) and attempts to avoid the painful situation. The extent to which each of these features is salient varies depending on the circumstances. For example, a dental patient will typically choose to not avoid a painful but necessary dental procedure despite fear and concern (manifested as thoughts) about the risks of the procedure.

In the encoding phase (B), expressive behavior is represented by two smaller solids (see Figure 12.1). The top solid represents verbal expressions of pain that are primarily dependent on cognitive executive mediation (represented by a larger side of the solid) although automatic processes such as reflexes (represented by a smaller side of the solid) can also exert an influence. The bottom solid of phase (B) represents non-verbal expressions of pain (e.g., grimaces, a reflexive withdrawal of a limp) that are primarily reliant on reflexive automaticity, although they can, to some extent, be voluntarily suppressed or exaggerated (e.g., Hill and Craig 2002; Campbell et al. 2008; France et al. 2002) which is why a smaller side of the solid shows a cognitive executive mediation component. According to the CMP, the dimension of reflexive automaticity vs. cognitive executive mediation also affects message clarity with verbal messages being, on average, easier to decode by observers than non-verbal behaviors (e.g., paralinguistic vocalizations) which may be more ambiguous.

During the decoding phase (C), represented by the last large solid, the behavioral, cognitive and motivational responses of the observer (e.g., actions to palliate the pain experience) are shown at the top side of the solid (Hadjistavropoulos et al. 2011). In turn the actions of the observer have the capacity to affect the pain experience. The brain regions that are highlighted in the decoding solid (see Figure 12.1) are those that have been shown to become activated when observing another person's pain (Singer et al. 2006).

The CMP is best construed as a systematic synthesis of a very extensive and complex empirical literature. For example, research has demonstrated that in addition to stimulus intensity and physical factors, social and psychological parameters have a significant impact on the experience of pain (e.g., Craig and Weiss 1971; Coan et al. 2006; Chambers et al. 2002). These studies show, for example, that factors such as social support, presence of pain-tolerant models, and communicative actions of others can influence pain responses and report. Similarly, the encoding of pain is also affected by a variety of physical, social and psychological factors. For example, despite some inconsistency across studies, the empirical literature suggests that catastrophic thinking about pain is associated with a propensity to display increased pain reactivity (Sullivan 2008; Vervoort et al. 2009a, 2009b, 2008). As a second example, Dworkin and Chen (1982) have shown that people who undergo a dental procedure in a clinic report greater pain than those who undergo the same procedure in the experimental laboratory.

Finally, the third main step of the CMP (decoding) has also been shown to be influenced by a wide variety of biopsychosocial determinants. For example, social stereotypes based on characteristics that are not relevant to the pain expression (e.g., physical attractiveness, sex and participant age) have been found to affect observer judgements of pain (Hadjistavropoulos et al. 1996). Similarly, observer characteristics, such as professional background, also affect the decoding of pain (e.g., Hadjistavropoulos et al. 1998). Finally, observer psychological tendencies, such as the tendency to catastrophize about pain, affect interpretations of others' pain signals (e.g., Goubert et al. 2009; Pincus and Morley 2001). For example, Martel et al. (2008) showed that a higher level of observer catastrophizing was associated with a lower discrepancy between observers' and sufferers' pain estimates.

Despite a great deal of literature consistent with the biopsychosocial formulations described in the CMP, much of what we know about social influences in the pain experience is based on studies recreating an analogue of the clinical setting (e.g., studies showing photographs or vignettes to health professionals or to students studying the health professions rather than the study of how personal patient characteristics influence professional judgements in clinical settings) (Hadjistavropoulos et al. 2011). More research on the influence of psychosocial parameters in clinical situations is needed. It is important to note, however, that studies of psychological parameters (e.g., such as fear and anxiety; e.g., Koho et al. 2011; Lemay et al. 2011) are more often conducted in clinical settings than studies of social influences.

3 Clinical applications of biopsychosocial ideas

Biopsychosocial ideas have led to the development of psychosocial interventions designed to improve the pain experience and quality of life. The primary focus of such interventions has been on people who suffer from chronic pain, although psychosocial interventions for acute pain (e.g., labor pain, post-operative pain) have also been developed (e.g., Koranyi et al. 2014). These interventions are typically administered in conjunction with other modalities of therapy (e.g., pharmacological, physiotherapy) rather than as stand-alone approaches. In fact, consistent with the biopsychosocial perspective, single-modality treatments (e.g., physiotherapy alone, psychotherapy alone, medication alone) tend to be less effective in the treatment of persistent chronic pain problems than interdisciplinary, multidimensional approaches (Turk et al. 2011). Cognitive-behavioral therapy (CBT) and mindfulness-based approaches, including Acceptance and Commitment Therapy (ACT), are commonly employed interventions that are, ultimately, based on the broad biopsychosocial model of pain (for discussion, see also Chapter 11, this volume). That is, while these interventions recognize the biological basis of pain problems, they emphasize the psychological (e.g., emotion, behavior and cognition) as well as social influences on the pain experience.

3.1 Cognitive-behavioral therapy

The CBT perspective emphasizes the view that pain as well as related emotions and behaviors are affected by interpretation of and inferences about the sensory information and associated circumstances. The following are central assumptions of this perspective (Skinner et al. 2012):

a   Individuals interpret stimuli, and their responses are based on appraisals and expectations. These interpretations may not necessarily be accurate reflections of reality.

b   Beliefs can affect emotion and physiological arousal (e.g., if a situation is believed to be threatening in terms of potential for pain elicitation, it may lead to physiological arousal and fear; such reactions may not be elicited if the situation is not perceived as threatening).
c   Emotion, arousal and behavior may influence thinking.
d   Behavior is reciprocally affected both by the person and the environment.
e   People may have learned maladaptive ways of interpreting and responding (e.g., some people may perceive a pain problem as devastating to one's well-being whereas others may perceive the same pain problem as an inconvenience that can be tolerated and managed).
f   People are capable of changing maladaptive ways of thinking and responding to pain.

CBT emphasizes a variety of techniques designed to change people's maladaptive interpretations (e.g., using a Socratic approach to examine the validity of a person's pain-related beliefs) and replacing these with more adaptive ones. An example would be the thought that "unless my pain is completely gone, there is nothing worthwhile that I can do" which could be replaced with the belief that "there are effective strategies to manage my pain and there are worthwhile activities that I can pursue that would help improve the quality of my life despite my injury."

CBT also targets maladaptive behaviors through the use of approaches such as problem solving around challenges, pacing of activity, and relaxation training. Psychoeducation around the impact of social/psychological factors on pain is also emphasized. The effectiveness of CBT in contributing to the treatment of chronic pain is well supported. That is, it has been shown to have beneficial effects on pain intensity, catastrophizing, mood, pain-related disability and activity interference. These beneficial effects, although found consistently, have been estimated as being moderate in some areas (e.g., mood and catastrophic thinking) and small in other areas (e.g., level of pain and disability) (Ehde et al. 2014).

3.2 Mindfulness and acceptance and commitment approaches

Mindfulness-based approaches have also been gaining popularity in the treatment of chronic pain. Such approaches are based on principles of meditation and focus on attending to the present moment and on observing pain and associated negative thoughts/emotions in a non-judgemental and non-reactive way (Rosenzweig et al. 2010). According to Martin (1997) mindfulness is "a state of psychological freedom that occurs when attention remains quiet and limber, without attachment to any particular point of view" (Martin 1997: 291). The view is that much of the psychological distress associated with chronic pain stems from efforts to control and manage pain-related cognitions and emotions rather than to simply accept them. This contrasts with CBT approaches that emphasize the goal of changing maladaptive cognitions.

Acceptance and commitment approaches to chronic pain incorporate mindfulness. In contrast to CBT, thoughts and feelings associated with pain are neither viewed as helpful nor as unhelpful. Instead of encouraging the client to battle these feelings and thoughts, the client is encouraged to observe them and accept them while focusing on behavior change (committed action) designed to alter the context of the psychological experience (rather than altering its content). The therapy is present-focused (i.e., change does not rely on interpretations of past behavior) and consistent with mindfulness ideas (Hayes et al. 1999; McCracken and Jones 2012). Approaches that primarily emphasize mindfulness as well as acceptance and commitment therapies have shown a great deal of promise in the management of chronic pain with beneficial effects on the pain and associated depression as well as on improving life satisfaction, self-esteem and other related variables (Thorsell et al. 2011; Wicksell et al. 2013, 2008; Wetherell et al. 2011; Dahl, Wilson & Nilsson 2004; Buhrman et al. 2013; McCracken et al. 2013; Yang and McCracken 2014; Morone et al. 2008). The magnitude of the beneficial effects of ACT for chronic pain patients appears to be at least comparable to those of CBT (Wetherell et al. 2011; Veehof et al. 2011; Ost 2014).

4 Conclusion and future directions

Pain is a psychological, physical and social experience. The biopsychosocial formulations of the pain experience are consistent with the most widely accepted conceptualization of the physiological mechanisms involved in the pain experience (the gate-control theory of pain; see Chapters 6 to 10). These formulations enjoy empirical support and explain a variety of phenomena involving social and psychological influences on pain. Despite this, there are challenges. These challenges open directions for future research. For example, more studies of biopsychosocial influences on pain are needed in clinical settings in order to replicate laboratory findings (e.g., that stereotypes based on irrelevant factors, such as sufferer physical attractiveness, affect judgements of another's pain; Hadjistavropoulos et al. 1996). Similarly, more longitudinal investigations are needed to study phenomena over time in order to examine theoretical assumptions that have been tested primarily through correlational research. For example, although associations of catastrophic thinking and disability have been found in correlational research (e.g., Cook et al. 2006), additional longitudinal study is necessary to demonstrate clearly the temporal sequence associated with such phenomena in order to improve our understanding of psychological influences in pain-related disability.

Biopsychosocial formulations are not only of theoretical importance but have also formed the basis for the development of effective psychosocial interventions such as CBT and mindfulness-based approaches including ACT. Consistent with biopsychosocial models, these types of interventions emphasize the role of social (e.g., efforts to optimize social support networks for pain patients) and psychological parameters (e.g., beliefs and attitudes about pain) in the pain experience while, at the same time, accepting the importance of biological factors. Nonetheless, not all patients benefit from such interventions and there are individual differences with respect to the outcomes achieved. As such, future research is likely to focus on researching predictors of differential responsiveness to treatment (possibly facilitating the tailoring of specific interventions for specific patients) and on finding better ways of maintaining treatment gains in the longer term (Ehde et al. 2014; Sturgeon 2014).

Another exciting avenue for future study involves the use of technology in the delivery of psychosocial pain management interventions. In recent years, evidence has begun to emerge that shows that CBT and ACT can be delivered effectively via Internet, allowing for increased access and cost-effectiveness (Trompetter et al. 2015; Law et al. 2012). It is highly probable that we will see a steep increase in the number of investigations focusing on the optimization of the delivery of Internet-delivered psychosocial interventions for chronic pain (e.g., ways of minimizing dropout rates, increasing participation of societal groups who may have more limited access to technology).

Related topics

Chapter 5: Fault lines in familiar concepts of pain (Hill)
Chapter 6: Advances in the neuroscience of pain (Apkarian)
Chapter 7: Neuromatrix theory of pain (Roy and Wager)

References

Beecher, H.K. (1959) *Measurement of Subjective Responses: Quantitative Effects of Drugs.* New York: Oxford University Press.

Buhrman, M., Skoglund, A., Husell, J., Bergström, K., Gordh, T., Hursti, T., Bendelin, N., Furmark, T., and Andersson, G. (2013) Guided Internet-delivered acceptance and commitment therapy for chronic pain patients: a randomized controlled trial. *Behaviour Research and Therapy* 51(6): 307–315.

Burckhardt, C.S. (1985) The impact of arthritis on quality of life. *Nursing Research* 34(1): 11–16.

Campbell, C.M., France, C.R., Robinson, M.E., Logan, H.L., Gefken, G.R., and Fillingim, R.B. (2008) Ethnic differences in the nociceptive flexion reflex (NFR). *Pain* 134: 91–96.

Chambers, C.T., Craig, K.D., and Bennett, S.M. (2002) The impact of maternal behavior on children's pain experiences: an experimental analysis. *Journal of Pediatric Psychology* 27(3): 293–301.

Coan, J.A., Schaefer, H.S., and Davidson, R.J. (2006) Lending a hand: social regulation of the neural response to threat. *Psychological Science* 17(12): 1032–1039.

Cook, A.J., Brawer, P.A., and Vowles, K.E. (2006) The fear-avoidance model of chronic pain: validation and age analysis using structural equation modeling. *Pain* 121: 195–206.

Craig, K.D. (1986) Social modeling influences: pain in context. In R.A. Sternbach (ed.), *The Psychology of Pain*, 2nd ed. New York: Raven Press, pp. 67–96.

Craig, K.D. and Weiss, S.M. (1971) Vicarious influences on pain-threshold determinations. *Journal of Personality and Social Psychology* 19(1): 53–59.

Crombez, G., Vlaeyen, J.W., Heuts, P.H., and Lysens, R. (1999) Pain-related fear is more disabling than pain itself: evidence on the role of pain-related fear in chronic back pain disability. *Pain* 80(1–2): 329–339.

Crombez, G., Eccleston, C., Van Damme, S., Vlaeyen, J.W., and Karoly, P. (2012) Fear-avoidance model of chronic pain: the next generation. *Clinical Journal of Pain* 28(6): 475–483.

Dahl, J., Wilson, K.G., and Nilsson, A. (2004) Acceptance and commitment therapy and the treatment of persons at risk for long-term disability resulting from stress and pain symptoms: a preliminary randomized trial. *Association for Advancement of Behavior Therapy* 35: 785–801.

Day, M., Thorn, B., and Burns, J.W. (2012) The continuing evolution of biopsychosocial interventions for chronic pain. *Journal of Cognitive Psychotherapy* 16(2): 114–129.

Ditre, J.W., Zale, E.L., Kosiba, J.D., and Zvolensky, M.J. (2013) A pilot study of pain-related anxiety and smoking-dependence motives among persons with chronic pain. *Experimental and Clinical Psychopharmacology* 21(6): 443–449.

Dworkin, S.F. and Chen, A.C. (1982) Pain in clinical and laboratory contexts. *Journal of Dental Research* 61(6) 772–774.

Ehde, D.M., Dillworth, T.M., and Turner, J.A. (2014) Cognitive-behavioral therapy for individuals with chronic pain: efficacy, innovations, and directions for research. *American Psychologist* 69(2): 153–166.

Engel, G.L. (1977) The need for a new medical model: a challenge for biomedicine. *Science* (New York) 196(4286): 129–136.

Faucett, J.A. and Levine, J.D. (1991) The contributions of interpersonal conflict to chronic pain in the presence or absence of organic pathology. *Pain* 44(1): 35–43.

France, C.R., France, J.L., Absi, M.A., Ring, C. , and McIntyre, D. (2002) Catastrophizing is related to pain ratings, but not nociceptive flexion reflex threshold. *Pain* 99: 459–463.

Goubert, L., Vervoort, T., Cano, A., and Crombez, G. (2009) Catastrophizing about their children's pain is related to higher parent–child congruency in pain ratings: an experimental investigation. *European Journal of Pain* (London, UK) 13(2): 196–201.

Hadjistavropoulos, T. and Craig, K.D. (2002) A theoretical framework for understanding self-report and observational measures of pain: a communications model. *Behavior Research and Therapy* 40(5): 551–570.

Hadjistavropoulos, T., McMurtry, B., and Craig, K.D. (1996) Beautiful faces in pain: biases and accuracy in the perception of pain. *Psychology and Health* 11: 411–420.

Hadjistavropoulos, T., LaChapelle, D., MacLeod, F., Hale, C., O'Rourke, N., and Craig, K.D. (1998) Cognitive functioning and pain reactions in hospitalized elders. *Pain Research and Management* 3: 145–151.

Hadjistavropoulos, T., Craig, K.D., Duck, S., Cano, A., Goubert, L., Jackson, P.L., Mogil, J.S., Rainville, P., Sullivan, M.J., de C. Williams, A.C., Vervoort, T., and Fitzgerald, T.D. (2011) A biopsychosocial formulation of pain communication. *Psychological Bulletin* 137(6): 910–939.

Hale, C. and Hadjistavropoulos, T. (1997) Emotional components of pain. *Pain Research and Management* 2: 217–225.

Hayes, S.C., Strosahl, K., and Wilson, K.G. (1999) *Acceptance and Commitment Therapy: An Experiential Approach to Behavior Change*. New York: Guildford Press.

Hill, M.L. and Craig, K.D. (2002) Detecting deception in pain expressions: The structure of genuine and deceptive facial displays. *Pain* 98: 135–144.

Koho, P., Orenius, T., Kautiainen, H., Haanpaa, M., Pohjolainen, T., and Hurri, H. (2011) Association of fear of movement and leisure-time physical activity among patients with chronic pain. *Journal of Rehabilitation Medicine* 43(9): 794–799.

Koranyi, S., Barth, J., Trelle, S., Strauss, B.M., and Rosendahl, J. (2014) Psychological interventions for acute pain after open heart surgery. *Cochrane Database Systematic Reviews*, no. 5: CD009984. doi:10.1002/14651858.CD009984.pub2.

Kosambi, D.D. (1967) *Scientific American* 216 (February): 105–114.

Law, E.F., Murphy, L.K., and Palermo, T.M. (2012) Evaluating treatment participation in an internet-based behavioral intervention for pediatric chronic pain. *Journal of Pediatric Psychology* 37(8): 893–903.

Lemay, K., Wilson, K.G., Buenger, U., Jarvis, V., Fitzgibbon, E., Bhimji, K., and Dobkin, P.L. (2011) Fear of pain in patients with advanced cancer or in patients with chronic noncancer pain. *Clinical Journal of Pain* 27(2): 116–124.

McCracken, L.M. and Jones, R. (2012) Treatment for chronic pain for adults in the seventh and eighth decades of life: a preliminary study of Acceptance and Commitment Therapy (ACT). *Pain Medicine* (Malden, MA) 13(7): 860–867.

McCracken, L.M., Sato, A., and Taylor, G.J. (2013) A trial of a brief group-based form of Acceptance and Commitment Therapy (ACT) for chronic pain in general practice: pilot outcome and process results. *Journal of Pain* 14(11): 1398–1406.

Martel, M. O., Thibault, P., Roy, C., Catchlove, R., Sullivan, M. J.L. (2008) Contextual determinants of pain judgments. *Pain* 139: 562–568.

Martin, J.R. (1997) Mindfulness: a proposed common factor. *Journal of Psychotherapy Integration* 7(4): 291–312.

Melzack, R. (1973) *The Puzzle of Pain*, 1st ed. New York: Basic Books.

Melzack, R. (2001) Pain and the neuromatrix in the brain. *Journal of Dental Education* 65(12): 1378–1382.

Melzack, R. and Chapman, C.R. (1973) Psychologic aspects of pain. *Postgraduate Medicine* 53(6): 69–75.

Mendell, L.M. (2014) Constructing and deconstructing the gate theory of pain. *Pain* 155(2): 210–216.

Merskey, H. and Bogduk, N. (eds.) (1994) *Classification of Chronic Pain*, 2nd ed. Seattle: IASP Press.

Morone, N.E., Greco, C.M., and Weiner, D.K. (2008) Mindfulness meditation for the treatment of chronic low back pain in older adults: a randomized controlled pilot study. *Pain* 134(3): 310–319.

Murphy, S., Creed, F., and Jayson, M.I. (1988) Psychiatric disorder and illness behaviour in rheumatoid arthritis. *British Journal of Rheumatology* 27(5): 357–363.

Ost, L.G. (2014) The efficacy of Acceptance and Commitment Therapy: an updated systematic review and meta-analysis. *Behaviour Research and Therapy* 61: 105–121.

Pincus, T. and Morley, S. (2001) Cognitive-processing bias in chronic pain: a review and integration. *Psychological Bulletin* 127(5): 599–617.

Pincus, T., Smeets, R.J., Simmonds, M.J., and Sullivan, M.J. (2010) The fear avoidance model disentangled: improving the clinical utility of the fear avoidance model. *Clinical Journal of Pain* 26(9): 739–746.

Prkachin, K.M. and Craig, K.D. (1995) Expressing pain: the communication and interpretation of facial pain signals. *Journal of Nonverbal Behavior* 19: 191–205.

Quartana, P.J., Campbell, C.M., and Edwards, R.R. (2009) Pain catastrophizing: a critical review. *Expert Review of Neurotherapeutics* 9(5): 745–758.

Rosenthal, R. (1982) Conducting judgement studies. In K. Scherer and P. Ekman (eds.), *Handbook of Methods in Nonverbal Behavior Research*. New York: Cambridge University Press, pp. 287–361.

Rosenzweig, S., Greeson, J.M., Reibel, D.K., Green, J.S., Jasser, S.A., and Beasley, D. (2010) Mindfulness-based stress reduction for chronic pain conditions: variation in treatment outcomes and role of home meditation practice. *Journal of Psychosomatic Research* 68(1): 29–36.

Singer, T., Seymour, B., O'Doherty, J. P., Stephan, K. E., Dolan, R. J., and Frith, C. D. (2006) Empathic neural responses are modulated by the perceived fairness of others. *Nature* 439: 466–469.

Skinner, M., Wilson, H.D., and Turk, D.C. (2012) Cognitive-behavioral perspective and cognitive–behavioral therapy for people with chronic pain: Distinctions, outcomes, and innovations. *Journal of Cognitive Psychotherapy* 26(2): 93–113.

Sturgeon, J.A. (2014) Psychological therapies for the management of chronic pain. *Psychology Research and Behavior Management* 7: 115–124.

Sullivan, M.J. (2008) Toward a biopsychomotor conceptualization of pain. *Clinical Journal of Pain* 24: 281–290.

Sullivan, M.J., and Stanish, W.D. (2003) Psychologically based occupational rehabilitation: the Pain-Disability Prevention Program. *Clinical Journal of Pain* 19(2): 97–104.

Sullivan, M.J., Rodgers, W.M., and Kirsch, I. (2001a) Catastrophizing, depression and expectancies for pain and emotional distress. *Pain* 91(1–2): 147–154.

Sullivan, M.J., Thorn, B., Haythornthwaite, J.A., Keefe, F., Martin, M., Bradley, L.A., and Lefebvre, J.C. (2001b) Theoretical perspectives on the relation between catastrophizing and pain. *Clinical Journal of Pain* 17(1): 52–64.

Sullivan, M.J., Adams, H., and Sullivan, M.E. (2004) Communicative dimensions of pain catastrophizing: social cueing effects on pain behaviour and coping. *Pain* 107(3): 220–226.

Sullivan, M.J., Feuerstein, M., Gatchel, R., Linton, S.J., and Pransky, G. (2005) Integrating psychosocial and behavioral interventions to achieve optimal rehabilitation outcomes. *Journal of Occupational Rehabilitation* 15(4): 475–489.

Swinkels-Meewisse, J.E.J., Roelofs, J., Schouten, E.G.W., Oostendorp, R.A., and Vlaeyen, J.W. (2006) Fear of Movement/(re) injury predicting chronic disabling low back pain: a prospective inception cohort study. *Spine* 31: 658–664.

Thorsell, J., Finnes, A., Dahl, J., Lundgren, T., Gybrant, M., Gordh, T., and Buhrman, M. (2011) A comparative study of 2 manual-based self-help interventions, Acceptance and Commitment Therapy and applied relaxation, for persons with chronic pain. *Clinical Journal of Pain* 27(8): 716–723.

Trompetter, H.R., Bohlmeijer, E.T., Veehof, M.M., and Schreurs, K.M. (2015) Internet-based guided self-help intervention for chronic pain based on Acceptance and Commitment Therapy: a randomized controlled trial. *Journal of Behavioral Medicine* 38(1): 66–80.

Turk, D.C., Wilson, H.D., and Cahana, A. (2011) Treatment of chronic non-cancer pain. *Lancet* (London) 377(9784): 2226–2235.

Turner, R.J. and Noh, S. (1988) Physical disability and depression: a longitudinal analysis. *Journal of Health and Social Behavior* 29(1): 23–37.

Veehof, M.M., Oskam, M.J., Schreurs, K.M., and Bohlmeijer, E.T. (2011) Acceptance-based interventions for the treatment of chronic pain: a systematic review and meta-analysis. *Pain* 152(3): 533–542.

Vervoort, T., Goubert, L., Eccleston, C., Verhoeven, K., De Clercq, A., Buysse, A., and Crombez, G. (2008) The effects of parental presence upon the facial expression of pain: the moderating role of child pain catastrophizing. *Pain* 138(2): 277–285.

Vervoort, T., Goubert, L., and Crombez, G. (2009a) The relationship between high catastrophizing children's facial display of pain and parental judgment of their child's pain. *Pain* 142(1–2): 142–148.

Vervoort, T., Goubert, L., Eccleston, C., Vandenhende, M., Claeys, O., Clarke, J., and Crombez, G. (2009b) Expressive dimensions of pain catastrophizing: an observational study in adolescents with chronic pain. *Pain* 146(1–2): 170–176.

Vlaeyen, J.W. and Linton, S.J. (2000) Fear-avoidance and its consequences in chronic musculoskeletal pain: a state of the art. *Pain* 85(3): 317–332.

Wetherell, J.L., Afari, N., Rutledge, T., Sorrell, J.T., Stoddard, J.A., Petkus, A.J., Solomon, B.C., Lehman, D.H., Liu, L., Lang, A.J., and Atkinson, J.H. (2011) A randomized, controlled trial of Acceptance and Commitment Therapy and cognitive-behavioral therapy for chronic pain. *Pain* 152(9): 2098–2107.

Wicksell, R.K., Ahlqvist, J., Bring, A., Melin, L., and Olsson, G.L. (2008) Can exposure and acceptance strategies improve functioning and life satisfaction in people with chronic pain and whiplash-associated disorders (WAD)? A randomized controlled trial. *Cognitive Behaviour Therapy* 37(3): 169–182.

Wicksell, R.K., Kemani, M., Jensen, K., Kosek, E., Kadetoff, D., Sorjonen, K., Ingvar, M., and Olsson, G.L. (2013) Acceptance and Commitment Therapy for fibromyalgia: a randomized controlled trial. *European Journal of Pain* (London, UK) 17(4): 599–611.

Yang, S. and McCracken, L.M. (2014) Acceptance and Commitment Therapy for chronic pain case study and commentary. *Journal of Clinical Outcomes Management* 21(3): 134–144.

13

PSYCHOGENIC PAIN

Old and new

Mark D. Sullivan

1 Introduction

The concept of psychogenic pain has a long and hoary history in both the clinical and philosophical literature on pain. Sensible modern scholars are now expected to reject the concept of psychogenic pain with a quick toss of the head. However, I believe it is time for a serious reconsideration of psychogenic pain and the dualistic assumptions about physical and mental causation within which it is usually situated. Many of these assumptions are not compatible with the presentation of pain as a clinical problem or with contemporary research into the neuroscience of pain.

In modern medicine, the concept of psychogenic pain is poorly defined. Rather than clearly define psychogenic pain, clinicians often oppose it to something clearer and more definite (Portenoy 1989). Most crudely, psychogenic pain is opposed to "real pain" or pain that can be associated with observable tissue damage in the body. Here, psychogenic pain is implied to be "unreal" or "imaginary" pain, though no one ever explains what that is. I don't think I have ever met a patient who was complaining of unreal or imaginary pain. In more sophisticated contexts, psychogenic pain is opposed to "somatogenic pain" (APA 1994).

This is a purely physical or physiological pain produced by the body and brain, without any involvement of psychological processes.

Philosophers have been fascinated by this form of pain since Descartes proposed his mechanical model of pain perception. He illustrated this model with the famous image of the boy with his foot in the fire. (See Figure 6.1.) The damage produced by the fire tugged on a nerve that ran from the boy's foot, through his spinal cord, and up into his brain where pain was produced, much like someone ringing a church bell. In the 1970s and 1980s, materialist philosophers told us that we would soon stop expressing pain through terms like "ouch!" that referred to the subjective experience of pain. We would replace these antiquated folk psychology concepts with modern scientific descriptions of the physiological processes that produce pain such as "my C-fibers are firing." Unfortunately for these philosophers, it turns out that activation of C-fibers by peripheral nociceptors is neither necessary nor sufficient for the experience of pain (Moseley and Vlaeyen 2015). Needless to say, we have not replaced reference to pain with reference to C-fibers firing (Bickle 2012).

But the dream of finding a purely objective "neurological signature" for pain lives on. For example, in 2013, the *New England Journal of Medicine* published "An fMRI-Based Neurologic Signature of Physical Pain" by Wager et al. (2013). This paper described a pattern of brain activation produced by experimental heat stimuli that predicted pain intensity in individual persons with high sensitivity and specificity (for further discussion, see Chapter 7, this volume). The title of this paper makes its agenda clear: it is describing a neurological signature of physical pain. This is about access to pain independent of subjectivity or psychological processes. Wager et al. argue that this purely objective access to pain will allow us to bypass the flawed and mediated access to pain provided by patient self-report. This ideal of a fully objectified and "de-psychologized" pain is the concept against which psychogenic pain is now generally defined. This is a pain without personal interpretation. But this is a trap. Only when we escape the dualistic opposition between purely psychogenic and purely somatogenic pain, will we achieve a clinically useful and philosophically robust concept of pain.

2 History of psychogenic pain concepts

The recent history of the psychiatric diagnosis of "psychogenic pain" is instructive. Before 1980, psychologically caused pain was understood in terms of psychodynamic processes. These concerned the dynamic interaction of emotional and motivational forces that affect behavior and states of mind. Sigmund Freud drew upon the work of Anton Mesmer and Jean Charcot that showed hypnosis could reverse paralysis and other conversion symptoms such as blindness or deafness. Freud interpreted these effects of hypnosis as evidence that powerful unconscious processes could cause physical symptoms like pain (Breuer and Freud 1966). He used hypnosis and free association to uncover and resolve these unconscious conflicts. In the nineteenth and twentieth centuries, psychodynamic forces were used to explain pain and other physical symptoms that could not be explained by observable changes in the body. For example, in 1889 Hermann Oppenheim developed the concept of traumatic neurosis that wedded elements of hysteria and neurasthenia (syndrome of lassitude, fatigue, headache) to explain physical symptoms as the result of physical reactions to fright (Holdorff 2011). In a 1959 paper, "Psychogenic Pain and the Pain-Prone Patient," George Engel proposed that psychogenic pain arose from guilt and an intolerance of success (Engel 1959). He argued that pain functioned as a substitute for loss or a replacement for aggression. In the 1968 second edition of the American Psychiatric Association's *Diagnostic and Statistical Manual* (DSM-II), psychogenic pain was codified as part of psychophysiological disorders and described under "painful conditions caused by emotional factors" (APA 1968).

In 1980, DSM-III introduced a new diagnostic category for pain problems, "Psychogenic Pain Disorder" (APA 1980). To qualify, a patient needed to have: severe and prolonged pain inconsistent with neuroanatomical distribution of pain receptors or without detectable organic cause or observable tissue damage. Related organic pathology was allowed, but the pain had to be "grossly in excess" of what was expected on the basis of physical exam. Difficulties in establishing that pain was psychogenic led to changes in the diagnosis for DSM-IIIR, published in 1987 (APA 1987). Here, the diagnosis was renamed "Somatoform Pain Disorder," and three major changes were made in the diagnostic criteria. The requirements for etiologic psychological factors and lack of other contributing mental disorders were eliminated and a requirement for "preoccupation with pain for at least six months" was added. In DSM-IIIR, therefore, Somatoform Pain Disorder becomes purely a diagnosis of exclusion. The diagnosis is not made on the basis of a clear set of signs and symptoms, but when medical disorders are excluded in a patient "preoccupied" with pain.

When it came time to revise these criteria for DSM-IV, the subcommittee on pain disorders found that, despite these changes to improve the diagnosis in DSM-IIIR, "Somatoform Pain Disorder" was rarely used in research projects or clinical practice. They identified a number of reasons for this: (1) the meaning of "preoccupation with pain" is unclear, (2) whether pain exceeds that expected is difficult to determine, (3) the diagnosis does not apply to many patients disabled by pain where a medical condition is contributory, (4) the term "somatoform pain disorder" implies that this pain is somehow different from organic pain, and (5) acute pain of less than six months duration was excluded (King and Strain 1992).

Psychogenic pain survived in DSM-IV as a subtype of the psychiatric diagnosis of Pain Disorder (APA 1994). This diagnosis requires (a) pain in one or more anatomical sites is of sufficient severity to warrant clinical attention, (b) pain causes clinically significant distress or impairment in social, occupational, or other important areas of functioning, (c) psychological factors are judged to have an important role in the onset, severity, exacerbation, or maintenance of the pain, (d) the symptom of pain is not intentionally produced or feigned (as in Factitious Disorder or Malingering), (e) the pain is not better accounted for by a Mood, Anxiety, or Psychotic Disorder and does not meet criteria for Dyspareunia. Though great efforts were made to overcome the shortcomings of the DSM-III and DSM-IIIR definitions, DSM-IV Pain Disorder remained a diagnosis of exclusion founded upon unclear notions of medically unexplained pain and psychologically caused pain. No clear criteria were provided for when pain was medically unexplained or exceeded what was expected given a certain amount of tissue damage. Nor were clear criteria or mechanisms provided for the psychological causation of pain (Creed and Gureje 2012).

The most current, fifth edition of the *Diagnostic and Statistical Manual* was issued in 2013 (DSM-5) (APA 2013). It does not include a pain specific disorder. Instead, it includes Somatic Symptom Disorder (SSD), a single diagnosis that replaces three of the DSM-IV somatoform disorders (Somatization Disorder, Pain Disorder, and Undifferentiated Somatoform Disorder). The diagnostic criteria for SSD require the presence of one or more physical symptoms lasting six months or longer that are associated with excessive thoughts, feelings, or behaviors. Three specifiers describe the nature (e.g., with predominant pain), duration (e.g., persistent, if longer than six months), and severity (e.g., mild, moderate, or severe) of the symptoms. The diagnosis of SSD in DSM-5 thus abandons criteria requiring that pain be medically unexplained or psychologically caused in favor of a focus on excessive concern. But critics have argued that this makes the diagnosis far too inclusive and risks mislabeling medical illness as mental disorder (Frances and Chapman 2013; Frances 2013; Hauser and Wolfe 2013). These critics propose reintroducing the former criteria concerning medical and psychological causation which had disappeared from the DSM by 1994.

How are we to escape this oscillation between psychogenic pain criteria that are too nonspecific and criteria that are too specific? Either all pain without adequate medical explanation is psychogenic by default, or a specific pain is attributed to a specific psychological conflict (e.g., by Franz Alexander [1950]). We are drawn to the concept of psychogenic pain because it fills the gaps left when our attempts to explain clinical pain exclusively in terms of tissue damage fail. But the concept of psychogenic pain as it has been laid out in recent editions of the DSM is an empty concept. Positive criteria for the identification of psychogenic pain, mechanisms for the production of psychogenic pain, and specific therapies for psychogenic pain are lacking (Sullivan 2000). The diagnosis of many psychiatric disorders, such as depression and post-traumatic stress disorder, can be very helpful to clinicians caring for patients with chronic pain by pointing toward specific effective therapies. But the diagnosis of psychogenic pain too often only serves to stigmatize further the patient who

Mark D. Sullivan

experiences chronic pain. Patients feel as if they are being told their pain is not real, is not caused by an injury, and will not be covered by their medical insurance or worker's compensation claim.

3 Modern pain psychology

Over the past forty years, cognitive-behavioral therapy (CBT) has become the most popular and well-tested psychological approach to managing patients with chronic pain. CBT grew out of behavioral therapies for chronic pain which sought to promote adaptive behavior using principles of learning theory. As it came to be recognized that cognitive processes determined which environmental events were reinforcing for a behavior and which were not, treatment was expanded to address the patient's thoughts, beliefs, and appraisals as well as behaviors. (For further discussion, see Chapter 11, this volume.)

CBT is often justified through reference to the gate-control theory of pain that describes the modulation of nociception in the spinal cord by descending influences from the brain. These influences include psychological processes such as threat, depression, and anxiety. Though the gate-control theory provides a scientific rationale for a fully biopsychosocial model of pain (see Chapter 12, this volume), where psychological processes affect pain itself as well as the suffering and disability that arises from pain, this is not how CBT is generally focused in clinical practice. The usual clinical focus of CBT is summarized by the maxim: "pain is unavoidable, but suffering is optional" (Moseley and Butler 2015).

The primary focus of CBT is thus on the appraisal of pain and coping with pain rather than the causation of pain. In practice, a CBT therapist usually approaches pain as something given to the patient by a physiological process unaltered by psychological or personal factors. In contrast, the suffering and disability that accompany this pain are approached as constructed out of psychological as well as physiological processes. CBT thus focuses on helping patients live well despite pain, rather than reducing the amount of pain that they feel. Therefore, this most popular psychological treatment for chronic pain does not challenge the somatogenic model of pain causation. I believe one principal reason for this is that the psychologists who developed CBT for pain and utilize it in medical settings did not want to defend a psychogenic model of pain causation or directly challenge the reigning biomedical somatogenic pain causation model (Moseley and Butler 2015).

Recently, an adaptation of CBT called Acceptance and Commitment Therapy (ACT) has been developed. Rather than the CBT focus on challenging and controlling cognitions, the ACT focus is on accepting pain and discomfort while remaining committed to values-based action (McCracken and Vowles 2014; see also Chapters 11 and 12, this volume, for review).

A number of features of ACT are worth noting here. First, the feasibility and utility of pain acceptance is not determined by pain intensity. That means acceptance and mindfulness can be useful even when pain is severe. Although some ACT studies have shown modest reductions in pain intensity, this is decidedly not the focus of ACT treatment. ACT urges adoption of a mindful, accepting stance toward pain and a dedication to acting in accord with one's most deeply held values. ACT is therefore agnostic about whether pain is somatogenic or psychogenic. Because it is not focused on pain reduction, it does not address pain causation. Pain reduction may occur incidentally, because, as Bill Fordyce was fond of saying, people who have something better to do don't hurt as much.

In summary, current psychological therapies for chronic pain are well-proven and widely used, but they do not utilize or address the concept of psychogenic pain. CBT accomplishes this by focusing on the suffering and disability that result from pain rather than pain itself.

ACT remains agnostic about the cause of pain as it urges acceptance of pain and a renewed commitment to valued action. This stands in contrast to psychodynamic and psychoanalytic therapies for pain which sought to address the psychological causes of pain.

4 Role of psychological trauma in chronic pain

One important example of psychogenic pain is pain that follows psychological trauma. Exposure to events that pose a threat to personal integrity can be psychologically traumatic. It is estimated that 70 percent of adults living in the US have been exposed to traumatic events (Norris 1992; Resnick et al. 1993). Most people who experience traumatic events do not experience lasting effects, though people exposed to motor vehicle accidents, sexual assault, and military combat appear more likely to have lasting effects of trauma. The most prominent lasting effect of psychological trauma is Post-Traumatic Stress Disorder (PTSD). The lifetime prevalence of PTSD in the US population is 7.8 percent. PTSD symptoms emerge in 30 percent of those exposed to extreme stressors within days of the exposure, but usually resolve in a few weeks. For 10–20 percent of those exposed, PTSD symptoms persist with impairment in functioning. Of patients with PTSD, 50 percent improve without treatment in one year, while a third develop a chronic disorder that lasts for years (Kessler et al. 1995). PTSD is defined in DSM-5 as having seven components: (1) exposure to severe trauma, such as threatened death, (2) re-experiencing of the traumatic event through intrusive memories, nightmares, or flashbacks, (3) avoidance of trauma reminders, (4) negative alterations in cognition and mood such as inability to remember traumatic event as well as negative beliefs and emotions regarding the event, (5) altered arousal and reactivity such as irritable or self-destructive behavior, (6) persistence for over one month, and (7) significant distress or functional impairment (APA 2013). Physical trauma may be one component of the psychological trauma, but need not be.

Chronic pain is reported by 35–50 percent of patients with PTSD, regardless of the trauma experienced (Asmundson et al. 2002). The most common kinds of pain associated with PTSD are pelvic pain, low-back pain, facial pain, bladder pain, and fibromyalgia (widespread musculoskeletal pain). PTSD is also common among patients presenting for care of chronic pain, with 7–50 percent meeting criteria (Otis et al. 2003). PTSD is especially prevalent in some subsets of the population with chronic pain. It is seen in 39 percent of motor vehicle accident survivors who present for care of pain, as well as 39 percent of assault victims, and 35 percent of injured workers sent for rehab. Among patients with fibromyalgia, 20 percent currently meet criteria for PTSD, while 42 percent have met criteria at some point in their life. In young adults, PTSD is the psychiatric disorder most strongly associated with medically unexplained pain (Andreski et al. 1998).

PTSD and chronic pain may reinforce each other in multiple ways. Severe acute pain can be traumatic. Acute pain level after trauma predicts PTSD (Norman et al. 2008). Chronic pain may function as a reminder of the trauma, setting up a cycle of mutual maintenance between pain and PTSD. PTSD also prompts the re-experiencing of trauma, which itself triggers arousal that leads to avoidance and pain through muscle tension. This can lead to perpetual avoidance. In a prospective study, baseline re-experiencing and avoidance predicted arousal and pain at three months, which then predicted re-experiencing, avoidance, arousal, and pain at twelve months (Liedl et al. 2010). If the original injury is seen as the result of injustice or unfair treatment, both PTSD and pain are likely to persist (Sullivan et al. 2009).

PTSD is not only common in patients with chronic pain. It changes the experience of chronic pain and the treatment received. Chronic pain patients who have PTSD report more intense pain and affective distress as well as higher levels of disability than those without PTSD. In a landmark study of 141,029 Iraq/Afghanistan veterans with chronic pain treated in VA hospitals, it was noted that approximately 10 percent received opioid therapy (e.g., morphine, oxycodone). This included 6.5 percent of veterans without mental health disorders, 11.7 percent with non-PTSD mental health disorders, and 17.8 percent of veterans with PTSD. Thus, mental health disorders doubled the rate of opioid therapy and PTSD tripled the rate of opioid therapy compared to veterans without mental health disorders. Furthermore, veterans with PTSD were more likely to receive: higher-dose opioids, two or more opioids, concurrent sedative-hypnotics, and early opioid refills. They also showed the highest rates of adverse clinical outcomes from opioid therapy (Seal et al. 2012).

This PTSD research suggests that psychological trauma may play as important a role as physical trauma in the development, severity, course, and treatment of chronic pain. This suggests that much of chronic pain may be simultaneously somatogenic and psychogenic. Indeed, in a sample of 1,206 patients seen at the University of Washington Center for Pain Relief, endorsement of 0–4 PTSD symptom domains was linearly related to the severity of all pain clinical outcomes monitored, including not only depression and anxiety, but pain intensity, activity interference, sleep interference, disability, global health, and opioid risk (personal communication, paper in preparation).

There is research that suggests that the importance of physical and psychological factors in the causation of chronic pain may shift over time. A prospective study of patients with low-back pain using multiple fMRI (functional magnetic resonance imaging) brain scans showed that as back pain evolves from acute and subacute to chronic, the associated brain activity shifts from nociceptive regions involved in acute pain to emotion-related circuitry (Hashmi et al. 2013). Importantly, this back pain usually feels the same to the patient when it is acute (less than three months' duration) and when it is chronic (more than three months' duration). Thus, the brain is involved in both acute back pain that we are likely to label somatogenic due to its frequent association with physical trauma, and the brain is involved in chronic back pain that we are likely to label psychogenic due to our inability to identify any associated damage to the back. In contrast to the experimental pain studied by Wager et al., it appears that clinical pain does not have a single "neurological signature." Hence, our opposition of somatogenic and psychogenic pain may be based on outdated neuroscience and not clinically useful.

We are not only inclined to distinguish pain with physical causes from pain with psychological causes, we are inclined to dismiss psychogenic pain as less real and important than somatogenic pain. This is most apparent in medicolegal contexts where psychological trauma is much more difficult to verify and much less likely to result in compensation in tort or workers' injury cases. But physical pain and social pain may be more similar than we think.

5 Physical and social pain arise from similar neurophysiological processes

Most people would rather have a broken bone than a broken heart. We experience social rejection, exclusion, or loss as among the most "painful" experiences that we endure. Research, largely out of the laboratory of Naomi Eisenberger at UCLA, suggests that painful feelings produced by social disconnection share the same neurobiological substrates as experiences of physical pain (Eisenberger et al. 2003). She has hypothesized that "threats to social connection may be just as detrimental to survival as threats to basic physical safety and thus may be processed by some of the same underlying neural circuitry" (Eisenberger 2012: 422). She suggests that in social primates "the social attachment system may have piggybacked onto the opioid substrates of the physical pain system to maintain proximity with others, eliciting distress upon separation (through low opioid receptor activity) and comfort upon reunion (through high opioid receptor activity)." Hence the brain processes somatogenic and psychogenic pain in similar ways. (Cf. Chapter 7, this volume.)

Other research suggests clinical parallels between social and physical pain. Sensitivity to social and that to physical pain tend to vary together. In clinical studies, patients with chronic pain are more sensitive to social pain as evidenced by greater fear and avoidance of social interactions (Eisenberger et al. 2011). Conversely, heightened sensitivity to social pain (e.g., anxious attachment style) is associated with more physical symptoms, including pain (Ciechanowski et al. 2002). In experimental studies, individuals who are more sensitive to physical noxious stimuli also report more social pain in response to social exclusion (Eisenberger et al. 2006). Finally, social and physical pain respond to the same treatments. It is well known that opioids relieve social pain as well as physical pain (Panksepp et al. 1978). It is perhaps more surprising that the over-the-counter pain reliever acetaminophen (Tylenol) was shown to reduce social pain in a double-blind placebo-controlled study (Dewall et al. 2010). Hence, the same treatments relieve somatogenic and psychogenic pain.

6 Explaining pain without reference to psychogenic or somatogenic categories

Clinical pain is caused by some combination of nociception (detection of noxious stimuli by specialized peripheral receptors) and personal threat (Wall 2002). If nociception is accompanied by a reduction rather than an increase in personal threat, the person may experience no pain. This is what Henry Beecher famously reported after observing soldiers with traumatic injuries on the beach at Anzio in the Second World War. Because injury was a ticket out of this highly lethal battlefield, it increased rather than decreased personal safety and was associated with little pain and few requests for morphine (Beecher 1946). As described above, nociception is generally more important in acute and experimental pain, while threat is more important in chronic pain. Contrary to general belief, nociception is probably less necessary for much of clinical pain than personal threat or a sense of danger. Many patients with common chronic pain syndromes such as fibromyalgia and low-back pain do not show evidence of tissue damage or nociception. Thus for the most common chronic pain syndromes, the "psychogenic" elements are more important than the "somatogenic" elements.

Lorimer Moseley and David Butler from Australia have incorporated these insights into their Explaining Pain program. "Explaining Pain (EP) refers to a range of educational interventions that aim to change someone's understanding of the biological processes that are thought to underpin pain as a mechanism to reduce pain itself … .The core objective of the EP approach to treatment is to shift one's conceptualization of pain from that of a marker of tissue damage or pathology, to that of a marker of the perceived need to protect body tissue" (Moseley and Butler 2015: 807, abstract). The core insight transmitted to patients by the EP program is that the pain system is not a damage-detection system. It is a danger-detection system. Not all danger is experienced as pain; often we feel anxiety or fear. But danger to bodily tissue is an important, often necessary, component of clinical pain. While damage can be detected on physical examination and MRI scans, danger cannot. Many features of the person's situation beyond the amount of tissue damage determine how much pain he or she will feel. This attention to the importance of context in understanding pain experience takes us well beyond the classic opposition between psychogenic and somatogenic pain (Moseley and Arntz 2007). The central role of context means that purely somatogenic pain is rare in clinical practice. Indeed, the importance of context emphasizes something about the under-lying biological mechanisms of pain that is ignored by "neurophilosophers": pain is funda-mentally dependent on meaning (Dennett 1981; Arntz and Claassens 2004; see also Chapter 9, this volume).

"EP emphasizes that any credible evidence of danger to body tissue can increase pain and any credible evidence of safety to body tissue can decrease pain" (Moseley and Butler 2015: 808). Use of EP in a wide variety of formats has been proven to improve patients' pain and disability when added to other programs that aim to increase mobility and exercise (Moseley et al. 2004). Key messages in the EP program include: the variable relationship between nociception and pain, the potent influence of context on pain, up-regulation in the danger-detection system as pain persists, the influence on pain of several interacting protective sys-tems, and above all, the adaptability and trainability of our pain biology. Unlike CBT and ACT, EP does challenge the reigning biomedical model concerning the causation of pain. EP moves beyond the opposition of psychogenic and somatogenic pain not only in theory, but in practice. It has fashioned a clinically effective treatment that shifts patients' conception of pain from damage detection to danger detection.

7 Conclusion

Psychogenic pain makes no sense in the biomedical and mechanical approach to pain still prevalent in much of professional allopathic medicine – other than as a way to dismiss and stigmatize patients' pain as imaginary or exaggerated. We are right to discard this old concept. But the most informed and effective conceptions of clinical and chronic pain have moved beyond the opposition between psychogenic and somatogenic pain to focus on danger rather than damage as the cause of pain. This new conception of clinical and chronic pain as both psychogenic and somatogenic is more compatible with modern pain neuroscience and with the presentation of pain as a clinical problem.

Related topics

References

Alexander, F. (1950) *Psychosomatic Medicine: Its Principles and Applications*. New York: Norton.
Andreski, P., Chilcoat, H., and Breslau, N. (1998) Post-traumatic stress disorder and somatization symptoms: a prospective study. *Psychiatry Research* 79: 131–138.
APA (American Psychiatric Association). (1968) *Diagnostic and Statistical Manual of Mental Disorders*. Washington, DC: APA.
APA (American Psychiatric Association). (1980) *Diagnostic and Statistical Manual of Mental Disorders*. Washington, DC: APA.
APA (American Psychiatric Association). (1987) *Diagnostic and Statistical Manual of Mental Disorders: DSM-III-R*. Washington, DC: APA.
APA (American Psychiatric Association).. (1994) *Diagnostic and Statistical Manual of Mental Disorders: DSM-IV*. Washington, DC: APA.
APA (American Psychiatric Association). (2013) *Diagnostic and Statistical Manual of Mental disorders: DSM-5*. 5th ed. Arlington, VA: APA.

Arntz, A. and Claassens, L. (2004) The meaning of pain influences its experienced intensity. *Pain* 109: 20–25.

Asmundson, G.J., Coons, M. J., Taylor, S., and Katz, J. (2002) PTSD and the experience of pain: research and clinical implications of shared vulnerability and mutual maintenance models. *Canadian Journal of Psychiatry* 47: 930–937.

Beecher, H.K. (1946) Pain in men wounded in battle. *Bulletin of the US Army Medical Department* 5: 445–454.

Bickle, J. (2012) The philosophy of neuroscience. In E.N. Zalta (ed.), *Stanford Encyclopedia of Philosophy*. <http://plato.stanford.edu/entries/neuroscience/>.

Breuer, J.F. and Freud, S. (1966) *Studies in Hysteria*. New York: Avon Books.

Ciechanowski, P.S., Walker, E.A., Katon, W.J., and Russo, J.E. (2002) Attachment theory: a model for health care utilization and somatization. *Psychosomatic Medicine* 64: 660–667.

Creed, F. and Gureje, O. (2012) Emerging themes in the revision of the classification of somatoform disorders. *International Review of Psychiatry* 24: 556–567.

Dennett, D. (1981) *Brainstorms* Brighton: Harvester.

Dewall, C.N., Macdonald, G., Webster, G.D., Masten, C.L., Baumeister, R.F., Powell, C., Combs, D., Schurtz, D.R., Stillman, T.F., Tice, D.M., and Eisenberger, N.I. (2010) Acetaminophen reduces social pain: behavioral and neural evidence. *Psychological Science* 21: 931–937.

Eisenberger, N.I. (2012) The pain of social disconnection: examining the shared neural underpinnings of physical and social pain. *Nature Reviews Neuroscience* 13: 421–434.

Eisenberger, N.I., Lieberman, M.D., and Williams, K.D. (2003) Does rejection hurt? An FMRI study of social exclusion. *Science* 302: 290–292.

Eisenberger, N.I., Jarcho, J.M., Lieberman, M.D., and Naliboff, B.D. (2006) An experimental study of shared sensitivity to physical pain and social rejection. *Pain* 126: 132–138.

Eisenberger, N.I., Master, S.L., Inagaki, T.K., Taylor, S.E., Shirinyan, D., Lieberman, M.D., and Naliboff, B.D. (2011) Attachment figures activate a safety signal-related neural region and reduce pain experience. *Proceedings of the National Academy of Sciences of the United States of America*, 108: 11721–11726.

Engel, G.L. (1959) Psychogenic pain and pain-prone patient. *American Journal of Medicine* 26: 899–918.

Frances, A. (2013) The new somatic symptom disorder in DSM-5 risks mislabeling many people as mentally ill. *British Medical Journal* 346: f1580.

Frances, A. and Chapman, S. (2013) DSM-5 somatic symptom disorder mislabels medical illness as mental disorder. *Australian & New Zealand Journal of Psychiatry* 47: 483–484.

Hashmi, J.A., Baliki, M.N., Huang, L., Baria, A.T., Torbey, S., Hermann, K.M., Schnitzer, T.J., and Apkarian, A.V. (2013) Shape shifting pain: chronification of back pain shifts brain representation from nociceptive to emotional circuits. *Brain* 136: 2751–2768.

Hauser, W. and Wolfe, F. (2013) The Somatic Symptom Disorder in DSM 5 risks mislabelling people with major medical diseases as mentally ill. *Journal of Psychosomatic Research* 75: 586–587.

Holdorff, B. (2011) The fight for "traumatic neurosis," 1889–1916: Hermann Oppenheim and his opponents in Berlin. *History of Psychiatry* 22: 465–476.

Kessler, R.C., Sonnega, A., Bromet, E., Hughes, M., and Nelson, C.B. (1995) Posttraumatic stress disorder in the National Comorbidity Survey. *Archives of General Psychiatry* 52: 1048–1060.

King, S.A. and Strain, J.J. (1992) Revising the category of somatoform pain disorder. *Hospital and Community Psychiatry* 43: 217–219.

Liedl, A., O'Donnell, M., Creamer, M., Silove, D., McFarlane, A., Knaevelsrud, C., and Bryant, R.A. (2010) Support for the mutual maintenance of pain and post-traumatic stress disorder symptoms. *Psychological Medicine* 40: 1215–1223.

McCracken, L.M. and Vowles, K.E. (2014) Acceptance and commitment therapy and mindfulness for chronic pain: model, process, and progress. *American Psychologist* 69: 178–187.

Moseley, G.L. and Arntz, A. (2007) The context of a noxious stimulus affects the pain it evokes. *Pain* 133: 64–71.

Moseley, G.L. and Butler, D.S. (2015) Fifteen years of explaining pain: the past, present, and future. *Journal of Pain* 16: 807–813.

Moseley, G.L. and Vlaeyen, J.W. (2015) Beyond nociception: the imprecision hypothesis of chronic pain. *Pain* 156: 35–38.

Moseley, G.L., Nicholas, M.K. and Hodges, P.W. (2004) A randomized controlled trial of intensive neurophysiology education in chronic low back pain. *Clinical Journal of Pain* 20: 324–330.

Norman, S.B., Stein, M.B., Dimsdale, J.E., and Hoyt, D.B. (2008) Pain in the aftermath of trauma is a risk factor for post-traumatic stress disorder. *Psychological Medicine* 38: 533–542.

Norris, F.H. (1992) Epidemiology of trauma: frequency and impact of different potentially traumatic events on different demographic groups. *Journal of Consulting and Clinical Psychology* 60: 409–418.

Otis, J.D., Keane, T.M., and Kerns, R.D. (2003) An examination of the relationship between chronic pain and post-traumatic stress disorder. *Journal of Rehabilitation Research Development* 40: 397–405.

Panksepp, J., Herman, B., Conner, R., Bishop, P., and Scott, J.P. (1978) The biology of social attachments: opiates alleviate separation distress. *Biological Psychiatry* 13: 607–618.

Portenoy, R.K. (1989) Mechanisms of clinical pain. Observations and speculations. *Neurologic Clinics* 7: 205–230.

Resnick, H.S., Kilpatrick, D.G., Dansky, B.S., Saunders, B.E., and Best, C.L. (1993) Prevalence of civilian trauma and posttraumatic stress disorder in a representative national sample of women. *Journal of Consulting and Clinical Psychology* 61: 984–991.

Seal, K.H., Shi, Y., Cohen, G., Cohen, B.E., Maguen, S., Krebs, E.E., and Neylan, T.C. (2012) Association of mental health disorders with prescription opioids and high-risk opioid use in US veterans of Iraq and Afghanistan. *Journal of the American Medical Association* 307: 940–947.

Sullivan, M.D. (2000) DSM-IV Pain Disorder: a case against the diagnosis. *International Review of Psychiatry* 12: 91–98.

Sullivan, M.J., Thibault, P., Simmonds, M.J., Milioto, M., Cantin, A.P., and Velly, A.M. (2009) Pain, perceived injustice and the persistence of post-traumatic stress symptoms during the course of rehabilitation for whiplash injuries. *Pain* 145: 325–331.

Wager, T.D., Atlas, L.Y., Lindquist, M.A., Roy, M., Woo, C.W., and Kross, E. (2013) An fMRI-based neurologic signature of physical pain. *New England Journal of Medicine* 368: 1388–1397.

Wall, P. (2002) *Pain: The Science of Suffering*. New York: Columbia University Press.

14

PAIN, VOLUNTARY ACTION, AND THE SENSE OF AGENCY

Brianna Beck and Patrick Haggard

A primary function of pain is to guide behavior that helps the organism avoid injury. This implies a tight coupling between the neural systems underlying pain perception and those underlying action control. Indeed, it is well known that painful stimulation triggers protective spinal reflexes (e.g., Willer 1985; Willer and Bussel 1980). Moreover, it has been shown that pain simultaneously inhibits cortical control of movement, allowing those spinal reflexes to take precedence over higher-level motor control (for a review, see Farina et al. 2003). In addition to the pain-related inhibition of cortical motor control, other studies (to be reviewed below) have shown reciprocal effects of the cortical motor system on pain perception. Together, these findings suggest there may be important links between pain processing and the physiological circuits underlying voluntary action.

Of course, other sensory experiences can also trigger protective reflexes that override higher-level motor control (e.g., sudden loud noises, or the sight of something rapidly approaching). However, those sensory channels also provide detailed information that allows more sophisticated interactions with our surroundings. For example, when we see a cat, we can discern physical characteristics such as its shape, size, and color, as well as its behavioral patterns and emotional expressions. For pain, on the other hand, the motor response seems to follow directly from the sensory stimulation, without intermediate steps of perceptual analysis, recognition and representation of the external object. Because pain often signals an imminent threat, the priority of pain processing may be to motivate immediate protective action rather than to provide finer details about the nature of the threat. (Cf. discussion concerning pain and motivation in Chapters 3 and 4, this volume.)

Voluntary action is normally accompanied by a distinctive subjective experience, or "sense of agency" (Haggard 2008). This refers to the feeling of control over one's own actions, and over the sensory consequences of those actions in the external world. The sense of agency is thus relevant both to action control, and to the feeling that one is capable of enacting change upon one's environment. In goal-directed action, one selects a course of action in order to bring about a desired consequence, for example, by achieving a positive outcome or avoiding a negative one. In this light, pain is likely to strongly interact with the sense of agency. Pain is a highly salient and motivationally significant stimulus, signaling threat of imminent damage to the body (cf. Chapter 4, this volume). Because the avoidance and minimization of pain are high priorities, one might expect the sense of agency to be especially sensitive to painful outcomes. In particular, painful action outcomes might enhance the implicit sense of agency because of the importance of learning associations between one's own behavior and potentially injurious consequences. To date, however, few studies have investigated the link between pain and the sense of agency.

In this chapter, we will begin by reviewing findings that show an inhibitory effect of voluntary action on pain processing. We will then discuss two possible mechanisms by which this inhibition may occur: (1) voluntary action might generally inhibit the processing of any concurrent painful stimulation (e.g., tapping your foot might inhibit an entirely unrelated pain in your hand), perhaps through connections between motor and somatosensory cortices (Nakata et al. 2004), or (2) voluntary action might specifically inhibit the processing of painful stimuli that are a consequence of the action itself, by enhancing their controllability or their predictability. For example, controlling a device that delivers a noxious stimulus might make that stimulus feel less painful, compared to a situation in which someone else controls the device. Finally, we will outline the need for implicit measures of the sense of agency in considering the relation between agency and valenced events such as pain.

1 Self-administration of pain

Several studies have shown that self-administration of a painful stimulus, relative to administration of the same stimulus by external means, reduces perceived pain intensity and unpleasantness (Müller 2012; Wang et al. 2011) and modulates pain-related processing in the anterior cingulate cortex (Mohr et al. 2005; Wang et al. 2011), the primary somatosensory cortex (Helmchen et al. 2006; Wang et al. 2011), and the posterior insula and prefrontal cortex (Mohr et al. 2008). However, the detailed mechanism by which self-produced pain is attenuated remains unclear.

The reduction in the perceived intensity of self-administered pain is reminiscent of the classic sensory attenuation effect found in other modalities, including vision (Hughes and Waszak 2011; Schafer and Marcus 1973), audition (Aliu et al. 2009; Baess et al. 2009, 2011; Hazemann et al. 1975; Schafer and Marcus 1973), and touch (Blakemore et al. 1998, 1999, 2000; Claxton 1975; Weiskrantz et al. 1971), when the sensation is caused by one's own action. For example, self-produced tactile stimuli are perceived as less intense and less "tickly" than externally produced tactile stimuli of objectively equal magnitude (Blakemore et al. 1999; Claxton 1975; Weiskrantz et al. 1971). Further, the size of this sensory attenuation effect in the tactile domain varies with the degree to which the tactile stimulation matches the sensation predicted by the action (Blakemore et al. 1999). This finding suggests that such sensory attenuation effects may derive from an internal forward model of the motor system, as conceptualized by computational models of motor control (Wolpert et al. 1995). These models predict that, when a voluntary movement is made, an "efference copy" of the motor command is issued so that the actual motor output can be compared to the planned movement. According to such models, the efference copy of a motor command may be used to predict the sensory consequences of the voluntary movement via a "forward model." The forward model account of sensory attenuation would predict that if the efferent motor prediction closely matched the actual sensory consequences, then processing of the resulting sensations would be inhibited (Blakemore et al. 1999).

Interestingly, this sensory attenuation itself has been proposed to be an implicit marker of the sense of agency, as it may be one mechanism by which the brain determines whether a sensory outcome was self-produced or externally generated (Blakemore et al. 1999; Gentsch and Schutz-Bosbach 2011; Sato and Yasuda 2005). If a sensory event was predicted by the forward model, it must have been self-caused, and a consequence of one's own action. The suppression of sensory reafference in the immediate spatio-temporal context of voluntary movements is well established (Williams et al. 1998). It has the plausible functional role of preventing sensory systems from overload by self-caused reafference, which can in any case be predicted from motor commands. However, sensory attenuation may be less plausible as a model of sense of agency during goal-directed action. For example, it may seem paradoxical to suppress sensory processing of a goal, because that sensory input would generally be the desired outcome. It seems paradoxical that the very fruits of one's own endeavor should be tantalizingly suppressed. Further, the goals of voluntary actions may be spatially and temporally remote from the motor act itself. That is, when we flip a switch to turn on a light, the immediate sensory consequence of the movement is the sensation of the finger touching the switch. However, the perceptual event that we really care about is the one related to the goal, namely, being able to see the room. That may entail a short delay, and involve spatial locations other than the light switch. Similarly, when pain is the remote outcome of a goal-directed action rather than an immediate consequence of the movement itself, it is unclear whether any resulting sensory attenuation would be caused by efferent motor prediction.

2 Effects of voluntary movement and motor preparation on pain processing

Motor control models predict that sensory reafference is suppressed only to the extent that it is a directly predictable consequence of the motor command.[1] However, several studies have shown that voluntary movement can inhibit pain processing even when the pain sensations are not directly related to the motor action. Performing arbitrary voluntary movements during painful radiant heat stimulation increases pain thresholds, reduces subjective pain intensity, and decreases the amplitude of LEPs (laser-evoked potentials), which are considered a neurophysiological index of pain processing (Kakigi et al. 1993; Kakigi and Shibasaki 1992; Nakata et al. 2004; Vrana et al. 2005). Voluntary movement also modulates activity in S1 (primary somatosensory) and S2 (secondary somatosensory) cortices (Nakata et al. 2004; Vrana et al. 2005). Notably, it has been proposed that the operculo-insular cortex, a region of the brain encompassing the S2 and posterior insula, may be the primary sensory cortex for pain (Garcia-Larrea 2012a, 2012b; Mazzola et al. 2012a, 2012b). (Please see Chapters 6–10 on neural pain-processing models.) Therefore, these studies indicate that the neural centers for voluntary movement have an effect on primary sensory centers for pain processing. Further, these links are reciprocal. An immediate consequence of pain is the inhibition of cortical motor control in favor of involuntary motor reflexes (Farina et al. 2003).

Other studies have shown that mere motor preparation, in the absence of actual movement, can reduce perceived pain intensity and modulate neurophysiological markers of pain processing (Le Pera et al. 2007; Nakata et al. 2009; Stancak et al. 2012). In these studies, the painful stimulus occurred while the participant was in a state of motor readiness but had not yet executed a movement. The results suggest that – in certain situations, at least – it is the neural activity underlying the *intention* to act that influences pain processing, over and above any influence of movement execution. This interaction may involve the operculo-insular cortex and/or the anterior cingulate cortex, both of which are engaged during motor readiness and pain processing (Ball et al. 1999; Wasaka et al. 2005; Nakata et al. 2009; Stancak et al. 2012; Garcia-Larrea and Peyron 2013). As mentioned earlier, the operculo-insular cortex participates in primary sensory processing of painful stimuli (Garcia-Larrea 2012a, 2012b; Mazzola et al. 2012a, 2012b). The anterior cingulate cortex, on the other hand, seems to be more involved in the affective dimension of pain perception (Foltz and White 1962; Rainville et al. 1997). Motor preparation may thus reduce perceived pain either by inhibiting sensory processing of painful stimuli, by lessening the feeling of unpleasantness associated with the pain, or by a combination of both these mechanisms.

Considering these findings, an internal forward model of the motor system does not seem to fully account for the attenuation of self-administered pain. Both voluntary movement and motor preparation are able to inhibit processing of painful stimuli with which they have no causal or predictive relationship. By contrast, efferent motor prediction could only explain the attenuation of sensations that are caused by – or at least appear to be caused by – the participant's voluntary action. The forward model invoked by computational motor control models to predict the likely consequences of action might not simply be a model of the motor effectors themselves, but could involve a more general model of all sensory and motor events present in any given context. Moreover, the studies reviewed above describe attenuations of pain perception that are largely specific to voluntary action, as well as the intention to act in the absence of any actual movement. While the theoretical interpretation of this pain–action relation remains unclear, these findings show an interaction between the neural processes underlying intentional action and the processes underlying pain perception.

3 Effects of control and predictability on pain processing

In the studies described above, voluntary movement and motor preparation inhibited the processing of concurrent pain sensations, irrespective of any causal relationship between the action and the painful stimulation. However, other lines of research suggest that causal or predictive links between actions and pain sensations may influence pain processing in more specific ways. For example, some studies have shown that the degree of control one has over the termination of a painful stimulus affects both subjective ratings of pain intensity and pain anxiety, and neural measures of pain processing (Mohr et al. 2012; Salomons et al. 2004, 2007; Wiech et al. 2006). Generally, these studies have found that actual or perceived control over the offset of the painful stimulus attenuates pain perception, although individual differences in coping style also seem to mediate the effect (Salomons et al. 2007). Because these studies compared an externally controlled pain termination condition to a condition in which participants pressed a button to stop the painful stimulus, it is possible that motor readiness might partially account for the reduction in perceived pain intensity when participants themselves controlled pain offset. Importantly, however, one of these studies (Wiech et al. 2006) held motor readiness constant by requiring participants to also press a button as soon as they detected pain offset in the external control condition. Having control over pain offset still reduced participants' perceived pain levels, indicating that the effect of control cannot be entirely explained by differences in preparatory motor activity.

The analgesic effects of control over pain could have important implications for clinical settings. Patient-controlled analgesia has already been established as an effective method for providing efficient post-operative pain relief while avoiding excessive dosages of analgesic medications (Grass 2005). It allows the patients themselves to deliver small intravenous doses of analgesics as needed, typically by pressing a button connected to a programmable infusion pump. Interestingly, the effectiveness of patient-controlled analgesia is influenced by a psychological factor called "locus of control." People who believe that their own actions determine their health experience lower levels of pain and are more satisfied with patient-controlled analgesia, compared to people who believe that their health is determined by external causes beyond their own control (Johnson et al. 1989). Because the effectiveness of patient-controlled analgesia depends upon the patient initiating voluntary actions to produce pain relief, those who believe in their own ability to control their circumstances are better able to utilize this method than those who believe that they are not in control (Reynaert et al. 1995). While these studies focused on explicit evaluations of pain control, the implicit sense of agency might also have a role in patient-controlled analgesia. Specifically, factors that boost the sense of agency over pain levels should also lead to greater pain relief. Based on previous studies of intentional binding, these would include a short and consistent interval between action and outcome (Haggard et al. 2002), as described in further detail below. A pain management program that enhances agency may benefit post-operative patients by helping them to optimize their utilization of patient-controlled analgesia. In addition to this indirect effect of the sense of agency on pain, the studies on self-termination of pain described above suggest that the sense of being in control might directly boost the effects of self-administered analgesics, over and above any differences in the actual anesthetic usage (Mohr et al. 2012; Salomons et al. 2004, 2007; Wiech et al. 2006). (For further discussion, see Chapter 32 on pain and placebo effects, and Chapter 33 on pain management.)

Do effects of control on pain reflect a specific mechanism linked to voluntary motor control, or a more general expectation of the painful stimulus? A noxious stimulus is perceived as less painful when it has been cued than when it is unexpected (e.g., Carlsson et al. 2006; Crombez et al. 1994; Lin et al. 2014). Agency over pain could therefore attenuate perceived pain intensity by making the occurrence, the intensity, or some other property of the painful stimulus more predictable. A valuable aim for future research would be to determine whether there are effects of control on pain perception which rely on endogenous motor predictions, over and above any effects of predictability based on external cues. For example, one study found that activity in somatosensory cortex differed between self-administered painful stimuli and externally applied stimuli of equal physical intensities, *independently* of stimulus onset predictability (Helmchen et al. 2006). However, that particular study found no effects of self-administration on pain perception.

The studies described here suggest that the sense of being in control can reduce perceived pain levels, beyond any effects of voluntary movement or motor preparation on pain processing. One outstanding question is whether painful outcomes, as opposed to non-painful outcomes, affect the sense of being in control over the action that caused the pain. This feeling of control over one's own actions and their outcomes is known as the sense of agency.

4 Pain and the sense of agency

Acute pain typically signals bodily harm, or the imminent threat of such harm. For this reason, efficient perception of painful stimuli and appropriate responses to pain are vital to an organism's well-being. In the short term, pain stimulates actions such as avoidance and withdrawal from the source of pain, when this is possible. Moreover, one can often learn from previous painful experiences to avoid potentially harmful situations in the future. Because pain signals harm, and the avoidance of harm is crucial to survival, it is perhaps not surprising that pain affects both voluntary and involuntary motor systems (Farina et al. 2003; Willer 1985; Willer and Bussel 1980). In both these cases, actions are responses to pain. However, pain may also be the consequence of one's own action, rather than a purely exogenous event. Thus, an important part of acquiring efficient, functional control over one's own behavior must be learning which of one's own actions produce painful outcomes (e.g., putting one's hand in a flame), and which do not (e.g., grasping a shiny coin). That is, one needs to acquire a sense of agency with respect to pain in order to select actions that avoid pain. This point may seem obvious, but it is fundamental. Only by experiencing the action–pain link can organisms avoid reactivating this link through their operant actions. Despite the foundational nature of the action–pain link for directing behavior, very little is known about how pain might affect the sense-of-agency which normally accompanies voluntary action.

One implicit marker of the sense of agency is a perceived compression of the temporal interval between a voluntary action and its sensory outcome, often called "intentional binding" (Haggard and Clark 2003; Haggard et al. 2002). In the intentional binding paradigm, a voluntary action, such as a key press, is followed by a sensory outcome, such as an auditory tone, after a brief delay. Using a rotating clock hand as a reference, the participant reports either the time when they made the action, or the time when the sensory outcome occurred. The timing judgments in this "operant" condition are compared to judgments the participant makes when either the action or the sensory outcome occurs alone. When the sensory outcome is caused by the participant's voluntary action, the perceived time of the outcome shifts backwards in time towards the action. Likewise, the perceived time of the action shifts forwards in time towards the outcome. Together, these temporal binding effects shorten the perceived delay between the action and its sensory consequence.

Because temporal binding is either absent or significantly reduced for passive, involuntary movements (Haggard and Clark 2003; Haggard et al. 2002), it is considered a plausible measure of the sense of agency. Some have proposed that efferent motor prediction (i.e., the internal forward model) is one mechanism behind intentional binding (Haggard et al. 2002; Waszak et al. 2012). However, several recent studies have demonstrated that intentional binding is underpinned both by predictive motor processes (e.g., the posterior probability of an outcome given the action) and by postdictive, outcome-dependent processes (e.g., whether the outcome, and which outcome, does in fact occur; Moore and Haggard 2008; Moore et al. 2009; Synofzik et al. 2013; Takahata et al. 2012). It is therefore conceivable that the nature of the action outcome might influence the implicit sense of agency, particularly when that outcome has affective or motivational relevance to the agent.

Although no published study to date has investigated the effect of painful outcomes on intentional binding, some have revealed effects of emotionally valenced outcomes on the magnitude of binding. Using positive and negative emotional vocalizations (Yoshie and Haggard 2013) or monetary wins and losses (Takahata et al. 2012), these studies found reduced intentional binding when the outcome of the participant's action was negatively valenced. This effect may constitute an implicit analogue to the self-serving attribution bias, in which people tend to attribute negative outcomes to external sources rather than to their own actions (e.g., Bradley 1978; Greenberg et al. 1982; Mezulis et al. 2004). Pain is generally considered an unpleasant, negatively valenced experience. Consequently, one might expect a painful outcome to reduce the implicit sense of control over the painful event and the action that produced it.

On the other hand, the primary function of pain in guiding adaptive behavior suggests an alternative prediction for how painful outcomes might affect intentional binding. An optimally behaving organism would use past painful experiences to guide future behavior, thereby learning how to avoid or minimize pain whenever possible. For example, a young child who touches a hot stove and consequently feels a burning pain sensation will quickly learn not to touch the stove again. A reduction in intentional binding for painful outcomes could impede this learning process by weakening the association between the action that was made and the painful sensation it produced. Therefore, one might alternatively predict *stronger* intentional binding when action outcomes are painful.

There are two key differences between the situations giving rise to these competing predictions: (1) whether one can choose between alternative actions, and (2) whether those alternative actions have different likely outcomes. The first point determines one's freedom to act, and the second determines how meaningful one's actions are. Prior studies that investigated intentional binding in the context of valenced outcomes only allowed participants to make one action (Takahata et al. 2012; Yoshie and Haggard 2013). The reduction in the sense of agency that they found may have resulted not only from the negative valence of the outcome, but from participants' helplessness to avoid that outcome. Given the opportunity to choose between actions with higher or lower probabilities of causing pain, this decrease in intentional binding for negatively valenced outcomes might be reversed.

Assuming that effects of painful outcomes on intentional binding are found, would these effects be specific to pain, or generalizable to any negatively valenced outcome with motivational significance? If the effect of pain on intentional binding derives from its role in signaling threat, then one might expect, for example, that loud, startling sounds or threatening images would have similar effects on the implicit sense of agency. On the other hand, prior research has demonstrated specific interactions between neural systems underlying the processing of the sensory component of pain, voluntary movement (Farina et al. 2003; Nakata et al. 2004; Vrana et al. 2005), and action preparation (Le Pera et al. 2007; Stancak et al. 2012). These studies suggest that there may be a special relationship between pain, specifically, and the first-person experience of agency that accompanies voluntary action.

5 Conclusions

Self-administration of painful stimulation is known to attenuate both perceived pain levels and neural processing of pain (Helmchen et al. 2006; Mohr et al. 2005, 2008; Müller 2012; Wang et al. 2011). Although the exact mechanisms behind this effect are still unknown, the studies reviewed in this chapter suggest that it may arise from a combination of at least two factors: executing a voluntary movement, and being able to control (or predict) the painful outcome of that movement. Future studies should systematically manipulate these factors to determine the relative contributions of motor execution and outcome control to the sensory attenuation effect. Notably, motor execution control and outcome selection control constitute two key features of the concept of the sense of agency, so a finding that both contribute to the attenuation of self-administered pain may support the use of sensory attenuation as an implicit measure of the sense of agency.

Furthermore, though the relationship between acute experimental pain and clinical pain is complex, the results of studies on pain, voluntary action, and the sense of agency could potentially be applied to designing better pain management programs or more effective methods of administering analgesic treatments. For example, electrical stimulation of the motor cortex is already being used to treat some cases of chronic pain, but the reason for its effectiveness in pain relief is not well understood (for a review, see Lima and Fregni 2008). Treatment of chronic pain might thus benefit from further research into the connections between cortical motor activity and pain processing. Moreover, procedures that enhance the explicit or implicit sense of agency might also boost the efficacy of existing analgesic interventions, such as patient-controlled analgesia. Chapters 32 and 33 in this volume discuss such analgesia effects in more detail.

While previous studies revealed that having control over a noxious stimulus can make it feel less painful, it remains to be seen whether this relationship is reciprocal. Future studies could investigate whether pain, in turn, affects the implicit sense of control over one's own actions and their consequences – namely, the sense of agency. Further, it should be determined whether such an effect, if found, is specific to pain or general to any negatively valenced, motivationally significant sensory outcome. A painful experience has a strong affective component in addition to its sensory properties (Melzack and Casey 1968), and either the sensory or the affective dimension could underpin the proposed effects of pain on the sense of agency. If pain is shown to influence the implicit sense of agency, this would support the idea of a close link between the neural systems for pain processing and voluntary action, further extending it to the associated sense of control over one's actions, and, consequently, over outcomes in the external world.

Related topics

Chapter 3: Evaluativist accounts of pain's unpleasantness (Bain)
Chapter 4: Imperativism (Klein)
Chapter 6: Advances in the neuroscience of pain (Apkarian)
Chapter 7: Neuromatrix theory of pain (Roy and Wager)
Chapter 8: A neurobiological view of pain as a homeostatic emotion (Strigo and Craig)
Chapter 9: A view of pain based on sensations, meanings, and emotions (Price)
Chapter 10: Pathophysiological mechanisms of chronic pain (Thacker and Moseley)
Chapter 32: Pain and "placebo" analgesia (Moerman)
Chapter 33: Pain management (Berryman, Catley, and Moseley)

Acknowledgements

The authors wish to thank Nura Sidarus for her helpful comments on an earlier version of this chapter.

Note

1 Note that we do not imply a high-level, conscious prediction here, but a prediction that occurs implicitly and automatically within the sensory and motor systems.

References

Aliu, S.O., Houde, J.F., and Nagarajan, S.S. (2009) Motor-induced suppression of the auditory cortex. *Journal of Cognitive Neuroscience* 21: 791–802.

Baess, P., Widmann, A., Roye, A., Schroger, E., and Jacobsen, T. (2009) Attenuated human auditory middle latency response and evoked 40-Hz response to self-initiated sounds. *European Journal of Neuroscience* 29: 1514–1521.

Baess, P., Horvath, J., Jacobsen, T., and Schroger, E. (2011) Selective suppression of self-initiated sounds in an auditory stream: an ERP study. *Psychophysiology* 48, 1276–1283.

Ball, T., Schreiber, A., Feige, B., Wagner, M., Lucking, C.H., and Kristeva-Feige, R. (1999) The role of higher-order motor areas in voluntary movement as revealed by high-resolution EEG and fMRI. *Neuroimage* 10: 682–694.

Blakemore, S.J., Wolpert, D.M., and Frith, C.D. (1998) Central cancellation of self-produced tickle sensation. *Nature Neuroscience* 1: 635–640.

Blakemore, S.J., Frith, C.D., and Wolpert, D.M. (1999) Spatio-temporal prediction modulates the perception of self-produced stimuli. *Journal of Cognitive Neuroscience* 11: 551–559.

Blakemore, S.J., Smith, J., Steel, R., Johnstone, C.E., and Frith, C.D. (2000) The perception of self-produced sensory stimuli in patients with auditory hallucinations and passivity experiences: evidence for a breakdown in self-monitoring. *Psychological Medicine* 30: 1131–1139.

Bradley, G.W. (1978) Self-serving biases in attribution process – re-examination of fact or fiction question. *Journal of Personality and Social Psychology* 36: 56–71.

Carlsson, K., Andersson, J., Petrovic, P., Petersson, K.M., Ohman, A., and Ingvar, M. (2006) Predictability modulates the affective and sensory-discriminative neural processing of pain. *Neuroimage* 32: 1804–1814.

Claxton, G. (1975) Why can't we tickle ourselves? *Perceptual and Motor Skills* 41: 335–338.

Crombez, G., Baeyens, F., and Eelen, P. (1994) Sensory and temporal information about impending pain: the influence of predictability on pain. *Behaviour Research and Therapy* 32: 611–622.

Farina, S., Tinazzi, M., Le Pera, D., and Valeriani, M. (2003) Pain-related modulation of the human motor cortex. *Neurological Research* 25: 130–142.

Foltz, E.L. and White, L.E. Jr. (1962) Pain "relief" by frontal cingulumotomy. *Journal of Neurosurgery* 19: 89–100.

Garcia-Larrea, L. (2012a) Insights gained into pain processing from patients with focal brain lesions. *Neuroscience Letters* 520: 188–191.

Garcia-Larrea, L. (2012b) The posterior insular-opercular region and the search of a primary cortex for pain. *Clinical Neurophysiology* 42: 299–313.

Garcia-Larrea, L. and Peyron, R. (2013) Pain matrices and neuropathic pain matrices: a review. *Pain* 154 (suppl. 1): S29–S43.

Gentsch, A. and Schutz-Bosbach, S. (2011) I did it: unconscious expectation of sensory consequences modulates the experience of self-agency and its functional signature. *Journal of Cognitive Neuroscience* 23: 3817–3828.

Grass, J.A. (2005) Patient-controlled analgesia. *Anesthesia & Analgesia* 101(5 suppl.): S44–S61.

Greenberg, J., Pyszczynski, T., and Solomon, S. (1982) The self-serving attributional bias – beyond self-presentation. *Journal of Experimental Social Psychology* 18: 56–67.

Haggard, P. (2008) Human volition: towards a neuroscience of will. *Nature Reviews Neuroscience* 9: 934–946.

Haggard, P. and Clark, S. (2003) Intentional action: conscious experience and neural prediction. *Consciousness and Cognition* 12: 695–707.

Haggard, P., Clark, S., and Kalogeras, J. (2002) Voluntary action and conscious awareness. *Nat Neurosci* 5: 382–385.

Hazemann, P., Audin, G., and Lille, F. (1975) Effect of voluntary self-paced movements upon auditory and somatosensory evoked potentials in man. *Electroencephalography and Clinical Neurophysiology* 39: 247–254.

Helmchen, C., Mohr, C., Erdmann, C., Binkofski, F., and Buchel, C. (2006) Neural activity related to self- versus externally generated painful stimuli reveals distinct differences in the lateral pain system in a parametric fMRI study. *Human Brain Mapping* 27: 755–765.

Hughes, G. and Waszak, F. (2011) ERP correlates of action effect prediction and visual sensory attenuation in voluntary action. *Neuroimage* 56: 1632–1640.

Johnson, L.R., Magnani, B., Chan, V., and Ferrante, F.M. (1989) Modifiers of patient-controlled analgesia efficacy. I. Locus of control. *Pain* 39: 17–22.

Kakigi, R. and Shibasaki, H. (1992) Mechanisms of pain relief by vibration and movement. *Journal of Neurology, Neurosurgery & Psychiatry* 55: 282–286.

Kakigi, R., Matsuda, Y., and Kuroda, Y. (1993) Effects of movement-related cortical activities on pain-related somatosensory evoked potentials following CO_2 laser stimulation in normal subjects. *Acta Neurologica Scandinavica* 88: 376–380.

Le Pera, D., Brancucci, A., De Armas, L., Del Percio, C., Miliucci, R., Babiloni, C., Restuccia, D., Rossini, P.M., and Valeriani, M. (2007) Inhibitory effect of voluntary movement preparation on cutaneous heat pain and laser-evoked potentials. *European Journal of Neuroscience* 25: 1900–1907.

Lima, M.C. and Fregni, F. (2008) Motor cortex stimulation for chronic pain: systematic review and meta-analysis of the literature. *Neurology* 70: 2329–2337.

Lin, C.S., Hsieh, J.C., Yeh, T.C., and Niddam, D. M. (2014) Predictability-mediated pain modulation in context of multiple cues: an event-related fMRI study. *Neuropsychologia* 64C: 85–91.

Mazzola, L., Faillenot, I., Barral, F.G., Mauguiere, F., and Peyron, R. (2012a) Spatial segregation of somato-sensory and pain activations in the human operculo-insular cortex. *Neuroimage* 60: 409–418.

Mazzola, L., Isnard, J., Peyron, R., and Mauguiere, F. (2012b) Stimulation of the human cortex and the experience of pain: Wilder Penfield's observations revisited. *Brain* 135: 631–640.

Melzack, R. and Casey, K.L. (1968) Sensory, motivational, and central control determinants of pain. In D.R. Kenshalo (ed.), *The Skin Senses*. Springfield, IL: Thomas.

Mezulis, A.H., Abramson, L.Y., Hyde, J.S., and Hankin, B.L. (2004) Is there a universal positivity bias in attributions? A meta-analytic review of individual, developmental, and cultural differences in the self-serving attributional bias. *Psychological Bulletin* 130: 711–747.

Mohr, C., Binkofski, F., Erdmann, C., Buchel, C., and Helmchen, C. (2005) The anterior cingulate cortex contains distinct areas dissociating external from self-administered painful stimulation: a parametric fMRI study. *Pain* 114: 347–357.

Mohr, C., Leyendecker, S., and Helmchen, C. (2008) Dissociable neural activity to self- vs. externally administered thermal hyperalgesia: a parametric fMRI study. *European Journal of Neuroscience* 27: 739–749.

Mohr, C., Leyendecker, S., Petersen, D., and Helmchen, C. (2012) Effects of perceived and exerted pain control on neural activity during pain relief in experimental heat hyperalgesia: a fMRI study. *European Joural of Pain* 16: 496–508.

Moore, J. and Haggard, P. (2008) Awareness of action: Inference and prediction. *Consciousness and Cognition* 17: 136–144.

Moore, J.W., Lagnado, D., Deal, D.C., and Haggard, P. (2009) Feelings of control: contingency determines experience of action. *Cognition* 110: 279–283.

Müller, M.J. (2012) Will it hurt less if I believe I can control it? Influence of actual and perceived control on perceived pain intensity in healthy male individuals: a randomized controlled study. *Journal of Behavioral Medicine* 35: 529–537.

Nakata, H., Inui, K., Wasaka, T., Tamura, Y., Tran, T.D., Qiu, Y., Wang, X., Nguyen, T.B., and Kakigi, R. (2004) Movements modulate cortical activities evoked by noxious stimulation. *Pain* 107: 91–98.

Nakata, H., Sakamoto, K., Honda, Y., Mochizuki, H., Hoshiyama, M., and Kakigi, R. (2009) Centrifugal modulation of human LEP components to a task-relevant noxious stimulation triggering voluntary movement. *Neuroimage* 45: 129–142.

Rainville, P., Duncan, G.H., Price, D.D., Carrier, B., and Bushnell, M.C. (1997) Pain affect encoded in human anterior cingulate but not somatosensory cortex. *Science* 277: 968–971.

Reynaert, C., Janne, P., Delire, V., Pirard, M., Randour, P., Collard, E., Installe, E., Coche, E., and Cassiers, L. (1995) To control or to be controlled? From health locus of control to morphine control during patient-controlled analgesia. *Psychotherapy and Psychosomatics* 64: 74–81.

Salomons, T.V., Johnstone, T., Backonja, M.M., and Davidson, R.J. (2004) Perceived controllability modulates the neural response to pain. *Journal of Neuroscience* 24: 7199–7203.

Salomons, T.V., Johnstone, T., Backonja, M.M., Shackman, A. J., and Davidson, R. J. (2007) Individual differences in the effects of perceived controllability on pain perception: critical role of the prefrontal cortex. *Journal of Cognitive Neuroscience* 19: 993–1003.

Sato, A. and Yasuda, A. (2005) Illusion of sense of self-agency: discrepancy between the predicted and actual sensory consequences of actions modulates the sense of self-agency, but not the sense of self-ownership. *Cognition* 94: 241–255.

Schafer, E.W. and Marcus, M.M. (1973) Self-stimulation alters human sensory brain responses. *Science* 181: 175–177.

Stancak, A., Johnstone, J., and Fallon, N. (2012) Effects of motor response expectancy on cortical processing of noxious laser stimuli. *Behavioural and Brain Research* 227: 215–223.

Synofzik, M., Vosgerau, G., and Voss, M. (2013) The experience of agency: an interplay between prediction and postdiction. *Frontiers in Psychology* 4: 127.

Takahata, K., Takahashi, H., Maeda, T., Umeda, S., Suhara, T., Mimura, M., and Kato, M. (2012) It's not my fault: postdictive modulation of intentional binding by monetary gains and losses. *PLoS One* 7: e53421.

Vrana, J., Polacek, H., and Stancak, A. (2005) Somatosensory-evoked potentials are influenced differently by isometric muscle contraction of stimulated and non-stimulated hand in humans. *Neuroscience Letters* 386: 170–175.

Wang, Y., Wang, J.Y., and Luo, F. (2011) Why self-induced pain feels less painful than externally generated pain: distinct brain activation patterns in self- and externally generated pain. *PLoS One* 6: e23536.

Wasaka, T., Nakata, H., Akatsuka, K., Kida, T., Inui, K., and Kakigi, R. (2005) Differential modulation in human primary and secondary somatosensory cortices during the preparatory period of self-initiated finger movement. *European Journal of Neuroscience* 22: 1239–1247.

Waszak, F., Cardoso-Leite, P., and Hughes, G. (2012) Action effect anticipation: neurophysiological basis and functional consequences. *Neuroscience & Biobehavioral Reviews* 36: 943–959.

Weiskrantz, L., Elliott, J., and Darlington, C. (1971) Preliminary observations on tickling oneself. *Nature* 230: 598–599.

Wiech, K., Kalisch, R., Weiskopf, N., Pleger, B., Stephan, K. E., and Dolan, R. J. (2006) Anterolateral prefrontal cortex mediates the analgesic effect of expected and perceived control over pain. *Journal of Neuroscience* 26: 11501–11509.

Willer, J.C. (1985) Studies on pain. Effects of morphine on a spinal nociceptive flexion reflex and related pain sensation in man. *Brain Research* 331: 105–114.

Willer, J.C. and Bussel, B. (1980) Evidence for a direct spinal mechanism in morphine-induced inhibition of nociceptive reflexes in humans. *Brain Research* 187: 212–215.

Williams, S.R., Shenasa, J., and Chapman, C.E. (1998) Time course and magnitude of movement-related gating of tactile detection in humans I: Importance of stimulus location. *Journal of Neurophysiology* 79: 947–963.

Wolpert, D.M., Ghahramani, Z., and Jordan, M. I. (1995) An internal model for sensorimotor integration. *Science* 269: 1880–1882.

Yoshie, M. and Haggard, P. (2013) Negative emotional outcomes attenuate sense of agency over voluntary actions. *Current Biology* 23: 2028–2032.

SECTION II

THEORETICAL IMPLICATIONS

Why does pain matter, theoretically?

PART II-I

Pain in philosophy of mind

15

THE LIVES OF OTHERS

Pain in non-human animals

Paula Droege

Humans are wired to be empathetic. Our emotional response to the pain of others is rooted in evolutionarily tuned systems for infant care and social bonding (Churchland 2012). We rush to a crying infant, wince when an actor is wounded, gasp as a race car flips and rolls. We even respond empathetically to robots and simple geometric figures.[1] So it's not surprising that we should read the behavior of non-human animals (hereafter, "animals") as indicating pain: we really do feel their pain (de Vignemont and Jacob 2012). The feeling of empathy compels us to identify with the pain of others and motivates the response to alleviate their pain. But empathy is triggered by things it was not designed to identify with: geometric figures do not feel pain and therefore do not need help. In this case, the empathetic response is a mistake, and moral action is unwarranted. While empathy is an important motivator for moral action, it is an inadequate guide. We need a fuller picture of the role of pain as part of a system for attending to and responding to threat (Haggard et al. 2013; Chapter 9, this volume). In this chapter, I define pain as the representation of bodily damage and draw on insights from neurophysiology, comparative cognitive ethology, and consciousness theory to provide a functional description of the conditions for different forms of pain processing in animals. A better understanding of pain in the life of an animal, including the human animal, is necessary to guide moral action.

1 The problem of evidence across alternative taxonomic groups

The first challenge is to establish a definition of pain that is not designed exclusively for humans. I take the word "pain" very broadly to mean the representation of bodily damage. As I will argue in Section 2, the representational function of pain usefully supports comparison among the different sensory processing systems that represent damage, and allows a continuity from simple nociceptive reaction to more articulated forms of response. While nociception alone does not involve the conscious feeling of hurtfulness that we humans associate with pain (see Section 4), there are good reasons to consider both processes to be forms of pain. Along the same vein, Section 3 will discuss the emotional and cognitive aspects of pain without any implication that consciousness is required. In short, "pain" is characterized as the representation of damage, and different forms of representation (nociception, emotion, consciousness) are ways that pain serves its representational function.

The second challenge of this chapter is to take into account the diversity of animal groups and species. Due to the variety of ecological pressures, animals have widely different anatomical systems and behavior. Consequently, there will be no one-size-fits-all answer to the question of pain. With operational definitions of terms such as pain, emotion, and consciousness, we can coherently compare responses among animals. However, we should not expect that any animal feels pain just like us, or just like other animals. Each species has evolved a representational system suited to its environmental niche, so what it's like to be a bat will not be what it's like to be a rat, or a fish or even a fly. Nonetheless, analytical tools can shed light on ways that bat experiences are similar to and different from rat experiences. One of the goals of this chapter is to provide some of the necessary tools.

2 Nociception in animals

The first step in meeting these two challenges is to clarify the role of nociception in the mental life of animals. Though some philosophers restrict attribution of mentality to consciousness, accumulating evidence of unconscious sensation, emotion, thought, and action-initiation argue for a broader understanding of the mind. My view is that the mind is a representational device; mental states and processes just are representations. For reasons of brevity, I will consider only my favored theory of representation.[2] According to Ruth Millikan's teleosemantic theory, a representation is an item that varies isomorphically in relation to another item because that relation has served other useful functions in the past (Millikan 1989, 2004). Called a *consumer theory*, the critical element that specifies meaning is the adaptive function that the representation serves in the mental economy of the animal. A mental state does not represent because it is a picture or a copy or a simple causal effect of the item it represents. A frog's representation means fly, for example, because varying in accord with flies has helped the frog's food-catching systems function properly. Other dark, moving objects that trigger the system count as misrepresentations because they have not been the reason that the representation has been reproduced (Millikan 1993).

By thinking of the mind in terms of representation, we can see how different physical systems perform similar representational functions, and we can differentiate mental capacities according to their distinct functions. In relation to pain, function accounts for the relations between nociceptive response, negative affect, and conscious hurtfulness in terms of increasingly articulated representations of damage. Even the most basic stimulus–response reflex counts as mental if the system has the function of responding adaptively to stimuli.[3] For example, eye blinks represent danger to the eye, because the successful response to danger explains why genes that contribute to promoting the eye-blink reflex have been reproduced. Eye blinks are also selective; they do not occur in response to stimuli like variations in color or shape, for example. Yet they can misrepresent and so occur in the absence of potential damage. In fact, most eye blinks fail to serve their proper function, because the cost of blinking is so low relative to the risk of damage.

Though many, perhaps most, readers may be inclined to classify sensory reflex as mechanical rather than mental, a satisfying explanation of the mind needs to incorporate the deeply integrated levels of world-responsiveness that constitute a functional organism. To take a human example, pain from a paper cut begins with the activation of nociceptors that send a signal to the spinal column and a reflex response is initiated. This response is quick and unconscious. Next, the signal travels up to the brain where it is modulated by cognitive and affective processes that guide action in light of past associations. This more complex response may also be unconscious, particularly if the wound is not serious and other activities absorb attention. Only when the cut becomes conscious does the characteristic feeling of hurtfulness occur. All of these levels of response function together to represent the damage of the cut and to determine appropriate action. To try to explain conscious pain separately from these other forms of response is to segregate consciousness from the rest of the mind, and by extension from the rest of the animal kingdom whose minds are similar to and different from human minds in various ways. Evolution operates by adapting structures to new challenges rather than inventing something entirely new.[4] Pain, as the representation of damage, connects mental processes from simple nociceptive responses through to the exclusively human ability to report the character of our pains through language.

Converging evidence demonstrates strong similarities in nociceptive systems across the animal kingdom (Smith and Lewin 2009). Very simple animals such as sea anemones respond to column stimulation, however the response is undifferentiated and so better characterized as "nociceptive-like" (Braithwaite 2010). Somewhat more complex invertebrates such as leeches have neurons dedicated to responding to noxious stimuli. These neurons have the same basic physiological structure as nociceptors in fruit flies, fish, chickens, rats, and humans (Smith and Lewin 2009; Kavaliers 1988). Another form of nociceptor modulation is opioid dampening of activation. This systemic response couples sensory signaling with a mechanism for reducing that signal to avoid overloading the organism. Because nociceptor activation triggers appropriate withdrawal and avoidance behavior, it is the most basic and common form of pain processing.

3 Learning and emotion

While all animals need to represent damage in some way, some are so well-adapted to their environmental niche that nociceptive responses are sufficient. Animals in more complex environments need to learn from their sensory interactions with the world, so they require a more articulated form of representation. Rather than simply responding to noxious stimuli with a genetically fixed action, an animal can come to associate a secondary stimulus with the noxious stimulus in order to respond more quickly. This is basic Pavlovian conditioning and requires only a simple coupling of sensory and motor neurons in the spine to effect training (Grau 2014). A somewhat more complex structure is needed in order to evaluate the range and variety of environmental cues that lead to appropriate response. One important element in this evaluative process is emotion. By "emotion" I mean an affective response that indicates the positive or negative value of a stimulus or set of stimuli (Rolls 2014; Panksepp 2011). On this definition, emotions need not be conscious; they function broadly to provide a common currency for an animal to assess different sorts of stimuli along a scale from positive rewards to negative punishments. Pain is a form of punishment when nociception initiates a negative affective response that helps the animal learn what causes damage and should be avoided.

In Millikan's fanciful terminology, the animal forms a *pushmipullyu representation*, which associates the description of an environmental condition (bad) with the directive of appropriate response (avoid) in a single, undifferentiated representational unit (Millikan 2004). In other words, pain at this level is generally the representation of damage as bad and to be avoided (cf. Chapter 3, this volume),[5] where the specific content is determined by the location and sort of damage (tear on gill, burn on paw) as well as the kind of response required (flee, treat the wound, attack). Appropriate responses are learned based on past conditioning and can be quite finely tuned, despite the inability to separate how things are (description) from what to do (direction). The interdependence of emotion and cognition is best appreciated at this intermediate evolutionary stage between simple reflex and conscious evaluative response.

When the system is functioning well, a negative affective response conditions action that aids survival. Pain functions as part of the affective system whereby stimuli are associated with bodily damage so that the animal learns to respond better to those stimuli in the future.

Of course nature does not always function smoothly, and pathological cases can illuminate ways in which components of the affective system can be studied independently. In their work on pleasure, Kent Berridge and Morten Kringelbach (Berridge and Kringelbach 2011) have proposed three dissociable elements: "liking" is an affective response that can be either positive or negative ("dislike"); "wanting" is the motivation to approach or avoid a stimulus; and "learning" involves the various ways behavior is affected by past experience.[6] While it might seem essential to pleasure that anything liked is wanted and vice versa, drug addiction shows that people often reach a point where they want drugs without either liking or learning from the experience. Berridge and Kringelbach suggest objective ways to measure each element independently in order to better understand how the affective system functions and malfunctions. In addition to subjective reports which are applicable only to humans, objective measures can be used comparatively to assess animal emotions (Braithwaite et al. 2013; Kringelbach and Berridge 2009). Body movements such as facial expression, tail twitches, rocking, and rubbing can indicate like/dislike. Conditioned place preference and maze tests gauge motivation. Bias tasks and other instrumental tests assess learning. This behavioral evidence combines with evidence that these functions are subserved by similar neuroanatomical circuits, suggesting the basic structures for pain were selected for phylogenetically early and conserved in later species (Berridge and Kringelbach 2011).[7]

In the previous section I described the most basic function of pain as nociceptive response to avoid further damage. The evaluative response described in this section shows how nociception can lead to the representation of a stimulus or set of stimuli as negative and motivate avoidance. The evaluative response builds on the nociceptive response in precisely the stepwise way one would expect natural selection to proceed. Thinking about pain in terms of function also helps to explain malfunctions. We already considered the problems that occur when elements in an affective system come apart. There are also cases where a stimulus is misrepresented as nociceptive in the absence of sensory activation, such as phantom pain and chronic pain. While these cases are difficult and require further study, recent research suggests that misrepresentation of body image contributes to pain perception (Haggard et al. 2013).

In sum, pain figures as one of several affective systems that, when working properly, help an animal regulate its internal states in relation to the environment. (Cf. Chapter 8, this volume.) These systems – others include fear, anger, desire, play (Panksepp 2011) – are common among diverse animal groups and operate in tandem to guide the animal toward adaptively beneficial conditions and away from aversive ones.

4 The question of consciousness

But why think nociception, even accompanied by a negative evaluation, is "pain"? Isn't conscious feeling necessary for pain? (Cf. discussion on this question in Chapter 17, this volume.) Unlike sensations such as vision or hearing which represent environmental conditions, pain indicates a bodily condition. When you consciously experience your pain, its function to represent *your own private body* gives the impression that nothing outside your body could possibly indicate when pains are occurring. Moreover, the conscious feeling of hurtfulness seems essential to pain from the subjective perspective, rendering unconscious pain incoherent. What I have been arguing in this chapter is that the view of pain as limited to conscious hurtfulness is too narrow. By thinking of pain as part of an affective system, we gain a better understanding of how pain functions in human and non-human animals and how it evolved to fulfill those functions.

In fact, an explanation of how conscious pain evolved from unconscious forms of pain processing is much more plausible than a hypothesis that conscious pain is an entirely separate process. This section will propose an account of conscious pain as a further articulated form of the representation of damage. This argument involves several steps, each of which could be contested. What I hope to convey is not that this particular theory must be the answer to the question of consciousness, but that there *can* be an answer, and that the answer is important to understanding pain in animals. Two of the steps in the argument have already been discussed: representation is the mark of the mental, and pain is the representation of tissue damage. The next step is to describe the representational content of consciousness, using examples of human consciousness to motivate the theory. Toward the end of the section, I show how this theory applies to non-human animals.

According to my *temporal representation theory*: consciousness represents the present moment (Droege 2009). A careful examination of the content of conscious states reveals its essential spatio-temporal structure (Husserl 1990/1905). As I write, my experience shifts and drifts as I glance at the leaf-filtered light, notice the soft whoosh of nearby traffic, disappear into a thought. This is consciousness: at each moment, representations are selected and coordinated to compose the best approximation of the world as it is now, where "best" is determined by past adaptive success relative to me as species and individual in the particular context, and "world" is whatever internal or external states of affairs are selected. The world is represented as present in sensation and thought to me as now, now, now, in a continuous, serial order. On this view, consciousness is a representation of the present moment, because it serves the function of varying in accord with the world as it is now.

To represent presence in this biologically adaptive way is a peculiar thing. Because representations have functions on a teleosemantic theory, the requirement is not simply that "now" is represented in any sort of way, such as the word in this sentence. Of all the sensory and cognitive representations that *occur* now, only a selection are coordinated into a representation *of* now. The fact that only some of the current representations are conscious is one of the most convincing reasons to believe that pain can be unconscious. The chronic pain caused by my hip injury ceases to hurt when I am deeply absorbed in work or while sleeping. "Now" does not include the representation of damage when I am absorbed, and does not exist at all when I am in dreamless sleep. That pain representations continue is evidenced by the way my body favors the injured area. Further evidence of a common representational structure between conscious and unconscious pain is their shared neural structure. The first two stages of pain processing remain the same: nociception and cortical sensorimotor response.[8]

The fourth critical step is to explain *why* some representations are conscious, what *function* a representation of the present moment might serve. I suggest that pushmipullyu representations function unconsciously, because the descriptive input (pushmi) is tied to a specific directive output (pullyu). This form of representation may be quite complex when chains of learned responses form what is known as *fixed action patterns*. Though any sequence involves temporal order, no position in that order needs to be represented as "now." Pushmipullyu representations are activated according to environmental (or bodily) cues, so there need not be a representation of that cue as present.[9]

A representation of the present moment is needed when alternative responses are possible, that is, when pushmipullyu representations come apart and an animal can choose different actions in response to a situation. Representing how the world is now informs the animal of unexpected dangers and opportunities and allows it to track progress toward particular goals.

Maybe things are going well, or maybe a change is in order. Flexible response requires a representation of the present moment as distinct from past situations in order to identify unique combinations that may be relevant to future goals. Consciousness, according to the temporal representation theory, just is a representation of the present moment. While the contents of human consciousness can be quite elaborate,[10] fundamentally, consciousness represents the present so as to facilitate flexible response.

The final step in the argument, then, is to apply the theory to animals in order to show when animal pain is conscious. If consciousness is a representation of presence, and a representation of presence is necessary for flexible action, then flexible action is sufficient to demonstrate consciousness. That is, animals capable of flexible response are conscious animals, animals that feel conscious pain. However, distinguishing flexible from fixed response is not a simple matter. The basic idea behind flexibility is that an animal no longer simply acts based on past associations; it generalizes on past learning to anticipate which sort of action is best. For example, an animal may choose to eat food with an analgesic when it is lame but choose different food when well. Key to distinguishing flexibility from trial-and-error learning is to see whether the animal acts appropriately in response to different sorts of pain.[11] Provided good measures for flexible response can be formulated, we can use these acts to provide evidence of conscious pain.

Where philosophers have constructed principled obstacles to the investigation of conscious pain in animals, we now have a way forward. (1) Take teleosemantic representation as definitive of mental states and processes, where (2) pain is the representation of damage, and (3) consciousness is the representation of the present moment. (4) Consider that the function of consciousness is to facilitate flexible action, and (5) look for flexibility in animal responses to pain.

5 Pain and animal welfare

The final and most vital issue to consider is what ethical consequences follow from the identification of consciousness in animals. One perfectly reasonable answer is: none. Marian Dawkins has persuasively argued that animal welfare research would be more effectively pursued if the question of consciousness were put to the side (Dawkins 2012). Assessments of animal health and preference can be determined according to objective, behavioral criteria without the distracting objection that consciousness is inaccessible to scientific investigation.

This strategy is a good pragmatic approach, but the question of consciousness remains relevant to debates about animal welfare. Utilitarians place special weight on conscious pain in calculating the sum total good and bad of an act as well as in determining the sort of beings subject to moral consideration. Because conscious pleasure is especially valuable to me and conscious pain is abhorrent to me, one argument goes, moral action demands that I account for similar states in others (Varner 2012). Animal rights advocates make similar arguments when the inherent value of animals is rooted in their capacity to experience the world in ways humans do (Regan 2004). The problem with both arguments is that ethical response is grounded in the way animals are "like us." Instead, ethical response should be grounded in the way pain functions in the animal's own behavior and physiology. Yet recent attempts to develop moral theory entirely out of the biological basis for empathy and altruism (Churchland 2012) do not go far enough. Biology is descriptive, not prescriptive. In addition to understanding the cause and function of action, we need to know why these sorts of actions are *good*. More fundamentally, a theory should say when natural action is *bad* and how future action can be changed. My proposal is in line with the Aristotelian value of well-being developed through action and reflection (Aristotle, trans. 2000).

All of nature aims toward well-being in the sense that behavior conducive to survival and reproduction is selected for in evolution. Strictly speaking, natural selection operates on genes, so the care of offspring counts toward well-being in the evolutionary sense, even if there is considerable cost to the parent. Care toward members of a group likewise makes sense when care is reciprocated. The mechanisms that underlie these forms of care are fairly well understood and widespread among social animals (de Waal 2009). Humans certainly share the emotional equipment that grounds caring emotions, an assertion with which this chapter began. The question is when this empathetic response is warranted.

The answer to this question depends on the capacity for abstraction gained through the use of symbols. Language allows humans to sort the world into categories and submit those categories to rational and empirical tests. The importance of empirical as well as rational criteria for assessing value is one way that an Aristotelian approach to ethics is distinctive.[12] Well-being is determined by action and reflection on the results of that action, and reflection provides the resources for future changes in action. With respect to care for the well-being of others, we can begin by considering how the action affects the function of others.

Various means for assessing the function of animals have been the focus of this chapter. Ways in which animals process pain differ. Some have only a nociceptive response; others incorporate an emotional response where the evaluation of stimuli facilitates learning; and others feel conscious pain as a way to track progress toward goals. These different forms of pain processing call for different sorts of treatment. Even when we know which animals are capable of consciousness and which are not, there will still be reasons to care for the health and preferences of animals that do not experience conscious pain just as there are reasons to care for forests and other natural resources. The kinds of biological considerations scouted in this chapter motivate a reconfigured form of the golden rule: Do unto others appropriate to their function as you would have things done appropriate to your own function.[13]

Obviously too unwieldy to be a good slogan, the statement nonetheless captures the *mutatis mutandis* character of the ethical guideline I am recommending. Our evolutionary, behavioral and physiological continuity with animals calls for a continuity of ethical treatment. Yet continuity is not identity; relevant differences apply as well. Differing needs and capacities among groups and individuals should be taken into account in assessing moral action, as should differences in contexts. Much more would need to be said to flesh out this sketch, but I hope at least the general approach is comprehensible.[14]

6 Conclusion

In the end as at the beginning, the human empathic response to the pain of others forms the foundation of our concern about animals. To help answer the question of when other animals perceive pain and what humans should do about it, I have suggested a functional approach. Various elements in pain perception are relevant: nociception, learning, emotion, and flexibility. Careful scientific investigation can determine the ways these elements interconnect, and these interconnections can in turn illuminate similarities and differences in functional capacity among animal groups. Though pain is by no means unique to human animals, we are in a unique position to respond to pain in a reflective way to promote well-being.

Related topics

Chapter 17: Pain and consciousness (Pereplyotchik)
Chapter 36: Fetal pain and the law: abortion laws and their relationship to ideas about pain
(Derbyshire)

Acknowledgements

This chapter would not have been possible without Victoria Braithwaite, who started me wondering about animal pain and has provided invaluable inspiration, information, and criticism as my views have developed. The Institute for Advanced Study (*Wissenschaftskolleg*) in Berlin provided the ideal environment for thinking about complex, interdisciplinary problems as I worked on this chapter. Finally, I am grateful to Jennifer Corns whose thoughtful and constructive comments make her an exemplary editor.

Notes

1 Heider and Simmel (1944) showed that a simple video of two triangles and a circle was sufficient to motivate attribution of intentionality, emotion, and character. See the video, "Heider and Simmel Movie," *YouTube*, <https://www.youtube.com/watch?v=76p64j3H1Ng>.
2 Theories of representation range from computational approaches (Fodor 1990) to informational theories (Dretske 1981) to embodied cognition (Clark 1997). One reason to favor Millikan's theory is its aptitude for addressing issues like animal pain.
3 As already mentioned, the term "representation" is deeply contested, and I cannot do justice to the many controversial issues it raises. For example, Millikan herself initially resisted the application of the term to the most rudimentary forms of intentional content (Millikan 1989). Whether or not one approves of the word, I will try to define my usage as clearly as possible to indicate how "representation" is useful in the study of animal minds. For more on the relation between representation and pain, see Cutter (Chapter 2, this volume).
4 This description of pain processing as a series of events is adapted from Braithwaite (2010: 27–33)
5 That is, the damage is to be avoided, not necessarily the situation that brought on the damage.
6 Each of these elements requires more precision than space here allows. "Liking" and "wanting" are likely scalar, for example, and the "liking" scale may split into separate pleasure and pain scales (Shriver 2014). I leave it to the specialists to work out these details as well as to specify necessary and sufficient conditions for pain when these components come apart. A good place to begin is Corns 2014.
7 To whatever extent I have been able to convey the role of liking, wanting, and learning to pain and animals, I am entirely indebted to the excellent comments of Jennifer Corns.
8 While the neural correlate for consciousness remains in debate, there is wide agreement that sensorimotor activations are common to unconscious and conscious processing of stimuli.
9 A fixed sequence may involve very long temporal intervals, regulated by diurnal or lunar cycles or other means of oscillatory mechanisms. In this case temporal mechanisms are used by the representational system to perform its function even though time does not figure as part of the content of the representations.
10 Most importantly, conscious memory, and imagination involve an embedded temporal structure (the past or future is brought into the present) that may be exclusively human (Droege 2013).
11 Much more needs to be said in order to flesh out this proposal into a research program. For a start, see Droege and Braithwaite 2014.
12 This approach is distinctive but not unique. Pragmatists argue for a similar, results-oriented view.
13 My hint about proper care of forests and natural resources suggests that "function" can be taken quite broadly here. A sustainable ecosystem requires more care about the treatment of disposable plastics (reduce, reuse, recycle) as well as industrial fishing practices, even if the recipient of care is artificial and therefore has only functions derived from human needs and desires.
14 For example, does this approach entail vegetarianism? The answer depends on how you think about function. In any case, it would be inconsistent to be concerned only about consciousness and disregard all other considerations of function. Cf. discussion of fetal pain in Chapter 36, this volume.

References

Aristotle (2000) *Nicomachean Ethics*. Indianapolis: Hackett Publishing Co.

Berridge, K.C. and Kringelbach, M.L. (2011) Building a neuroscience of pleasure and well-being. *Psychology of Well-Being: Theory, Research and Practice* 1(1): 3.

Braithwaite, V.A. (2010) *Do Fish Feel Pain?* Oxford: Oxford University Press.

Braithwaite, V.A., Huntingford, F., and Bos, R. van den (2013) Variation in emotion and cognition among fishes. *Journal of Agricultural and Environmental Ethics* 26(1): 7–23.

Churchland, P.S. (2012) *Braintrust: What Neuroscience Tells Us about Morality*. Princeton: Princeton University Press.

Clark, A. (1997) *Being There: Putting Brain, Body and World Together Again*, Cambridge, MA: MIT Press.

Corns, J. (2014) Unpleasantness, motivational oomph, and painfulness. *Mind & Language* 29(2): 238–254.

Dawkins, M.S. (2012) *Why Animals Matter: Animal Consciousness, Animal Welfare, and Human Well-Being*. Oxford: Oxford University Press.

de Vignemont, F. and Jacob, P. (2012) What is it like to feel another's Pain?. *Philosophy of Science* 79(2): 295–316.

de Waal, F. (2009) *The Age of Empathy: Nature's Lessons for a Kinder Society*. New York: Crown.

Dretske, F. (1981) *Knowledge and the Flow of Information*. Cambridge, MA: MIT Press.

Droege, P. (2009) Now or never: how consciousness represents time. *Consciousness and Cognition* 18(1): 78–90.

Droege, P. (2013) Memory and consciousness. *Philosophia Scientiae* 17(2): 171–193.

Droege, P. and Braithwaite, V.A. (2014) A framework for investigating animal consciousness. In G. Lee, J. Illes, and F. Ohl (eds.), *Ethical Issues in Behavioral Neuroscience*. Current Topics in Behavioral Neurosciences. Berlin/Heidelberg: Springer, pp. 79–98.

Fodor, J.A. (1990) *A Theory of Content and Other Essays*. Cambridge, MA: MIT Press.

Grau, J.W. (2014) Learning from the spinal cord: how the study of spinal cord plasticity informs our view of learning. In A.R. Delamater and K.M. Lattal (eds.), *Associative Perspectives on the Neurobiology of Learning*, special issue of *Neurobiology of Learning and Memory* 108: 155–171.

Haggard, P., Iannetti, G.D., and Longo, M.R. (2013) Spatial sensory organization and body representation in pain perception. *Current Biology* 23(4): R164–R176.

Heider, F. and Simmel, M. (1944) An experimental study of apparent behavior. *American Journal of Psychology* 57(2): 243–259.

Husserl, E. (1990/1905) *On the Phenomenology of the Consciousness of Internal Time (1893–1917)*. Husserliana: Collected Works. Dordrecht: Kluwer Academic.

Kavaliers, M. (1988) Evolutionary and comparative aspects of nociception. *Brain Research Bulletin* 21(6): 923–931.

Kringelbach, M.L. and Berridge, K.C. (2009) Towards a functional neuroanatomy of pleasure and happiness. *Trends in Cognitive Sciences* 13(11): 479–487.

Millikan, R.G. (1989) Biosemantics. *Journal of Philosophy* 86(6): 281–297.

Millikan, R.G. (1993) *White Queen Psychology and Other Essays for Alice*. Cambridge, MA: MIT Press.

Millikan, R.G. (2004) *Varieties of Meaning*. Cambridge, MA: MIT Press.

Panksepp, J. (2011) The basic emotional circuits of mammalian brains: do animals have affective lives?. In H.C. Cromwell and V. Bingman (eds.), *Pioneering Research in Affective Neuroscience: Celebrating the Work of Dr. Jaak Panksepp*, special issue of *Neuroscience & Biobehavioral Reviews* 35(9): 1791–1804.

Regan, T. (2004) *The Case for Animal Rights*. Oakland, CA: University of California Press.

Rolls, E.T. (2014) Emotion and decision-making explained: a précis. *Cortex* 59: 185–193.

Shriver, A.J. (2014) The asymmetrical contributions of pleasure and pain to animal welfare. *Cambridge Quarterly of Healthcare Ethics* 23(2): 152–162.

Smith, E.S.J. and Lewin, G.R. (2009) Nociceptors: a phylogenetic view. *Journal of Comparative Physiology A* 195(12): 1089–1106.

Varner, G.E. (2012) *Personhood, Ethics, and Animal Cognition: Situating Animals in Hare's Two Level Utilitarianism*. New York: Oxford University Press.

16

ROBOT PAIN

Pete Mandik

1 Introduction: suffering robots

What if the painful but necessary experiments that are conducted on animals and people could instead be conducted on elaborate robots? This would be an ethical boon, but only if the robotic surrogates weren't so elaborate as to themselves suffer real pain. Aside from the potential benefits to medical research, there might be other motives – some benign, some nefarious – for creating robots with the potential of themselves suffering pains. It might increase the usefulness of a robot servant if it took care to prevent damage to itself; and the resultant self-monitoring system may turn out to implement pain. Some humans may seek to purchase pain-feeling robots for the purpose of torturing them – a sad fact about some humans. Plausibly, there's an ethical imperative for making sure avoidable robot pains are not inflicted.[1] But there's a metaphysical question of whether such pains – robot pains – *could* be inflicted. Further, there's an epistemological question of how we would ever know. As our technologies advance, this special version of the problem of other minds – the problem of robot pain – becomes increasingly pressing.

Can robots feel pain? I intend this question as shorthand for a much more elaborate question, and the sequence of elaborations I intend proceed along two lines, one of which goes beyond "robots" and the other of which goes beyond "feel pain."

More than robots, I want to ask about a broader class of entities, a class that includes technological artifacts – such as artificially intelligent computers (AI), and computer simulations of human and non-human animals – including so-called "mind uploads," simulations based directly on brain scans (for more specifically on the feasibility of mind uploading, see Mandik 2015a). Unless it matters for some particular point, I will continue to use "robot" as a handy label for the sort of entity in question, whose resemblance to humans is sufficiently incomplete as to leave interesting and special questions open about whether they feel pain.

About the phrase "feel pain," there are two sorts of pain phenomena or aspects of pain one might indicate by use of that phrase, but only one of those sorts is my primary focus in this chapter and only one of those is what I primarily aim to pick out by "feel pain." To be very brief, we might sort these aspects into the first-person aspects and the third-person aspects, and it is the first-person aspects that I primarily intend to pick out by "feeling pain" and related.

The bifurcation I have in mind can be conveyed in terms of the classic other-minds problem. The third-person aspects of pain are those aspects of pain upon which I base my confidence that someone else is in pain, whereas the first-person aspects of pain are the ones which I might, in a certain philosophical frame of mind, find myself doubting that anyone but me ever feels. These first-person aspects of pain are my primary focus here. (See also, in the present volume, Chapters 17, 18, and 20.) To elaborate my description of them even further, they are pains as they appear to the one who is having them. They are consciously experienced pains. There may be even further elaborations needed in nailing down the target here, but I will address them as further needs arise. It should suffice for now to say that the question "Can robots feel pain?" is shorthand for my real question, "Can robots and their ilk (e.g., computer simulations) consciously suffer pains, pains of the sort that I have little doubt that I myself suffer when I appraise my own pains from my first-person point of view?"

Echoing Chalmers' (1996) taxonomy of sorting problems of consciousness into the "easy" and the "hard," we might say that the question of present concern is far harder than the question of whether there could be a robot that, to all outward appearances, was in pain. When we turn to the hard question of robot pain, the question of whether there can ever be pains that feel "from the inside" to robots the way pains feel to us, we encounter a question that does not seem straightforwardly empirical. It may very well ultimately turn out to be an empirically decidable question, but it seems that further philosophical reflection is needed before we know how to proceed empirically here.[2]

To my mind, it seems that the strongest and most convincing lines of thought relevant to the question of robot pain are two arguments, one of which offers a negative answer and the other of which offers a positive one. The first argument, the one whose conclusion is that robots cannot feel pain, is an adaptation of John Searle's famous Chinese room argument against artificial intelligence (Searle 1980). Searle develops his own argument in terms of the mental state of understanding, though it seems to me to be readily adaptable to pain states. The second argument, the one concluding that robots can feel pain, is an adaptation of a prosthetic neurons argument, perhaps most well known in the work of Chalmers (1996), but earlier versions of which may be found at least as far back as Harman (1973: 38–39).[3]

In the next section, I'll further explore the Chinese room argument against robot pain. I'll turn then in the section after that to explore the prosthetic neurons argument in favor of robot pain. Finally, in the concluding section I'll offer a comparative assessment of the two arguments.

At the heart of my assessment is a comparison between premises in each argument that relate the ways things seem with respect to conscious pain phenomena to conscious pain phenomena themselves. The respective premises differ in their logical structure – one is the logical converse of the other. Putting this very briefly: At the core of the argument for robot pain is a premise that moves from the ways thing seem first-personally to the ways they are, whereas at the core of the argument against robot pain is a premise that moves in the opposite direction, that is, from the ways things are to the ways they first-personally seem. This logical difference, I'll suggest, makes a difference in the respective likelihoods of the soundness of each argument.

2 Chinese rooms and the case against robot pain

At the heart of Searle's famous argument is the thought experiment that gives the argument its name. We are invited to imagine Searle inside of a room running a program – that is, following a set of instructions – that would result in observers outside of the room concluding that someone inside the room understands Chinese.

The program in question is structurally equivalent to a program that, when run on a digital computer, would allow someone to have a convincing conversation in Chinese with it, perhaps via an exchange of text messages. In the room scenario, observers outside of the room send and receive messages via printed cards going into and out of slots in the room's walls. Inside of the room is John Searle, who is stipulated to understand absolutely no Chinese himself. He understands English, and follows a set of instructions printed in English in a manual that also contains pictures of a variety of Chinese symbols. The English text does not provide translations from Chinese into English, but instead directs Searle to select appropriate output cards for each given input card. We can imagine the instructions having something like the general form of "If receiving symbol ABC, then reply with symbol XYZ," which would be an instruction that a monolingual English reader can follow well enough without having any clue what the appropriate translation of ABC and XYZ into English would be.

We can see at this point the relevance of Searle's thought experiment for AI: If Searle can run the program without himself understanding Chinese, then an AI or robot that gives the outward appearance of understanding Chinese might nonetheless be running a program without itself thereby understanding Chinese.

We are in a position, too, to see how to adapt the Chinese room argument to pertain to pain. The program in question can be one the running of which convinces outside interlocutors that they are conversing with an entity undergoing some degree of pain. And if we imagine the room in the head of a large robot, instead of just card outputs that say things in Chinese about being in pain, the robot's outputs might additionally involve moving its body in ways consistent with, for instance, suffering the pains associated with a sprained ankle. I'll postpone further discussion of pain for now, and return to the version of the thought experiment focused on understanding a language.

This thought experiment is not itself an argument, but instead serves as a part of an argument. To briefly indicate some of the main parts of the larger argument, we can make do for now with the following points. First, we need to suppose a version of the thesis of AI – the thesis that robots, computers, and their ilk can have genuine mental states – that is stated in terms of the running of programs. We might put the crucial point like this: If AI is possible, then something or someone could understand Chinese merely by running a program. We can put essentially the same point in a different, contrapositive form. The following should serve our purpose: If it is possible for something or someone to run any arbitrarily selected program without themselves *thereby* understanding Chinese, then AI is not possible. The "thereby" here is important – a Chinese/English bilingual person running Searle's program suffices for Chinese understanding, but they don't understand Chinese *because* (or *in virtue of*) of the running of the program.

The role of the Chinese room thought experiment is to establish the truth of the claim that it is indeed possible for something or someone to run any arbitrarily selected program without thereby understanding Chinese. It should be clear that, given the above formulation of what AI entails about programs, if the thought experiment succeeds, then AI fails.

However, the thought experiment does not succeed. As even Searle himself notes (Searle 1980: 419–42), one of the most natural responses available to the defender of AI is the now famous "systems reply": While the defenders of AI can readily grant that Searle himself does not understand Chinese, they need not grant that Searle himself is running the program. Instead, says the systems reply, Searle is a proper part of a larger system – a system including other contents of the room, including the cards and instruction manual – and it is this larger system that runs the program. It's open, then, for the AI defender to assert that the larger system understands Chinese, and Searle's stipulated ignorance is powerless to cast doubt on this.

Searle introduces a second thought experiment to shore up his argument against the threat posed by the systems reply. In this second thought experiment, he dispenses with the room and the other external props – the cards, the instruction manual. We are invited now to imagine Searle memorizing the program, including all of the pictures of the symbols. We might even imagine Searle memorizing sounds and instructions for which sounds to offer in reply to other sounds. Hypothetically, at least, Searle could run the program at such a speed that an outside observer/interlocutor might think Searle himself could both speak and write Chinese. But, again, we are invited to imagine Searle running this program without himself actually understanding Chinese. The systems reply now seems impotent, for it is not a larger system that is running the program, but Searle himself. And if he also does not understand Chinese, then this would be a case in which running a program does not thereby give rise to understanding.

We can imagine adapting Searle's thought experiment to pain states by imaging Searle undergoing a procedure – involving perhaps local anesthetics, analgesics, or some combination thereof – so that he cannot feel pain, while nonetheless remaining awake and alert. Numb to pain, he might nonetheless, by memorizing a set of instructions and observing by sight, etc., various pokes and prods to his flesh, give a convincing performance that would enable him to pass a Turing test for being in pain. He would be running a program that would, if run by a robot, give every outward aspect of being in pain. But he wouldn't thereby be in pain by running the program. Or so we are invited to imagine. If Searle can run the program without thereby being in pain, there seems little reason to believe, then, that a robot running what's essentially the same program would thereby feel pain.

But the question we must now contemplate is this: Is it indeed the case that Searle can run the program without thereby being in pain? What reason is there to believe that this is the case? What reason is there for not instead believing that, in running the program, Searle must thereby indeed be in pain?

To get a feel for what the underlying reasoning must be here, it helps to contrast the Searlean argument with some arguments that are decidedly *not* the Searlean argument. One argument that is certainly not the present argument is one where the opponent of AI presents an actual modern-day computer and declares it to be evident that it fails to be in pain. They would be correct in their claim that it is evident that computer is pain-free. Most AI proponents would likely grant that current computers exhibit none of what we take to be the third-person accessible evidence for the presence of pain states. This would be a very weak argument against the possibility of robot pain, and I think that the Searlean argument is better than that.

Another argument that is decidedly not the Searlean argument is a version of Leibniz's *Monadology* argument for the simplicity of minds. Leibniz imagines shrinking down and examining a complex mechanism – he seems clearly to have a brain in mind – and discovers nothing therein that would explain perception. We can easily modify the Leibnizian argument to involve a similar failure to explain pain. A shrunken explorer might make an incredible journey through the entire course of a brain and remain puzzled as to whether this complex system must give rise to any felt pain. Note that what our miniaturized Leibniz accesses are third-personal aspects of pain. Despite being physically inside of a brain, there remain senses of "inside" and "outside" whereby Leibniz remains outside. For all that he observes, the possibility remains that there is something it's like to be the complex mechanism, and the complex mechanism itself feels what it's like "from the inside."

The improvement that the Searlean argument offers over these other two arguments is the way it attempts to access things "from the inside" in the relevant senses of the terms. We can see the Searlean argument as attempting to marshal first-person evidence in the service of his anti-AI conclusion. In conducting the Searlean thought experiment ourselves we must imaginatively inhabit a point of view that puts us in a position to access first-personal evidence. But what is this so-called first-person evidence? It can be nothing else besides its seeming to the person in question that they are not in pain – I have no idea what it could mean for someone to have first-person evidence that they are not in pain without it seeming to that person that they are not in pain. And from this first-person evidence about how things seem, the Searlean attempts to draw a conclusion about how things are, namely that one is not in pain.

We are in a position now to lay out the main logical structure of the full Searlean argument.

1   If robot pain is possible, then there ought to be some program in virtue of which one would be in pain solely by running that program.
2   Searle can run any arbitrarily selected program without it seeming to him from the first-person point of view that he is in pain.
3   If it doesn't seem to one from the first-person point of view that one is in pain, then one is not in pain.
4   It's true of every possible program that Searle could run it without himself thereby being in pain.

Therefore, robot pain is not possible.

The conclusion follows straightforwardly from premises (1) and (4). Premise (1) seems an obvious entailment of the basic idea of robot pain. Premise (4) follows straightforwardly from premises (2) and (3). Premise (2) is the core idea of the Searlean thought experiment, especially the one designed to avoid the systems response. Premise (3), which I'll hereafter refer to as the *Searlean conditional*, is the one that strikes me as the most questionable part of the whole argument. But I'll postpone my critical remarks for the section after the next. It is time now to turn to the case in favor of believing in robot pain.

3 Prosthetic neurons and the case for robot pains

If robots could indeed feel pain, how might we go about building such a robot? One approach that suggests itself is that we identify systems we know to already feel pain – namely ourselves – and we copy as much as we can from the human case into a robotic form. One way to construct a robotic copy of a human is by gradually transforming a human into a robot by a sequence of prosthetic replacements of the human's naturally occurring parts, especially parts of the nervous system, with artificial analogs.

Like all physiological systems in the human body, the nervous system is composed of causally interacting cells. The most significant cells in the nervous system are neurons. The causal interactions between the cells together serve in the causal mediation between sensory stimulus to, and behavioral response of, the entire organism. The interactions between cells also serve to constitute those aspects of cognition that can be characterized causally. One such aspect is memory, which can be characterized in terms of changes in an organism that underwrite its ability to give different responses to instances of the same type of stimulus presented at different times (as when a ringing bell at one time doesn't cause salivation but when presented at a later time does). Another aspect of cognition that can be characterized causally is the ability to make discriminations, as when one discriminates a paint chip's color from the color of the background. Part of such a capacity must involve the different causal effects that the respective colors of the chip and background have on the discriminating organism.

Hypothetically, the causal influence that one naturally occurring cell exerts on another can also be exerted by a device that is not a naturally occurring cell, but is instead an artificial prosthesis, perhaps a microchip that has the same input–output profile as a neuron. Imagine a sequence of surgeries that transforms a human into a robot by gradual replacement of components. We will make the simplifying assumption that all that matters for present discussion is located in the nervous system, and so we will imagine the sequence of prosthetic replacements as involving a sequence of procedures whereby, during each procedure, a single cell of the nervous system is replaced by a chip that has the same causal effects and sensitivities vis-à-vis other cells as the cell that the chip replaces. Note that we are not supposing that the chip has *all* of the same causal properties as a neuron. If it did, it would be impossible to distinguish by any experiment or observation a neuron from a chip. But chips are made largely of silicon, and neurons are not, and the chemical differences involve causal differences. Nonetheless, we are supposing that a neuron is not causally sensitive to all of the causal properties of another neuron. And we are further supposing that the limited range of causal properties that characterize interneuron interaction can be fully replicated by chip–neuron interaction, which in turn can be fully replicated by chip–chip interaction. The result of transforming NaturalPete into RobotPete by a sequence of chip replacements will be that RobotPete is what I'll call a "coarse-grained causal isomorph" of NaturalPete.

NaturalPete feels pain. A natural thing to suppose goes hand-in-hand with the very idea of robot pain is that, given that NaturalPete feels pain, in being NaturalPete's coarse-grained causal isomorph, RobotPete feels pain too. (We assume throughout that when each is awake, they are each in the same environment in all relevant respects.) For the purposes of the central argument in this section, the most important connection between the thesis of robot pain and the neural prosthesis scenario can be stated thusly: If, by being the coarse-grained causal isomorph to an entity that feels pain, the isomorph feels pain, then robot pain is possible.

The thought experiment serves the larger argument in favor of robot pain in the following manner. We are invited to imagine ourselves undergoing the sequence of prostheses replacements without it ever, at any point, thereby ceasing to seem to ourselves that we have pain. The "thereby" here is important: It may be prudent to administer a general anesthetic for the duration of the surgery, and thus any pain would, arguably, cease for the duration. Nonetheless, it isn't here supposed that the pain is temporarily abated *because* one or more neurons were replaced by chips, but instead because an anesthetic was administered. At every point in the sequence at which the subject is neither anesthetized nor asleep, it seems to the subject that they are in pain despite how many of their neurons have been replaced by chips.

Important in thinking through the thought experiment of the transformation of NaturalPete into RobotPete is the sequence $n + 0$, $n + 1$, $n + 2$, ..., where $n + m$ equals the number of neurons so far replaced at that point by prostheses, $n + 0$ corresponds to NaturalPete, and $n + z$ corresponds to RobotPete. Throughout this sequence, there is something that uncontroversially remains constant, namely the coarse-grained functional structure. Each respective entity in the sequence, then, is a coarse-grained functional isomorph of its sequential predecessor.

But why is it important to the argument that there's a gradual transformation of a human into a robot? It helps here to contrast the present argument with one that depends only on the consideration of a robot that has the same coarse-grained functional structure as a human. In this latter case, all we are imaginatively presented with, being humans ourselves, is third-person evidence concerning whether the robot is in pain. It exhibits all the outward behavioral evidence that we would utilize in determining that some human other than ourselves is in pain. And minus the very fine details that distinguish neurons from microchips, it has the same third-person-accessible internal causal structure as well. In contrast, the advantage of the neural prosthesis argument is the way in which it marshals the first-person point of view. We imaginatively put ourselves in the position of NaturalPete, and imagine ourselves living through the sequence of surgeries and post-operative occasions. Throughout the sequence, what we are invited to imagine is that it would seem to us, from the inside, as it were, that our pains neither fade nor suddenly disappear. For the thought experiment to serve its role in the larger argument, we need additionally a linking principle from how things *seem* with respect to one's own pain states to how things actually *are* with regard to one's pain. We need, then, a premise in the argument along the lines of this: If it seems to one that one is in pain, then one is indeed in pain.

Assembling the pieces sketched so far, we are in a position now to consider the structure of the larger prosthetic neurons argument, noting a rough structural similarity to the adapted Chinese room argument.

1   If, by being the coarse-grained causal isomorph to an entity that feels pain, the isomorph feels pain, then robot pain is possible.
2   Via a sequence of neuro-prosthetic replacements, you can be transformed into your coarse-grained causal isomorph without it ever ceasing to seem to you from the first-person point of view that you are in pain.
3   If it seems to one from the first-person point of view that one is in pain, then one is in pain.
4   By being your coarse-grained causal isomorph, an entity thereby feels pain.

Therefore, robot pain is possible.

The conclusion of this argument follows straightforwardly from premises (1) and (4). Premise (1) is a highly natural thing to suppose about the relation between the idea of robot pain and the notion of a being who is a coarse-grained causal isomorph of a normal human being. Premise (4) follows straightforwardly from premises (2) and (3). Premise (2) is a condensed statement of the prosthetic neurons thought experiment. Premise (3) is the one that strikes me as the one most in need of further comment, and I turn to that issue in the next section, where I'll also remark on a counterpart premise from the Searlean argument.

4 Concluding comparative assessment

The above arguments cannot both be sound, for their conclusions cannot both be true. One or both arguments must be unsound. Unfortunately a full discussion would far exceed the allotted space. In this remaining section, I give a very brief account of one possible view of both arguments, one whereby the third premise of the adapted Chinese room argument is false and the third premise of the prosthetic neurons argument is true. Of course, this falls far short of establishing the soundness of the one argument and unsoundness of the other. I hope the present discussion to nonetheless be useful for further thought on the matter.

Before remarking on the merits of premise (3) of the prosthetic neurons argument, it is worth noting its logical relationship to its counterpart premise from the Searlean argument. Recall that the third premise from the adapted Chinese room argument is this:

The Searlean conditional: If it doesn't seem to one from the first-person point of view that one is in pain, then one is not in pain.

The Searlean conditional is logically equivalent, by contraposition, to this conditional (which I'll hereafter call *the thesis of self-intimation*):

The thesis of self-intimation: If one is in pain, then it seems to one from the first-person point of view that one is in pain.

The thesis of self-intimation is logically distinct from its converse, a conditional we can call *the thesis of incorrigibility*:

The thesis of incorrigibility: If it seems to one from the first-person point of view that one is in pain, then one is in pain.

Note that the thesis of incorrigibility is one and the same as the third premise of the prosthetic neurons argument. The remainder of my commentary on the two arguments will focus on these two theses, *self-intimation* and *incorrigibility*.[4]

The merits of the thesis of self-intimation can be regarded as one and the same as the merits of the claim that pains never occur unconsciously. Unconscious pains, if there are such things, are pains one is in without it seeming to one that one is in pain. See David Pereplyotchik's Chapter 17 in the present volume for an overview of the case for unconscious pains. As Pereplyotchik points out, one basis for acknowledging unconscious pain is a version of a Higher-Order representational account of consciousness, in particular the Higher-Order Thought (HOT) account as spelled out by Rosenthal (2005, 2011).

Being very brief here: according to Rosenthal's HOT theory, one and the same pain can be unconscious at one time, and conscious at another. The relevant difference between the two different times boils down to whether or not there's a suitable accompanying HOT about the pain state. Putting it in a very simplified manner, when there's a HOT about the pain state, the pain state is conscious, and when there is no such HOT, the pain state is unconscious. So, on this view, there are two ways of being in pain: one way is to be in pain consciously, and the other is to be in pain unconsciously.

The view additionally allows for two different ways of consciously being in pain. The first is the way just mentioned above, a way involving two actual mental states, one of which is the pain, the other of which is a HOT about the pain. A second way one may count as being in a conscious pain state is when one is simply in a HOT about a pain. The pain the HOT is about need not actually exist; it is, in this case, merely notional. There are then, three ways of being in pain: one unconscious way and two conscious ways, and the two conscious ways are when the state the HOT is about is actual and when the state the HOT is about is merely notional (Rosenthal 2011: 433–434).

This may seem an unintuitive way of reading HOT theory. One might prefer to read it instead as entailing that one is in a conscious pain only when one has both of two states: a pain and a HOT about it. On such a reading, in the case where one has only the HOT, one is not in pain even though it seems to oneself that one has a pain. And thus, on such a reading, *incorrigibility* would turn out false.[5]

Whatever the merits of this latter reading of HOT theory, it goes against the one that Rosenthal emphasizes (as well as the interpretations favored by other HOT theorists, see, for example, Weisberg 2010, 2011). One way of unpacking these distinct readings of the HOT theory is, as I spell out in further detail in Mandik (2015b: especially 194–195), as a non-relational reading of HOT theory, as opposed to a relational one. In favor of this non-relational reading of HOT theory, Rosenthal writes "[a]ll that matters for a state's being conscious is its seeming subjectively to one that one is in that state. On the HOT theory, that's determined by a HOT's intentional content" (Rosenthal 2011: 436). On this non-relational reading of HOT theory, the HOT alone suffices for being in a conscious state and thus is consciousness non-relational, for it does not consist in a relation borne between a HOT and another state.

The upshot of all this for the present chapter is that, insofar as Rosenthal's HOT theory and the non-relational reading of it are coherent, we thereby have a coherent basis for rejecting the thesis of self-intimation while at the same time affirming the thesis of incorrigibility. HOT theory allows us to reject self-intimation on the grounds that there can indeed be pains without accompanying HOTs about them (see again Pereplyotchik's chapter for details). HOT theory allows us to affirm incorrigibility on the grounds that, when there is a HOT to the effect that one is in pain, one is in pain, at least in a notional sense of "is in pain."

A converse move seems unavailable to the Searlean. The Searlean seems to lack any basis for rejecting incorrigibility while at the same time affirming self-intimation. The Searlean lacks, as far as I can tell, any basis for saying that while it is true that if one is in pain, then it seems from the first-person point of view that one is in pain, it is nonetheless false that if it first-personally seems to one that one is in pain, then one is. The Searlean may try to bolster their case along such lines by arguing that all pains are conscious pains, but now the dialectic shifts to the one covered in Pereplyotchik's chapter, and space does not permit further pursuing it here. (See also Chapter 15, this volume.)

Insofar as we are focusing critique only upon the third premise of each of the two main arguments concerning robot pain (the premises that comprise the theses of *incorrigibility* and *self-intimation*), we now have a basis for rejecting the Chinese room argument, while retaining the prosthetic neurons argument. Of course, the arguments contain other premises, and while I have tried to indicate somewhat why I think those other premises are the most secure parts of the arguments, other thinkers may focus their critiques on exactly those points. Such lines of thought cannot be further pursued in the present space.

In this chapter, I have laid out what seem to me to be the most promising arguments on opposing sides of the question of whether what humans regard as the first-person accessible aspects of pain could also be implemented in robots. I have emphasized the ways in which the thought experiments in the respective arguments attempt to marshal hypothetical first-person accessible evidence concerning how one's own mental life appears to oneself. In the Chinese room argument, a crucial premise involves the thesis that from a lack of it seeming that one is in pain, one can conclude that one is not in pain. There's a counterpart thesis playing a crucial role in the prosthetic neurons argument, one asserting an entailment from its seeming that one is in pain to one's being in pain. I further suggested that by adopting a HOT theory of consciousness, of the sort reviewed in Pereplyotchik's chapter in the present volume, one is thereby in a better position to endorse the prosthetic neurons argument over the Chinese room argument than to make the opposite appraisal.

Related topics

Acknowledgements

For especially helpful discussions of earlier versions I am enormously grateful to Jennifer Corns and David Pereplyotchik. Thanks too are due for comments from David Bain and Olivier Massin, and also from attendees of presentations I made at The Role of Phenomenal Consciousness Workshop at the University of Glasgow's Value of Suffering Project.

Notes

1 For an excellent survey on the distinctively ethical dimensions of robot pain, see Sandberg 2014.
2 The problem under present consideration is a less general version of what Schneider and Mandik (forthcoming) identify as the Hard Problem of AI Consciousness.
3 See also Pylyshyn 1980, Zuboff 1981, 2008, 1994, and Cuda 1985.
4 See Chapter 20, this volume, for more on incorrigibility.
5 I am grateful to Jennifer Corns for pressing this concern in response to an earlier version of the present material.

References

Chalmers, D.J. (1996) The conscious mind. In *Search of a Fundamental Theory*. Oxford: Oxford University Press.
Cuda, T. (1985) Against neural chauvinism. *Philosophical Studies* 48: 111–127.
Harman, G. (1973) *Thought*. Princeton, NJ: Princeton University Press.
Mandik, P. (2015a) Metaphysical daring as a posthuman survival strategy. *Midwest Studies in Philosophy* 39 (1): 144–157.
Mandik, P. (2015b) Conscious-state anti-realism. In C. Muñoz-Suárez and F. de Brigard (eds.), *Content and Consciousness Revisited: With Replies by Daniel Dennett*. Berlin: Springer.
Pylyshyn, Z. (1980) The "causal power" of machines. *Behavioral and Brain Sciences* 3: 442–444.
Rosenthal, D.M. (2005) *Consciousness and Mind*. Oxford: Clarendon Press.
Rosenthal, D.M. (2011) Exaggerated reports: reply to Block. *Analysis* 71(3): 431–437.
Sandberg, A. (2014) Being nice to software animals and babies. R. Blackford and D. Broderick (eds.), *Intelligence Unbound: The Future of Uploaded and Machine Minds*. Hoboken, NJ: Wiley Blackwell.
Schneider, S. and Mandik, P. (Forthcoming) How philosophy of mind can shape the future. In Amy Kind (ed.), *Philosophy of Mind in the Twentieth and Twenty-First Centuries*. London: Routledge.
Searle, J.R. (1980) Minds, brains, and programs. *Behavioral and Brain Sciences* 3: 417–457.
Weisberg, J. (2010) Misrepresenting consciousness. *Philosophical Studies* 154(3): 409–433. doi:10.1007/s11098-010-9567-3.
Weisberg, J. (2011) Abusing the notion of what-it's-like-ness: a response to Block. *Analysis* 71(3): 438–443. doi:10.1093/analys/anr040.
Zuboff, A. (1981) The story of a brain. In D.R. Hofstadter and D.C. Dennett (eds.), *The Mind's I*. New York: Basic Books.
Zuboff, A. (1994) What is a mind? *Midwest Studies in Philosophy* 19(1): 183–205.
Zuboff, A. (2008) Thoughts about a solution to the mind–body problem. *Think* 6(17–18): 159–171.

17

PAIN AND CONSCIOUSNESS

David Pereplyotchik

1 Introduction

A useful taxonomy of personal-level mental properties will include qualitative character, conceptual content, and affective valence. Qualitative character is the distinctive feature of sensations – the mental property in virtue of which they facilitate a creature's ability to discriminate between perceptible properties, such as odors, sounds, textures, and bodily conditions (Clark 1993). The qualitative properties of sensations are intimately related to the conceptual contents of the perceptual judgments that they elicit; a sensation of red will typically give rise to a perceptual judgment that deploys the concept RED. Finally, it is commonly agreed that the distinctive feature of emotions is their affective valence, which is associated in various ways with both evaluative judgment and motivational force (Barrett 2006; Lerner and Keltner 2000).

Pain has been thought of in all of these ways. (See the chapters in Section I, this volume.) It has been characterized as a sensation (Kripke 1980), a perception (Cutter and Tye 2011), an imperative (Klein 2015), an emotion (Craig 2003), and a combination of these (Clark 2005). Whichever view one prefers, it should be clear that any *informative* account of pain – any account that goes beyond the unhelpful thought that "we know it when we feel it" – will characterize the mental properties of pain in terms of its functional role. For instance, those who view pain as including a sensory component will stress its role in discriminating potentially harmful thermal, mechanical, and chemical stimuli, as well as the associated bodily conditions (Clark 2005; Grahek 2007). Those who view pain as a perceptual judgment likewise stress its discriminative function, but they take the deployment of concepts to be a necessary condition on the relevant type of discrimination (Hill 2005). Similarly, in characterizing the intentional content and mental attitude of pain, imperativists stress the role that pain plays in guiding withdrawal, escape, and avoidance responses (Grahek 2007), as well as the intentions, plans, and behaviors that facilitate healing (Klein 2015). In fleshing out the functional characterization of pain, one might also mention its contribution to the production of behaviors such as complaining, groaning, grimacing, and screaming, as well as autonomic effects, such as tachycardia, hypertension, sweating, and mydriasis. Finally, theorists who view pain as an emotional state will concentrate on both its motivational power and its central role in evaluative judgment, as well as its relationship to distress, anxiety, anger, fear, and depression (see Chapter 8, this volume). In all of these cases, the aim is to illuminate the nature of pain by appeal to its relations to environmental stimuli, behavioral responses, and other mental states. A comprehensive theory of pain would extend these functional characterizations to include the effects of pain on attention, learning, and other cognitive processes.

Reference to such functional relations is evidently the only means that we have of securing a notion of pain that is useful in guiding neurocognitive investigation and medical treatment. While some accounts of pain are constructed solely for the purpose of bolstering one or another distinctively metaphysical or epistemological thesis (Aydede 2005; Kripke 1980), it is not clear what practical or social value this might have. If one's aim is the kind of theoretical understanding that contributes to the development of compassionate, effective treatment, then one's very notion of pain should be conditioned by the deliverances of behavioral and neurocognitive research, as well as the needs and methods of medical and pharmacological practice. Given the stakes, it is both irrational and irresponsible to rely on sources of information that are known to be inferior in their epistemic credentials. This includes unreflective intuition, philosophical prejudice, and casual first-person reflection on one's own case (Kahneman 2011). The broadly pragmatist perspective adopted here puts social concerns and empirical findings well ahead of metaphysical predilections and armchair pronouncements. This, in turn, guides the methodology of the present discussion, whose central topic is the relationship between pain and consciousness.

Many assume that pain, whatever else it is, *must* be a conscious state. My goal in what follows is to challenge this assumption. I shall argue that pain can occur non-consciously, whether construed as a sensation, perception, emotion, mental imperative, or a combination of these. Making the case for this claim involves getting clear on the nature of consciousness. To that end, I draw distinctions between different senses of the term "conscious," homing in on the central phenomenon of *state consciousness*. After a brief survey of the available theories, I go on to discuss the consequences of applying the most promising ones – *global workspace* and *higher-order* theories – to the case of pain.

Other chapters in this volume develop competing accounts of pain. Though I remain neutral on which of these best meets scientific and philosophical criteria of adequacy, my discussion does proceed under two substantive assumptions.

First, I assume that pain is a real psychological phenomenon that can be characterized in respect of one or another of the mental properties surveyed above. This sets aside eliminativist views (Hardcastle 1999) that would render otiose the question of whether pain can occur non-consciously. While I do not find our common-sense notion of pain to be irredeemably incoherent (Dennett 1978), I take no stand on the related but distinct question of whether the personal-level phenomenon that we call "pain" maps on to any unique set of subpersonal mechanisms. It may well be that Corns (2012) is right that pain is not a "natural kind" – i.e., that neither pain, nor any subtype of pain, is susceptible to a mechanistic explanation that would provide the scientist or clinician with useful tools for generalization, prediction, and treatment. Still, legitimate questions can be asked even about "folk kinds," such as teacups and Tuesdays, and cluster-concepts, such as "limb." So even if pain – or, for that matter, consciousness – falls into such a class, the central question that animates the present discussion may still admit of a principled answer.

Second, in keeping with the above remarks, I will be concerned exclusively with accounts of pain that characterize it in functional terms, broadly construed. Alongside visual sensations, pain has often been seen by philosophers as a paradigm case of a state that cannot be exhaustively described in functional terms (Kripke 1980; Nagel 1974). This view stems from relying on dubious sources of information – armchair pronouncements about what pain and vision *must* be – which themselves typically rest on casual first-person reflections on one's own case, as well as imaginative extensions to the case of other sentient beings. In the case of vision, as philosophers caught up with the relevant science, it became increasingly clear that various surprising but robust phenomena put severe pressure on the idea that visual states are best characterized from the first-person point of view. Indeed, it is now known that such states need not be conscious (Berger 2014), and can thus *only* be described in functional terms, from the third-person perspective. This in turn gave rise to a functional characterization of visual states that is *conceptually independent* of "what it's like" for a creature to be in those states – independent, that is, of consciousness (Clark 1993; Rosenthal 2005; Chapters 5 and 6, this volume). In what follows, I argue that analogous considerations are operative in the case of pain. The central message of this chapter is that, in spelling out the functional role of pain, we should be prepared to find that the connection between pain and consciousness is entirely contingent.

2 Consciousness

The term "conscious" is used in a number of different ways. We distinguish beings that are conscious, for a given stretch of time, from those who are asleep, comatose, or otherwise incapacitated; in this sense, "consciousness" means roughly the same as "wakefulness." We may call this *creature consciousness*.

Adaptive engagement with an environment requires a creature to be conscious *of* various things. Here, the use of "conscious" is grammatically transitive, requiring the preposition "of." To be conscious *of* something, in this sense, is to have a mental representation of it – a sensory, perceptual, or intellectual awareness of it. Let us call this *transitive consciousness*.

Transitive consciousness of a stimulus, or of some feature of the environment, can occur consciously, but it can also occur non-consciously, as in cases of subliminal priming, blindsight, and hemineglect (Dehaene 2014). Here, the use of the term "conscious" pertains to one or another mental state, not a whole creature. It is in this sense that we speak of conscious and non-conscious desires, worries, fears, and the like. Let us use the term *state consciousness* to distinguish this notion from the others surveyed above. Thus, when we speak of a fully awake and vigilant creature non-consciously perceiving certain things, what we mean is that, while such a creature is *creature*-conscious, and *transitively* conscious *of* various things, some of its mental states are not *state*-conscious. For the remainder of this discussion, my topic will be state consciousness; when I use the term "consciousness," I intend it in this sense only.

Historically, philosophers and psychologists conflated consciousness with mentality, failing to recognize the existence of states that are genuinely mental but non-conscious (Locke 1959/1688). As the jargon of psychoanalytic theory permeated ordinary discourse, it became common to speak of unconscious desires, emotions, and intentions. More recently, work in cognitive science has made it clear that a wide range of mental states can occur non-consciously (Berger 2014; Dehaene 2014). Most scientifically informed philosophers now recognize that a central adequacy condition on any theory of the mind is that it provide an account of the difference between conscious and non-conscious mental states – a theory of state consciousness.

Philosophers in the naturalist camp are increasingly drawn to *representationalism* – a view according to which the mental properties of a state are determined entirely by its representational properties (Tye 2005). On this view, perceptions, thoughts, judgments, and other "assertoric" mental states represent how things are, while desires, preferences, intentions, emotions, and other "appetitive" or "motivational" states represent how things ought to be.

Representationalism in this sense aims at a uniform account of all mental properties. (See Chapter 2, this volume.) But it is not immediately clear how an appeal to representation can, by itself, provide an account of state consciousness. After all, some mental representations occur consciously, while others are non-conscious. Representationalism must be supplemented with an account of the difference.

Some representationalists (Dretske 2006) hold that a state's being conscious is a matter of our being able to cite it as a reason. But many of our reasons are non-conscious, hence unavailable for report. Though we could not supply them if asked to explicitly rationalize our behavior, they are reasons just the same. Indeed, they are *our* reasons, in virtue of playing a role in our overall cognitive economy. A latent pedophile's reasons for playing tag with the children at the family reunion are *his* reasons, even if he could not cite them – indeed, even if he adamantly and sincerely denied having them.

Drawing on recent work by Prinz (2012), a representationalist might instead appeal to attention in distinguishing conscious from non-conscious states. But there are now strong grounds for thinking that both spatial and object-based attention are dissociable from consciousness (Kentridge et al. 1999; Schurger et al. 2008; Norman et al. 2013).

A more promising route for the representationalist is to claim that the necessary supplement is entry into the "global workspace" – a hypothesized neurocognitive structure, whose function is to amplify and continuously broadcast information to disparate psychological mechanisms. A mental state can, on this view, start out below the threshold of consciousness, but then gain entry in the global workspace by winning a kind of neuronal competition for signal amplification (Dehaene 2014). Having won the race, a state's being conscious will consist in its content being projected, via long-range neural pathways, to a wide variety of psychological processing routines, including those that deal with memory, planning, reasoning, action-guidance, and speech production.

Although the global workspace theory (GWT) is motivated by a wide range of impressive empirical findings (Dehaene 2014), there is room for doubt about its conceptual underpinnings. In particular, it's arguable that some states are globally accessible but *not* conscious. As many theorists have stressed, state consciousness involves there being something that it's like *for the subject* to be in a particular state (Nagel 1974). Indeed, we would not count a mental state as conscious, in the relevant sense, if the subject who is in that state were in no way aware of herself as being in it. But many states that a subject is not aware of, or explicitly denies being in – i.e., states that do not figure in the subject's first-person subjective sense of her own state of mind – have been shown to have sophisticated and far-reaching cognitive effects, playing an important role in inference and decision-making (Berger 2014; Bergström and Eriksson 2014; Kahneman 2011). Insofar as global accessibility involves availability for report, GWT does capture the idea that state consciousness requires some form of self-awareness. For, reporting a state requires expressing a thought to the effect that one is in that state, and such a "higher-order" thought – e.g., *I am in pain* – is a plausible implementation of the relevant kind of self-awareness (Rosenthal 2005). But if a state can be widely accessible *without* being available for report – hence without the subject's awareness of it – then this would arguably constitute a counterexample to GWT.

A competing account of consciousness builds on what Rosenthal (2005) has called the "transitivity principle," according to which a state is conscious only if the subject of that state is aware of herself as being in it. Theories that espouse this principle see consciousness as *mental appearance* – a matter of how one's own mental life subjectively appears to one, from the first-person point of view. The transitivity principle explicitly codifies the pre-theoretical notion that no mental state can be conscious without the subject of that state being in some way aware of herself as being in it – without there being something that it's like *for her* to be in that state. This principle is at the heart of "higher-order" (H-O) theories of consciousness, so-called on account of their appeal to higher-order representations – ones whose content concerns one's own mental life.

Besides accommodating core pre-theoretical convictions, H-O theories do justice to the methodology of psychological research, which treats subjective report – an expression of self-awareness – as the most reliable measure of whether a given state is conscious. Moreover, like GWT, H-O theories provide plausible explanations of key psychological phenomena – e.g., subliminal priming, blindsight, change blindness, and the Sperling effect – and they make testable predictions at the level of neural implementation (Lau and Rosenthal 2011).

Alternative ways of implementing the transitivity principle will rest on differing characterizations of the relevant higher-order states (Gennaro 2004). For instance, some H-O theorists (e.g., Rosenthal 2005) treat such states as ontologically independent from the "first-order" states they purport to represent, while others (e.g., Gennaro 2012) see them as "integrated" or "unified" with their target states. The latter type of view is motivated by the perceived need to block the possibility of "empty" and mistaken higher-order representations – ones whose target first-order states either don't exist or fail to satisfy the relevant description (Block 2011; Gennaro 2012). Following up on Rosenthal (2011) and Pereplyotchik (2013), I shall argue that H-O theorists should instead *welcome* the possibility of higher-order misrepresentations. Drawing an appearance/reality distinction within the mind provides them with the resources to explain various puzzling pain experiences.

Proponents of GWT will argue that H-O theories are better seen as addressing introspection, self-awareness, or metacognition, rather than the target phenomenon of consciousness. On their view, consciousness need involve no self-awareness (Dehaene 2014: 24). But this claim is likely based on a first-person impression to the effect that consciously perceiving something need not involve thinking about oneself. H-O theorists explain away this impression by pointing out that the kind of self-awareness that is necessary for consciousness need not itself be apparent from the first-person point of view. The higher-order states that implement the relevant kind of self-awareness are not *themselves* conscious states, except in the relatively rare case of focused introspection (Rosenthal 2005). If this is right, then the first-person impressions that motivate this common objection are misleading.

3 Pain and consciousness

Reflection on one's own pain experiences frequently gives rise to the intuition that *that* kind of state cannot occur without its feeling *that* particular way – where the contents of the demonstratives are determined by the distinctive nature of a *conscious* experience, apprehended from the first-person point of view. Uncritical reliance on such impressions leads many theorists to insist that one cannot be *in* pain without being aware *of* one's pain. Such a view enjoys a distinguished philosophical pedigree, having been taken virtually for granted by generations of theorists who have little else in common (Locke 1959/1688; Kripke 1980; for discussion, see also Chapters 16, 18, and 27, this volume). But whatever the popularity and intuitive appeal of this view, in judging its merits, the pragmatist orientation adopted here counsels us to look at accounts of consciousness that are responsive to the available empirical findings. With that in mind, I propose to examine some of the consequences of applying GWT and H-O theories of consciousness to the case of pain.

GWT views a state's consciousness as its presence in the global workspace. A state that fails to gain entry into the global workspace may nevertheless have psychological effects on subsequent processing, but only in a limited manner and for only a brief period of time. The latter kind of condition has been both observed and induced in states of vision, hearing, touch, face perception, emotion, and volition (Dehaene 2014). GWT thus opens up the possibility that pain can likewise occur without being conscious. All that would be required is for the pain state to be implemented by a neural activation pattern that is too weak to set off the avalanche of activity that Dehaene calls "global ignition." Such a state could nevertheless serve to discriminate between noxious stimuli, to influence behavior, and to affect various emotional and cognitive processes – though, again, only within strict limits, both temporal and functional.

Turn now to H-O theories, on which a mental state is conscious insofar as it features in a creature's subjective representation of its own mental life. This self-awareness is implemented by higher-order representations, which, on standard versions of the theory, are numerically distinct from their target first-order states; the two kinds of state can occur independently, each without the other. Thus, when the first-order state is pain, and the higher-order awareness ("I am in pain") is wholly missing, the result is a non-conscious pain. Such a pain could still serve to discriminate noxious stimuli, to motivate the creature to protect and nurse a site of injury, and to cause distress, anxiety, and frustration, as well as a characteristic suite of autonomic and cognitive effects. All that would be missing is the creature's awareness *of* its own pain. There would thus be nothing that it's like for the creature to be in that state. Conversely, even in the absence of an actual first-order pain, a suitable higher-order state could represent its bearer as being in pain, giving rise to a conscious pain experience.

Both H-O and GWT agree, then, that pain – like any other state – can in principle occur non-consciously. And both theories supply accounts of the psychological and neural mechanisms that would be operative in such a case. Although they differ on the details, they agree that parietal and prefrontal regions are key sites for the neural activity that constitutes consciousness. Moreover, because self-awareness is one of the psychological processes that are triggered by instances of global broadcasting, the two theories will concur, in a wide range of cases, on whether a given pain state is conscious.

Despite these points of agreement, the two theories diverge in their commitments on three important issues: (i) the possibility of consciousness in the absence of self-awareness, (ii) the functionality of consciousness, and (iii) the consequences of a creature's misrepresenting its own mental life. The first of these has already been discussed: H-O theories view self-awareness as a necessary condition for consciousness, whereas GWT treats it as a contingent correlate. The other two points will require elaboration.

Regarding the issue of functionality, GWT rests on the idea that the capacity for state consciousness is a useful and adaptive trait (Dehaene 2014). With regard to pain, GWT predicts that consciousness renders pain more efficacious, by globally broadcasting it to a variety of psychological mechanisms, thus allowing it to mobilize a broader range of adaptive resources. H-O theories, by contrast, remain neutral on this point, holding that consciousness may well add nothing to the functionality that is already possessed by a first-order state (Rosenthal 2008). They are thus consistent with the possibility that conscious and non-conscious pains are *equally* efficacious and adaptive, when other factors are carefully controlled for. There is some evidence that this is true in the case of vision and other psychological domains (Bergström and Eriksson 2014; Lau and Rosenthal 2011). Whether it is true also in the case of pain remains to be seen. (For further discussion of the functionality of consciousness, see also Chapter 15, this volume.)

Consider now the issue of misrepresentation. Both H-O and GWT hold that self-awareness is the product of fallible interpretive processes, which can (and often do) provide a distorted picture of one's own mental life. For instance, one might have a visual sensation of scarlet, but misrepresent oneself as having a coarser-grain sensation – e.g., of generic red – or, in rarer cases, an entirely different state. Pain is no different in this regard. Both H-O and GWT entail that one's awareness of a concurrent pain can mis-characterize its duration, intensity, location, and other qualities. The two theories differ, however, on whether such errors determine the contents of consciousness. According to GWT, when a state triggers "global ignition," its *actual* contents become conscious, even if one's self-monitoring mechanisms – and hence self-reports – are inaccurate with regard to that state. Distortion can occur, at most, during the amplification process that facilitates global access. By contrast, H-O theories take self-representation to be *constitutive* of what it's like for a creature to be in some particular state. Thus, they entail that the conscious experience of a creature whose subjective take on its own mental life is erroneous will be determined by the contents of its inaccurate higher-order representations, not by the mental properties of its first-order states.

Let us now consider several cases in which it is plausible to describe subjects as misrepresenting their own pains, or mistaking non-pain states for pain. Such test cases are particularly revealing about the relation between pain and consciousness.

4 Relevant cases

Let's begin with long-lasting headaches. (Usage note: not all pains are aches, but the reverse inclusion holds.) An interesting case to consider is the anecdotal headache that persists throughout the day, without being conscious at every single moment. Is such a thing possible? Can there be *non-conscious headaches*? Intuitions differ. Some say yes, while others insist that a headache must always be conscious, if only in the manner of a "background hum." By themselves, such intuitions cut no ice. For, suppose we ask *why* people have different intuitions about this. Do their mental lives really differ in the relevant respects? Though logically possible, this is most unlikely. More plausibly, the differences in people's intuitive judgments track differences in their background theoretical predilections. If that is so, it should lead us to suspect that such judgments are not the authoritative deliverances of direct introspective access, but, rather, the outputs of a fallible interpretative mechanism for forming intuitive judgments (Kahneman 2011). Addressing the matter in a more careful fashion, then, let us survey some relevant empirical findings.

Particularly germane is the phenomenon of pain catastrophizing, wherein "an exaggerated negative mental set [is] brought to bear during actual or anticipated painful experience" (Sullivan et al. 1995; see also Chapter 12, this volume). The Pain Catastrophizing Scale has been developed to measure what effect one's "mental set" – beliefs, preferences, goals, and the like – has on pain ratings. The scale takes into account patients' degree of pain-rumination, pain-magnification, and their judgments of helplessness. A key finding is that pain can seem subjectively better or worse when accompanied by a correspondingly optimistic or pessimistic assessment of its likely duration into the future, its effects on ongoing projects, the severity of the underlying injury or illness, and other such factors. A related phenomenon occurs in post-cingulotomy patients, as well as those undergoing reactive dissociation under morphine, in whom diminished concern about the persistence and severity of a pain causes it to be consciously experienced as less awful (Grahek 2007).

H-O theories predict these effects, by identifying patients' conscious pain experiences with how their pains *seem* to them. On this view, the patients' "mental set" influences their higher-order representations of their pain, and these in turn determine the character of their conscious experience. Proponents of GWT can tell a similar story, claiming that the amplification process that facilitates global access distorts the character of the input state, perhaps as an effect of the subject's prior mental set. While this would not be a case of misrepresentation – the global workspace does not *represent* the input states – the distortion could nevertheless propel a mild non-conscious pain into an intense conscious pain experience, or vice versa.

Consider now a fraternity hazing ritual in which pledges are made to believe that they will be lashed on their backs with a whip. They then report feeling pain when their backs are touched lightly with an ice-cube. It is reasonable – though by no means mandatory – to interpret this as a case in which the pledges have, if only momentarily, a conscious experience of pain, without actually being in pain. The same can be said for other expectation-driven effects (Koyama et al. 2005), of which daily life provides abundant examples. Consider, for instance, the phenomenon of "dental fear," wherein patients respond to the loud sound and vibration of a dentist's drill by reporting being in pain, despite being under local anesthesia or lacking a nerve at the relevant site (Chapman and Kirby-Turner, 1999; Sullivan et al. 1995). Interestingly, after being apprised of the effect, patients come to agree that what they are now experiencing is something other than pain, though they still classify their earlier experiences as painful. Here again, higher-order representations can be seen as determining the character of a conscious pain experience, though not one's memory of a prior experience.

Also relevant is the "nocebo" effect, wherein conscious pain experiences occur in the absence of any relevant physical stimulation. For instance, participants report headaches when led to falsely believe that an electric current is passing through their heads (Schweiger and Parducci 1981). In the related placebo analgesia effect, false beliefs about, e.g., a sugar pill lower subjects' ratings of what may well be a pain of constant intensity (Price 2015, Chapter 9, this volume). This may be why adherents of the Lamaze method of childbirth claim that "by giving a mother a meaningful task to perform, the input that would otherwise be perceived as pain is endowed with a complex action-directing significance; since the patient is not merely a passive or helpless recipient of this input, but an interested recipient, a user of the input, it is not perceived as pain" (Dennett 1978: 437). Related findings support the idea that the *subjective* intensity of a pain can be manipulated independently of its *actual* intensity. For instance, subjects who believed, of a pain of a fixed intensity, that it was caused by someone with an intention to hurt them, tended to rate their conscious pain experiences as more intense than subjects who didn't have this belief (Gray and Wegner 2008). Studies of how hypnosis affects pain reports can be interpreted along similar lines. The experiments reported in Rainville et al. (1997, 1999) seem to show that a pain state can be consciously experienced as more or less intense or painful, depending on which beliefs have been hypnotically induced. The H-O theorist would once again appeal to the distinction between first-order and higher-order states – between mental appearance and mental reality – to account for these effects.

The examples surveyed above can all be interpreted in a number of different ways. Plainly, one's interpretations will be a function of one's antecedent commitments concerning the nature of both pain and consciousness. A theorist who insists on collapsing the appearance/reality distinction in the case of pain will construe the above findings as showing that pain is subject to influences that we had not previously known. But this interpretation is entirely optional. A competing account, according to which the appearance/reality distinction applies to pain as much as to anything else, is a live option, and it derives from a theory of consciousness that enjoys independent support. By viewing first-order pain states as distinct from higher-order self-representations, the H-O theory distinguishes between the actual features of a pain and one's subjective awareness of it. Likewise, proponents of GWT can point to the distorting effects of the amplification process that facilitates global access in explaining how conscious pain experiences can differ, sometimes dramatically, from the first-order states that cause them. It is less clear, though certainly possible, that the GWT can explain how those experiences can arise even in the absence of pain – a phenomenon that H-O theorists can readily account for, as we saw above.

The GWT and H-O accounts of consciousness open promising avenues of research in pain science. If taken seriously, these two perspectives may even assist in the treatment of chronic pain – a condition that has been described as affecting "about four-fifths of all people" (Hardcastle 1999: 9–10; Chapter 10, this volume). There is a possibility that some cases of chronic pain are analogous to a rare version of Charles Bonnet Syndrome, in which visual hallucinations appear to originate not in the visual system, but in the prefrontal cortex – a likely location of higher-order representations. Lau and Brown (forthcoming) convincingly argue that this condition is not plausibly seen as involving confabulation or mistaken introspection; the patients are entirely cogent and aware that their visual hallucinations are a consequence of neural damage. If something similar is true of any sufferers of chronic pain, then the treatment options should include targeting activity in the prefrontal cortex – or whatever brain region is found to support the relevant kind of self-awareness or global access – rather than the mechanisms that underlie first-order pain.

5 Conclusion

The arguments in this chapter have been driven primarily by theoretical considerations – i.e., the general implications of two of the most promising available theories of consciousness. On the basis of robust empirical findings, both theories hold that a wide variety of mental states and processes occur in the absence of consciousness. Pending an argument to the effect that pain is relevantly different from visual, auditory, and tactile perception, face recognition, emotion, memory, reasoning, planning, and language processing, we should expect that what is true of these psychological phenomena is true also of pain. The resulting conception of the relation between pain and consciousness goes well beyond the uncontroversial claim that nociceptive activity sometimes results in non-conscious execution of nocifensive behaviors. Rather, it forces us to reconsider the very nature of pain, thus opening up new avenues of thought, not only about the traditional mind–body problem, but, more importantly, about how best to deliver effective treatment.

Related topics

Chapter 1: A brief and potted overview on the philosophical theories of pain (Hardcastle)
Chapter 2: Pain and representation (Cutter)
Chapter 3: Evaluativist accounts of pain's unpleasantness (Bain)
Chapter 4: Imperativism (Klein)
Chapter 5: Fault lines in familiar concepts of pain (Hill)
Chapter 6: Advances in the neuroscience of pain (Apkarian)
Chapter 7: Neuromatrix theory of pain (Roy and Wager)
Chapter 8: A neurobiological view of pain as a homeostatic emotion (Strigo and Craig)
Chapter 9: A view of pain based on sensations, meanings, and emotions (Price)
Chapter 10: Pathophysiological mechanisms of chronic pain (Thacker and Moseley)
Chapter 12: Bisopsychosocial models of pain (Hadjistavropoulos)
Chapter 13: Psychogenic pain: old and new (Sullivan)
Chapter 14: Pain, voluntary action, and the sense of agency (Beck and Haggard)

Acknowledgements

Thanks to Jacob Berger, Wesley Buckwalter, Jennifer Corns, and David Rosenthal for helpful comments on previous drafts. Thanks also to the audience at the Cognitive Science Symposium at the CUNY Graduate Center, where I presented a version of this paper in July 2015 – especially Ben Abelson, Anthony Dardis, Jesse Rappaport, and Henry Shevlin.

References

Aydede, M. (ed.) (2005) *Pain: New Essays on Its Nature and the Methodology of Its Study*. Cambridge, MA: MIT Press.

Barrett, L.F. (2006) Valence is a basic building block of emotional life. *Journal of Research in Personality* 40: 35–55.

Berger, J. (2014) Mental states, conscious and nonconscious. *Philosophy Compass* 9(6): 392–401.

Bergström, F. and Eriksson, J. (2014) Maintenance of non-consciously presented information engages the prefrontal cortex. *Frontiers in Human Neuroscience* 8: 1–10.

Block, N. (2011) The higher-order approach to consciousness is defunct. *Analysis* 71: 419–431.

Chapman, H.R. and Kirby-Turner, N.C. (1999) Dental fear in children – a proposed model. *British Dental Journal* 187(8): 408–412.

Clark, A. (1993) *Sensory Qualities*. Oxford: Clarendon Press.

Clark, A. (2005) Painfulness is not a quale. In M. Aydede (ed.), *Pain: New Essays on Its Nature and the Methodology of Its Study*, Cambridge, MA: MIT Press, pp. 177–197.

Corns, J.R. (2012) *Pain Is Not a Natural Kind*. PhD diss. City University of New York.

Craig, A.D. (2003) A new view of pain as a homeostatic emotion. *Trends in Neurosciences* 26(6): 303–307.

Cutter, B. and Tye, M. (2011) Tracking representationalism and the painfulness of pain. *Philosophical Issues* 21(1): 90–109.

Dehaene, S. (2014) *Consciousness and the Brain: Deciphering How the Brain Codes Our Thoughts*. New York: Viking Press.

Dennett, D.C. (1978) Why you can't make a computer that feels pain. *Synthese* 38(3): 417–456.

Dretske, F. (2006) Perception without awareness. In T.S. Gendler and J. Hawthorne (eds.), *Perceptual Experience*. Oxford: Clarendon Press.

Grahek, N. (2007) *Feeling Pain and Being in Pain*, 2nd ed. Cambridge, MA: MIT Press.

Gray, K. and Wegner, D. (2008) The sting of intentional pain. *Psychological Science* 19(12): 1260–1262.

Gennaro, R. (ed.) (2004) *Higher-Order Theories of Consciousness*. Philadelphia: John Benjamins.

Gennaro, R. (2012) *The Consciousness Paradox: Consciousness, Concepts, and Higher-Order Thoughts*. Cambridge, MA: MIT Press.

Hardcastle, V.G. (1999) *The Myth of Pain*. Cambridge, MA: MIT Press.

Hill, C.S. (2005) Ow! The paradox of pain. In M. Aydede (ed.), *Pain: New Essays on Its Nature and the Methodology of Its Study*, Cambridge, MA: MIT Press, pp. 75–98.

Kahneman, D. (2011) *Thinking, Fast and Slow*. New York: Farrar, Straus & Giroux.

Kentridge, R.W., Heywood, C.A., and Weiskrantz, L. (1999) Attention without awareness in blindsight. *Proceedings of the Royal Society B: Biological Sciences* 266: 1805–1811.

Klein, C. (2015) *What the Body Commands: The Imperative Theory of Pain*. Cambridge, MA: MIT Press.

Koyama, T., McHaffie, J.G., Laurienti, P.J., and Coghill, R.C. (2005) The subjective experience of pain: where expectations become reality. *Proceedings of the National Academy of Sciences of the United States of America* 102(36): 12950–12955.

Kripke, S. (1980) *Naming and Necessity*. Cambridge, MA: Harvard University Press.

Lau, H. and Rosenthal, D.M. (2011) Empirical support for higher-order theories of conscious awareness. *Trends in Cognitive Sciences* 15(8): 365–373.

Lau, H. and Brown, R. (Forthcoming) The emperor's new phenomenology? The empirical case for conscious experience without first-order representations. In A. Pautz and D. Stoljar (eds.), *Themes from Block*. Cambridge, MA: MIT Press.

Lerner, J.S. and Keltner, D. (2000) Beyond valence: toward a model of emotion-specific influences on judgment and choice. *Cognition and Emotion* 14(4): 473–493.

Locke, J. (1959/1688) *An Essay on Human Understanding*. New York: Dover.

Nagel, T. (1974) What is it like to be a bat? *Philosophical Review* 83: 435–450.

Norman, L.J., Heywood, C.A., and Kentridge, R.W. (2013) Object-based awareness without attention. *Psychological Science* 20(10): 1–8.

Pereplyotchik, D. (2013) Some HOT family disputes: a critical review of *The Consciousness Paradox* by Rocco Gennaro. *Philosophical Psychology* 28(3): 434–448.

Price, D.D. (2015) Unconscious and conscious mediation of analgesia and hyperalgesia. *Proceedings of the National Academy of Sciences of the United States of America* 112(25): 7624–7625.

Prinz, J. (2012) *The Conscious Brain: How Attention Engenders Experience*. Oxford: Oxford University Press.

Rainville, P., Duncan, G.H., Price, D.D., Carrier, B., and Bushnell, M.C. (1997) Pain affect encoded in human anterior cingulate but not somatosensory cortex. *Science* 277(5328): 968–971.

Rainville, P., Carrier, B., Hofbauer, R.K., Bushnell, M.C., and Duncan, G.H. (1999) Dissociation of sensory and affective dimensions of pain using hypnotic modulation. *Pain Forum* 82(2): 159–171.

Rosenthal, D.M. (2005) *Consciousness and Mind*. Oxford: Clarendon Press.

Rosenthal, D.M. (2008) Consciousness and its function. *Neuropsychologia* 46: 829–840.

Rosenthal, D.M. (2011) Exaggerated reports: reply to Block. *Analysis* 71: 431–437.

Schurger, A., Cowey, A., Cohen, J.D., Treisman, A., and Tallon-Baudry, C. (2008) Distinct and independent correlates of attention and awareness in a hemianopic patient. *Neuropsychologia* 46(8): 2189–2197.

Schweiger, A. and Parducci, A. (1981) Nocebo: the psychologic induction of pain. *Pavlov Journal of Biological Science* 16(3): 140–143.

Sullivan, M.J.L., Bishop, S., and Pivik, J. (1995) The Pain Catastrophizing Scale: development and validation. *Psychological Assessment* 7(4): 524–532.

Tye, M. (2005) Another look at representationalism about pain. In M. Aydede (ed.), *Pain: New Essays on Its Nature and the Methodology of Its Study*, Cambridge, MA: MIT Press, pp. 99–120.

18

PAIN

Perception or introspection?

Murat Aydede

Is feeling pain in a bodily location, say, in one's elbow, a form of *perception* or something that essentially involves *introspection*? Am I perceiving something in my elbow when I feel pain there? Or am I engaged in some form of introspection about my awareness of something there?

In popular culture or even among scientists, the term "perception" is often used in a very broad sense to designate any kind of ongoing epistemic access to (or, some form of awareness of) *something* (anything) in real time. Used in this sense, the common practice of using expressions like "pain perception" or "perception of pain" (popular among pain scientists)[1] may be unobjectionable. Indeed, the term "perception" in this broad sense may also be used to characterize introspection itself. Whatever ultimately the nature of introspection turns out to be, it is by definition a form of direct *first-person* access (subjective, from inside) to one's own *mental* states, processes, events, or to their mental features. In this minimal sense, it is something that may already be covered by the broad sense of "perception" just mentioned. But there is a narrower sense of "perception" with which "introspection" is to be *contrasted*. In the narrower sense, perception is ongoing epistemic access to something that is *other* than one's own mental states or features. This is the familiar epistemic activity that occupies most of our ordinary waking lives when we see, hear, smell, taste, or touch something in or outside of our bodies. In this sense, perception is access to something *extramental* in the sense of being beyond our own mental states. This is typically access to worldly objects (including our own bodies), their physical properties, states, or conditions. When I see a lemon in front of me, touch it, smell it, taste it, I am perceiving the lemon and its physical features, its color, shape, sounds it makes when I take a bite or tap on it, its texture, odor, taste, etc. In other words, in perception I am getting information about the physical objects in the environment surrounding me and my body, and this information is typically made available to me for recognition, identification, categorization, etc. – or more generally, for cognizing and further mental processing or motor action. In all this, and what is essential for the narrow sense of "perception," the mental activity is world-directed. In introspection, it is internally (mind-) directed. This is not to deny that perception in the narrow sense and introspection can co-occur – or perhaps even always co-occur. Indeed, when I perceive the lemon in front of me, I may also be simultaneously attending to the way I sense or experience it. This is epistemic access to the peculiar *way* in which the lemon *feels* to me in seeing, touching, tasting, or sniffing it. I may be *introspectively* attending, in other words, to the very character

221

(the phenomenology) of my perceptual experience of the lemon in the very act of *perceiving* it. The point, rather, is that perception (in the narrow sense) and introspection are different mental activities even when they co-occur. In this chapter, when I use "perception" I will always mean it in the narrow sense.[2]

Returning to the opening question: is my feeling pain in my elbow a form of perception or something involving introspection? Given that perception and introspection may not be mutually exclusive and may co-occur, at the end of the day, we may answer the question by saying that it is both. We may also answer it by saying it is neither. But, let us try to understand the question as asking what feeling a pain is *in the first place* (primarily, or perhaps, even essentially). A natural reaction to the question is to say something like the following:

> Look, if I feel a pain in my elbow, I am clearly aware of *something in my elbow*. Whatever this is, it has a bodily location – it is *in my elbow*. Does it make sense to talk about a "thing" in my elbow as something other than a physical condition of my elbow? Does it make sense to talk about a mental condition or experiential condition of elbows? Can a mental item be literally located in elbows? Add to this the fact that when we feel pain in bodily parts, most often there is some kind of physical insult (actual or impending), disturbance, or disorder located roughly in or around those bodily parts, it becomes clear that the intuitively correct answers to these questions are in the negative. This rules out that my feeling pain in my elbow is a form of introspection and makes a compelling case for the claim that it is a form of perception (interoception) of a physical/objective condition of my elbow – to the effect that there is something physically wrong with my elbow. Feeling pain in a bodily location, in other words, is *perceiving* some kind of physical disorder or disturbance or damage (actual or potential) in, on, or around, those bodily locations.

This view has come to be known as the Perceptual/Representational Theory (PRT) of pain, and there are various versions of it in the literature.[3] PRT has many virtues. It does justice to the intuition that in feeling pain in body parts, we are often getting very useful information about the physical condition of these parts. Thus, just like other perceptual modalities, pain perception is epistemic access to one's physical environment – in this particular case, to one's own body and its states. This access has immediate and often almost hard-wired motivational consequences about what to do with this information: move (or stop moving, as the case may be) the body or body parts in certain ways. In this respect, it resembles smell, taste, and touch more than vision and hearing. Thus, the fact that pain has a very pronounced affective-motivational aspect (pains feel bad, unpleasant, and almost always motivate) may not take away from its being a perceptual phenomenon (sensory-discriminative). When viewed this way, it makes little sense to think of feeling pain in a bodily part as a form of introspection: what would be the point of accessing one's mental states, experiences, feelings, sensations, when the important issues lie with what is happening to the body and what to do about it? Thus, there is a lot going for a view that treats feeling pain in a body part as a form of perception – especially when combined with an account of the affective-motivational aspect of pains.

Nevertheless, there are genuine puzzles and problems with PRT whose appreciation points in the opposite direction. PRT naturally suggests that when we attribute pains to body parts, we attribute (believe and report the existence of) some objective/physical condition of those body parts – for ease of use, let us abbreviate this physical condition of body parts as D (actual or impending physical disorder, disturbance, damage, or some such). D is the *object* of our perception – what it is that we perceive. The nature of D may differ from case to case, but in all cases it is meant by perceptualists to be an objective condition of bodily parts. When we perceive a pain in a bodily location, according to PRT, we perceive D. Are pains identical to D, then? Is the pain in my elbow the same thing as the swollen/bruised condition of my elbow – the same thing as whatever physical damage exists there?

The answer is: No. We understand the physical disorder (D) in my elbow to be the *cause* of my pain there – if there is indeed some kind of disorder there. But we don't identify pain with physical disorder. (In general: for any x and y, if x is a cause of y, $x \neq y$.) This could easily be seen when you reflect on the following scenario. Suppose there is in fact no tissue damage or any kind of physical disorder or disturbance in my elbow. I feel pain in there because I have a pinched nerve in the relevant part of my spine. This would not make my belief/report that there is a pain in my elbow incorrect. It would still be true that there is a pain in my elbow if I truly happen to feel a pain there. Compare a similar scenario in a genuinely perceptual case: if I come to believe that there is an apple in front of me on the basis of my visual experience (if I seem to see an apple and report the presence of an apple on that basis), when in fact there was no apple and I was simply hallucinating, my belief/report would be *incorrect* and my visual experience would be non-veridical, hallucinatory. But no such thing happens in cases where we *feel pain in a bodily part in the absence of any physical disorder in those parts*. In such cases, we still continue to *correctly* judge that we have pain *in those bodily parts*. Thus, we don't have pain hallucinations.

This is not simply a result of how we *ordinarily* think and talk about pains. Pain scientists and clinicians themselves have been insisting on this point for decades. Here is the IASP (International Association for the Study of Pain) definition of "pain" with a profoundly anti-perceptualist note added[4]:

> Pain: An unpleasant sensory and emotional experience associated with actual or potential tissue damage, or described in terms of such damage.

> *Note*: … Pain is always subjective. Each individual learns the application of the word through experiences related to injury in early life … It is unquestionably a sensation in a part or parts of the body … Many people report pain in the absence of tissue damage or any likely pathological cause … There is no way to distinguish their experience from that due to tissue damage if we take the subjective report. If they regard their experience as pain and if they report it in the same ways as pain caused by tissue damage, it should be accepted as pain. This definition avoids tying pain to the stimulus. Activity induced in the nociceptor and nociceptive pathways by a noxious stimulus is not pain, which is always a psychological state, even though we may well appreciate that pain most often has a proximate physical cause.

It follows, *a fortiori*, that any physical or objective condition of tissue or body parts is not pain either, even though "we may well appreciate that pain most often has" such a condition as its (distal?) physical cause.[5]

Despite the ordinary or clinical practice of locating pains in body parts, the dominant ordinary opinion (not *just* the scientific opinion) is that pains are subjective experiences. As experiences, they don't admit an appearance/reality distinction: this is why there are no pain hallucinations. In having a pain in my elbow, I am essentially having a pain experience that nevertheless manages to say something about my elbow. If this is correct, then coming to know that one is in pain or is feeling pain in a bodily part is necessarily coming to know that one is having a (mental, what else?) experience. But this is to engage in introspection – one is having epistemic access to one's experience – a paradigm mental occurrence. Note that there is no parallel in cases like vision: if, on the basis of my visual experience, I come to know that there is an apple in front of me, then this knowledge (that there is an apple in front of me) is perceptual, not introspective – it is epistemic access to the extramental (worldly) reality. Of course, I may *also* come to know that I am having a visual experience about an apple. This piece of knowledge would be introspective, yes, but this is extra, something in addition to my perceptual knowledge.

How are we to answer our opening question then? My own view is that there is no serious alternative to identifying pains with experiences. This fact is acknowledged even by most perceptualists themselves: on their view, pains are experiences – but, they say, these experiences are perceptual. If pains are experiences, however, our epistemic access to them is, by definition, introspective. For knowledge of one's own pain is knowledge of one's own experience, and this is introspective knowledge.

Unfortunately, this settles very little. Deep puzzles remain. If pains are subjective experiences, it is not at all clear what it is that we are doing when we attribute pains to bodily parts. When I feel a sharp pain in my elbow, does it make sense to talk about introspecting a mental item in my elbow?

Compare the situation to seeing the apple in front of me as round. On the basis of my visual experience I make a perceptual judgment "*this* is round," where "this" refers to the apple. I am attributing roundness to the apple in front of me. The roundness of the apple won't be affected when I stop seeing it. Not so with the pain *in my elbow*. Seeing roundness is perceptual. Awareness of one's seeing roundness is introspective. In principle, it seems, one can have the former without having the latter: one can see the roundness of an apple without being introspectively aware that one is doing so. The puzzle is that this distinction seems to collapse in the case of feeling a pain in my elbow. The act of locating pain in a bodily location (in the extramental space) argues for an understanding of pains as perceptual, but the robust resistance to identifying pains with anything physical in those locations (thus making located pains awareness-dependent) exerts pressure for an understanding of pains as introspective. If we follow the dominant understanding of pains as subjective experiences, as I think we should, we need to find a way to make the following claim intelligible:

> (P) When I feel a pain in my elbow, the pain in my elbow is both literally *located in my elbow* and *mental* so that the proprietary epistemic access to it is introspective, rather than perceptual.[6]

It is the pessimism about making (P) intelligible in naturalistic terms that has kept philosophers busy and driven away from non-perceptualist and non-representationalist views of pain for fear of quantifying over irreducibly mental objects (sense-data) or mental/phenomenal qualities (qualia).[7]

The standard perceptualist and representationalist way of making sense of our practices of attributing pains to bodily parts is to reinterpret the logical structure of first-person judgments when one locates a pain in one's body. So suppose that I truly judge now that

> (1) I feel pain in my elbow.

What makes this true, according to PRT, is not, as one would normally have expected, that

(2) I stand in some perceptual relation to some objective condition (D) of my elbow,

but rather it is the fact that

(3) I am having an experience with the intentional content that
(3a) some D is occurring in my elbow.[8]

Note that if, when I judge (1) I am in fact judging (3) and that this is typical, as PRT says, then my ordinary pain-attributing judgments are introspective judgments. By contrast, on the natural reading of (2), it is made true in virtue of obtaining a perceptual relation between me and the physical condition (D) of my elbow. In other words, PRT denies that when I truly judge (1), *I* am making an attribution *to my elbow* – an attribution of pain, or even D, for that matter. On PRT, no such attributions are being made: instead, I attribute an experience *to myself* with a certain intentional content. On PRT, whether or not this content (3a) is true is irrelevant to the correctness of my introspective judgment.

Another way to put the PRT proposal is this. Suppose (1) is merely true, whether or not I judge or happen to think (1). Then what makes (1) true is the mere fact that I have a pain experience, which, according to PRT, is in fact perceptual in that it (non-conceptually) represents my elbow as having something physically wrong with it – as having D. For brevity, in case (1) is true, I am undergoing a perceptual experience *as of* D in my elbow. This experience, according to PRT, may be a misperception or non-veridical if my elbow has nothing physically wrong with it. So, we may have genuine pain experiences that are hallucinatory in this respect. So far so good: the case seems parallel to genuine perception like vision. But according to PRT, this perceptual experience never gives rise to perceptual judgments about D. Our pain-attributing beliefs and judgments formed on the basis of these pain experiences are never directly (*de re*) about D's being instantiated in a body part: they always report the experience itself. It is puzzling why the defenders of PRT think that pain experiences are perceptual when these experiences always give rise to introspective judgments, and never to perceptual judgments. This is in stark contrast to genuinely perceptual experiences like seeing an apple in front of me as round: these typically give rise to *de re* perceptual judgments such as "this is round," which may be true or false depending on what the actual objective facts are with the apple. In other words, the epistemic value of genuinely perceptual experiences is typically transferred to the perceptual judgments they normally give rise to.[9]

The puzzle PRT generates, then, is that if pain experiences are perceptual, we never seem to think of their objects as perceptual objects, i.e., extramental objects (D), that we perceive through these experiences. As a matter of course, we treat both the objects of these experiences (pains in body parts) and the experiences themselves as mind-dependent, hence, not as extramental objects of perception (in the narrow sense). If pain experiences were genuinely perceptual, they would normally give rise to *de re* judgments about their (extramental) objects as such (this is what happens in all genuinely perceptual experiences). But we never see that! It becomes puzzling why perceptual theorists insist that the pain experiences are nevertheless perceptual.[10]

There are further difficulties with PRT: the proposed analysis of pain-attributing judgments, intuitively, doesn't capture the phenomenological import of these first-person introspective judgments. When I am sensorially aware of a sharp pain in my elbow, intuitively, I seem to be presented with an essentially phenomenal item or quality somehow instantiated in my elbow. Otherwise, why resist identifying this quality with anything physical that may be instantiated in my elbow? But it is precisely this phenomenal presence that gets lost in the proposed analysis by PRT. Recall that, on this view, my introspective report about my awareness of this pain is simply a report of an experience as of some sort of physical disturbance (D) in my elbow. But when I attribute pain to my elbow, as a matter of fact, like everybody else, I both mean to literally locate pain in my elbow and resist identifying this pain with any physical condition of my elbow. In fact, I mean more: I mean this pain to be awareness-dependent. Hence, I positively conceive of this pain in my elbow as a mind-dependent presence. But if PRT is true, I am massively confused in what I mean, indeed, in what I *can* mean – not just me, of course, pretty much *everybody* is so confused. This doesn't seem right.

In light of this, I think that PRT should be rejected: pain experiences are not perceptual. In fact, I am inclined to believe, they are not *fully* representational either. Rejecting PRT doesn't, of course, commit one to denying the obvious, namely, the mundane observation that feeling pain in a body part often conveys very useful, sometimes crucial, information about the physical condition of that part and allows one to be immediately motivated in appropriate ways to act to protect one's body. This observation is a truism and not in dispute, but the view that feeling pain in a body part is a perceptual experience with a representational content is a *recent* development by historical standards: up until the early1960s, it had been (almost) unheard of. In fact, arguably the contemporary silent majority may still not be friendly to such a view.[11]

It was David Armstrong and George Pitcher in the 60s and 70s who proposed the perceptualist view of pains and other "intransitive" bodily sensations such as itches, tickles, tingles, orgasms, etc.[12] Unsurprisingly, this was in accordance with their naturalist (materialist) program in philosophy of perception and mind. We noted above the difficulty of making naturalistic sense of (P) which is about pains. But exactly the same puzzles remain for other intransitive bodily sensations, of course. The traditional anti-PRT view had taken (P) for granted and didn't worry much about its alleged non-naturalistic metaphysical implications: most were at home with dualism, idealism, sense-datum theories, indeed with any form of non-materialism. Thanks to the likes of Armstrong, Pitcher, and other pioneers, most of us these days do, and ought to, worry about the alleged non-naturalistic metaphysical implications of our views and seek ways to address them.

By rejecting PRT,[13] we will be returning to the historically dominant view of pains as bodily sensations that sets them apart from genuinely perceptual experiences involved in standard perceptual modalities. If we reject PRT, however, can we make sense of (P) without falling into a metaphysical abyss? Here is a rough outline of a naturalist proposal that comports well with the core traditional understanding of pains as both locatable items and subjective experiences. The proposal is weakly intentionalist, qualia-friendly, but fully naturalist, which has close affinities with adverbialism in philosophy of perception.[14]

Pains are sensory and affective experiences. I will focus on the sensory aspect in what follows. I will start with the assumption that sensory experiences have an intentional structure in that they have both a referential and a predicative structure. This is to say that these experiences have a structure that picks out particulars in space-time and then *typically* attributes features, properties, or relations to these particulars. The picking-out bit is referential, and the property attribution is handled by the predicates proprietary to the sensory modality, probably structured according to the organization of the sensory quality space for that modality.[15]

As an analogy, think of a paper marine chart of a certain lake. The points or regions on the paper chart, as fixed by the horizontal/vertical coordinates of the chart, will pick out or refer to actual points or regions on the lake. This is the referential aspect. What colors, lines, or marks there are on those points or regions of the paper chart will then tell us what oceanographic or geographic properties (e.g., depth, currents rates or directions, submerged rocks, etc.) are true of the corresponding places on the lake. Here we have a representational vehicle (the paper chart) with a syntactic structure roughly corresponding to referential and predicative functions. The claim is that sensory experiences as intentional structures have a similar referential/predicative divide. Despite the presence of a predicative structure, however, the representational format of sensory experiences is not conceptual – similar to the way the chart is *not* a discursive or sentential representation.

Presumably, in the case of pains, the *referential* structure of the experience is physiologically realized by a body map or a map-like representation (a somatotopically organized body image or schema, perhaps) whose referring elements pick out or refer to points or regions in one's somatosensory field – to body parts. But the "properties"[16] that are placed in or attributed to the regions picked out by these referential elements are handled by the sensory *predicates* involved in pain processing. The qualitative phenomenology of sensory experiences is determined by the predicative structure of these experiences.[17]

Pain experiences just like other sensory experiences feed into a conceptual system wherein introspective and perceptual *judgments* are made based on these experiences. I claim that the judgments made in locating pains in bodily locations track what sensory predicates are deployed, and not what sensible properties/conditions, if any, are thereby attributed to these locations by these predicates. Thus, whatever property (if any) is attributed to bodily locations, our judgments are about the *ways* these properties are experienced or sensorially registered – they are not about the *properties* these ways may attribute. Because these ways are *ways* in which certain "properties" are sensorially attributed to extramental particulars (bodily locations), we cannot help but attend to these *ways* by attending to the locations (picked out by the referential elements) instantiating these properties. These *ways* are the phenomenal qualities of our experiences, whose knowledge is thus knowledge of the *ways* in which certain "properties" or conditions are sensorially attributed to body parts.[18] Thus when I judge I have a pain in my elbow, my judgment is correct in virtue of my undergoing a pain experience attributing a "property" to my elbow in a certain way. My judgment thus correctly reports an experience – it is an introspective judgment.

What is the property (or range of properties/conditions) that seems to be attributed by my experience? In genuinely perceptual modalities, the predicative structure of sensory experiences attributes sensible properties to physical objects. These are often complex but objective (physical) features or conditions of extramental objects that we sense, such as colors, chemical constitution, surface textures, temperature, pressure, etc. In the case of pain experiences, unlike a perceptualist or representationalist, we are not theoretically constrained in thinking of what these attributed properties ought to be. In fact, we may *legitimately* draw a blank – just as the folk and scientists do. But there are various options. I will first mention a conciliatory option, and then, briefly explore the option I am more attracted to.

One option about what the attributed properties might be is to follow representationalists by identifying them with some sort of physical disturbance (D). If we do this, our pain-attributing *judgments* (analyzed as introspective judgments about experiences with a certain intentional content) would still come out as correct, as desired, but our *experiences* now may *not* be veridical. I may correctly report pain in my elbow when in fact there is nothing physically wrong with it and my pain is a referred pain due to a pinched nerve in my upper spine. My pain *experience* would thus be illusory but my pain *judgment* would still be correct. I suppose we can live with this result – even though, as I have argued, the lack of relevant *de re* perceptual judgments would make these experiences non-perceptual. This is a non-perceptualist weak representationalist position that allows for widespread non-veridical experiences to be still genuine pain experiences. Although we can live with this, I don't find this option very satisfying. Furthermore, as complained before, the proposed analysis of introspective judgments doesn't do justice to the pain phenomenology and the conception of pains as occurring in body parts.

On the second option, pain experiences are not fully representational because there are no genuine property attributions made, despite successful reference. The "properties" that the sensory predicates involved in pain experiences appear to attribute to body parts are *mental* in the following sense: a body part has pain in it just in case it is the intentional target of a sensory predicate predicating a dummy property to that location – it is the inverse intentional property of being the target of a sensory predicate *being used with respect to a referential position* in the sensory experience that in fact picks out that target. In other words, as long as sensory reference succeeds, the reference is guaranteed to have the mental/intentional property insofar as the system makes a prediction with respect to that reference. Accordingly, the metaphysics of pain experiences consists of sensory representations making dummy property attributions to bodily parts. We can then distinguish between informative pains, referred pains, and phantom limb pains.

- *Informative pains* are those in which the predication actually signals or indicates actual or impending physical disturbance/damage (D) at the location to which reference is successfully being made. Correlations between physical disturbances and firing of a predicate have been claimed to be fairly poor – but perhaps when the channel conditions are right, there is information flow after all, even though this may not be enough for genuine representation.
- *Referred pains* are those in which reference is successfully made to actual body parts with respect to which a predicate is causally activated by some disturbance in some other part of the body, but the activation does not indicate disturbance in the part of the body to which the reference is actually being made.
- *Phantom limb pains* are those where attempted reference to a body part fails but with respect to which a sensory predicate is activated.

If the "property" attributed to body parts is *mental* in this sense, then there are no representational mistakes anywhere in the intentional nociceptive system. Our pain experiences are intentional because there is either successful or failed reference. But the pain experiences do not make genuine property attributions to bodily locations, so they do not have full veridicality conditions. Thus they are not *fully* representational.[19] However, our *judgments* prompted by them are correct in intuitively the right way. These judgments usually correctly locate the mental properties in those bodily regions (pains in body parts) when the relevant mental properties are understood in the above way. When I correctly report a pain in my elbow, I am introspectively reporting pain (a certain phenomenal quality) as literally being in my elbow. For my elbow is the intentional target of a sensory predicate being used with respect to a referential position that picks out my elbow. Although my introspective *judgments* fully represent the instantiation of such mental properties in my body parts or regions, these mental properties are not represented by the pain *experiences* themselves; as said, pain experiences, although intentional (*de re* reference), are not fully representational (no genuine property attribution generating accuracy conditions). Folk and the pain scientists (including clinicians) do routinely attribute pains and other sensations to bodily locations after all – come to think of it: *sensations* (paradigmatic mental episodes) in body parts! This story about how to account for the pain qualities attributed to body parts explains how to make sense of such practices.[20]

The above proposal, especially with the second option in mind, needs to be supplemented with an account of introspection and the role of negative affect in pain experiences.[21] The proposal assumes a largely intentionalist framework in helping itself to its representational resources, along with its syntactic apparatus. The assumption is that such a framework is fully realizable in purely physical systems, thus fully naturalistic. No doubt, in philosophy (and in cognitive science as a whole) there is a sense of optimism that in the last fifty years or so we have made progress in understanding intentional systems (natural or artificial) in mechanistic/computational terms, systematically interacting with their natural or engineered environments. My proposal builds on these naturalistic foundations.

Related topics

Chapter 1: A brief and potted overview on the philosophical theories of pain (Hardcastle)
Chapter 2: Pain and representation (Cutter)
Chapter 3: Evaluativist accounts of pain's unpleasantness (Bain)
Chapter 4: Imperativism (Klein)
Chapter 5: Fault lines in familiar concepts of pain (Hill)
Chapter 8: A neurobiological view of pain as a homeostatic emotion (Strigo and Craig)
Chapter 9: A view of pain based on sensations, meanings, and emotions (Price)
Chapter 15: The lives of others: pain in non-human animals (Droege)
Chapter 17: Pain and consciousness (Pereplyotchik)
Chapter 27: Bad by nature: an axiological theory of pain (Massin)
Chapter 31: An introduction to the IASP's definition of pain (Wright)

Acknowledgements

Many thanks to Andrew Wright and Jennifer Corns for helpful comments.

Notes

1 Just run a Google search with these expressions to see how popular and seemingly unavoidable their uses are.
2 Perception in the narrow sense is sometimes divided into *exteroception* and *interoception*. The latter is typically meant to apply only to the perception of one's own bodily states, position, or its various physiological or regulatory conditions. The former is perception of worldly conditions beyond one's skin. See, for instance, Craig 2003; Chapters 8 and 9, this volume. Also, in what follows, when I talk about perception and perceptual experiences, I will have in mind conscious perception and conscious experiences. I don't, of course, deny that there may be non-conscious perceptual states. For more discussion, see Chapters 15 and 17, this volume.
3 For perceptualist views, see Armstrong 1962, 1968; Pitcher 1970, 1971; Hill 2005, 2009, Chapter 5, this volume. For representationalist views, see (among others) Harman 1990; Dretske 1981, 1995; Byrne and Hilbert 1997, 2003; Byrne and Tye 2006; Tye 1995, 1996, 1997, 2005a, 2005b; Bain 2003, 2007, 2013, Chapter 3, this volume; O'Sullivan and Schroer 2012; Cutter, Chapter 2, this volume. Perceptualists and representationalists are natural allies but the views, strictly speaking, don't entail each other. The kind of representationalism I associate with PRT is sometimes known in the literature as strong representationalism usually promoted as a metaphysical thesis about the nature of perceptual phenomenology. Its main thesis is that perceptual phenomenology is entirely determined by the (non-conceptual) wide representational content of experiences. The differences between perceptualists and representationalists won't matter for the purposes of this entry – but see Aydede 2009, 2013 for a detailed critical discussion of these views and how they are related.

4 First published in 1979 in IASP's official journal, *Pain*, and endorsed again in 1986, 1994, and 2011. The definition, along with other pain related terms, is now available through the website of IASP (under "IASP Taxonomy"): <http://www.iasp-pain.org/Taxonomy?navItemNumber=576#Pain>. For further discussion of the IASP definition of pain, see Chapter 31 in this volume by Andrew Wright, and Aydede, forthcoming-b.

5 Interestingly, almost all perceptual theorists also agree with this point, except Chris Hill (2005, 2009, Chapter 5 of this volume), who explicitly identifies pains with disordered conditions of bodily parts, although he also claims that the common concept of pain is confusing two distinct notions of pain. With the exception of Hill, all perceptualists claim that pains are experiences, not physical disorders or the like, but these experiences, they say, are nevertheless perceptual. (See also Chapter 27, this volume.) They think that our ordinary (or scientific, for that matter) ways of talking about pains as things that are locatable in body parts are just confused. Perceptualists generally tend to give an intentionalist reading of pain-attributing practices as pain locations being merely *intentional* locations within the representational content of pain experiences; see below for more discussion. See Aydede 2013 for a more detailed discussion.

6 Cf. Hardcastle's discussion of the purported puzzle of pain in Chapter 1.

7 George W. Pitcher, an early and influential perceptual theorist, is explicit: "The obstacles [to a direct realist version of the perceptual view of pain] are some features of pain that seem to rule out [such a view], since they seem to demand either (a) that pains be mental (or at any rate non-physical) particulars, or (b) that the awareness of pains be the awareness of subjective 'sense-contents' that are not identical with anything in the physical world. My aim in the paper is to show that these obstacles are merely illusory, and there are no features of pains that force on us the mental-particulars view of pain. So although my attack on [this view] is only indirect, I nevertheless regard it as lethal" (Pitcher 1970: 369). Frank Jackson (1977), on the other hand, happily embraces a non-naturalist sense-datum theory.

8 The content (3a) would be more correctly expressed with a referential expression such as "this [part of the body] is [undergoing] D" – see below.

9 See Aydede 2009 for a more detailed elaboration of this line of criticism.

10 Surprisingly, to the best of my knowledge, no perceptualists have ever addressed this problem. Here is another way to state the problem. A perceptualist who claims that pains in bodily locations (L) *are* physical disturbances in those locations should explain why the truth-values of the following two extensional sentences sometimes come apart: (a) "there is pain in L," (b) "there is disturbance in L," if pain in L = disturbance in L. It's not clear on what non-question-begging grounds, perceptualists who take this line can stipulate away that they never come apart. Try to explain to a patient with a heart condition who claims to feel pain in his left arm that he is dead wrong – that there is in fact no pain in his left arm that he feels – and see what happens … A doctor may correctly say, of course, that he has no disturbance in his left arm, but not that he has no pain in his arm. An empirically adequate model of pain should shed light on this fact, not stipulate it away as merely confused ways of talking. See my proposal below.

11 See for instance, Colin McGinn (among many others): "bodily sensations do not have an intentional object in the way that perceptual experiences do. We distinguish between a visual experience and what it is an experience of; but we do not make this distinction in respect of pains. Or again, visual experiences represent the world as being a certain way, but pains have no such representational content" (McGinn 1982: 8). For many other references for endorsement of the traditional view, see Bain 2003: 502. To be sure, since antiquity, many thinkers (including Galen and Avicenna) regarded pain as informative of tissue disturbance. They talked of pain as typically *caused* by such and such disturbances, or as *signs* of damage or illness, and studied or used them in the service of proper diagnosis and prognosis (see Rey 1995; Cohen 2010). But this is not necessarily to hold a perceptualist view of pain. As said, any non-perceptualist would acknowledge the informative role of pain.

12 Armstrong 1962, 1968; Pitcher 1970, 1971. There were others, to be sure – see my *Stanford Encyclopedia* article (Aydede 2013) for a more detailed history. Pitcher was quite aware of how his perceptualist view would be received: "I shall defend the general thesis that to feel, or to have, a pain, is to engage in a form of sense perception, that when a person has a pain, he is perceiving something. This perceptual view of pain will strike many as bizarre. But sense-datum theorists, at least, ought not to find anything at all odd in it: indeed, I am puzzled why philosophers of that school do not subscribe to the perceptual view of pain *as a matter of course*. Since I am not a sense-datum theorist, however, but a direct realist, I espouse what must at first appear to be an irremediably perverse position – namely, a

direct realist version of the perceptual view of pain" (Pitcher 1970: 368). There is much to be said, of course, about why the sense-datum theorists didn't hold a perceptual view of pain; see Aydede 2013.

13 And ignoring a few other options such as Colin Klein's imperativism (Klein 2015, Chapter 4, this volume) and other purely motivational theories of pain (see also Chapter 8, this volume). However, I am increasingly inclined to think that Klein's imperativism can be seen as a notational variant of PRT; see Aydede, in preparation-b.

14 For more details, see my "Is the Experience of Pain Transparent? Introspecting Phenomenal Qualities" (Aydede, in preparation-a).

15 The quality space for pain may not be completely proprietary to pain: it may overlap with that of touch and perhaps other connected modalities such as proprioception. This is largely an empirical issue better left open. For the notion of the quality space for sensory modalities and the science behind it, see Clark 1996, 2000.

16 The reasons for scare quotes will be clear shortly below.

17 Plus affect – to be handled as further (second-order) adverbial modification of the instantiations of sensory predicates. See Aydede 2014, forthcoming-a for details.

18 In genuinely perceptual cases, these *ways* are ways of sensing the sensible properties in the natural environment (realized by the deployment of sensory predicates) and need to be explicated within a qualia-friendly adverbialist framework. Introspective judgments about sensory experiences track what predicates are activated, but introspective mechanisms don't have their own referential devices singularly picking out these activations. This explains the so-called transparency of sensory experiences. If we want to introspectively focus on the phenomenal qualities of our experiences, our focus seems to go right through our experiences to the extramental particulars that are the objects of these experiences and have the properties attributed by these qualities/predicates. Our introspective judgments are thus about the experiential *ways* in which extramental particulars are represented as being (as having certain properties), without singularly referring to these ways. See Aydede, in preparation-a, for more details, and Aydede and Güzeldere 2005 for the dual informational structure of sensory/phenomenal concepts (predicates used in perceptual and introspective *judgments* and acquired directly from sensory experiences).

19 Consider an apprentice among alchemists in the premodern world pointing to the vapor coming out of boiling water. He utters, "this is phlogiston." Given my Russellianism and the fact that there is no property of being phlogiston, the apprentice is not making a genuine property attribution, although his reference is successful. But although his utterance is not strictly speaking true or false, there are nevertheless appropriateness or suitability conditions to his utterance that are not satisfied in this particular case. And that is what would be pointed out to him when his tutors point out his "mistake" – this description is of course from the perspective of a semanticist. Pain experiences, on the option I am exploring now, are like this utterance. We might say that they do not make *genuine property* attributions, or we might say that they do not *genuinely make* property attributions – either way, they are not fully representational.

20 Note that this is not a form of projectivism – there are no representational mistakes anywhere in the system. One robust mark of projectivism is that it makes experiences under consideration and our judgments based on them massively illusory or somehow mistaken.

21 Projects I take up elsewhere (Aydede and Güzeldere 2005; Aydede 2014, forthcoming-a, in preparation-a).

References

Armstrong, D.M. (1962) *Bodily Sensations*. London: Routledge & Kegan Paul.

Armstrong, D.M. (1968) *A Materialist Theory of the Mind*. New York: Humanities Press.

Aydede, M. (2009) Is feeling pain the perception of something? *Journal of Philosophy* 106(10): 531–567.

Aydede, M. (2013) Pain. In E.N. Zalta (ed.), *The Stanford Encyclopedia of Philosophy* (Spring 2013 ed.). <http://plato.stanford.edu/archives/spr2013/entries/pain/>.

Aydede, M. (2014) How to unify theories of sensory pleasure: an adverbialist proposal. *Review of Philosophy and Psychology* 5(1): 119–133.

Aydede, M. (Forthcoming-a) A contemporary account of sensory pleasure. In L. Schapiro (ed.), *Pleasure: A History*. Oxford: Oxford University Press.

Aydede, M. (Forthcoming-b). Defending the IASP definition of pain. *Monist*.

Aydede, M. (In preparation-a) Is the experience of pain transparent? Introspecting phenomenal qualities.

Aydede, M. (In preparation-b) Review of *What the Body Commands*, by C. Klein.

Aydede, M. and Güzeldere, G. (2005) Cognitive architecture, concepts, and introspection: an information-theoretic solution to the problem of phenomenal consciousness. *Noûs* 39(2): 197–255.

Bain, D. (2003) Intentionalism and pain. *Philosophical Quarterly* 53(213): 502–522.

Bain, D. (2007) The location of pains. *Philosophical Papers* 36(2): 171–205.

Bain, D. (2013) What makes pains unpleasant? *Philosophical Studies* 166 (suppl. 1): S69–S89.

Byrne, A. and Hilbert, D.R. (1997) Colors and reflectances. In A. Byrne and D.R. Hilbert (eds.), *Readings on Color*, vol. 1. Cambridge, MA: MIT Press.

Byrne, A. and Hilbert, D.R. (2003) Color realism and color science *Behavioral and Brain Sciences* 26(1): 3–21.

Byrne, A. and Tye, M. (2006) Qualia ain't in the head. *Noûs*, 40(2): 241–255.

Clark, A. (1996) *Sensory Qualities*. New York: Oxford University Press.

Clark, A. (2000) *A Theory of Sentience*. New York: Oxford.

Cohen, E. (2010) *The Modulated Scream: Pain in Late Medieval Culture*. Chicago: University of Chicago Press.

Craig, A. (2003) Interoception: the sense of the physiological condition of the body. *Current Opinion in Neurobiology* 13(4): 500–505.

Dretske, F. (1981) *Knowledge and the Flow of Information*. Cambridge, MA: MIT Press.

Dretske, F. (1995) *Naturalizing the Mind*. Cambridge, MA: MIT Press.

Harman, G. (1990) The intrinsic quality of experience. *Philosophical Perspectives* 4: 31–52.

Hill, C. (2005) Ow! The paradox of pain. In M. Aydede (ed.), *Pain: New Essays on Its Nature and the Methodology of Its Study*. Cambridge, MA: MIT Press.

Hill, C. (2009) *Consciousness*. Oxford: Oxford University Press.

Hilbert, D.R. (1987) *Color and Color Perception*. Stanford, CA: CSLI Publications.

Jackson, F. (1977) *Perception*. Cambridge: Cambridge University Press.

Klein, C. (2015) *What the Body Commands*. Cambridge, MA: MIT Press.

McGinn, C. (1982) *The Character of Mind*. Oxford: Oxford University Press.

Pitcher, G.W. (1970) Pain perception. *Philosophical Review* 79: 368–393.

Pitcher, G. (1971) *A Theory of Perception*. Princeton: Princeton University Press.

O'Sullivan, B. and Schroer, R. (2012) Painful reasons: representationalism as a theory of pain. *Philosophical Quarterly* 62: 737–758.

Rey, R. (1995) *The History of Pain*. Cambridge, MA: Harvard University Press.

Tye, M. (1995) *Ten Problems of Consciousness: A Representational Theory of the Phenomenal Mind*. Cambridge, MA: MIT Press.

Tye, M. (1996) The function of consciousness. *Noûs*, 1(3): 287–305.

Tye, M. (1997) A representational theory of pains and their phenomenal character. In N. Block, O. Flanagan, and G. Güzeldere (eds.), *The Nature of Consciousness: Philosophical Debates*. Cambridge, MA: MIT Press.

Tye, M. (2005a) Another look at representationalism about pain. In M. Aydede (ed.), *Pain: New Essays on Its Nature and the Methodology of Its Study*. Cambridge, MA: MIT Press.

Tye, M. (2005b) Reply to commentaries. In M. Aydede (ed.), *Pain: New Essays on Its Nature and the Methodology of Its Study*. Cambridge, MA: MIT Press.

PART II-II

Pain in epistemology

19

PAIN AND RATIONALITY

Jonathan Cohen and Matthew Fulkerson

> [B]ecause he suffers hunger or cold or other pain he is only the more determined
> to persevere and conquer. His noble spirit will not be quelled until he either slays
> or is slain; or until he hears the voice of the shepherd, that is, reason, bidding his
> dog bark no more.
>
>

Plato, Republic *IV, 440d*

1 Introduction

Pain plays many roles in our mental lives.[1] It motivates, protects, and is often a source of negative moral and pragmatic value. Moreover, and perhaps more surprisingly, pain has a number of interesting, and interestingly incomplete, connections with rationality.

A few caveats are in order before we begin to survey some of these connections. First – and though we intend to remain as agnostic as we can about the nature of pain, so as to make our discussion maximally general – we will assume in what follows that pains are complex states, and that they involve sensory-discriminative, affective-motivational, and cognitive components. We'll also be assuming that pains ordinarily involve a negatively valenced affect, which we refer to as painfulness, though we set aside the question of what account of pain best accounts for its painfulness.[2]

One of the most important reasons for thinking of pain as importantly connected to human rationality is that experienced pains seem to provide reasons to the subjects in whom they occur – reasons that can be both practically motivating and rationally justifying (at the personal level).[3]

In saying that pains provide justifying (or, sometimes, normative) reasons, we mean that they provide considerations that objectively count in favor of an action for a subject (whether or not they are appreciated by the subject). Even if Sasha believes sunscreen is unnecessary and has no intention or desire to use it, one might think there is still a very good justifying reason for her to do so (to prevent UV skin damage). In saying that pains provide motivating (or, sometimes, explanatory) reasons, we mean that they provide the (often causal) explanations for why an action was undertaken, given from the perspective of the agent. Perhaps Sasha sprays herself with sunscreen at the beach mistakenly thinking that it's insect repellent. While she still has a justifying reason for putting on the sun screen, that wasn't her motivating, explanatory reason. The motivating reason was something like: she wanted to put on insect repellent and she believed that the sun screen was insect repellent.

As we say, it is pre-theoretically plausible that pains can supply both of these sorts of reasons for the subjects in whom they occur. Thus, consider Lucy the distracted machinist, who strikes her thumb hard with a ballpeen hammer. First, the pain Lucy feels provides her with a motivating reason to tend to her injured thumb – perhaps holding or squeezing it, or applying ice to it. After all, without the pain she wouldn't have undertaken these actions, and that she does undertake them is a direct consequence of her experienced pain. Additionally, however, Lucy's pain seems to count as a justifying reason for Lucy. Whether or not Lucy holds her thumb and applies ice to it, her pain justifies her doing so: that is what she objectively ought to do in the circumstance, given the pain, but not otherwise.

In this entry we will explore some of the connections between pain and rationality in terms of these two sorts of reasons that pain plausibly provides. We'll begin by considering the nature of the connection between pain and motivation, principally by reference to long-standing philosophical disputes about the nature of the connection between reasons and motivation (Section 2). And then we'll ask whether and in what ways pains are like other justification-providing rational elements of our psychologies in being responsive to reasons and rationally evaluable (Section 3).

2 Motivational internalism: from reasons to pain?

We begin with pain's capacity to provide motivational reasons. It seems hard to deny that pains do provide highly salient reasons of this type: indeed, the most natural person-level explanations of why Lucy shakes, presses, or ices her thumb after hitting it with a hammer will advert to her pain. But this leaves open a suite of interesting questions about the nature of the connection between pain and motivation. We can begin to probe this connection indirectly by reference to the more widely discussed issue of what connections to motivation are exhibited by (not pain, but) reasons.

On a family of views we'll call motivational internalism about reasons (also sometimes referred to by the less than perfectly perspicuous label 'reasons internalism'), there is an essential, or constitutive, connection between justifying reasons and practical motivation.[4, 5] While there are many versions of motivational internalism about reasons, perhaps the most widely discussed version of the view is the so-called Humean Theory of Reasons (HTR), according to which there is a constitutive connection between reasons and desires. HTR claims, for example, that if Tony has a justifying reason to ϕ, then Tony must also have a desire to ϕ. (Note that the opposite entailment is clearly false – and not assumed by HTR: having a desire to ϕ does not secure a justifying reason to ϕ.)

HTR is controversial both as a substantive thesis (see Setiya 2004; Smith 1995; Williams 1979), and as an interpretation of Hume's own views (see Persson 1997; and the essays in Pigden 2009). We want to put these debates aside for now in order to ask a different question suggested by the consideration of HTR in the present setting: might there be an analogous motivational internalist view about pains, on which there is a similarly constitutive connection between pain and desire?

2.1 Two forms of motivational internalism about pain

We can imagine answering this question affirmatively in at least the following two different ways, corresponding to different articulations of motivational internalism about pain. A first, indirect, affirmative answer would begin with the assumption, bruited above, that being in pain automatically confers on a subject justifying reasons (as it might be, a justifying reason to φ). If (controversially) this assumption is not only true but necessary, and if we additionally accept HTR, then this would yield the affirmative conclusion we were after, that being in pain necessarily/constitutively confers on the subject a desire (as it might be, a desire to φ).[6] Alternatively, one might accept motivational internalism about pain independently of any connections to justifying reasons: one might simply think that genuine pains could not occur without the presence of concomitant desire-like internal states.

While both of these possibilities would end up connecting pains to desires or desire-like states, and so sustaining forms of motivational internalism about pain, the first possibility makes this connection indirectly, via (alleged) constitutive links both pain and motivation bear to justifying reasons. Accordingly, we'll call this view indirect motivational internalism about pain so as to contrast it with the latter view, which we'll call direct motivational internalism about pain.

2.2 Motivations for motivational internalism about pain

As we sketched the view, indirect motivational internalism about pain depended on assuming a theory like HTR or some other form of motivational internalism about reasons. One possible attraction of this position is that it could be used to argue for particular accounts of the nature of pains that are suited to the provision of justifying reasons. For example, some writers (Bain 2013, Chapter 3, this volume; Helm 2002; O'Sullivan and Schroer 2012) have argued on such grounds against theories on which pains are identified with mere causes or motivating reasons; the thought is that pains, construed as mere causes, would not, by themselves, provide the justifying reasons that they must. Such theorists have typically, therefore, advocated an alternative evaluative theory of pains as rich states with evaluative contents which, when veridical, are suitably poised to provide the needed justifying reasons. However, as Cohen and Fulkerson (2013) urge, this line of argument presupposes two controversial theses: (i) that HTR is true, and (ii) that pains qua mere causes cannot amount to justifying reasons. Moreover, since the latter of these theses is typically rejected both by proponents of causal accounts of pain and even by evaluativists themselves, the argument in question is probably of limited utility in actually changing anyone's views about the nature of pain. Still, it does highlight a rich set of dependencies between one's theories of pains, reasons, and motivation.

A different possible attraction of motivational internalism about pain (of either indirect or direct flavors) is that such views make available an especially simple explanation of the apparent fact that pains do seem to come with practical motivation. Thus, to return to the example above, it is extremely plausible that when Lucy undergoes pain after hitting her thumb with a hammer, she has a practical motivation for her subsequent action of icing her thumb. The pain internalist will have a ready explanation of this co-occurrence in Lucy's psychology: she will claim that pains and practical motivations co-occur necessarily, because the two sorts of state are constitutively linked. Indeed, one way of working out (direct) pain internalism might be found in so-called "attitudinal" views of pain (e.g., Heathwood 2006), according to which pains (more precisely, painfulness) just is the result of a motivational attitude (typically a desire or similar con-attitude) being directed towards a noxious sensation.[7]

2.3 Motivational internalism about pain reconsidered

Unfortunately, and whatever one thinks of the motivations discussed above, it is unclear whether pains and practical motivation are constitutively linked in the way envisaged by motivational internalism about pain.

To bring this issue into relief, it may be helpful to consider a parallel question about the relation between moral judgment and moral motivation. It is more or less uncontroversial that a subject in normal circumstances who judges (sincerely, reflectively) that she ought to φ will have a moral motivation to φ; this is to say that these two states of the subject seem to co-occur. But it is much more controversial whether this co-occurrence should be explained by positing a constitutive connection between the two types of states. Some (e.g., Smith 1994) hold that it's essential to moral judgments that subjects who have them *ipso facto* have (possibly defeasible) moral motivation; extending the terminology we've been using in the obvious way, we can call this view motivational internalism about moral judgment. Other theorists, however, hold the view, which we can call motivational externalism about moral judgment, that moral judgment is only contingently (though perhaps universally) connected to moral motivation (Brink 1997; Railton 1986; Shafer-Landau 2000; Svavarsdottir 1999). Thus, on the latter sort of view, a subject who judges that she ought to φ will only be morally motivated to φ in the presence of some numerically distinct conative state – say, a disposition to do what she judges to be right – that is typically but inessentially linked to her judgment.

Much of the dispute between motivational internalists and externalists about moral judgment has centered on the possibility of what Brink (1997) labels an "amoralist" – a subject who, after undergoing frontal lobe trauma, makes all of the same moral evaluative judgments as before the brain damage, but no longer feels motivated to act appropriately on the basis of these judgments. Such cases, if indeed possible, seem to provide a serious impediment to any robust internalism about moral motivation. As Brink notes, "[w]here there is such physical and psychological interference, practical judgment does not produce motivation. If so, we must deny that judgments of practical reason entail motivation" (Brink 1997: 17).

Given this backdrop, what should we say about the relation between pain and practical motivation? When Lucy undergoes her pain, most theorists would agree that she will evaluate her bodily state negatively, and that she will be motivated to act in certain ways. But by analogy to the dispute about moral motivation, we can imagine two different understandings of how this instance of practical motivation is related to Lucy's practical evaluation. On the one hand, we have seen that motivational internalists about pain will hold that it's essential to Lucy's undergoing pain – including having a negatively valenced practical evaluation of her bodily state – that it bring about in Lucy a (possibly defeasible) practical motivation to act. That is to say that, without bringing about this motivation, the pain wouldn't include the sort of negative evaluation that such motivational internalists take to be essential to a state's being a pain. On the other hand, a motivational externalist about pain will hold that practical evaluation is only contingently (though perhaps universally) connected to practical motivation. Thus, for a motivational externalist about pain, Lucy's negatively valenced evaluation of her bodily state will only practically motivate Lucy to undertake remediative action in the presence of some numerically distinct conative state – say, a disposition to remediate those states of her body she evaluates negatively – that is typically but inessentially linked to her evaluation.

As before, we can bring out this disagreement by considering the possibility of what we might call an "apracticalist" who, after brain trauma, forms all of the same practical evaluations of her bodily condition as before the injury, but who no longer feels motivated to act appropriately on the basis of these evaluative states. Motivational internalists will hold that an apracticalist of this sort is impossible, while motivational externalists will hold that the apracticalist is possible.

These concerns can easily be applied to pain.

There are several well-known pathologies, similar in structure and scope to the sorts of amoralist and apracticalist cases considered above, that involve a clear disconnect between pain experience, pain evaluation, and pain motivation. The most discussed of these pathologies is *pain asymbolia*. The pain asymbolic is indistinguishable from control subjects in assessing and describing painful stimuli. For instance, an asymbolic can clearly discriminate between a sharp, shooting pain, and a dull, burning ache. More impressively, when asked to rate the intensity of the pain on a scale (from 1 to 10, say), an asymbolic will rate the pains in a manner indistinguishable from that of control subjects. Unlike control subjects, however, the asymbolic claims not to care or to be motivated by these pain experiences, even when they rate them as extremely intense. Asymbolics suffer immense practical disadvantage from this condition, since they remain completely unconcerned even while undergoing extremely damaging interactions with the world. For instance, when cooking they will simply reach out and touch hot foods, completely unconcerned by the resulting skin damage. They also fail to move appropriately when sleeping in awkward or stressful positions, often resulting in severe injuries and even disfigurement. An asymbolic thus seems to experience and undergo pain, form judgments about the nature and severity of the signal, and to understand the connection of such signals to the actual damage it portends, and yet find him- or herself with no motivation to act in ways typical of pain experiences. *Prima facie*, this suggests that painful experiences and even painful evaluations (if we choose to consider intensity judgments as a kind of evaluation) can in these cases become disconnected from the motivations typically generated by painful episodes.[8]

Some have indeed taken these and similar cases to be straightforward counterexamples to motivational internalism about pain (see especially Grahek 2007). Others have urged that the cases at issue are not counterexamples to the latter view, but only cases in which the subjects experience a mitigated, incomplete, or inauthentic form of pain. Still others (Klein 2015) have defended motivational internalism about pain by holding that asymbolics robustly undergo pain, but simply lack a capacity to show care or concern for their own well-being.

Asymbolia is not the only interesting pathology, of course. In addition to asymbolia, cases of interest include congenital insensitivity to pain, allodynia, morphine pain, and certain diseases like leprosy (cf. Hardcastle 1999). Each of these cases suggests a way in which pain experiences and motivation can come apart. While appeal to such cases doesn't settle the issue immediately (as above), they do raise interesting questions and offer some novel ways of putting pressure on motivational internalism about pain.

3 Pain and justifying reasons

So far our discussion has centered on pain's capacity to provide motivating reasons. In this section, we want to consider pain's capacity to provide normative, justifying reasons.

3.1 Reasons-responsiveness and pain

As noted, it is pre-theoretically plausible that pains do provide justifying reasons for creatures like us, and that this counts as an interesting way in which pains are connected to our rationality. Interestingly, however, though pains are (justifying) reasons-providing in subjects who have them, such as Lucy, pains also tend to be stubbornly resistant to rational considerations – they are not reasons-responsive in the way that other reasons-providing states typically are. Thus, when Lucy undergoes pain as a result of eating a modestly pungent curry, her (correct) belief that her pain is not signaling any imminent danger – that she is not under threat of any further bodily harm as a result of eating the food – is strangely ineffective in mitigating either the intensity of her pain or its action-guiding force.

Of course, Lucy can ordinarily reason herself out of being guided by other kinds of justi-fying reasons. For example, Lucy might hold a desire for relaxation and a belief that going to the beach would afford relaxation, and these might be counted a reason for Lucy to go to the beach. But when reflections about impending deadlines lead her to stay at home and work, she (by an exercise of her practical deliberation) brings it about that other considerations overwhelm the first reason, and consequently (unlike in cases involving pain) makes the latter cease to be action-guiding for her. Pains (and other forms of suffering) stand in contrast to these ordinary cases of rational mitigation of (justifying) reason-providing states because pains are much less robustly responsive to other reasons.

Now, we don't want to overstate this point. Our claim is not that pain is completely unresponsive to other reasons: on the contrary, there is good evidence of certain kinds of reasons-based modulation of suffering (e.g., through anticipation or social context, and perhaps some forms of therapy). Still, this sort of modulation is strikingly different from the modulation of others of our reasons-providing internal states: in cases of suffering in particular, modula-tion by reasons is relatively limited in its efficacy, relatively effortful (whence the need to seek out professional help), and relatively temporary (whence the need to continue the ther-apeutic interventions). It is this apparent break in kind between the two types of influence by reasons that we have in mind in saying that pains are not reasons-responsive in the way that other justifying reasons-providing states typically are.

It would seem, then, that pains, despite providing justifying reasons for subjects, are sticky in the face of countervailing considerations in a way that other reasons(/reason-providing states) are not.[9] Moreover, as we have argued elsewhere (Fulkerson and Cohen, forth-coming), it's not plausible that this very stickiness is itself deeply disturbing – that it can lead creatures like us to a kind of further, second-order harm, over and above the first-order pain, which can be extremely serious and deleterious to the creatures in whom it arises.[10]

3.2 Rational evaluability

A final consideration concerns the question of whether pains can be rationally evaluable.

It is standard to suppose that we can rationally evaluate our ordinary doxastic and conative states. For instance, consider Ashley, who, with no evidence, forms the belief that Elvis Presley is alive and living secretly in Germany. Her belief is evaluable with respect to its rationality: given that she has no evidence for forming this belief, we can evaluate it negatively. It is irrational for her to hold this belief. This means, on many plausible accounts of responsibility, that we can hold her responsible for this belief, at least to the extent that her holding of this belief impacts her overall rationality. She her-self is in part irrational to the extent that she holds irrational beliefs like the one described above. The evaluability of this belief and the assessment of irrationality does not depend on the truth of doxastic voluntarism, the idea that our beliefs are formed voluntarily. Given the nature of belief, we can and do hold subjects rationally responsible for their beliefs.

Similarly, it is natural to think our conative states like desires and wishes can be targets of rational evaluation. Thus, Davidson (1963: 686) gives the example of Paul, a man who has had a yen his whole life to drink a can of paint. This yen, like a belief, seems rationally evaluable: we can say with confidence that Paul has no good reason for this yen and there-fore evaluate it negatively. We can say it is an irrational desire that Paul has, and that he himself is irrational in part because of his possession of this desire. And we can imagine here a range of desires and wishes that fail a test of rationality.[11]

These considerations invite us to ask: can we, similarly, treat a subject's pain state as rationally evaluable, and can we hold the subject rationally responsible for that state?

One possible avenue to an affirmative answer to this question comes from extending to the case of pain arguments offered by Corns (submitted) to the effect that at least some affective states can indeed be rationally evaluated. Corns invites us to consider a subject with an irrational desire for symmetry; and she imagines that, if this subject is presented with a highly asymmetric flower arrangement, the non-satisfaction of her (*ex hypothesi*, irrational) desire might cause her extreme distress. Corns goes on to urge that, given its etiology in irrational desire, the subject's distress is also rationally evaluable. We can, just as with false and unsupported beliefs and irrational wants and desires, hold this subject responsible for her distress. We can say, like a caring parent, that her distress is inappropriate to the circumstances, that it arises from a lack of adequate coping strategies or supporting beliefs on the part of the subject, and that it doesn't, in some straightforward sense, cohere with the subject's other mental states. And this lack of coherence gives us a robust sense of (negative) rational evaluation that applies to the subject's distress even if we don't construe the latter in overtly/overly intellectualist terms. If we are sympathetic to this treatment of Corns' subject's distress, we might extend similar conclusions to pain. After all, we might imagine (as Corns does not) that the presentation of the asymmetric flower arrangement produces in the symmetry-lover not only distress, but an experience of diffuse pain. If so, then all the considerations offered about the distress will apply to the pain as well. It, too, has an irrational source. We would reasonably hold the subject responsible for the pain, might think of the pain as circumstantially inappropriate, as something that arises from a lack of coping strategies, and as something that fails to cohere with her other mental states. Thus, these considerations appear to make available a good (but not intellectualized) sense in which the subject's pain, too, is rationally evaluable.

Evidence from child development and pain learning may also support an affirmative answer to our question. Thus, when a young child has a modest fall or slight injury, parents often suggest an evaluation of the pain itself, in terms of the appropriate amount of hurt the noxious stimuli should have generated (note the normative language throughout). For instance, suppose a child touches a warm but not hot cup of coffee. Perhaps because of previous warnings and expectations, the child responds to this mild thermal insult with extreme wincing, screams, and distress. A parent, confirming the mere warmth of the cup, might gently suggest that the child is overreacting, with soothing admonitions that "it doesn't really hurt so much," and "it's not that bad, the cup was just a little warm," etc. This seems initially to be a case where a parent is rationally evaluating his child's pain – suggesting that some pain states are irrational, without reason in a straightforward sense, while allowing that other pains can be more appropriate to the circumstances (for discussion of such cases, see Helm 2001).

On the other hand, one might respond that in these sorts of cases, rather than evaluating the rationality of pain states themselves, we're instead evaluating numerically distinct negative emotional reactions (say, sadness, upset, worry, concern) to the pain. Brady (2009) argues plausibly that these and other felt emotions can be rationally evaluable (like beliefs and desires). If so, then perhaps the locus of evaluation in the asymmetric flower arrangement case or the parental soothing case is not the pain, but instead the causally downstream emotional and other secondary reactions pain produces.[12]

A further line of support for the idea that pains may be rationally evaluable comes from recent studies suggesting that learned coping strategies for dealing with painful episodes can generate strong differences in pain tolerance and subjective reports of pain intensity (Lu et al. 2007; Piira et al. 2002; see also Chapters 11 and 12, this volume). Subjects who have learned self-efficacy and cognitive intervention strategies (e.g., subjects who have strong beliefs in their ability to cope with pains and who have learned to distract themselves during pain) typically have much higher pain tolerances than subjects who (for example) catastrophize their pains (for instance, subjects who express pain reactions in order to trigger emotional and other support from others). Seeking aid from others instead of managing it oneself tends to decrease pain tolerance and increase subjective reports of discomfort.[13]

It's tempting to read these results as showing evaluations and learning can have a strong impact on pain itself (as measured by pain tolerance and self-reports of pain intensity) rather than pain behaviors. However, this evidence is open to a version of the reply we already considered in connection with the asymmetric flower arrangement case or the parental soothing case. Namely, one might insist that what subjects rationally evaluate here, and what shows up in measures of their pain tolerance and self-reports of pain intensity, is not the pain itself, but reactions to the pain.

(We can see a rough parallel here with accounts of the rational evaluability of perceptual states, though the point is rarely put in these exact terms. Many theorists have held that perceptual states have contents that can be assessed for truth and falsity [e.g., Byrne 2002; Siegel 2010]. If so, then their having such contents provides one natural way of thinking about the states themselves as being rationally evaluable. There are views of perception, however, that deny that perceptual states have content or are subject to such evaluation [e.g., Martin 2006; Travis 2004]. On these views – Travis especially – it is not the perception itself that is the locus of assessment but the downstream judgments and beliefs formed on the basis of the perceptual experience. So, too, those who treat pains as having truth-evaluable contents will hold that the pains themselves can be rationally assessed in terms of their content; however, one might reject this view by holding that rational assessment applies to downstream psychological consequences of pains rather than pains themselves.)

It would seem, then, that there is suggestive evidence of the rational evaluability of pains, but that the evidence to date is so far not completely decisive by itself.

Related topics

Chapter 1: A brief and potted overview on the philosophical theories of pain (Hardcastle)
Chapter 2: Pain and representation (Cutter)
Chapter 3: Evaluativist accounts of pain's unpleasantness (Bain)
Chapter 4: Imperativism (Klein)
Chapter 5: Fault lines in familiar concepts of pain (Hill)
Chapter 6: Advances in the neuroscience of pain (Apkarian)
Chapter 7: Neuromatrix theory of pain (Roy and Wager)
Chapter 8: A neurobiological view of pain as a homeostatic emotion (Strigo and Craig)
Chapter 9: A view of pain based on sensations, meanings, and emotions (Price)
Chapter 11: Psychological models of pain (Williams)
Chapter 12: Biopsychosocial models of pain (Hadjistavropoulos)

Notes

1 This work is fully collaborative; authors are listed alphabetically.
2 For more discussion of such questions about the proper characterization of pain itself, see Chapters 1–9, 11, and 12 of this volume.
3 We won't worry here about whether pain provides one reason that is both motivating and justifying, or whether it provides two separate reasons (one motivating, one justifying). Nor will we enter into the many complicated disputes about the structure and nature of action explanations, motivating

reasons, and rational justification (for an entry into this literature, see, e.g., Mele 2003; Parfit and Broome 1997; Smith 1987). See also Chapter 3, this volume. We hope what we say here about these issues will be sufficiently truistic to be accepted by all sides.

4 Caution: 'internalism' is used in various ways in the literature; our usage is slightly idiosyncratic.

5 It is perhaps worth observing that this is, in fact, a substantive thesis. Whereas it is trivially true that there is a necessary connection between motivating reasons and motivation (since, after all, motivating reasons just are whatever actually motivated a subject to act), it is not so obvious that there is a similar connection between justifying reasons and motivation.

6 Of course, appealing to HTR will produce a view that links pains constitutively to desires as opposed to other motivating states; slotting in other versions of reasons internalism will result in views on which pains are linked to other intrinsically motivating states or dispositions.

7 There are of course many details and subtleties to be worked out in such views, and some ways might fall outside the proper scope of the internalism we're considering here.

8 This makes asymbolia doubly interesting, for it puts pressure both on views according to which the motivational aspect is internal to pain itself (our direct views), and also on views that connect motivation to a state related to but distinct from the pain.

9 To be fair, pain is plausibly not unique in being reasons-providing but not reason-responsive (or, at any rate, not reasons-responsive to the extent typical of states that are reason-providing). On many views, such extrapsychological entities as states, events, facts, and states of affairs can share this combination of features: thus, if Theo is thirsty and heads to the fridge because he knows there is water there, there's a good, if minimal, sense in which the water's being in the fridge counts as a reason for his action; but of course, the water's being in the fridge is completely immune to influence by Theo's broader reasons and motivational profile. But the case of pains is more interesting than the case of the water's being in the fridge (etc.) because it reveals that there can be failures of reasons-responsiveness in elements internal to (and, indeed, highly salient and intense in) the thinker's own psychology.

10 There are a number of other types of cases in which our reason-providing states are or seem to be oddly resistant to the influence of our reasons; these would include (at least) cases of akrasia, non-intentional actions, rapid redeliberation, and failures of deliberative decisiveness. Fulkerson and Cohen (forthcoming) introduce and consider these cases, and argue that the reason-resistance exhibited by pains is interestingly different from each of them, hence that it deserves its own explanation.

11 There are, of course, different accounts of what it is in virtue of which such states are evaluable. On some views, for instance, what makes them irrational is that an ideal subject under rational reflection would disavow such a desire or wish. On another view, such a state counts as irrational because it fails to cohere with a subject's other sincerely held beliefs and desires.

12 In the case of the asymmetrical flower arrangement, we might additionally evaluate the upstream desire for symmetry that, when violated, is a partial cause of the subject's pain.

13 Indeed, it appears that parents can significantly increase their children's pain tolerance and decrease their reports of pain intensity by employing distraction and empowerment responses, while parents who treat even minor stimuli as serious matters tend to cause their children to have lower pain tolerance and an increase in subjective intensity ratings (cf. Bearden et al. 2012; Gonzalez et al. 1993).

References

Bain, D. (2013) What makes pains unpleasant? *Philosophical Studies* 166 (suppl. 1): S69–S89.

Bearden, D.J., Feinstein, A., and Cohen, L.L. (2012) The influence of parent preprocedural anxiety on child procedural pain: mediation by child procedural anxiety. *Journal of Pediatric Psychology* 37(6): 680–686.

Brady, M.S. (2009) The irrationality of recalcitrant emotions. *Philosophical Studies* 145(3): 413–430.

Brink, D.O. (1997) Moral motivation. *Ethics* 108(1): 4–32.

Byrne, A. (2002) Intentionalism defended. *Philosophical Review* 110: 199–240.

Cohen, J. and Fulkerson, M. (2013) Affect, rationalization, and motivation. *Review of Philosophy and Psychology* 4(4): 1–16. doi10.1007/s13164-013-0173-0.

Corns, J. (Submitted) Hedonic rationality.

Davidson, D. (1963) Actions, reasons, and causes. *Journal of Philosophy* 60(23): 685–700.

Fulkerson, M. and Cohen, J. (forthcoming) The agony of reason: the unsteady bond between suffering and human rationality. In D. Bain, M. Brady, and J. Corns (eds.), *The Nature of Pain*.

Gonzalez, J.C., Routh, D.K., and Armstrong, F.D. (1993) Effects of maternal distraction versus reassurance on children's reactions to injections. *Journal of Pediatric Psychology* 18(5): 593–604.

Grahek, N. (2007) *Feeling Pain and Being in Pain*, 2nd ed. Cambridge, MA: MIT Press.

Hardcastle, V.G. (1999) *The Myth of Pain*. Cambridge, MA:MIT Press.

Heathwood, C. (2006) The reduction of sensory pleasure to desire. *Philosophical Studies* 133(1): 23–44.

Helm, B.W. (2001) *Emotional Reason: Deliberation, Motivation, and the Nature of Value*. Cambridge: Cambridge University Press.

Helm, B.W. (2002) Felt evaluations: a theory of pleasure and pain. *American Philosophical Quarterly* 39(1): 13–30.

Klein, C. (2015) What pain asymbolia really shows. *Mind* 124(494): 493–516.

Lu, Q., Tsao, J.C.I., Myers, C.D., Kim, S.C., and Zeltzer, L.K. (2007) Coping predictors of children's laboratory-induced pain tolerance, intensity, and unpleasantness. *Journal of Pain*. 8(9): 708–717.

Martin, M.G.F. (2006) On being alienated. In T.S. Gendler and J. Hawthorne (eds.), *Perceptual Experience*. Oxford: Oxford University Press, pp. 354–410.

Mele, A.R. (2003) *Motivation and Agency*. Oxford: Oxford University Press.

O'Sullivan, B. and Schroer, R. (2012) Painful reasons: representationalism as a theory of pain. *Philosophical Quarterly* 62(249): 737–758.

Parfit, D. and Broome, J. (1997) Reasons and motivation. *Proceedings of the Aristotelian Society* 71: 99–146.

Persson, I. (1997) Hume – not a "Humean" about motivation. *History of Philosophy Quarterly* 14(2): 189–206.

Pigden, C.R. (ed.) (2009) *Hume on Motivation and Virtue: New Essays*. London: Palgrave Macmillan.

Piira, T., Taplin, J.E., and Goodenough, B. (2002) Cognitive-behavioural predictors of children's tolerance of laboratory-induced pain: implications for clinical assessment and future directions. *Behaviour Research and Therapy* 40(5): 571–584.

Railton, P. (1986) Moral realism. *Philosophical Review* 95(2): 163–207.

Setiya, K. (2004) Against internalism. *Noûs* 38(2): 266–298.

Shafer-Landau, R. (2000) A defense of motivational externalism. *Philosophical Studies* 97: 267–291.

Siegel, S. (2010) *The Contents of Visual Experience*. New York: Oxford University Press.

Smith, M. (1987) The Humean theory of motivation. *Mind*, n.s., 96(381): 36–61.

Smith, M. (1994) *The Moral Problem*. Oxford: Blackwell.

Smith, M. (1995) Internal reasons. *Philosophy and Phenomenological Research* 55(1): 109–131.

Svavarsdottir, S. (1999) Moral cognitivism and motivation. *Philosophical Review* 108(2): 161–219.

Travis, C. (2004) The silence of the senses. *Mind* 113(449): 57–94.

Williams, B. (1979) Internal and external reasons. In R. Harrison (ed.), *Rational Action*. Cambridge: Cambridge University Press, pp. 101–113.

20

PAIN AND INCORRIGIBILITY

Peter Langland-Hassan

1 Introduction

Could Jane be in pain, while believing she is not? Could Shane feel *no* pain, while believing that he does? If our beliefs about our own current pains are *incorrigible*, the answer to both questions must be no.

To be *incorrigible* on a topic is equivalent to being *infallible*: any belief one forms simply cannot be wrong. At least, that is how I will understand incorrigibility. Some in philosophy understand incorrigibility as a mere *unwillingness* to have one's beliefs corrected, or an inability of others *to convincingly show* that one's belief is incorrect (see Schwitzgebel 2014 for discussion). That sort of incorrigibility is consistent with a person *in fact* being wrong about the matter at hand.

Yet my interest is in the strong thesis that we simply *cannot be wrong* about our own current pains. Whether or not one finds it immediately plausible that we are incorrigible about our pains in this strong sense, reflection on the question reveals interesting tensions and ambiguities in the ordinary notion of pain, and in our understanding of mental processes and sensations generally.

Speaking for myself, I came to this essay highly skeptical that we have incorrigibility with respect to any of our mental or bodily states; yet I leave it thinking that, in the case of pain, matters are not so straightforward.

2 The incorrigible and the self-intimating

The question of incorrigibility is fundamentally a question about beliefs. We want to know whether a certain class of beliefs – beliefs about whether we are in pain – can ever be wrong. There are two ways we could err in such beliefs. We might believe that we are in pain when we are not. Let us call this a *false positive*. And we might believe we are not in pain when we are in pain. Let us call this a *false negative*. We can then understand the *incorrigibility thesis* as holding that there can be no false positives and no false negatives with respect to one's own current pains.

Note that the question of *whether* we are in pain is different from the question of what *kind* of pain we are in. The incorrigibility thesis is most plausible, and of most interest, when taking the relevant judgments to be about whether one is in *some* kind of pain or other,

245

regardless of type (where the type could specify a certain *quality* or *location* of the pain, for instance). I will therefore focus on the "some kind or other" reading here. It is worth considering, however, whether an ability to be wrong with respect to what type of pain we are having also entails or suggests an ability to be wrong about being in pain *tout court*. If we could mistake a throbbing pain for a burning pain, for instance, it might seem we could also mistake an intense itch for a sharp pain. The latter possibility would speak against our incorrigibility with respect to pain judgments.

We should also keep in mind that even if the incorrigibility thesis were true, it would not entail that we always know when we are in pain. The incorrigibility thesis is compatible with our having pains that we never form beliefs about one way or the other. A different thesis holds that *if* we are in pain, we necessarily know that we are. To accept this thesis is to hold that pains are *self-intimating*. Unlike the incorrigibility thesis, the self-intimating thesis is compatible with there being false positives.

In what follows, I will maintain focus on the question of incorrigibility. Most of the important points to be made with respect to the self-intimating thesis can be made in addressing the question of incorrigibility as well.

3 Consciousness

The relationship of pain to consciousness is a matter of controversy. Of particular dispute is whether pains are always conscious or if, instead, they can occur non-consciously. (See Chapter 17 of this handbook.) The question of incorrigibility is distinct from the question of whether pains can occur non-consciously. For *even if* pains are always conscious, it need not follow that our beliefs with respect to our pains are incorrigible. It might be that, in certain circumstances, we simply make false judgments about the contents of our conscious minds (Schwitzgebel 2008).

Nevertheless, we should expect interaction between views on the relationship of consciousness to pain and the incorrigibility thesis. Views on the relationship of introspection to pain (discussed in Chapter 18) will also likely interact with views concerning incorrigibility. Because the relationships of introspection and consciousness to pain are discussed separately in this volume, I will set aside considerations relating specifically to consciousness and introspection for the remainder of this entry. This will allow our conclusions concerning pain and incorrigibility to serve as independent data points in considerations concerning the relationship of pain to consciousness and introspection.

4 Pains-as-sensations versus pains-as-tissue-damage

As elsewhere remarked in this volume, there are at least two different phenomena commonly referred to in ordinary uses of the word "pain" (see, e.g., Chapter 5 of this volume). On the one hand, "pain" can serve to refer to certain kinds of tissue damage or nerve stimulation. When I hit my thumb with a hammer, it seems true to say that there is literally a pain *in my thumb*. This suggests that "pain" refers to a certain kind of bodily trauma or tissue damage present in my thumb. When the word "pain" is used in this way, we are speaking of *pains-as-tissue-damage*, or what I will call *T-Pains*. On the other hand, when I put my injured thumb in a bucket of ice, we are not inclined to say that there is a pain in the bucket (to paraphrase an old joke). This is because the word "pain," in a more fundamental use, also serves to refer to a certain kind of unpleasant sensory experience typically *caused by* tissue damage or nerve stimulation. Something can only be "in pain" in this sense if it is having a sensory experience of the right kind; and this is something buckets cannot do. We can call these *pain sensations,* or *S-Pains*. Yet we should leave open the possibility that S-Pains have cognitive and affective components *in addition to* certain distinctive sensory features (Hardcastle 1999; Corns 2014; earlier chapters in this volume, e.g., Chapter 9). Further, we should leave open, for the time being, whether one or more of these components is *essential* to S-Pain and others only contingently associated with S-Pain. (This question becomes central later.) Cases of phantom limb pain – where an amputee feels pain in a limb no longer possessed – make vivid the distinction between the two senses of "pain." The person suffering phantom limb pains has very real S-Pains, without the normal T-Pains that typically cause or accompany them. In such cases, an S-Pain seems to indicate or represent the presence of a T-Pain in one's limb, even though one no longer has the limb (or the relevant T-Pain). A common view is that S-Pains are representations of T-Pains (see Chapter 2, this volume); S-Pains indicate the presence of T-Pains in specific bodily locations, though are perhaps not exhausted by this representational role.[1]

The most interesting questions with respect to pain and incorrigibility concern S-Pains. For it is not hard to see how there might be false positives and false negatives with respect to T-Pains. *Referred pains*, for instance, occur when a person reports pain at a location other than where the tissue damage or trauma responsible for the pain has occurred. Such reports can be seen as evidence that one falsely believes oneself to have a certain kind of T-Pain – they are false positives with respect to T-Pains. And phantom limb pains suggest the possibility of believing oneself to have a T-Pain in the absence of any relevant tissue damage at all. By the same token, if a certain type of tissue damage or nerve stimulation in a localized area is considered sufficient for a T-Pain, then it is easy to imagine false negatives for T-Pains, such as when a local anesthetic prevents one from noticing a surgical incision.[2] For these reasons, I will focus on S-Pains going forward, using "pain" exclusively to refer to S-Pains unless otherwise noted.

5 An argument from the appearance/reality distinction

Here is a quick argument for the impossibility of false positives for one's own pains. A corresponding argument can be run against the possibility of false negatives, by inserting "not" before each instance of "in pain":

> Premise 1: If you believe that you are in pain, then it appears to you that you are in pain.
> Premise 2: If it appears to you that you are in pain, then you *just are* in pain.
> Conclusion: Therefore, if you believe that you are in pain, then you *just are* in pain.

The argument form is valid. If we accept the premises, we must accept the conclusion. Taking the premises in reverse order, why would someone accept premise (2)? It is sometimes remarked that, in the case of pain, there is no appearance/reality distinction. Hiking through the desert, I might seem to see an oasis … but no, it is only a mirage. The appearance is one thing, the reality another. But could I, similarly, seem to have a pain, yet it be only a pain-mirage – the mere appearance of a pain? No, one might say, for to have a pain *just is* for it to appear that you are in pain. There is, one might insist, no distinction between the appearance and the reality in this case, precisely because a pain *just is* the appearance of pain (Cf. Searle 1992: 122; see also Chapter 18, this volume.)

However, the plausibility of premise (2) is due in part to an equivocation on the meaning of "pain." It is common to allow for the possibility of perceptual experiences in the absence of the things they represent, as in hallucinations and illusions. If the perceptual experience of an apple can be considered "the appearance" of an apple, then it is easy to see how such an appearance can obtain in the absence of the reality it aims to represent. Supposing that S-Pains also offer perceptual appearances, what are they appearances *of?* A reasonable answer is that they are appearances of pains-as-tissue-damage (i.e., T-Pains). Presumably, the amputee suffering phantom pains appears to have a pain-as-tissue-damage in his right foot, in virtue of having a certain type of pain-as-sensation. However, this would suggest that there *is* an appearance/reality distinction with respect to pain after all: S-Pains are appearances of T-Pains. And, like visual experiences and the apples they are experiences *of,* one can occur in the absence of the other. Thus, if we read "pain" as referring to T-Pain in the consequent of premise (2), the premise is clearly false. (Cf. the discussion of incorrigibility in Chapter 27, this volume.)

The defender of premise (2) will therefore need to insist that the kind of pain mentioned in the consequent of premise (2) is an S-Pain. To make this understanding clear, we can rewrite the premise as:

(2★) If it appears to you that you are in pain, then you just are having an S-Pain.

But now there is a more serious form of equivocation present in both premises (2★) and (1) that we must consider. So far we have discussed one kind of appearance, what we might call *sensorial appearances.* Both a visual experience of an oasis and an S-Pain can be thought of as sensorial appearances, insofar as they are states with sensory character that indicate or represent the presence of some responsible stimulus (an oasis and a T-Pain, respectively). However, there are also *doxastic appearances,* which are appearances grounded in a person's beliefs.[3] Frowning into the empty cookie jar, it *appears* to me – in this non-sensory, doxastic sense – that John ate the last cookie. In this same sense of appearances, the stammering defendant *appears* guilty during testimony. Quite generally, a belief that *p* is sufficient for its appearing to you that *p,* in this sense of appearances.

It is standardly (though not unanimously [Byrne 2012]) assumed that sensorial appearances are psychologically distinct from doxastic appearances. To take a shopworn example, the parallel lines of the Müller-Lyer illusion look to be of different lengths, even if one is convinced (through measuring them) that they are in fact the same length (see Figure 20.1). A natural way to describe the situation is to say that the lines sensorily appear to be of different lengths while doxastically appearing to be the same length. In other words, we visually represent the lines as being of different lengths, while believing that they are the same length.

Now recall premise (1) above, which holds that if you believe you are in pain, then it appears to you that you are in pain. If the sense of "appears" in the consequent is the doxastic sense, then this premise becomes a tautology. It asserts: If you believe you are in pain, then

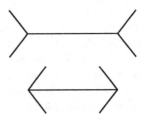

Figure 20.1 The Müller-Lyer optical illusion.

you believe that you are in pain. This presents a problem for the argument as a whole. In order for the argument to be valid, the sense of "appears" must be the same in *both* premises. But interpreting the "appears" of (2★) doxastically turns (2★) into: "If you believe that you are in pain, then you are having a pain-as-sensation." Premise (2★) is now simply asserting the principle that there are no false positives with respect to pain, which was the intended conclusion of the argument. Thus (2★) cannot be used as part of an argument for that conclusion.

What if we interpret the "appears" of premise (1) in the *sensorial appearance* sense and not the doxastic sense, and do the same for (2★)? In that case, premise (1) would read: "If you believe that you are in pain, then you are having a pain-as-sensation." Now premise (1) has become equivalent to the argument's intended conclusion. It therefore cannot be used in an argument for that conclusion. Doing so is begging the question.

6 Sensations and beliefs

We have seen that simple appeals to the lack of an appearance/reality distinction in the case of pain cannot serve as *arguments* for the incorrigibility thesis. They either equivocate on two distinct senses of "appearance," or assume the very point in question. Thus, if one is inclined to accept the incorrigibility thesis, it cannot be *for the reason* that there is no appearance/reality distinction in the case of pain. Yet this is not to say that there are no *other* reasons one might have for accepting *both* the incorrigibility thesis and the version of the appearance/reality claim that assumes it.

Before considering those reasons, let us first air some skepticism concerning incorrigibility. The mere fact that beliefs are not themselves S-Pains – the fact that the two are "distinct existences," as philosophers say – might seem enough by itself to undermine the incorrigibility thesis. One could grant that we don't *normally* form a belief that we are in pain when we are not in pain, and vice versa; but, given that the belief that I am in pain is one thing, and the pain another, why should it be absolutely impossible for one to occur without the other?

Now, for an *intense* pain – caused, say, by slamming your hand in a door – it might seem *bizarre* to think that someone could sincerely deny feeling it. But consider delusions. Delusions are plausibly characterized as *beliefs*, however strange they may be (Bortolotti 2009). It is not uncommon for a person with schizophrenia to believe that another person's thoughts have been inserted into his mind, or that aliens are secretly monitoring his activities (Langland-Hassan 2008). If, in general, people are capable of having highly irrational and bizarre false beliefs of this kind, it is hard to see why mistaken beliefs about pains would be an exception.

But there remain a number of possible replies for the defender of the incorrigibility thesis. One is to hold that beliefs about pain can have a causal influence on the presence or absence of pains. If a belief that one is in pain is sufficient to *cause* a pain, and if a belief that one is not in pain were sufficient to *extinguish* a pain, then there would be no false positives or false negatives. Of course, in considering the Müller-Lyer illusion above, we saw a reason for thinking that beliefs cannot, in general, have this sort of effect on sensory-perceptual states; we continue to visually represent the two lines as being different lengths even after we believe that they are equivalent. This is just one instance of the so-called *cognitive impenetrability* of sensations and perceptual states by cognitive states such as beliefs and desires.

However, blanket endorsements of cognitive impenetrability have come under fire. Arguably, there are some cases where one's background beliefs, for instance, exert an influence on the nature of one's current perceptual states (Lupyan 2015; Macpherson 2012).

(Though see Firestone and Scholl, forthcoming.) This may seem to open the door for a defense of the incorrigibility thesis. For if pains are cognitively penetrable, perhaps a firm belief that one is in pain is sufficient to give rise to a pain after all – such as when a dental patient, fearing the approaching drill, cries out in pain despite the removal of any nerve the drill might hit. Likewise, perhaps the power of positive thinking – "I am *not* in pain! I am mighty!" – is strong enough to make some pains disappear. (See also Chapters 22 and 32, this volume.) Yet we have to bear in mind the strength of the incorrigibility thesis. It does not merely state that a belief *can* cause a pain, or make one go away, but that there can *never* be a false positive or false negative. Whatever exceptions to cognitive impenetrability there may be, they do not seem pervasive enough to warrant belief in the incorrigibility thesis.

Another response on behalf of the incorrigibility thesis would be to hold that some concepts are partly *constituted by* sensory states. A number of philosophers have recently posited that there is indeed such a class of concepts – *phenomenal concepts* – that are partly constituted by the very sensory states to which they refer (Balog 2012; Papineau 2007). A motivation for positing this class of concepts is that certain sensory experiences seem necessary for having certain beliefs. For instance, it may seem that one cannot know what it is like to see red if one never has had a sensation of red (Jackson 1982). Similarly, it could be argued that one can only know what pain is if one has felt a pain. A possible explanation of this tight coupling of past sensation and current knowledge is that the very concept of pain involves, as a proper part, a faint version of pain itself – one that can only be summoned by those who have felt pain. If this were the case, it is easy to see how there could not be any false positives: one could not *think* that one is in pain without in fact having a pain. (Though, by the same token, it would make all judgments of the form "I am not in pain" false!) Yet it seems clear that we often think about pains without experiencing even a faint pain, such as when reading this paragraph (I hope). This suggests that even if some (phenomenal) concepts of pain contain instances of pain within them, others do not. Thus, if phenomenal concepts offer a means for defending the incorrigibility thesis, it is only a weaker version of the thesis, relativized to beliefs involving a special *phenomenal concept* of pain.[4]

7 Pain as assessment-dependent

In what remains of this essay I will consider a different sort of argument that, in my view, offers the best case for the incorrigibility thesis. The statement "I am in pain" typically functions to alert listeners to the occurrence of a sensory state in the speaker – one that the speaker finds to be unpleasant. If we were to give this typical function of such statements pride of place, we might go so far as to say that "I am in pain" is an appropriate statement when and only when the speaker is in a sensory state that she deems to be unpleasant. But then, what else is it to be in a sensory state we deem to be unpleasant than to believe, of one of our sensory states, that it is a pain? If the two come to the same thing, then our beliefs that we are in pain are infallible just because they themselves make it true that we deem ourselves to be in an unpleasant sensory state. The idea here is that, while we are always in sensory states of various kinds, we are only having a *pain* when we judge one of those states to be unpleasant. A natural corollary would be that, whenever we do *not* judge one of our sensory states to be unpleasant, we are *ipso facto* not having a pain. (We can remain neutral on whether the person judges the unpleasant sensory state to be located in a body part – as in T-Pains – or whether she judges it to be in his mind or brain – as in S-Pains.) Note that I am distinguishing between sensory states that are *intrinsically* unpleasant – if such are possible – and those which are *believed* to be unpleasant. The idea being considered is that simply being in a sensory state one *believes to be* unpleasant is necessary and sufficient for having a pain. If pains were assessment-dependent in this manner, we would avoid both false positives and false negatives.

An immediate objection is that "I am in pain" simply does not mean the same thing as "I am in a sensory state that is unpleasant." The latter might be true when one feels nausea, for instance, but no pain. Yet here the defender of the incorrigibility thesis can maintain that unpleasant states such as nausea are indeed particular *kinds* of pain. After all, it is uncontroversial that there are pains with differing sensory characters – from throbbing pains, to sharp pains, to burning pains, and so on. It is not clear that they share any robust characteristics over and above being unpleasant and indicative of unfavorable internal conditions. Nausea shares those features. So there is no obvious barrier to including nausea among them. On this approach, two people could conceivably be in sensory states that are intrinsically the same, while only one of them is in pain *just because* only he judges the sensory state to be unpleasant.[5]

But why should a negative assessment have any bearing on what type of mental state is in fact occurring? In most cases, it would indeed be a mistake to type a sensory state according to how it is appraised. And yet, bearing in mind the typical function of statements like "I am in pain," there is some reason to think that this kind of judgment-dependency makes sense for pain. Consider a favorite example of the British Empiricists: as we move our hand closer to an open fire, the pleasant sensation of warmth gradually shifts to a feeling of pain. Plausibly, two people approaching the fire in unison might judge themselves to be in pain at different times, even if they were at each instant in sensory-discriminative states of the same kind. What one takes to be painful the other still finds toasty and soothing. In short, they disagree about whether their current sensory state is one of pain. When such a disagreement occurs, one response would be to hold that only one person can be correct. But a more natural response might be to allow that one may indeed be in pain when the other is not, simply because a sensory state is only a pain once it is judged to be unpleasant. After all, there is not obviously any *less* arbitrary boundary on this spectrum between what is pain and what is not. And drawing the line in this way meshes with the independently plausible idea that the central role of the word "pain" in public discourse is to mark those, and only those, sensory states that the subject finds to be unpleasant. That "pain" plays this communicative role explains why we *care* that a person is in pain in a way that goes beyond our interest in her sensory states generally.

In response, one may insist that it still seems coherent to suppose that someone might believe himself to be in pain and fully *enjoy* the feeling (as in masochism), or that, more commonly, one might have a mild pain – from a paper cut, or a lingering headache, say – that one simply doesn't pause to assess one way or the other. If such people are indeed in pain, then being in pain must dissociate from judging oneself to be in an unpleasant state. I will address the masochism objection below in considering the neurocognitive diagnosis of pain asymbolia. In response to the objection that some pains may go by without one's assessing them either way, one can hold that a state is a pain just in case one is *disposed* to judge it unpleasant. This *dispositional*-assessment view of pain would hold that a state is a pain just in case one would judge it unpleasant, were one's attention drawn to it. This allows there to be pains we never bother to assess, while ensuring that our judgments that we are (or are not) in pain are always true.

8 Pain as a complex phenomenon: implications for incorrigibility

As earlier noted, it is common to conceive of pain as a *complex* mental phenomenon, with distinct sensory-discriminative, affective-emotional, and cognitive-evaluative components

(Corns 2014; Grahek 2007; Hardcastle 1999). We can conclude our reflections on the incorrigibility thesis – and the assessment-dependency view I have outlined – by considering it in light of possible dissociations among these features. Such dissociations help focus attention on the question of which (if any) aspects of pain are truly essential to pain, and which are merely associated with it.

In the phenomenon of pain asymbolia, patients with particular neural lesions[6] seem to experience the sensory-discriminative aspect of pain upon harmful stimulation, without its cognitive or affective aspect (Berthier et al. 1988). As Grahek puts it in an extended treatment of the issue, "these patients do not mind pain at all; indeed, they may even smile or laugh at it" (Grahek 2007: 2–3). Patients with pain asymbolia tend to describe their perceived pains as hurtful – showing awareness of the sensory aspect – yet show no avoidance behavior, nor any related anxiety with respect to the painful stimulus.

Are people with pain asymbolia truly *in pain*? We can certainly see some grounds for saying that they are: they share an important sensory-discriminative state with people who are more obviously in pain. And they would seem to be in pain at least in the same sense as the (idealized) masochist. On the other hand, once we see how cleanly the sensory-discriminative aspect of pain can dissociate from its normal cognitive and affective accompaniments, we might wonder whether we really ought to describe these people as in pain. For one could argue that they only experience the sensory-discriminative *part* of what pain really is, and that pain *proper* requires negative affective and cognitive components as well; these would include stress, anxiety, a desire to alleviate the sensation, a belief that the sensation is unpleasant, and so on. Declaring these components essential to pain would enable us to avoid the odd conclusion that someone could be in pain while laughing at the pain and lacking any desire to end it.

If we are willing to hold that pain has some cognitive and affective states as necessary components – that pain asymbolia is not pain *proper* – then the kind of assessment-dependent view of pain discussed above gains plausibility. For the belief that one is in an unpleasant state is a reasonable candidate for a necessary cognitive component of pain. Doing so allows for a principled means for marking the point at which a sensation of warmth shades into one of pain (as discussed above), and respects the particular role that talk of pain plays in public discourse.

However, if the sensory-discriminative aspect of pain is an equally necessary component of pain *proper*, false positives will still be possible. These would be cases where people judge themselves to be in pain (and in an unpleasant state) and have the negative affective components of pain, yet lack the sensory-discriminative aspect of pain. Interestingly, such dissociations have been reported. Ploner et al. (1999) describe a patient whose ability to spatially localize and qualitatively describe painful stimuli was greatly impaired. Nevertheless, the patient still showed clear signs of discomfort upon receiving normally painful stimuli and wished to avoid further stimuli of that kind. This suggested (in the words of Ploner and colleagues) "a loss of pain sensation with preserved pain affect" (211, as quoted in Grahek 2007). We can interpret this patient as having the cognitive and affective components of pain, without the normally associated sensory component. If such a patient is wrong to judge himself as being in pain – because he lacks the sensory-discriminative component of pain – then false positives remain possible.

But *would* such a patient be wrong to judge himself as being in pain? The answer is not obvious. Faced with someone with the full affective component of an intense pain, we may feel deeply inclined to grant that he is in pain, regardless of whether he is in the normally associated sensory-discriminative state. Clearly such a person – beset by stress, anxiety, and a strong desire to end the pain – would not be able to live what we normally take to be a happy and *pain-free* life until his situation changed. In this way, the cognitive and affective aspects of pain may trump its sensory components. Of course, our attention to the affective and cognitive components does not show that the *mere* cognitive judgment that one is in an unpleasant state is sufficient for pain. That judgment in the absence of any of the affective or sensory components of pain could reasonably be considered a false positive. Yet, on the other hand, the contents of states like beliefs and desires are typically ascribed on the basis of their causes and effects. And it is reasonable to think that the judgment that one is having an intense pain has, as one of its necessary cognitive *effects,* anxiety and negative affect of the kind associated with intense pain. That is, we might be warranted in saying that any cognitive state that does *not* cause anxiety and negative affect just isn't the belief that one is in intense pain. If *that* were true, and if we agreed that the sensory-discriminative aspect is not essential to pain, we can see how false positives would also be impossible (at least with respect to intense pains).

Nevertheless, it must be admitted that the reasons so far considered for holding a certain cognitive self-assessment to be necessary and sufficient for pain are less than conclusive. A reasonable opponent might still question whether any one component of pain – be it sensory, affective, or cognitive – is privileged in that manner. Perhaps each is typical or paradigmatic of pain, with none truly essential (Corns 2014). Granting the basic sobriety of such a view, we can still conclude that the best prospect for a vindication and *explanation* of the incorrigibility thesis's attraction lies in granting pain's assessment-dependency. It's surprising that there should be so reasonable a route to our own incorrigibility.

Related topics

Chapter 2: Pain and representation (Cutter)
Chapter 4: Imperativism (Klein)
Chapter 5: Fault lines in familiar concepts of pain (Hill)
Chapter 9: A view of pain based on sensations, meanings, and emotions (Price)
Chapter 13: Psychogenic pain: old and new (Sullivan)
Chapter 17: Pain and consciousness (Pereplyotchik)
Chapter 18: Pain: perception or introspection? (Aydede)
Chapter 22: Pain and cognitive penetrability (Jacobson)
Chapter 27: Bad by nature: an axiological theory of pain (Massin)
Chapter 32: Pain and "placebo" analgesia (Moerman)

Acknowledgements

Special thanks to Jennifer Corns for valuable feedback on drafts of this chapter.

Notes

1 Typically such representations are held to be non-conceptual in nature, insofar as the creatures having them need not possess the concepts needed to specify their accuracy conditions.
2 These examples raise the question of whether T-Pain is rightly equated simply with tissue damage of a certain sort (so that the damage is sufficient for the T-Pain) or if, instead, T-Pains are only instances of tissue damage that one is aware of *in the right way* (e.g., in virtue of an S-Pain that represents it). See Chapters 2 and 5, this volume, for discussion of this sort of distinction.

3 The distinction between sensorial and doxastic appearances, and the ensuing argument, is inspired by Schwitzgebel's (2008: 262–263) distinction between phenomenal and epistemic senses of "appears," which he puts to much the same ends.

4 For skepticism about the ability of phenomenal concepts to play this kind of role, see Tye 2009.

5 One might wonder whether animals could have pains on this view, if they lack the concepts needed to judge their states to be unpleasant. So long as animals have a means for negatively assessing their own states – be it through the use of concepts or some other mode of thought – the spirit of the view can be extended to allow animals pains. At the same time, it bears noting that to deny that animals have pain of the human sort is not to suggest that they cannot suffer (Carruthers 2004).

6 See also Rainville et al. 1999 for evidence of the dissociation in neurotypical individuals under hypnosis.

References

Balog, K. (2012) Acquaintance and the mind–body problem. In S. Gozzano and C.S. Hill (eds.), *New Perspectives on Type Identity: The Mental and the Physical*. Cambridge: Cambridge University Press, pp. 16–42.

Berthier, M., Starkstein, S., and Leiguarda, R. (1988) Asymbolia for pain: a sensory-limbic disconnection syndrome. *Annals of Neurology* 24(1): 41–49. doi:10.1002/ana.410240109.

Bortolotti, L. (2009) *Delusions and Other Irrational Beliefs*. Oxford: Oxford University Press.

Byrne, A. (2012) Knowing what I see. In D. Smithies and D. Stoljar (eds.), *Introspection and Consciousness*. Oxford: Oxford University Press, pp. 183–210.

Carruthers, P. (2004) Suffering without subjectivity. *Philosophical Studies* 121(2): 99–125. doi:10.1007/s11098-004-3635-5.

Corns, J. (2014) The inadequacy of unitary characterizations of pain. *Philosophical Studies* 169: 355–378.

Firestone, C. and Scholl, B.J. (Forthcoming) Cognition does not affect perception: evaluating the evidence for "top-down" effects. *Behavioral and Brain Sciences*.

Grahek, N. (2007) *Feeling Pain and Being in Pain*, 2nd ed. Cambridge, MA: MIT Press.

Hardcastle, V. (1999) *The Myth of Pain*. Cambridge, MA: MIT Press.

Jackson, F. (1982) Epiphenomenal qualia. *Philosophical Quarterly* 32(127): 127–136.

Langland-Hassan, P. (2008) Fractured phenomenologies: thought insertion, inner speech, and the puzzle of extraneity. *Mind & Language* 23(4): 369–401.

Lupyan, G. (2015) Cognitive penetrability of perception in the age of prediction: predictive systems are penetrable systems. *Review of Philosophy and Psychology* 6(4): 547–569. doi:10.1007/s13164-015-0253-4.

Macpherson, F. (2012) Cognitive penetration of colour experience: rethinking the issue in light of an indirect mechanism. *Philosophy and Phenomenological Research* 84(1): 24–62.

Papineau, D. (2007) Phenomenal and perceptual concepts. In T. Alter and S. Walter (eds.), *Phenomenal Concepts and Phenomenal Knowledge*. Oxford: Oxford University Press.

Ploner, M., Freund, H.-J., and Schinitzler, A. (1999) Pain affect without pain sensation in a patient with a postcentral lesion. *Pain* 81: 211–214.

Rainville, P., Carrier, B., Hofbauer, R.K., Bushnell, M.C., and Duncan, G.H. (1999) Dissociation of sensory and affective dimensions of pain using hypnotic modulation. *Pain* 82(2): 159–171.

Schwitzgebel, E. (2008) The unreliability of naive introspection. *Philosophical Review* 117(2): 245–273.

Schwitzgebel, E. (2014) Introspection. In E.N. Zalta (ed.), *The Stanford Encyclopedia of Philosophy* (Summer 2014 ed.).<http://plato.stanford.edu/archives/sum2014/entries/introspection/>.

Searle, J. (1992) *The Rediscovery of Mind*. Cambridge, MA: MIT Press.

Tye, M. (2009) *Consciousness Revisited: Materialism without Phenomenal Concepts*. Cambridge, MA: MIT Press.

21

CAN I SEE YOUR PAIN?

An evaluative model of pain perception

Frédérique de Vignemont

[O]ur way of knowing (or one of our ways of knowing) about other minds (e.g., that his finger hurts) is exactly the same as our way (or one of our ways) of knowing about other bodies (e.g., that his finger is in his mouth).

(Dretske 1973: 35)

According to Dretske's optimistic conception, there is no problem of other minds. More specifically, he argues that we can have perceptual knowledge of other people's pain, although pain is not an observable entity. To some extent, Dretske's claim seems to be relatively uncontroversial. We can easily say that we see that the other person is in pain. Furthermore, we can have sometimes a feeling of immediacy and of visual presence associated with our knowledge of other people's pains (Smith 2013). Hence, one may want to go further and claim that we have *direct perception* of their pains (Cassam 2007; Green 2007, McDowell 1978; Scheler 1954; Schutz 1967; Stout 2010; Zahavi 2011). After exploring various interpretations of this claim, I will show the difficulties that a direct model of third-person pain perception faces. I will then appeal to the evaluative theory of pain (Cutter and Tye 2011; Bain 2013, Chapter 3, this volume) to offer an indirect perceptual account of third-person pain perception.

1 How direct?

That one can directly access other people's mental states is a recurrent theme in the recent literature about mindreading. It is thus worth spending some time on what this means in this specific context.[1] In the phenomenological tradition, it may sometimes seem that direct perception only involves the lack of awareness of inferential processes. For instance, I can be said to directly see my friend's distress when I see her crying, because I am aware only of her tears, and not of any inferences that I draw on the basis of my perception of her tears. On this interpretation, however, many cognitive processes qualify as direct because we are rarely aware of the inferential steps that they involve. A more interesting interpretation is that I directly see her distress because there is simply no extra inferential step, conscious or unconscious one. Seeing her tears is seeing her distress. If so, one has a direct access to others' minds in the same way as one has a direct access to their bodily expressions through perception. One may try to be even more specific by distinguishing between three distinct claims:

i   I directly see your pain
ii   I directly see *that* you are in pain
iii I *indirectly* see that you are in pain.

The difference between (i) and (ii) follows from Dretske's (1969) distinction between epistemic and non-epistemic perception. Let us imagine that a dog is barking. I can hear that a dog is barking. This requires me to possess concepts, including the concepts of DOG and of BARKING, and to apply them. My perception is then said to be epistemic. I may be right or wrong, but in any case I hear the world in a certain way. Imagine, however, that I have heard the sound but without recognizing it. I definitely hear the dog barking since I turn my head towards it. Yet I do not recognize the dog barking as such. I simply acquire information about the world, which does not amount to my having a conceptually structured representation of the world. My perception is then said to be non-epistemic.

The difference between (ii) and (iii) follows from another distinction that Dretske made between direct and indirect epistemic perception. Although it involves recognitional processes, there is a sense in which my epistemic perception can be said to be direct when I hear that the dog is barking. More specifically, it can be said to be direct because all the information about the dog barking is embedded in the non-epistemic perception from which it follows. It just needs to be extracted and conceptually structured.[2] Let us now imagine that the dog barks each time that the postman comes. According to Dretske, one can say that I hear that the postman is coming. My perception, however, is only indirect. This is so because the information about the postman is not embedded in information from the more proximal object (the dog barking). It needs to be derived on the basis of further knowledge (about the dog barking each time that the postman comes). There is thus an extra inferential step.

Within this conceptual framework, we can ask the following two questions. First, can third-person pain perception be non-epistemic? As we shall see, it may sometimes seem that the phenomenological tradition claims that one can have a non-conceptual perceptual awareness of another individual's pain like in (i). I shall call this view the non-epistemic hypothesis. A weaker conception consists in claiming that one can have non-epistemic perception only of bodily expressions, and not of pain itself. The perception of pain is only epistemic. This raises the second question: is it direct or indirect?

2 The non-epistemic hypothesis of pain perception

We shall start by evaluating the non-epistemic hypothesis, according to which one can have non-conceptual awareness of other people's pains. One may then be said to *experience* their pains. However, one may be tempted to immediately rule it out on the basis of the following *reductio ad absurdum*.

1   Non-epistemic hypothesis: Knowledge of other people's pains is grounded in the immediate experience of their pains.
2   Knowledge of one's own pain is grounded in the immediate experience of one's own pain.
3   Thus, there is no epistemological difference between the knowledge of one's own pains and the knowledge of other people's pains.

4   (3) is false.
5   Hence, (1) is false.

The assumption underlying this reductio is that the knowledge of one's own pain is incorrigible. Arguably, if I believe that I am in pain because I feel it, everyone else is in a worse position than I with respect to the question whether I am in pain.[3] From its incorrigibility directly follows the corrigibility of the knowledge of other people's pains. Whatever the grounds you may have to believe me to be in pain, I will always be entitled to deny it. There is thus a fundamental asymmetry between the knowledge of one's pains and the knowledge of other people's pains. Hence, (3) is false. Yet the *reductio* fails. This is so because the epistemic asymmetry (3) does not follow from (1) and (2) since there is an equivocation of the term "experience." If one can experience other people's pain, it can be only under an experiential mode different from the one that one has when one experiences one's own pain. More specifically, according to the non-epistemic hypothesis, one can experience other people's pain, but only *from the outside*. The outside mode of experience is defined by contrast to the inside mode that characterizes bodily experiences. Typically, the inside mode refers to an internal privileged access to one's own bodily and mental properties, including pain. (See Chapter 16, this volume.) Whether this kind of experience from the inside is perceptual or not is a question that I will not address. Indeed, what is at stake here is whether one can experience pain from the outside, that is, on the basis of external senses such as vision and audition. And if one can, then it means that one can also experience *other people*'s pain from the outside because external senses give perceptual access to bodies other than one's own. However, at no point does the non-epistemic hypothesis entail that experiences from the outside are as reliable as experiences from the inside. The knowledge of one's own pain and the knowledge of other people's pains can be both rationally grounded in experiences, and these experiences can have different justificatory force. Hence, the epistemic asymmetry between the knowledge of one's own pain and the knowledge of other people's pains does not show that the latter is not experiential. The *reductio ad absurdum* thus fails.

The non-epistemic hypothesis, however, faces other difficulties. More specifically, I will show how challenging the task is to provide an adequate model for analyzing third-person pain in experiential terms, that is, to defend the view that we experience others' pains from the outside. A systematic review of the idiosyncrasies of each perceptual model is beyond the scope of this chapter, and I will focus only on one interpretation that one can give of the phenomenological tradition. Let us see how Zahavi and Overgaard describe the direct perception of other people's emotions:

> I obviously do not see the distress the same way I see the color of his shirt; rather I see the distress "in" his pained countenance (Stein 1989, 6). In this case it makes sense to say that I *experience* (rather than imagine or infer) his distress.
>
> (Zahavi and Overgaard 2012: 8, my emphasis)

They acknowledge the peculiarity of third-person pain perception. It should not be assumed that it is like any other kind of perception of mundane properties like color or shape. Still, they claim, it is experiential. This does not mean that one has no experience of the pained countenance itself. Rather, one experiences the other's pain *in* his pained expression. There is, however, no real account of what that means. Interestingly, one can find a description of the notion of "seeing-in" in some aesthetic theories. According to Wollheim's influential account, one sees the surface of a painting, and sees also, simultaneously, what is depicted "in" the surface. There is thus a double load for visual experiences of pictures.

> When I look at the Manet, my perception is twofold in that I simultaneously am visually aware of the marked surface and experience something in front of, or behind, something else – in this case, a woman in a hat standing in front of a clump of trees. These are two aspects of a single experience. They are not two experiences.
>
> *(Wollheim 2003: 3)*

The pictorial content is not inferred from the experience of the painting. It is itself experiential. It normally leads to the epistemic perception of what is depicted, but it can remain non-conceptual. One may then suggest that we experience pain *in* bodily expressions in the same way as we experience a woman in a hat *in* the marked surface of a portrait. In Wollheim's terms, when I see someone's expression of pain, my non-epistemic perception is twofold in that I am visually aware simultaneously of the marked face and of the pain behind. One can have a visual awareness of the bodily expressions of pain, and also, simultaneously, a visual awareness of the pain "in" the bodily expression. The experience of the facial expression does not disappear behind the experience of the person's pain.[4]

At first sight, the seeing-in model thus seems to be relatively promising to account for our access to other people's pains. Furthermore, it seems compatible with empirical findings that show that one can recognize emotions on the basis of the perception of facial expressions, especially if the visual stimuli are dynamic (Ekman and Friesen 1975). However, the fact that the participants in these studies can succeed in recognizing the emotional type in a facial pattern does not show that someone's emotional state is part of the content of their visual experience. Such empirical results cannot be taken as evidence for the seeing-in model, and more generally for the non-epistemic hypothesis. Actually it is not clear how any experimental findings could show that we have non-conceptual awareness of other people's pains. On the other hand, neither could they show that we do *not* have such awareness.

If we cannot assess the validity of the non-epistemic hypothesis with the help of empirical evidence, then how can we do it? At this stage, we might want to explore more thoroughly the notion of seeing-in and the parallel between the perception of pictures and the perception of emotional expressions.[5] According to Wollheim himself, there are limits to what one can see in a picture. More specifically, he claims that the notion of seeing-in does not apply to abstract paintings. One can have a visual experience in the marked surface of the objects, the landscapes, the individuals that are depicted, but not of abstract ideas. In particular, one cannot have a visual experience of the artist's intentions that the painting expresses. Although the artist's intentions set the standard relative to which the depicted content is evaluated, it is not part of the experiential content. Expression and depiction are two distinct functions of representation, and the notion of seeing-in exclusively applies to depiction. The problem for the seeing-in model is that pain should be compared to the intention rather than to the depicted content. The evaluation of the painful expression is done on the basis of what the person feels in the same way as the evaluation of the painting is done on the basis of what the artist intended to do. Pain determines what is expressed in the same way as the artist's intention. For instance, a painting would be considered by its artist as a failure if her intention was to paint a depressing landscape but ended up depicting a happy sunny spring afternoon. Even if the sunny landscape were well painted, the artist would still think that he had failed. Expression and depiction are thus different. And the pain grimace expresses rather than depicts pain.

To conclude, the seeing-in model fails to account for the peculiarities of third-person pain perception. There may be other non-epistemic models, but I suspect that they would face the same or other difficulties. I will now turn to epistemic models and see whether they fare better. They do not assume that one has a non-conceptual awareness of the other's pain. They only assume that one can see that someone is in pain. The question then is whether one sees it directly or not.

3 The epistemic hypothesis of pain perception

> We should not jibe at, or interpret away, the commonsense thought that ... one can literally perceive, in another person's facial expression or his behavior, that he is in pain, and not just infer that he is in pain from what one perceives.
>
> *(McDowell 1978: 136)*

What McDowell describes here is the possibility of being perceptually aware *that* another individual is in pain, that is, an epistemic model of pain perception. There are, however, two ways the epistemic hypothesis can be spelled out. According to the most cognitive version, one is *indirectly* aware that the other is in pain in virtue of being directly aware of her bodily expressions. To use Dretske's (1973) example, for me to see that your finger hurts involves recognizing that your finger is in your mouth and knowing that one puts one's finger in one's mouth when it hurts. On this version of the epistemic hypothesis, pain perception is grounded in epistemic bodily perception and in further knowledge. McDowell, however, rejects such extra inferential processes and defends a less cognitively demanding conception, according to which one is *directly* aware that the other is in pain. Recognizing the bodily expression is recognizing it as a manifestation – on this occasion – of pain. No further knowledge is required. How can one decide between these two versions? Is third-person pain perception direct or indirect?

According to Dretske, only the perception of a proper part of an object can ground the direct epistemic perception of the object. One can then suggest the following epistemic model of third-person pain perception, which I call the *mereological model*. It characterizes the relationship between bodily expressions and pain in terms of the part–whole relationship, as it has been defended by Green (2007), for instance:

> Let α be an object, event, or process that is perceptible. Then we may say that relative to an organism O and ecological situation E, a *characteristic component of* α is a part of α that, when perceived in E without any other part of α being perceived, enables O to perceive α.
>
> *(Green 2007: 87, italic in the original)*

According to the mereological model, a painful grimace is a part of what it is to be in pain. Seeing a part of pain is then seeing pain. In other words, the facial expressions are the tip of the iceberg of pain. When one is visually aware of the tip of the iceberg, then one is visually aware that there is an iceberg, although the rest of it is not visible. Likewise, when one sees the face, one sees that there is a back of the head. One may then say that when one sees the facial expression, one sees that there is pain. One of the interests of the mereological model is that it grants that one can be visually aware that there is pain without assuming that all the parts of painful experiences are visible.

However, one may question the hypothesis that painful experiences have parts, and if they have, that a painful grimace is one of those parts. It is true that according to a now classic conception, pain has *components*, the sensory-discriminative one, the affective one, and possibly the cognitive-evaluative one. (See, for instance, Chapter 9, this volume.) But on this conception, bodily expressions are the results of these components, and do not constitute an additional one. Another way to put it is to say that pain has a motivational force, which causes and justifies specific behaviors, including bodily expressions. The motivational force is constitutive of pain, but its behavioral consequences are not. To claim that bodily expressions are parts of pain would be to renounce the idea that pain causes bodily expressions.[6] But if they are not parts of pain, one cannot directly perceive that there is pain, at least on this definition of directness.

Putting aside the mereological model, there seems to be a fundamental obstacle to third-person pain perception being direct and this is the lack of one-to-one mapping between bodily expressions and emotions. For epistemic pain perception to be direct, the information about the pain must be embedded in the information that one gets in a direct way about the painful expression. However, information about the other's affective state often requires contextual information in addition to information about bodily expressions. Although most studies show that participants can recognize the expression of the six basic emotions, they are far from doing so with 100-percent accuracy. Just to give an example, Nico Frijda (1953), one of the leading social psychologists of emotions, reports a success rate of only 44 percent. Roughly speaking, without the context, one is most of the time not very good at decoding what the other feels. It is only when the emotion, and the corresponding expression, is very intense and vivid (intense rage or overwhelming happiness, for instance) that there is little room for interpretation.

Let us consider Dretske's example of a man frowning. We have a visual experience of his facial expression. If his facial expression is barely perceptible because the conditions of visibility are bad or because he does not show much of what he feels, we can be mistaken and believe that he is raising his eyebrows, for instance. But under good conditions, this does not happen. Our visual experience normally justifies us in forming the visual belief that he is frowning because it results from reliable visual processing. In addition, our visual experience can justify us in forming other beliefs, about the man's affective state. But a person's frown can express either anger or pain. Seeing that the man is frowning can then justify two perceptual beliefs: that he is angry and that he is in pain. There is a *one-to-many* mapping between bodily expressions and affective states. Even if the frown is clear and distinct, its emotional interpretation is open. Without the context, one may well fail to disambiguate between pairs of facial emotional signals (Dailey et al. 2002). It seems that it is only under some specific conditions that emotion recognition is reliable, but in these cases, the reliability often arises more from further knowledge of the context than from the perception of the bodily expression itself. Consequently, the idea that one perceives another's emotion *just* by perceiving her bodily expression loses its grip (Stout 2010).

Interestingly, even proponents of the direct perception theory acknowledge the absence of a one-to-one relationship between bodily expressions and affective states. Yet they do not believe that it precludes pain perception being direct:

> But is it impossible for something to be both direct and contextual at the same time? ... The problem, however, is that there is not one golden [*sic*] standard of what directness amounts to. As Bennett and Hacker (2003) recently remarked, we can speak of indirect evidence or of knowing indirectly only where it also makes

sense to speak of a more direct evidence, but there is no more direct way of knowing that another is in pain than by seeing him writhe in pain.

(Zahavi and Overgaard 2012: 13–14)

Here, there is a risk that such a liberal definition of directness trivializes the direct perception theory of other people's emotions. Let us consider the following example. There is no more direct way of knowing what the landscape on Mars looks like than looking at pictures sent by the NASA Exploration Rovers. Yet I can hardly claim that I directly see that the Martian sunrise is blue.[7] In other words, the fact that a way of knowing cannot be "more direct" does not preclude it involving many complex computational stages. Even if we did not have a gold standard of directness, it would still not be clear that we are ready to qualify such a complex process as being direct. I thus invite one to offer the explicit conditions under which epistemic perception of other people's pains can be direct that do not trivialize the notion of directness.

4 The evaluative model of pain perception

I will now conclude with an alternative epistemic model of pain perception, which I call the *evaluative model*. It does not assume that one can be directly aware that there is pain. It only assumes that one can be directly aware that there is something *bad*, and indirectly aware that someone could be in pain. It is inspired from the recent representationalist view of pain known as evaluativism (Cutter and Tye 2011; Bain 2013, Chapter 3, this volume).

A subject's being in unpleasant pain consists in his (i) undergoing an experience (the pain) that represents a disturbance of a certain sort, and (ii) that same experience additionally representing the disturbance as bad for him in the bodily sense.

(Bain 2013: S82)

If now we apply evaluativism to third-person pain perception, it leads to the following two claims: a subject's perceiving unpleasant pain consists in his (i) undergoing a visual or auditory experience that represents a disturbance of a certain sort, and (ii) that same experience additionally representing the disturbance as bad in the bodily sense. If this were to suffice to perceive other people's pains, it may seem that we have finally found a direct model of third-person pain perception. However, as I will later argue, these two conditions do not suffice and a third one is required: (iii) further knowledge about the context in order to compute the probability of pain.

Let us start with the first two conditions. As one may note, they cannot be strictly identical to the evaluative account of pain itself. Two further qualifications are needed. First, one needs to specify for whose body the disturbance is represented as bad. Secondly, one needs to specify the nature of the disturbance that is perceived as bad in the bodily sense. In pain, the disturbance is represented as bad for the subject having the experience. By contrast, in third-person pain perception, the disturbance is primarily represented as bad for the person undergoing the disturbance, rather than for the subject having the visual experience. Still, there is a sense in which the disturbance can also be seen as bad for the perceiving subject. To be in perceptual contact with the person in pain indeed generally involves sharing the same space, and thus sharing the same potential threats. For example, if I see you bitten by a mosquito, I can be the next victim. The evaluative property ascribed to the disturbance can then be conceived as an alarm signal, which is both other-oriented (bad for the person that one sees enduring the disturbance) and self-oriented (bad for the person that sees the disturbance).

One may then question the type of disturbance that the visual experience represents as bad. The notion of disturbance is actually quite vague. Does it refer to whatever normally causes pain, to homeostatic deficiency, or to activity in the nociceptive system? None of these replies seems to be satisfactory (Klein 2015). For the sake of the evaluative model of third-person pain perception, I will rather refer to what I call *warning properties*, whose scope is wider than what is generally assumed by the notion of disturbance. Warning properties are properties of objects or events that occur either in personal space or peripersonal space,[8] to which the perceptual system ascribes a negative value because they indicate the high probability of something bad happening to the body. They include not only bodily damage (e.g., blood pouring from the hand), but also what is upstream to the damage, like threats close to the body (e.g., a knife approaching your thigh), as well as what is downstream, like bodily and verbal expressions (e.g., pain grimace, tensed posture, "ouch") and bodily reactions (e.g., withdrawal).[9] For instance, if we go back to the case of the frowning man, our visual experience represents his frown as a warning property.

The hypothesis is thus that perception of warning properties *as* warning properties is evaluative because the perceptual system has ascribed a negative value to them. Such an evaluative perception gives direct awareness of other people's bodily situation being bad. Although there are some interesting similarities with the evaluative theory of pain, there are also dissimilarities. There is thus no risk of confusion between painful experiences and the perceptual experiences of warning properties.[10] As Bain (2013) notes, there is a fundamental difference between seeing and feeling injuries, and only the latter constitutes a painful experience. Still, one may wonder whether the perceptual experiences of warning properties are themselves unpleasant since they seem to meet the evaluativist characterization of the unpleasantness of pain. Indeed, according to evaluativism, an experience is unpleasant in virtue of representing disturbances as bad. However, it may not be enough for an experience to feel unpleasant to represent something as bad. It has to represent something as bad *for the subject* of the experience. This is the case of painful experiences. And, as already mentioned, it can be true in some circumstances in evaluative perceptual experiences, for instance if the threat that is close to you is not so far from me. But there are many contexts in which warning properties indicate only the probability of something bad happening to the other person only (when seeing you frowning, for instance). In these contexts, I would argue that evaluative perceptual experiences do not have to be unpleasant.

The question that interests us, however, is whether the perception of warning properties can ground beliefs about other people's pains, and if it does, whether it is in a direct or indirect manner. Let us compare three stages in the following scenario: I see a rock falling on you, I see your leg broken, and I see you frowning and screaming. According to the evaluative model, I see warning properties at each stage: I directly see that something bad is happening to you. But badness is different from pain. It is actually a relatively indeterminate notion. The perception of warning properties simply ascribes a negative value to the event, but it does not do much more. It is not more informative than an alarm signal. If it were more informative, arguably, it would require more complex inferences and information. One could then no longer claim that one can directly see that something bad is happening. How do I then go from badness to pain? My account is twofold. First, my evaluative perception can only justify me in forming a belief about *the probability* of your being in pain now or in the near future. Secondly, my evaluative perception contributes but does not suffice to compute the probability of pain. Arguably, the computation of the probability of pain can be relatively complex and require further knowledge of the context. For instance, I need to know whether you have noticed the rock falling and whether you have the ability to jump quickly enough to avoid it. Even at the second stage, when I see your leg broken, my belief that you are in pain will depend on whether you are anesthetized, having surgery to fix your leg. Finally, at the last stage, I need to know whether you have reasons to be in pain or to be angry that explain why you scream.

Hence, evaluative perception gives direct awareness that the bodily situation is bad. It does not give direct awareness that the person is in pain. It is only in virtue of being directly aware of the badness that one can become indirectly aware of the pain. This is so because perceptual experiences of warning properties do not suffice by themselves to fix the probability that the person is in pain. But they do suffice to alert that something bad is happening to the person. In other words, under normal circumstances, it suffices for me to see you frowning to know that there is something wrong, but it does not suffice for me to know that you are in pain. Further knowledge is required. This is our third condition of third-person pain perception.

To recapitulate, according to the evaluative model of third-person pain perception, one can experience warning properties from the outside, which grounds direct epistemic awareness that the bodily situation is bad, which in turn grounds the indirect epistemic awareness that the person is, or will be, in pain. Although the perception of warning properties does not give a direct access to other people's pain, it is still an efficient tool for motivating prosocial behaviors as well as attentional vigilance for the surrounding, and possibly avoidance behaviors. It is also an efficient tool for acquiring knowledge about the badness of other people's situations and the danger of the world around us.[11] From an evolutionary perspective, these functions actually seem more important than directly learning about other people's pain.

5 Conclusion

Our starting point was the feeling of directly apprehending other people's pains. I have argued that this feeling is illusory. Direct perceptual models, whether non-epistemic or epistemic, fail to successfully account for the relationship between bodily expressions and pain (see the table below). I do not see the pain in your eyes. What I see are warning properties that I represent as bad. In other words, I see an alarm signal, not your pain. My awareness of your pain is thus only indirect.

Third-person pain perception	*Direct*	*Indirect*
Non-epistemic	Seeing-in model	—
Epistemic	Mereological model	Evaluative model

Why, then, do I sometimes have a feeling of immediate acquaintance? Arguably, it reveals dysfunction at the meta-perceptual level that results in my being mistaken about what is directly perceived. But what is the origin of the error? I will briefly suggest two answers. The first possibility is that badness is mistaken for pain. Since my awareness of warning properties is evaluative like pain, one can easily conceive that the two can be confused. There is, however, another possibility.[12] On this alternative view, my pain is mistaken for your pain. More specifically, perceiving that another individual is in pain can sometimes induce a vicarious experience of pain (de Vignemont and Jacob 2012). This has been empirically confirmed in a series of studies on pain perception, which show activation of parts of the neural basis of pain (e.g., Singer et al. 2004). Hence, in pain perception, it is true that there is a direct acquaintance with pain, but it is with one's own, or more precisely, with one's own vicarious pain. This gives rise to a feeling of immediacy. Yet, because one is barely aware of the vicarious experience itself, one erroneously attaches the feeling of immediacy to the awareness of the other person's pain.

Related topics

Chapter 3: Evaluativist accounts of pain's unpleasantness (Bain)
Chapter 9: A view of pain based on sensations, meanings, and emotions (Price)
Chapter 16: Robot pain (Mandik)
Chapter 20: Pain and incorrigibility (Langland-Hassan)

Notes

1 There are other interpretations, especially in the epistemology of perception, which I will not discuss here.
2 This notion of direct perception should not be confused with Gibson's notion, for instance. Since it is epistemic, it involves recognitional processes.
3 A stronger claim would be to say that it is infallible, but this is more controversial and it is not required by the argument here. See Chapter 20, this volume.
4 The notion of seeing-in even allows some flexibility about the dual experiential content. It may happen that one sees only the surface, and not beyond, when one restores a damaged Renaissance painting, for instance. Likewise, even the phenomenological tradition would accept that in some circumstances, one sees only the tears and not the pain behind.
5 One may question the very notion of seeing-in, even for picture perception (for discussion, see Abell and Bantinaki 2010). This, however, goes beyond the scope of this chapter.
6 Such an option, however, may be open to functionalists and behaviorists.
7 Zahavi and Overgaard may reply that one day in the future there will be a more direct way to see Mars by actually going there. But one can make the same claim about pain. With the progress of neuroimaging techniques, we are actually not so far from seeing pain in the brain.
8 An object or event is perceived in peripersonal space if it occurs in the immediate surrounding of the body. Numerous findings indicate that the representations of this special area display specific sensorimotor properties. In particular, it has been shown to play a defensive function and can be conceived as a margin of safety.
9 But it does not include other signs indicating pain, whose interpretation is more cognitively demanding (e.g., a person taking Advil).
10 I shall come back to that point in the conclusion.
11 For instance, seeing that a conspecific's body is instantiating warning properties after eating a specific kind of berry motivates me both to help this person and to stay away from those berries. Furthermore, I can learn by proxy that this specific kind of berry is poisonous.
12 I would like to thank Pierre Jacob for his helpful suggestion.

References

Abell, C. and Bantinaki, K. (eds.) (2010) *Philosophical Perspectives on Depiction*. Oxford: Oxford University Press.
Bain, D. (2013) What makes pains unpleasant? *Philosophical Studies* 166 (suppl. 1): S69–S89.
Cassam, Q. (2007) *The Possibility of Knowledge*. Oxford: Oxford University Press.
Cutter, B. and Tye, M. (2011) Tracking representationalism and the painfulness of pain. *Philosophical Issues* 21(1): 90–109.
Dailey, M.N., Cotrell, G.W., Padgett, C., and Adolphs, R. (2002) EMPATH: a neural network that categorizes facial expressions. *Journal of Cognitive Neuroscience* 14(8): 1158–1173.
de Vignemont, F. and Jacob, P. (2012) What is it like to feel another's pain? *Philosophy of Science* 79: 295–316.
Dretske, F. (1969) *Seeing and Knowing*. Chicago: University of Chicago Press.
Dretske, F. (1973) Perception and other minds. *Noûs* 7: 34–44.
Ekman, P. and Friesen, W.V. (1975) *Unmasking the Face: A Guide to Recognizing Emotions from Facial Clues.* Englewood Cliffs, NJ: Prentice-Hall.

Frijda, N.H. (1953) The understanding of facial expression of emotion. *Acta Psychologica* 9: 294–362.

Green, M. (2007) *Self-Expression*. Oxford: Oxford University Press.

Klein, C. (2015) *What the Body Commands*. Cambridge, MA: MIT Press.

McDowell, J. (1978) On the reality of the past. In C. Hookway and P. Pettit (eds.), *Action and Interpretation*. Cambridge: Cambridge University Press.

Scheler, M. (1954) *The Nature of Sympathy*, trans. P. Heath. London: Routledge & Kegan Paul.

Schutz, A. (1967) *The Phenomenology of the Social World*. Evanston, IL: Northwestern University Press.

Singer, T., Seymour, B., O'Doherty, J., Kaube, H., Dolan, R., and Frith, C. (2004) Empathy for pain involves the affective but not sensory components of pain. *Science* 303: 1157–1162.

Smith, J. (2013) The phenomenology of face-to-face mindreading. *Philosophy and Phenomenological Research* 87(2): 274–293.

Stein, E. (1989) *On the Problem of Empathy*. Washington, DC: ICS Publishers.

Stout, R. (2010) Seeing the anger in someone's face. *Aristotelian Society, Supplementary Volumes*, 84(1): 29–43.

Wollheim, R. (2003). In defense of seeing-in. In H. Hecht, R. Schwartz, and M. Atherton (eds.), *Looking into Pictures*. Cambridge, MA: MIT Press/A Bradford Book, pp. 3–16.

Zahavi, D. (2011) Empathy and direct social perception: a phenomenological proposal. *Review of Philosophy and Psychology* 2(3): 541–558.

Zahavi, D. and Overgaard, S. (2012) Empathy without isomorphism: a phenomenological account. In J. Decety (ed.), *Empathy from Bench to Bedside*. Cambridge: Cambridge University Press.

22

PAIN AND COGNITIVE PENETRABILITY

Hilla Jacobson

The question of the cognitive penetrability (hereafter, CP) of experience is, roughly, the question whether cognitive states (e.g., beliefs, desires, expectations, and emotions) can influence, in some direct and non-trivial manner, one's experiences. Whereas the CP of *perception* has recently been widely discussed by philosophers, the parallel question regarding *pain* has been utterly neglected. This is despite ever-growing successful clinical practices and scientific findings that appear to support direct cognition-to-pain influences. The present chapter purports to begin filling in this lacuna in the philosophical literature. The first section will introduce the general notion of CP, as well as its epistemic import, focusing on visual experiences; the second section will apply the notion of CP to pains, presenting some initial reasons to think that pains are cognitively penetrable; and the third section will conditionally inquire what the implications of CP are, if it does apply to pains.

1 CP and perceptual experience – a general characterization

There is hardly any question that perception affects, in a direct manner, cognition: e.g., what we see influences what we believe. Seeing a ripe yellow banana on the table would standardly lead me to believe there is a yellow banana on the table. However, many think that a direct causal relation does not obtain in the opposite direction: e.g., what we see is not affected by what we believe. Standing with my eyes shut while falsely believing that there is a ripe yellow banana on the table would not lead me to see the green banana as yellow upon opening my eyes.

Moreover, it might be thought, it is quite fortunate that perception is thus immune to cognitive influences, for the claim that it is susceptible to them would undermine its epistemic status as a source of justification and knowledge. *Prima facie*, if what we believe, desire, and expect partly determines what we see, perceptual experiences would be poor guides to what we ought to believe. To briefly mention one dire specific challenge to perceptual justification, which is raised by Siegel (2012), such influences would seem to entangle us in a circular structure of belief-formation: they seem to allow cases in which beliefs give rise to perceptual experiences, which then appear to justify those very same beliefs. Surely, or so the challenge goes, the resulting beliefs are not justified by the experiences. Furthermore, argues Siegel, CP thus poses a challenge for dogmatist theories of justification (see, e.g., Pryor 2000), according to which (absent defeaters) an experience as of *p* provides some immediate justification for *p* in virtue of the experience's having a distinctive phenomenology with respect to p.[1,2] As the circularity problem appears to show, cognitively penetrated perceptual experiences, such as experiences as of p that are caused by beliefs that p, fail to provide justification, because due to CP they have epistemically improper etiologies. The relevant theories are hence undermined – they yield wrong predictions as to which perceptual experiences are justificatory.

Two central questions, then, are whether the phenomenon of CP exists, and, if so, what precisely are its epistemic implications. Both require a more precise characterization of CP. There are some trivial, unquestionable cases, in which cognitive states influence perceptual states, but the influence seems indirect. For example, wanting to get a better view of a magnificent picture may cause me to get closer, focus my attention on its upper part, or put on my glasses, and as an (indirect) result my visual experience of it would probably change. Putative cases of CP, however, are deemed more interesting. An important challenge, then, is to clarify, and make precise, the nature of the relevant notion of directness, by characterizing CP in a manner that would leave the trivial, indirect cases, outside its scope. Thus, standard attempts to provide a more restrictive and precise characterization are aimed at identifying, and then setting aside, differences between experiences that are due to the (mediated) intervention of the factors operative in the "less-interesting cases," by holding those operative factors fixed. The following is a characterization in this spirit, on which many participants of the debate agree.[3]

> CP of Perceptual Experience: A perceptual experience with phenomenal character c is cognitively penetrable if it is (nomologically) possible for two subjects (or for the same subject at different times) to differ with respect to whether their experience has c, and the difference is due to a causal process tracing back to cognitive states of the subject, where we hold fixed between the two subjects (or one subject at different times) the following: (i) the distal stimuli and perceptual conditions, (ii) the subjects' spatial attention, and (iii) the conditions of the subjects' sensory organs.

In this characterization, CP is said to hinge on whether the cognitive states influence, in the required manner, the perceptual experience's *phenomenal character* (i.e., the "what it is like" aspect of the experience, or the phenomenal way things "look" to the subject). It should be noted that other characterizations of CP allude (exclusively – see, e.g., Siegel 2012; or additionally – see, e.g., Macpherson 2012) to a change in the experience's *representational content*, and that when the characterization mentions either phenomenal character or representational content alone, it is followed by a clarification that the two at least typically go hand in hand (see, e.g., Macpherson 2015). That is, CP is standardly understood as requiring an influence of cognitive states on both phenomenal character and representational content: it should be manifest in the way things appear to us both sensuously and representationally.

The claim that representational content supervenes on phenomenal character and/or vice versa is controversial, but in the context of the CP debate that claim is often taken as an assumption. In any event, I believe that there are implicit motivations for this dual requirement on CP.[4] First, it is clearly more interesting, in itself, if our cognitive states affect not only the "what it is like" aspect of our perceptual experiences and our phenomenal world, but also the perceptual world we inhabit – what we experience rather than only the way it feels to have the relevant experiences. Second, it seems that the significant epistemic implications of CP, mentioned above, are due to the putative effects of cognitions on the *contents* of perceptual experiences, and to a large extent the interest in CP stems from an interest in its epistemic implications. Third, the notion of CP designates a causal relation;

however, part of its significance is that this relation is not a mere, brute, causal relation. Rather, it is a psychological relation, and, as such, it seems that it ought to be characterized by the sort of intelligibility characteristic of the relations among psychological states. It is hard to see, the thought might be, how the relation can enjoy such intelligibility, rather than appearing arbitrary (from a psychological point of view), unless the penetrated as well as the penetrating states are contentful, and there are some non-arbitrary semantic relations among them. This third motivation also supports a further requirement sometimes imposed on CP – namely, that it be a "semantically coherent" relation (see, e.g., Pylyshyn 1999). As Stokes (2013) notes, semantic coherence can be understood as an inference-supporting relation, or, less demandingly (and more plausibly), as requiring, in the spirit of the third motivation, only that the content of the penetrating state has some non-arbitrary effect on the perception.

To get a better grip on CP, consider two cases of visual perceptual experiences that putatively exemplify it.

(1) Red looks: In an experiment conducted by Delk and Fillenbaum (1965), participants were asked to match the color of orange-red cardboard cut-outs to a color-adjustable background. Some of the cut-outs had the shapes of objects associated with red (hearts, lips, and apples), whereas the shapes of others had no such associations (squares, bells, horse-heads). Cut-outs with shapes associated with red were matched to redder backgrounds than were cut-outs with shapes not associated with red (the latter were matched to more orange colors, which were, objectively, the more accurate matches).

The CP interpretation of this case is that subjects' knowledge of the typical colors of objects influenced the way the shape of the cut-outs looked to them – it made the cut-outs associated with red objects look (in both the phenomenal and the representational senses of "look") redder to them.

(2) Steepy looks: In an experiment conducted by Stefanucci and Proffitt (Stefanucci et al. 2008), participants were asked to estimate the slant of a hill. Participants who were induced to experience fear, tended to more greatly overestimate its slant (both in verbal report and visual matching task).

The CP interpretation of this case is that subjects' fear influenced the way the slant of the hill looked to them – it made it look (in both the phenomenal and the representational senses of "look") steeper.

It is possible to resist CP interpretations, while admitting that subjects' perceptual experiences are influenced by their cognitive states, by arguing that one (or more) of the factors that are to be held fixed according to CP's characterization actually varies. The other route to undermining such interpretations is to insist that the perceptual experiences are unaffected. Rather, the penetrating cognitive states influence cognitive states downstream of the perceptual experiences – notably, they affect judgments made on the basis of these experiences.[5] Thus, it isn't that the hill looks steeper due to the induction of fear. Rather, it looks exactly as it would have otherwise looked, but the subjects form a (false) first-order judgment that it is steeper. In addition (or, less plausibly, alternatively), it might be argued, the subjects form a (false) second-order judgment – the fear misleads their introspective judgments regarding their experiences.

2 Cognitive penetrability and pain – an initial application

Prima facie, and given the prevalent (though by no means univocally accepted) view that pain is (or involves) a sort of perceptual experience (specifically, an experience of some bodily condition), the question of whether perceptual experiences are cognitively penetrable is also applicable to pains.[6] Thus, by substituting, in the general characterization of CP, "pain" for "perceptual experience," as well as inserting the specific factors relevant to pains in the specification of the conditions that are to be held fixed, we get:

> CP-pain (hereafter CPP): A pain with phenomenal character c is cognitively penetrable if it is (nomologically) possible for two subjects (or for the same subject at different times) to differ with respect to whether their pain has c, and the difference is due to a causal process tracing back to cognitive states of the subject, where we hold fixed between the two subjects (or one subject at different times) the following: (i) the bodily condition or tissue damage, (ii) the subjects' spatial attention (the extent to which they attend to the relevant body part(s)), and (iii) the conditions of the subjects' nociceptive sensory system (or more precisely, of those "early" aspects of the system that are parallel to sensory organs).

We have noted that whereas there is hardly any question that perception directly affects cognition, a direct influence in the opposite direction is far from obvious. The same is apparently true regarding pain. Having an intense toothache would often lead me to believe that there is something wrong with my tooth and to desire that the pain cease; yet, it initially seems that wanting the pain to stop or believing that my dental condition is excellent would have no effect on my pain. Relatedly, the fact that certain illusions, such as the Müller–Lyer illusion, are resilient to simultaneous occurrent beliefs with contrary contents, appears at first blush to tell against the CP of visual experiences, and there are analogous phenomena that seem to raise doubts regarding CPP.[7] Thus, phantom pains are notoriously resilient to subjects' beliefs that the body parts in which they feel their pains are missing. Similarly, cases of allodynia, in which pains result from stimuli that are normally neither harmful nor painful (such as light touch), exhibit apparent impenetrability to beliefs about the harmfulness of the stimuli.

Nonetheless, there are initial reasons for thinking that pains are cognitively penetrable. Moreover, relative to experiences of other sorts, pains are known to exhibit enormous (intra- as well as inter-subjective variability vis-à-vis their "typical" causes – the same noxious stimuli seem to lead to pains of quite different intensities, and are sometimes experienced as not painful at all – and scientists believe that these variations are partly dependent on psychological variables. (In fact, whereas variability between perceptions that come hand in hand with a difference in cognitions is often taken to point to CP, the variability in the case of pains is so great that some take it to undermine the claim that pains are, or are exhausted by, perceptual experiences, in which case the standard notion of CP may be inapplicable to them.) Thus, there is a huge body of scientific, mainly clinical, research that lends *prima facie* support to the CPP hypothesis (for such research, see, e.g., Chapters 9 and 32). For example, some experiments reveal effects of anxious depression on chronic pain, but not vice versa (Lerman et al. 2015: 201; see also Chapters 8 and 12, this volume). Given that anxious depression is propelled, at least in part, by cognitive forces, this may support CPP (provided that the impact is shown to be "direct"). Similarly, pain catastrophizing – broadly defined as "an exaggerated negative 'mental set' brought to bear during actual or anticipated pain experience" (Sullivan et al. 2001: 53) – is widely argued to be associated with heightened pain. More specifically, following the development of the Pain Catastrophizing Scale (Sullivan et al. 1995), catastrophizing is now standardly conceptualized as comprising three dimensions: magnification (a tendency to magnify the threat value of pain and/or its stimulus), rumination (a relative inability to inhibit pain-related thoughts), and helplessness (a tendency to feel helpless in the face of pain). It appears to influence pain reports both when assessed as a dispositional variable (e.g., in numerous studies of subjects suffering from chronic pain), and (more controversially) when induced as an occurrent state in the context of a specific painful encounter, such as laboratory-based noxious stimulation. Relatedly, the very usefulness of multidisciplinary pain treatment programs, which are partly driven by cognitive-behavioral models and attempt to influence *inter alia* subjects' cognitions, appears to testify to the efficacy of cognitions (see, e.g., Kerns et al. 2011; see also Chapter 11, this volume).

Last but not least, the study of the physiology and neuroanatomy of pain also lends support to CPP, by describing neurophysiological mechanisms that can underlie it. Since the launching of the classic gate-control theory of pain, proposed by Melzack and Wall (1965), the brain is no longer regarded as a merely passive recipient of nociceptive signals. Rather, virtually all neuroscientific models of pain assign a crucial modulatory role in pain processing to downstream projections from cognitive, cortical areas, thus allowing brain areas subserving psychological factors to play a dynamic role in pain perception.

There are various challenges to interpreting the phenomena considered above as instances of CPP. For example, many of the reported findings are correlational, and correlational findings do not shed light on causal relationships. In addition, according to attentional models of pain, the influence of psychological factors on pain is mediated by attentional mechanisms. As mentioned, standard characterizations of CP require that at least some modes of attention (notably, spatial attention) are held fixed. In addition, there are notorious difficulties that pertain to the scientific, objective measurement of the subjective experience of pain.

What of the standard route to undermining CP interpretations in cases of, e.g., visual experiences, by arguing that the penetrating cognitive states do not affect the experiences, but rather influence only cognitions downstream of the experiences? On the face of it, it is available also in the case of pain. But here we should note an asymmetry, which will be elaborated on in the next section. We have seen that in the visual case two counter CP interpretations can be given: that the penetrating cognitions have influenced the first-order judgment regarding the objects and properties represented by the experience, or that they have influenced the second-order judgment regarding the experience. As we will shortly see, in the case of pains, it is judgments of the second sort – introspective judgments – that are standardly immediately prompted by the experience, and it is arguable that only such judgments are thus prompted. That is, the standard evidence for CPP, and hence the one that opponents of CPP should counter, is a report of the sort, "I feel such and such a pain," construed as a report about the experience of pain. Hence, on the assumption that introspective judgments are relatively resilient to error, objecting to CPP by taking those reports to express false judgments is a tall order (for a discussion of the infallibility of pain reports, see Chapter 20, this volume).

3 Cognitive penetrability and pain – implications

The question of whether pains are cognitively penetrable is still open. In this section, I will assume the CPP thesis, and focus on its implications. The discussion will revolve around three respects in which pains appear to differ from visual experiences.

The first asymmetry concerns *the sort of concepts that our visual experiences and pains immediately prompt us to apply, or the kind of recognitional beliefs to which they directly give rise* (see, e.g., Aydede 2009, and Chapter 18). We will begin by exploring the epistemological implications of CPP, assuming a broadly perceptualist framework of pains – namely, that feeling pain in a body region is, or involves, perceiving a (non-mental) property of that region, e.g., the obtaining of some sort of tissue damage, or that something is wrong in that region (hereafter, bp for "bodily property").[8] Given this framework, it seems that pains can have a significant (direct) epistemic role vis-à-vis bodily directed beliefs, a role equivalent to that played by other perceptual experiences vis-à-vis perceptual beliefs about the subject's proximate environment. The natural analogy here is with a visual experience of a secondary quality, such as red. Perceiving a red apple immediately prompts us (under certain standard circumstances) to apply the concept RED to the apple. The term "immediately" indicates that we apply that concept simply on the basis of having the experience (no further mediating beliefs are required). That is, the experience prompts us to have a perceptual belief in which RED is ascribed to the represented external object: that belief is true iff the apple is red. Perceiving a red apple can also lead (in rather special circumstances) to an introspective belief – a belief that I have an experience of redness – whose truth does not hinge on the existence of a red apple before me. Yet, as representationalists are the first to acknowledge, the (sensory) concept RED is, in the first instance, the concept of the represented external property.

Turning to pains, the first thing to note is that in their case, the standard beliefs that are prompted by the experience are not beliefs about the represented non-mental bp, but rather introspective beliefs about the experience of pain. The report "I feel a pain in my hand" (despite superficial resemblance to the report "I see a red apple") can be true even if the bp is not instantiated (e.g., if I suffer from phantom pain or allodynia), and it can be false even if the bp is instantiated (e.g., if I am under the influence of a strong analgesic).[9] But the question that is most relevant for our purposes is whether there are *any* occasions in which pain immediately – i.e., simply on the basis of having it – prompts us to apply a concept that ascribes to the relevant body part the non-mental property of bp. This is actually the question of whether we *ever* apply, on the basis of experiencing pain alone, a concept whose correct application is dependent only on the instantiation of bp – one whose extension is different from that of the concept of the experience of pain. If not, then it seems that there are no pain perceptual beliefs – no bodily directed beliefs that are immediately prompted by pains, but only pain introspective beliefs.

The above question is hard. The pain I feel in my hand, does seem to "convey to me" that something – and not at all a nice thing – is going on in my hand. But do I ever believe, on the basis of my feeling pain alone, that "'this' (referring demonstratively to what I feel in my hand) is going on in my hand," where the belief in question is one I retract upon discovering that there is nothing wrong with my hand? Is the belief that "there's something wrong with my hand" truly prompted, and based solely on, my experience of pain? Or is it mediated by, e.g., the (implicit) belief that pain is a good indication of bodily damage? I do not purport to answer those questions here, but I would like to point out their significance to the *epistemic implications* of CPP. (Cf. discussion in Chapter 30, this volume.)

Recall the epistemic threats that are posed by CP. Echoing Siegel's (2012) circularity worry, suppose that, due to my fear, my visual experience misrepresents the hill as steeper than it really is. This experience, in turn, may wrongly appear to warrant that very fear. It may seem that CPP leads to just such circularity – indeed, that this is precisely the predicament of some catastrophizing subjects. These subjects' fears and exaggerated beliefs about the severity of the bodily damage make their pains worse, and those pains, in turn, lead to beliefs about severe bodily damage. Surely, those pains do not justify the beliefs that gave rise to them in the first place. If there are perceptual beliefs concerning bp (hereafter, bp perceptual beliefs), then the analysis of this case is precisely similar to that of the visual case. Yet, if there are no such beliefs – if, that is, our pains never prompt us directly to have bp perceptual beliefs – then, at least under some prevalent conceptions of justification, the two cases are dissimilar from the outset: even in the standard case, which does not involve CP, pains, in contrast to visual experiences, do not justify, all by themselves, beliefs about the objects and properties that they represent. The reason for this is simply that no such beliefs are ever prompted directly by pains. And this seems to show that views (such as dogmatism) according to which experiences provide justification for beliefs about their intentional objects in virtue of their distinctive phenomenology – those views against which the epistemic challenge from CP was directed – are wrong-headed with respect to pains to begin with.

The assumption that pains do not give rise to bp perceptual beliefs has been used to argue against perceptualist views of pain. To highly simplify Aydede's (2009) intricate argument, one prime motivation for – possibly even a condition on – taking an experience to be a perceptual experience as of *p* is that its phenomenology may immediately prompt us to have beliefs with content *p*. The main reason for thinking that a sensory state is a perceptual, representational experience is that, in virtue of its phenomenology, it allows us to have immediate cognitive access to the world – it immediately prompts and justifies beliefs about those aspects that it allegedly represents. If the above-mentioned assumption is warranted, that reason is absent in the case of pain. This, indeed, is a formidable challenge, and proponents of perceptualist representationalist views of pains are thus hard pressed to deny that assumption. Note also that if they do not deny it, then, CPP turns out to be particularly strange: bp beliefs can immediately prompt certain pains (according to CPP); but pains do not immediately prompt bp beliefs. In the case of pains, bp-cognitions directly influence experiences, but experiences do not directly influence bp-cognitions. CPP may give us reason to think that pains do represent bp – otherwise why should they be affected by bp-cognitions? This makes it all the more surprising that CPP does not affect bp perceptual beliefs. As we have noted, in the case of perceptual experiences other than pains, whereas the perception–cognition direction is unquestionable, and instances of it can be found in abundance, it is the cognition–perception direction that is considered problematic and scarce.

The two further respects in which pains appear to differ from visual experiences are commonly thought to be closely related. First, *(at least standard) pains are valanced states that have a pronounced affective dimension – they feel bad and are unpleasant.* Second, *pains seem to bear special, intimate relations to certain actions – they appear to be intrinsically motivational, and to rationalize some of the actions to which they give rise.* According to a plausible conception, it is due to their being unpleasant that standard pains have a motivational, reason-giving force (the expression "hedomotive aspects" coined by Bain [2013], expresses the close link between these features). Some philosophers (see, e.g., Klein 2015, and Chapter 4) go as far as to suggest that pains have no informational, indicative roles, but only a practical, action-guiding role. But even if this claim is rejected, pains do seem to have a distinctive action-guiding role, and so it is interesting to examine whether CPP has implications vis-à-vis that role.

Consider, first, the relations that seem to obtain between pains and actions in standard, non-CPP cases. *Prima facie*, upon my hand being hit by a fast tennis ball, the pain I feel in my hand motivates me, as well as provides me with reasons for, performing certain actions. It can lead me to rub my hand, to search for ice, and for an analgesic cream. When I search for analgesic cream, the action is clearly experience-directed (hereafter "e-directed") – its target is to alleviate the experience of pain. When I seek ice and rub my hand the actions are plausibly both bp-directed – i.e., ones whose target is to lessen the bodily damage – and e-directed (see, e.g., Aydede 2009; Bain 2013; and Jacobson 2013). From my perspective as an agent, either lessening the bodily damage or alleviating the pain would render the action successful. Now, I believe that many of us share a strong and persistent intuition that applies at least to some such actions, specifically, to "basic," intuitively non-reflective actions, such as rubbing my hand: my pain *intrinsically and immediately* – i.e., just in virtue of its phenomenal character, and independently of further (bp-directed as well as e-directed) desires and beliefs – motivates me, and provides me with reasons for, performing some bp-directed as well as e-directed actions. Moreover, in some cases the relevant reasons are good reasons – they justify the relevant actions. I need not believe that I am in pain or that my hand is damaged in order to be motivated to rub my hand, nor do I need those beliefs to justify my action. My being in pain, by itself, provides a perspective from which that action is deemed intelligible and reasonable.[10, 11]

The interesting thing to note is that there is an apparent similarity between the claim that pains provide immediate motivation and justification vis-à-vis bp-directed actions (hereafter, the Pain Immediate Action Thesis or PIA) and the thesis that perceptual experiences provide immediate rationalization of, and justification for, perceptual beliefs about their intentional objects in virtue of their distinctive phenomenology. PIA provides a practical parallel to that epistemic thesis. By substituting in the epistemic thesis "perceptual experiences" for "pains," and "perceptual beliefs about their intentional objects" with "actions that are directed towards their intentional objects (i.e., bodily parts and properties)" we get the practical PIA.

Just as CP threatens the justification of perceptual beliefs, according to the epistemic thesis, CPP threatens the rationalization and justification of actions, according to PIA. This threat is exemplified by the following imaginary CPP case. A friend who is interested in CPP tells me he is about to briefly touch my hand with a scalding iron stick. The stick is in fact cold, but as a result of my belief that the stick is burning hot, I briefly feel a pain in my hand, and am momentarily led to blow on my hand. In the framework of PIA, this is a case in which the etiology of my pain gets in the way of its phenomenology playing one of its proper roles – namely, to provide an immediate rationalization of, and justification for, my bp-action.

Still, an important disanalogy, which does not even hinge on whether pains motivate and rationalize actions independently of e-beliefs, remains. Another role of the phenomenology of pain is to rationalize and justify *e-directed actions*. There is a strong intuition that the reasonableness of, and the justification for, those actions are dependent only on the negative, unpleasant phenomenal character of pain. The actions are reasonable and justified independently of whether bp obtains (e.g., those actions are justified in the case of phantom pains), or whether, as a result of the action, the bp will be changed (as is shown by the reasonableness of taking painkillers).[12] Clearly, CPP does not threaten the role of pains in rationalizing and justifying those actions – in this case, etiology is clearly of no importance – and this explains its obvious practical importance.

Finally, returning to pains and bp-directed actions, let us now revisit the anti-perceptualist argument that proceeds from the assumption that pains do not immediately prompt bp perceptual beliefs. Recall that the rationale underlying this argument is that this assumption implies that in the case of pain a condition on taking an experience to be perceptual, and to represent items that are external to itself, is not met: pain is not an experience such that, in virtue of its phenomenology, it allows us to have an immediate cognitive access to the world. Pain does not directly prompt and justify beliefs about those aspects that it allegedly represents. As mentioned, due to the plausibility of this condition, pain-representationalists are hard pressed to deny the assumption that pains do not immediately prompt bp perceptual beliefs. Yet, I suggest that the plausibility of PIA provides an alternative reply to the argument. There is an important grain of truth to the above-mentioned condition: to count as perceptual, an experience should be such that, in virtue of its phenomenology, it allows us to have immediate contact with the world. But that contact need not be epistemic – i.e., it need not consist in an immediate link between perceptual experiences and perceptual beliefs. It can instead be practical – the link can obtain between perceptual experiences and the intentional actions to which they immediately lead. Pains, in virtue of their phenomenology, immediately motivate and rationalize bp-directed actions, and this is just as good a motivation for taking them to be, or to involve, perceptions of bp.

Related topics

Notes

1 The justification being *immediate* means that the experience that *p by itself* suffices to provide justification for *p* – there need not be any further proposition that the subject must be justified in believing.
2 I ignore here and elsewhere the question of whether the contents of perceptions are conceptual. For a discussion of this question in the context of CP, see Macpherson 2015.
3 For such characterizations, see, e.g., Siegel 2012, Macpherson 2012, and Stokes 2013.
4 These motivations are to a large extent independent of whether the supervenience claim is accepted. It is important to note in this context that opponents of supervenience can hold that phenomenal character is intimately related to representational content. Their view is often that phenomenal characters (or at least some of them) are vehicles of representations, and so, in a given context – i.e., when the subject is embedded in a particular environment – the supervenience does hold and each phenomenal character represents a particular property (see, e.g., Block 2003).
5 For discussions of challenges to CP interpretations along these lines, see, e.g., Macpherson 2012, Siegel 2012, and Machery 2015.
6 For the view that pains are a sort of perceptual experiences, see, e.g., Chapters 2 and 3, this volume. For opponents of this view, see, e.g., Chapter 4, this volume.
7 In the Müller-Lyer illusion, two parallel lines of equal length, one of which ends in inward pointing arrows and the other ends with outward pointing arrows, are seen as having different lengths. The illusion persists in the face of subjects' beliefs that the lines are of equal length. In the present context it is worth nothing, though, that it has been shown that there is variation in susceptibility to the illusion, across cultures and age groups.
8 For perceptualist views of pain, see, e.g., Chapters 2, 3, and 5, this volume. Note that views on which the contents of pains are rich evaluative contents that represent the bodily condition as, e.g., bad, are also perceptualist views, according to the above characterization.
9 For an opposing view regarding the truth conditions of the relevant beliefs, see Chapter 27.

10 Another, less radical option is that when I perform an intentional bp-directed action I do have (implicit) bp-beliefs; but those beliefs are parasitic on my being motivated to perform this action on the basis of my pain. (This idea is similar to, e.g., the McDowellian notion that upon acting on the basis of an evaluative belief I also have a desire, but that desire is parasitic on the belief). This may suffice for my main point below (see last paragraph), namely, that in the case of pain it is action, rather than belief, that connects us to bp.

11 Perhaps cases of avoidance behavior – specifically, ones that involve simple, instinctual (though not merely reflexive) actions of moving away from noxious stimuli – are especially helpful in bringing this intuition concerning the immediate link between pains and rationalizations of action to the fore. As Bain (2013: 71) notes, actions such as lifting one's foot from the hot bathwater make available "a distinctively perspectival kind of explanation, unavailable in the case of reflexive behavior, for instance. To explain your lifting your foot from the bathwater in terms of your unpleasant pain is to explain your action in terms of the reason for which you performed it; it is to delineate the perspective from which that foot-lifting seemed rational to its agent." Bain goes on to emphasize that such behaviors are motivated by pains independently of further desires, but I believe a similar claim holds also with respect to beliefs: explaining your foot-lifting by mentioning your pain makes it intelligible and reasonable; completeness does not require me to add that furthermore you had any (occurrent) e or bp desires or beliefs.

12 In favor of these claims, see, e.g., Bain 2013 and Jacobson 2013; for their denial, see, e.g., Cutter and Tye 2014.

References

Aydede, M. (2009) Is feeling pain the perception of something? *Journal of Philosophy* 106(10): 531–567.

Bain, D. (2013) What makes pains unpleasant? *Philosophical Studies* 166 (suppl. 1): S69–S89.

Block, N. (2003) Mental paint. In M. Hahn and B. Ramberg (eds.), *Reflections and Replies: Essays on the Philosophy of Tyler Burge*, with replies by Burge. Cambridge, MA: MIT Press.

Cutter, B. and Tye, M. (2014) Pains and reasons: why is it rational to kill the messenger. *Philosophical Quarterly* 64(256): 423–433.

Delk, J.L. and Fillenbaum, S. (1965) Differences in perceived colour as a function of characteristic colour. *American Journal of Psychology* 78(2): 290–293.

Jacobson, H. (2013) Killing the messenger: representationalism and the painfulness of pain. *Philosophical Quarterly* 63: 509–519.

Kerns, R.D., Spellinger, J., and Goodin, B.R. (2011) Psychological treatment of chronic pain. *Annual Review of Clinical Psychology* 7: 411–434.

Klein, C. (2015) *What the Body Commands: The Imperative Theory of Pain*. Cambridge, MA: MIT Press.

Lerman, S.F., Rudich, Z., Brill, S., Shalev, H., and Shahar, G. (2015) Longitudinal associations between depression, anxiety, and pain-related disability in chronic pain patients. *Psychosomatic Medicine* 77(3): 333–341.

Machery, E. (2015) Cognitive penetrability: a no-progress report. In J. Zeimbekis and A. Raftopoulos (eds.), *The Cognitive Penetrability of Perception: New Philosophical Perspectives*. Oxford: Oxford University Press.

Macpherson, F. (2012) Cognitive penetration of colour experience: rethinking the issue in light of an indirect mechanism. *Philosophy and Phenomenological Research* 84: 24–62.

Macpherson, F. (2015) Cognitive penetration and nonconceptual content. In J. Zeimbekis and A. Raftopoulos (eds.), *The Cognitive Penetrability of Perception: New Philosophical Perspectives*. Oxford: Oxford University Press.

Melzack, R. and Wall, P.D. (1965) Pain mechanisms: a new theory. *Science* 150: 971–979.

Pryor, J. (2000) The skeptic and the dogmatist. *Noûs* 34: 517–549

Pylyshyn, Z.W. (1999) Is vision continuous with cognition? The case for cognitive impenetrability of visual perception. *Behavioral and Brain Sciences* 22: 341–423.

Siegel, S. (2012) Cognitive penetrability and perceptual justification. *Noûs* 46(2): 201–222.

Stefanucci, J.K., Proffitt, D.R., Clore, G.L., and Parekh, N. (2008) Skating down a steeper slope: fear influences the perception of geographical slant. *Perception* 37(2): 321.

Stokes, D. (2013) Cognitive penetrability of perception. *Philosophy Compass* 8(7): 646–663.

Sullivan, M.J., Bishop, S.R., and Pivik, J. (1995) The pain catastrophizing scale: development and validation. *Psychological Assessment* 7: 524–532.

Sullivan, M.J., Thorn, B., Haythornthwaite, J.A., Keefe, F., Martin, M., and Bradley, L.A. (2001) Theoretical perspectives on the relation between catastrophizing and pain. *Clinical Journal of Pain* 17: 52–64.

PART II-III

Pain in philosophy of religion

23

SACRED PAIN

The use of self-inflicted pain in religion

Ariel Glucklich

1 Introduction

Pain presents itself to religious individuals, and to sacred traditions, as a matter of great interest. But the religious concern with pain differs in dramatic ways from that of the patient and the doctor. For, while some patients turn to religion for counseling to alleviate their suffering, many others eye pain through a spiritual lens and develop a great interest in, and even attraction to, pain. Indeed, the religious life, considered historically through thousands of written documents, or by direct observation today, evaluates pain in a variety of positive ways.

This chapter will look at this widespread phenomenon. I present evidence for the complex and often positive evaluation of pain in religious ideas and practice, including the ritual inducement of painful states. When is pain regarded in a positive manner and when as negative? I also survey a number of possible explanations for this widespread state of affairs and outline a method for ensuring a precise and sophisticated understanding for what is an elaborate cultural practice with extreme physiological and psychological ramifications.

A sensible way to begin such a program is to draw the important distinction between voluntary and involuntary pain and between pain and suffering. Voluntary pain means self-hurting or hurting with the assistance of others with a clear-minded intent to experience the pain. Such pain is usually self-modulated – although not necessarily so. Practitioners may whip themselves or scratch their skin with nails, but a martyr may willingly accept the uncontrolled savagery inflicted upon his or her body while renouncing any possibility of controlling the intensity and duration of the pain. Involuntary pain is unwelcome: it is the domain of the medical patient, the victim of a crime, or the political prisoner, among others.

Although pain is largely a mental event, I use it here as "an unpleasant sensory and emotional experience which is primarily associated with tissue damage or described in terms of such damage, or both" (IASP 2014; see also Chapter 31, this volume). Suffering, in contrast, is used here as the judgment of one's condition as highly adverse and non-sustainable. Pain and suffering often go together, but this connection is not necessary or essential. Religious ideology has, at times, accepted involuntary pain as an opportunity to transform one's natural inclinations toward pleasure into a rarefied and highly prized welcoming of physical adversity.

2 Involuntary pain and suffering

Involuntary pain is familiar to every major religious tradition and has often been taken as one of the characteristics of life as humans. It raises the issue of suffering, justice, and the relationship of humans to the divine. Prometheus was freed from his horrible tortures when Heracles shot the griffon-vulture that was tearing at his liver as punishment from Zeus. "Woe, woe!" Prometheus would cry, "Today's woe and the coming morrows I cover with one groan" (Browning 1994: 558). Ironically, what made the liberation of Prometheus possible was the horrible suffering of the divine Cheiron, which made him wish to give up the gift of immortality and replace Prometheus in Tartarus (Graves 1990). It was better to be dead than suffer the everlasting pain of an incurable wound.

Considering that Job's is still the God of Jews and Christians today, Job's suffering in the Hebrew Bible is more familiar and certainly more arbitrary (dare we say modern?) than those of Prometheus: "So Satan … afflicted Job with painful sores from the soles of his feet to the crown of his head. Then Job took a piece of broken pottery and scraped himself as he sat among the ashes" (Job 2:7).

At this point he refused to complain, though his wife told him to curse God and die. But he was willing to accept the bad from God, just he had gladly accepted the good previously. He did, however, curse the day he was born and asked: "Why did I not perish at birth and die as I came from the womb?" (3:11). This is a psychological and deeply personal complaint – not truly the voice of a theologian. It is only later that he would complain to God about the injustice and the randomness of his deep suffering, thus raising his pain to the level of a philosophical matter (10:22).

The patient today looks to medical science rather than a random and mysterious God with whom to commune as he suffers the pain of some unexplained illness. Ivan Ilych is such a figure, as perhaps we all are. And so he engages himself with the biological enemy and his own body as the battlefield: "The pain only increased, despite good medical attentions, but Ivan forced himself to feel that he was getting better." But even the good graces of almost-modern medicine could not alleviate his illness and its pain: "It was all the same: the gnawing, unmitigated pain, agonizing pain, never easing for an instant, the consciousness of life inexorably waning but not yet extinguished" (Tolstoy 1886: 43).

In all of these cases, ancient and modern alike, involuntary pain is never just pain: it is complete suffering. It calls to mind one's humanity or mortality – either as a regretted fact or, if the pain is intolerable, as an invitation to relief offered by death. Pain can be so bad that death presents itself as welcome. But all of these examples are natural or caused by God. What if the cause of pain is human, if the pain is used as a political tool for suppression and control? What does the victim of political torture say about his or her pain? According to Elaine Scarry's work in *The Body in Pain* (Scarry 1985), the victim of pain says nothing at all. The world of meaning, dependent as it is on language, ceases to exist for the torture victim. Pain is an "objectless" experience on this theory, and only summons language as an act of imagination that responds to the nihilism of pain. It is for that reason, some religion scholars have argued, that mystics hurt themselves. The contents of the world are "canceled out in their minds" argues Maureen Flynn (1996) as she surveyed Spanish women mystics.

The most famous case of religious pain in the West – the crucifixion of Jesus on the cross – raises questions that touch on and possibly undermine the theory of pain as a silent phenomenon. Do we call the horrible death on the cross a political or juridical event? It was certainly involuntary and profoundly unwelcome. And yet, Jesus – if one is to go by the Gospels – did speak while on the cross (though not about pain as such). His seven last words were actually seven sentences or statements which included the following moral request: "Father, forgive them for they know not what they do" (Luke 23:34). Other expressions were more human and tormented: "My God, my God, why have you forsaken me?" (Mark 15:34) and the most touching of all: "I thirst" (John 19:28).

3 Voluntary pain

Deliberate self-harm is a widespread phenomenon, usually associated today with emotional and neurological conditions that call for medical attention (Favazza 2011). In religious literature and ethnographic observation, voluntary pain has been remarkably pervasive and remains persistent into the modern world. There are numerous rituals (initiation, passage, purification, pilgrimage, vows, exorcism, and others) and literary expressions describing and extolling self-inflicted pain. The following examples make the case clearly.

1 In Sparta, when human sacrifice for Artemis was forbidden by King Lycurgus, it was replaced by the flogging of boys until their blood flowed. Soon it became a contest for the boys to show who could tolerate the most blows and the flogger was encouraged to strike harder and harder (Graves 1990).

2 In imitation of Christ on the cross, many mystics subjected their bodies to horrific pains. Heinrich Suso (1290–1365) tortured himself by nailing a small crucifix into his own back, by wearing a special undergarment with nails pointing inward, and by wearing gloves with embedded nails in order prevent himself from seeking relief at night, in his sleep (McNeill and Gamer 1938). Such torments were familiar to other monks and nuns, including Maria Maddalena de' Pazzi (1566–1607) and others.

3 Just as the Spartan boys turned their ordeal into a voluntary contest, so too, early Christian martyrs acted as though in a contest. In many cases their execution took place in large arenas, but some of those martyrs (for example St. Perpetua or St. Peter Balsam) actively demonstrated contempt in allowing the Roman authorities to carry out the show with them. It was a contest between two types of faith or the will of two individuals:

Severus, on hearing these words, ordered him [St. Peter Balsam] to be stretched upon the rack, and whilst he was suspended said to him scoffingly, "What say you now, Peter; do you begin to know what the rack is? Are you willing to sacrifice?" Peter answered, "Tear me with hooks, and talk not of my sacrificing to your devils; I have already told you, that I will sacrifice only to that God for whom I suffer."

(Thurston 1990: 27)

4 Traditional forms of self-hurting persist in the contemporary world around the globe, including the United States. The Sun Dance is celebrated in a number of forms by several Native American nations, including Arapahos, Cheyennes, Crows, Blackfeet, Dakota, Plain Crees, Ojibwas, and others. The ritual has been widely and thoroughly described and analyzed: it includes self-sacrificial elements of some discomfort (prolonged dancing around the central pole, fatigue, thirst, extreme heat) but at its heart is an enormously painful performance: the insertion of hooks (made of wood or eagle claws) into the chest muscle and tying the performer to the central pole (Glucklich 2001: 238 n. 48). The performer must then run backwards and literally tear himself away from the pole. According to one account the pain of the insertion and the tearing is enormous:

They pinched my skin, and I felt as the knife went into my flesh. I felt a sharp, intense pain in my chest, as if somebody had put a red hot iron on my flesh. I lost all sense of time. I couldn't hear any sounds. I didn't feel the heat of the sun. I tried to grit my teeth, but I couldn't – my crown was in my mouth. I prayed to the Creator to give me strength, to give me courage …

But then, when the author ran backwards and tore himself away by ripping his chest muscles he writes: "I was so happy, I let out a big yell" (Twofeathers 1996: 89–94).

5   In the Hindu immigrant communities of Southeast Asia (Thailand, Malaysia, Indonesia) the ritual of Thaipusam (*kavadi attam*) involves widespread displays of self-inflicted pain such as the insertion of spears through the cheeks, suspension of objects like lemons and coconuts by hooks set into the back muscles. Volunteers do this ritually and they report ecstatic states of mind and either great stoicism or a complete transcendence of the pain (Kent 2007).

While such rituals are performed in order to promote a psychic identification with God (Murugan, the son of Shiva), there are many practitioners of ritually or athletically induced pain (piercing, suspension, competition) without the traditional theological ideology. For example:

6   *The Guardian* (Sunday, 10 November 2013) ran an article about Dave Navarro, the rock guitarist of Jaw's Addiction, "Body Suspension: Why Would Anyone Hang from Hooks for Fun?" Several hooks are inserted under the skin (the body weight is thus distributed) and the practitioner is then raised up on suspension ropes. Instead of theology the subjects speak of psychological benefits, as described by Allen Falkner: "If life had a dial to adjust volume, suspension has a way of accessing this invisible knob and turning it down." In a less dramatic fashion, bodybuilders and long-distance runners have also reported extremely positive evaluations of the painful states they undergo in training and competition. These include burning muscles, painful feet and joints, fatigue, and so forth.

Comparing the cases of involuntary and self-inflicted pain demonstrates that pain itself is hard to separate from mental suffering. Job despairs from the absence of meaning and lack of justice in his known world. Ivan Ilych experiences acute isolation and like Job, meaninglessness. The pain patient who injures himself working as an electrician (perhaps) may report depression and anxiety because he has lost his job, his income, and his self-respect. Pain is seldom an isolated phenomenon and the context largely defines its "feel." And for victims of involuntary pain, suffering covers a whole range of lived experiences. Contemporary pain clinics take this into account and seldom regard the "organic" cause of pain as an isolated target for treatment (Deer 2013: 939). The focus – broadly understood – begins with coping, which goes beyond pain medication to counseling in order to address emotional, family, economic, and even philosophical or ethical dimensions of pain.

In contrast, voluntary pain rarely enters human experience as a type of suffering. In fact, pain may actually serve as the redress of suffering, as the cure for some other trouble that can only be overcome by means of severe physical stimulation. For example, even the pain of self-cutters is often reported as empowering and as a coping mechanism, a solution to the stress, anxiety or PTSD (Post-Traumatic Stress Disorder) (Favazza 2011: 153). In religious life, certainly, voluntary pain serves to promote a variety of positive feelings and judgments. Pilgrims, to give one example, report increased self-worth, belonging to a community, overcoming isolation, deepening their sense of ideological meaning (Daniel 1987).

Self-inflicted pain in religious life thus calls not for coping but for ritual elaboration, theological rationale, and – for the researcher – scientific explanations. Why do religions utilize pain in a variety of contexts and how do religious descriptions of such pain contribute to the way we might understand its value? The answer to these questions begins with an examination of pain discourse and then moves to the relationship between pain and its religious goals.

There are several forms of discourse, which I call "models," by means of which pain, self-inflicted or otherwise, is conceptualized in religious literature and in ethnographic data. These include the judicial model (punitive, evidence, debts), medical (curative, preventive), military, athletic, magical (alchemy, purifying), shared (vicarious), psychotropic, and ecstatic (Glucklich 2001: 16–31). Each model encompasses hundreds of examples but two may be offered here in a bit more detail.

One of the most widely distributed models is the juridical view of pain as a punitive force. The model is particularly pervasive in the three Western monotheistic religions and has an early mythical launch in the narrative of Adam and Eve's transgressions: "To the woman He said: 'I will greatly increase your pangs in childbearing; in pain you shall bring forth children, yet your desire shall be for your husband, and he shall rule over you.'" (Genesis 3:16) Meanwhile, Adam was condemned to earn his bread in great toil and the rest of us humans, "[i]n Adam's fall sinn'd we all: human life became penal and world hostile" (Sahlins 1996: 396). However, punishment – however painful – is not vengeance. It follows a moral logic and is certainly not arbitrary. It obeys some moral rule: we hurt because we sinned, and thus it eliminates a potential source of suffering, that is, meaninglessness. Steven F. Brena, who worked at the University of Washington at Seattle with chronic pain patients reports on patients who refuse to let go of their pain because they "deserve to hurt." According to Brena, this is often due to a pervasive feeling of guilt, but it also provides an ideological or moral mechanism whereby the pain is better tolerated because of a morally predictable universe (Brena 1972).

The pain may not only repair some moral damage one has inflicted on God's world, it can also prevent a great (and longer-lasting) punishment in the afterlife. It is therefore a good thing. As Peter Balsam, the martyr, continues his speech: "I feel no pain: but this I know that if I be not faithful to my God I must expect real pain, such as cannot be conceived." The punishment may even be self-inflicted, for preventing the greater harm of eternal punishment.

Medical tropes are used to describe pain when it is regarded as a cure for some moral or spiritual failing – a disease of the spirit. Like the punitive pain, it hurts, but that is the source of its healing power. One example comes from the pen of Prudentius, a fourth-century Christian poet who attributes to Saint Romanus (the martyr) the following words: "You will shudder at the handiwork of the executioners, but are doctors' hands gentler, when Hippocrates' cruel butchery is going on? The living flesh is cut and fresh-drawn blood stains the lancers when festering matter is being scraped away." To those who grieve his imminent death and extreme suffering he adds: "That by which health is restored is not vexatious. These men appear to be rending my wasting limbs, but they give healing to the living substance within." And Epictetus, comparing the philosopher's teaching room to that of the surgeon, claimed, "[y]ou ought not to walk out of it in pleasure, but in pain" (Roberts 1993: 10).

Although pain, the noxious bodily feeling, may be horrible, the overall experience – and uppermost the mental evaluation of its merit – can be positive because both punishment and medicine are meaningful and moral. Both the punishment and the medicine may be self-administered to achieve highly valued goals. Given the wealth of evidence across virtually all religious traditions, and given how irrational this evaluation may seem to the modern reader, a critical question must be addressed: By what overarching criterion or criteria should pain be judged as positive? A Christological rationale would not account for the Muslim or the Hindu – the answer must be sought beyond any specific theology. And yet, we must not abandon the conscious theory provided by those who value pain. A mid-level descriptive criterion (between the scientific-reductive and the theological) may be offered as the first step on the path to a theory of religious pain.

4 The agent and the telos

It is doubtful whether a single reductive theory can explain every type – let alone every case – of religious self-hurting. However, every case of intentional pain implicates the actor as an agent of his or her own hurting. This implies, at the very least, a sense of identity in which the empirical body fits as some sort of meaningful entity and a target towards which the intent to hurt is directed. From a descriptive point of view, then, the phenomenological psychology of religious pain can precisely determine the relationship between agency and telos (purpose) and gather the relevant data for analysis.

Following this agenda it is possible to observe a strong pattern: As the gap between agency and valued telos narrows, the valuation of the pain – viewed as a mediating device – improves. In this context "agency" applies to the specific cultural view of the self and "valued telos" describes that same culture's vision of the highest good. Consider, for example, the hypothetical electrician who hurt his back at work and remains in bed or in therapy for several months. If "self" is understood as a socially and economically viable ego, a provider for his family who enjoys the respect of his family and colleagues, and if his purpose in life is to enhance the well-being of his family and his own self – pain will be described as a destructive and horrifying enemy. However, if the empirical-biographical self (the working man's ego) is not the culturally normative but a distortive mask covering over a truer self, the picture can change. For example, both Christian and Hindu mystics have regarded the socially constructed personality, with its desires, moods, selfish interests, and pursuits of pleasure as an undesirable cover over something quite sacred: the soul in one case and Atman in the other (Glucklich 2001: 208). Provided that the valued telos is consistent with the view of the "genuine" self – for example, intimacy with God, sacred community, ultimate reality, etc. – the pain that is used to shrink the distance between true agent and telos will be described as medical or transformative in other ways.

A briefer and technical way of describing this relationship is as follows: telic-centralizing pain is valued and telic-decentralizing pain is abhorred (Bakan 1968). Due to the way many religious traditions have viewed personal agency and the purpose of life, pain has been described in positive terms and has been sought out in a variety of ritual contexts. However, none of this explains how pain actually functions to bring individual agency into resonance with a broader telos. That is, how does the individual's willingness to undergo pain contribute to goals that are defined by his or her culture? Is the explanation a physiological and even neurological phenomenon? Is there a social or cultural component to this process? A number of theories have been proffered, ranging from neurological to economic, and a brief survey will clarify the conceptual options available for various levels of scientific reduction.

The majority of contemporary theories, and those that have attained the widest circulation are evolutionary. In that category one can situate the works of Harvey Whitehouse, Richard Sosis, Christopher Olivela and Eldar Shafir, Brock Bastian and his colleagues, Rob Nelissen, and several others. The overarching theme that emerges from all of these research programs is the thesis that voluntary pain contributes to sociality, to social solidarity, or to the cohesiveness of social and cultural groups. The relationship between the pain and the social benefit is not always direct, but social evolution is always there.

For example, Olivela and Shafir (2013) have demonstrated experimentally that anticipation of pain and/or effort increases prosocial behavior despite what appears to be a "hedonic puzzle." That is, the commonsensical expectation that it is pleasure or reward that would be more effective for improving prosocial behavior, rather than pain, turns out to be incorrect. One mechanism involved is suggested by Bastian et al. (2014). These researchers argue, based on experimental findings, that pain enhances sociality because it increases individual ability to exercise self-control, which is essential for eliminating antisocial impulses and actions.

Other social theories are more overtly evolutionary in focusing on dimensions of pain behavior that are nearly ethological in their simplicity. For instance, Richard Sosis with Candace Alcorta (Sosis and Alcorta 2003) have published a series of highly cited studies on ritual pain. This work has supported the familiar argument that painful ritual participation increases social bonds. According to Sosis, the mechanism is the trust and cooperation that develops between ritual participants who undergo pain. The toleration of pain acts as a costly signal of in-group commitment. The more painful or costly the ritual, the harder it becomes to fake the willingness to pay and hence the signal becomes compelling or persuasive.

Interestingly, Rob Nelisson (2012) has taken signaling theory a step further, arguing that pain can signal remorse for some antisocial conduct (however hidden). This is a solid step in linking self-harm and guilt, not just as a prosocial mechanism but as a psychologically satisfying event, perhaps because it triggers the anticipation of social approval by those to whom one is signaling in the act of self-hurting. The approval is for the demonstration of remorse, which is a socially integrative emotion.

The scientific theories on the socially constructive role of pain extend to culture as well. Harvey Whitehouse (1996) has conducted wide-ranging and large-scale studies of painful rituals. He began this project with the ethnography of a millenarian cult in Papua New Guinea. He subsequently divided religious groups into large- and small-scale organizations and came up with the concept of "modes of religiosity" to characterize the doctrinal mode, with its routinized orthodox approach, in contrast with the imagistic mode that has its own infrequent and arousing – often dysphoric – rituals. Both modes are largely concerned with the transmission of religious information. Repetitive and doctrinal content passes via the first mode and rare and climactic via the other. In his work, Whitehouse is particularly interested in memory, which he regards as episodic for the doctrinal mode and schematic for the imagistic mode. The overall framework for this theorizing is cognitive-evolutionary. It seeks to answer such questions as, what are the cognitive mechanisms that allow for the survival and prospering of religious groups? The answer is either endlessly repeated doctrine and re-enacted ritual practice or rare but traumatic "rituals of terror" like the painful initiatory rites of New Guinea. Ritual pain, to conclude, acts as a central tool in the transmission and retention of cultural information.

Other studies have backed up various aspects of these broad conclusions. Phillip A. Mellor (2010) has shown how the religious use of pain as a bodily technique contributes to the production of cultural meanings and identities by internalizing cultural norms. Andrew Crisilip (2012) focused on late ancient Christianity to explain how involuntary pain (illness) becomes ascetic practice and thus culturally meaningful as obedience to the advice of Jesus. Collectively, this body of research supports the thesis that religiously valorized self-hurting acts as a socially integrative technique (increasing cooperation, altruism, and even self-sacrifice) and reinforces cultural ideologies by enhancing the assimilation of values, providing explanatory or coping schemes (such as theodicy or explanation of evil; see also Chapter 26, this volume) and reinforcing moral codes (through remorse and penance).

But religious self-hurting also functions as a powerful tool in individual psychological ways. To be sure, when the sociocultural dimension – the telos – is ignored, such pain can be taken as a highly dysfunctional fact. For example, Roy Baumeister (1991) has placed ascetic pain in the same context as alcoholism and masochism as "flights from the burden of self-hood," because it undermines what he regards as healthy agency. Empirically, in regards to agency, Baumeister is correct. Glucklich's *Sacred Pain* (Glucklich 2001) proves a number of theories – such as that of Ronald Melzack (1993) – accounting for the ways that painful overstimulation undermines agency. (See also Chapter 14, this volume.) However, agency is a sociocultural construct and while self-hurting alters one's sense of self, if the pain directs the individual toward a prized telos (God, community) the agency of the self-hurter may actually be strengthened in some meaningful sense. It is therefore important to study the phenomenon of religious self-hurting on multiple levels – individual psychology (including neuropsychology), social dynamics, and even ideology – understood as those values that both rationalize the goals of pain and strengthen cultural norms through the display of painful behavior.

5 Conclusion

If one were to evaluate the self-hurting conduct of countless Christian, Muslim, and other religious technicians like Heinrich Suso, Maria Maddalena de' Pazzi, etc., the full range of theories summarized above would have to be utilized. Short of that, it would be too easy to fall into the trap of anachronism, that is, projecting backwards our own culture of individuality and medical economy. It is self-evident that most of us undergo pain as a medical problem, and even religious patients turn to religion for help in coping, not for ways of valorizing the pain or channeling it for some benefit. Nonetheless, the still widespread distribution of pain rituals such as pilgrimage, Shi'ite Ashura, Hindu Kavadi, or even the urban subculture of piercing and suspension, demonstrates that self-induced pain is not entirely archaic. Pain continues to serve religious actors on behalf of highly prized goals and understanding it is still a matter of understanding our world and that of our neighbors.

Related topics

Chapter 14: Pain, voluntary action, and the sense of agency (Beck and Haggard)
Chapter 26: The problem of pain in the philosophy of religion (Layman)
Chapter 31: An introduction to the IASP's definition of pain (Wright)

References

Bakan, D. (1968) *Disease, Pain and Sacrifice: Toward a Psychology of Suffering*. Chicago: University of Chicago Press.

Bastian, B., Jettern, J., and Stewart, E. (2013) Physical pain and guilty pleasures. *Social Psychological and Personality Science* 4: 215–219.

Bastian, B., Jetten, J., Hornsey, J., and Leknes, S. (2014) The positive consequences of pain: a biopsychosocial approach. *Personality and Social Psychology Review* 18: 256–279.

Baumeister, R. (1991) *Escaping the Self: Alcoholism, Spirituality, Masochism and Other Flights from the Burden of Selfhood*. New York: Basic Books.

Brena, S. (1972) *Pain and Religion: A Psychophysiological Study*. Springfield, IL: Charles C. Thomas.

Browning, E. (1994) *Aeschylus: Prometheus Bound*. Cambridge: Cambridge University Press.

Crisilip, A. (2012) *Thorns in the Flesh: Illness and Sanctity in Late Ancient Christianity*. Philadelphia: University of Pennsylvania Press.

Daniel, E. (1987) *Fluid Signs: Being a Person the Tamil Way*. Berkeley: University of California Press.

Deer, T. (ed.) (2013) *Comprehensive Treatment of Chronic Pain by Medical, Interventional, and Integrative Approaches*. New York: Springer.

Favazza, A. (2011) *Bodies under Siege: Self-Mutilation, Nonsuicidal Self-Injury and Body Modification in Culture and Psychology*. Baltimore: Johns Hopkins University Press.

Flynn, M. (1996) The spiritual uses of pain in Spanish mysticism. *Journal of the American Academy of Religion* 64: 257–278.

Glucklich, A. (2001) *Sacred Pain: Hurting the Body for the Sake of the Soul*. New York: Oxford University Press.

Graves, R. (1990) *The Greek Myths*, vol. 2. London: Penguin.

IASP (International Association for the Study of Pain) (2014) IASP Taxonomy. IASP. Updated 2014. <http://www.iasp-pain.org/Taxonomy>.

Kent, A. (2007) *Divinity and Diversity: A Hindu Revitalization Movement in Malaysia*. Singapore: NIAS Press.

McNeill, J. and Gamer, H. (eds.) (1938) *Medieval Handbooks of Penance*. New York: Columbia University Press.

Mellor, P. (2010) Saved from pain or saved through pain? Modernity, instrumentalization and the religious use of pain as a body technique. *European Journal of Social Theory* 13: 521–537.

Melzack, R. (1993) Pain: past, present and future. *Canadian Journal of Experimental Psychology* 47: 615–629.

Nelisson, R. (2012) Guilt induced self-punishment as a sign of remorse. *Social Psychological and Personality Science* 3: 139–144.

Olivela, C. and Shafir, E. (2013) The martyrdom effect: when pain and effort increase prosocial contributions. *Journal of Behavioral Decision Making* 26: 91–105.

Roberts, M. (1993) *Poetry and the Cults of Martyrs: The Liber Peristephanon of Prudentius*. Ann Arbor: University of Michigan Press.

Sahlins, M. (1996) The sadness of sweetness: the native anthropology of Western cosmology. *Current Anthropology* 37: 395–428.

Scarry, E. (1985) *The Body in Pain: The Making and Unmaking of Worlds*. New York: Oxford University Press.

Sosis, R. and Alcorta, C. (2003) Signaling, solidarity, and the sacred: the evolution of religious behavior. *Evolutionary Anthropology* 12: 264–274.

Thurston, H. (1990) *Butler's Lives of the Saints*, vol. 1. Westminster, MD: Christian Classics.

Tolstoy, L. (1886) *The Death of Ivan Ilych*, trans L. Maude and A. Maude. Electronic Classics, Pennsylvania State University. <http://opie.wvnet.edu/~jelkins/lawyerslit/stories/death-of-ivan-ilych.pdf>.

Twofeathers, M. (1996) *The Road to the Sundance: My Journey into Native Spirituality*. New York: Hyperion.

Whitehouse, H. (1996) Rites of terror: emotions, metaphor and meaning in Melanesian initiation cults. *Journal of the Royal Anthropological Society* 2: 703–715.

24

THE ROLE OF PAIN IN BUDDHISM

The conquest of suffering

Palden Gyal and Owen Flanagan

> Seeing our pain as it is, is a tremendous help. Ordinarily, we are so wrapped up
> in it that we don't even see it. We are swimming in oceans of ice water of
> anxiety, and we don't even see that we are suffering. That is the most funda-
> mental stupidity. Buddhists have realized that we are suffering, that anxiety is
> taking place. Because of that, we also begin to realize the possibility of salvation
> or deliverance from that particular pain and anxiety.
>
> Chögyam Trungpa, The Truth of Suffering and The Path
> of Liberation *(Chögyam Trungpa 2009)*

This chapter begins by contextualizing the notion of existential pain in Buddhism and the
Buddhist discourse. The first half of the chapter discussing and examining how pain is
understood in Buddhism with an emphasis on its philosophical assumptions in making sense
of pain. In the second half, it analyzes and explains the causal theory of pain in Buddhism,
which necessarily demands discussion of fundamental concepts like the doctrine of dependent
origination and no-self. It concludes by asserting that the realization of suffering, impermanence, and interdependence as features of existence inspires us to lead a more compassionate
and caring life.

Now, to investigate the role of pain in Buddhism, it is crucial to take care of potential
semantic confusions of the word "pain" or "suffering" in the context of Buddhism and
Buddhist philosophy. The notion of *duhkha* (Sanskrit; Pali: *dukkha*) in Buddhism is the central
idea of existential "suffering," "stress," "dissatisfaction," or "pain," i.e., rendered in these
terms, and it is the fundamental conception of the human condition in the Buddhist worldview. This chapter maintains the term "pain" to describe this important existential notion of
suffering in Buddhism, which refers to not just physical pain but also psychological afflictions.
The central project of this chapter is to investigate the role of this notion of existential pain in
Buddhism and Buddhist practice. As indicated, the notion of *duhkha* or existential pain in
Buddhism not only includes ordinary everyday physical and mental pain, but it refers to a
deeper feature of existence where even in moments of deep satisfaction there is the penumbra
that this too will pass, that suffering and loss are around the corner, that what I now possess is
ephemeral. In that sense, there is an aspect of inseparability between pain and pleasure,
samsara and nirvana, as we shall analyze in this chapter.

1 The Four Noble Truths

The Four Noble Truths stipulate the fundamental conception of the human condition and the nature of human existence according to the Buddhist worldview. The Four Noble Truths were given in the first teaching of the Indian prince, Gautama Siddhartha or widely known as the Buddha, which he expounded subsequent to his "awakening" or "enlightenment" as the ultimate state of perfect knowledge or wisdom combined with infinite compassion. It is the attainment of understanding the true nature of reality and existence. In doctrinal terms, it is to achieve a state of perfect realization of both ultimate and relative modes of existence or the two truths as discussed in the third section. To put it succinctly, the Buddha declared the following as he fully realized the Four Noble Truths:

a   All is suffering.
b   Suffering is caused by desire and attachment.
c   Suffering can be eliminated.
d   The Noble Eightfold Path can lead one to the end of suffering.

Now, even though a certain conception of pain or suffering seems to characterize all major religious traditions as an aspect of the human condition, for Buddhism, the idea of pain or *duhkha* is positioned at the foundation of its teachings. Ariel Glucklich examines the role of pain experiences across a wide range of religions in Chapter 23 of this volume. Buddhism seems to be one of the few religions that locate suffering or pain at the heart of its worldview. Suffering is not an attribute of life or human existence on earth. To exist as a sentient being is to suffer. Our desires exceed our capacity to satisfy our desires. Ego is rapacious. We desire not to be in "ordinary physical and mental pain," and we desire to get what we want, but there is ordinary pain and physical pain; we and our loved ones die. We get what we want and we no longer want it; it no longer satisfies us the way it once did, or the way we expected. There is disloyalty and betrayal. There are tsunamis and earthquakes, plagues, and wars. These experiences are of "ordinary physical and mental pain" in the sense that we experience them as immediate and conscious encounters. This is one of the three kinds in the typology of existential pain in Buddhism, as we shall explain in the following.

The first question that troubled the mind of the young Indian prince was "why does *duhkha* exist?" His second question was whether and how *duhkha* can be mitigated, possibly how it can be eliminated. Since suffering exists for sentient beings because sentient beings have egos, they want and desire things for themselves, the key to explaining why *duhkha* exists and how it might be mitigated or eliminated lies with ego. Ego is the sense of "self," "I," or self-identity that is the ground of all desires and attachments. The Noble Eightfold Path involves a threefold plan of action: the first two paths are right view and right intention ((1) and (2)) which fall under wisdom or *prajna* that requires the understanding of impermanence (*anitya*, Sanskrit; *annica*, Pali) and no-self (*anatman*, Sanskrit; *annata*, Pali); the prescription of right speech, right action, and right livelihood ((3), (4), and (5)) pertains to moral conduct or *sila*; and right effort, right mindfulness, and right concentration ((6), (7), and (8)) concern mental discipline or *samadhi* (Flanagan 2011). Different Buddhist traditions place differential but never exclusive emphasis on any of the three elements, and there is a general acceptance of their codependency in achieving proper human flourishing or *nirvana* (Flanagan 2011: 29). Thus one could maintain that the Noble Eightfold Path throws light on a Buddhist philosophy of education that emphasizes the training of both mind and heart/character aided by mindfulness for its instrumental import. A philosophy of education that is not just concerned with rational human intellect, but also equally attentive to human emotions. The threefold cord of wisdom, morality, and meditation offers an integrated method for leading a "flourishing" life in the Buddhist sense, and ultimately attend *nirvana*. This philosophy of education is inextricably linked to the notion of existential pain in Buddhism because it maintains that ignorance, desire, and jealousy are the root causes of existential pain. We can think of the Buddha as an educator, a psychologist, or a physician as he is often analogized to, and he began his forty-five years of teaching by contemplating the question: why do we suffer?

2 A study of existential pain

The Buddhist narrative of "The Great Departure" has it that the young Gautama Siddhartha resolves to leave the worldly pleasures of his palace following a series of exposures to sights of human suffering and mortality, and a commitment to finding a solution to end suffering (Strong 1995). Thus, it would not be wrong to approach Buddhism as a psychological study and investigation of existential pain (*duhkha*) as a fact about the human condition, and to think of the historical Gautama Buddha as a troubled mind trying to seek answers and a solution to the problem of suffering. As the fundamental teaching of Buddhism, the Buddha taught the Four Noble Truths as the first sermon, entitled "the first turning of wheel of *Dharma*" in the Deer Park of Varanasi, Benares, to the five ascetics (his former associates) who left Gautama Siddhartha in disgust when he began to pursue a path of moderation by giving up self-mortification and self-starvation in his quest for the supreme wisdom ("Setting in Motion of the Wheel of the Dhamma," in the *Saṃyutta Nikāya*, trans. Bhikkhu Bodhi 2000: 1844):

> Now this, bhikkhus, is the noble truth of suffering: birth is suffering, ageing is suffering, illness is suffering, death is suffering; union with what is displeasing is suffering; separation from what is pleasing is suffering; not to get what one wants is suffering; in brief, the five aggregates subject to clinging are suffering. Now this, bhikkhus, is the noble truth of the origin of the suffering: it is craving which leads to renewed existence, accompanied by delight and lust, seeking delight here and there; that is, craving for sensual pleasures, craving for existence, craving for extermination. Now this, bhikkhus, is the noble truth of cessation of suffering: it is the remainderless fading away and cessation of that same craving, the giving up and relinquishing of it, freedom from it, nonreliance on it. Now this, bhikkhus, is the noble truth of the way leading to the cessation of suffering: [l. 422] it is this Noble Eightfold Path; that is, right view … right concentration.

The Four Noble Truths are the foundation of Buddhism and the Buddhist worldview. They present the fundamental nature of human existence as one of pain or dissatisfaction (*duhkha*). The Buddha declares that his teaching is a "Middle Path" between the two extremes: the pursuit of desire and pleasure (hedonism) and the pursuit of pain and hardship (asceticism) – a path of moderation between the extremes of self-mortification and sensual indulgence. On the surface, the notion of the human condition as fundamentally pain or dissatisfaction (*duhkha*) may not appear to merit a wholly distinct philosophical and spiritual tradition or to be anything antithetical or antagonistic to Brahmanism, but it is the philosophical foundations of this worldview that shake the very foundations of the Brahmanical sociomoral worldview and establishes itself as a comprehensive philosophical system. For instance, the Buddhist analysis of self or the argument for *no-self* repudiates the fundamental notion of *atman* (self) in Brahmanism.

In explicating a thorough and comprehensive analysis of the notion, Buddhism offers a taxonomy or a hierarchy of different existential pains. The first Noble Truth, i.e., the truth of suffering, is explained and analyzed at three different levels or as three different forms against the background of and informed by the three characteristics or marks of existence. The three marks of existence are existential pain, impermanence, and no-self as the fundamental nature and characteristics of all phenomena. The three different levels or forms of the Buddhist investigation of existential suffering are: (a) the suffering of suffering; (b) the suffering of change; and (c) the pervasive suffering or the suffering of no-self (Garfield 2015: 7–8). The first (a) is the manifest suffering of all sentient beings, i.e., the physical suffering and discomfort that occur in events like death, ageing, hunger, thirst, and sickness, etc. It concerns physical pain as a condition or characteristic of existence which non-human beings too experience, as opposed to higher levels of pain in the psychological or mental realm. The suffering of suffering concerns a double or simultaneous encounter with two or multiple unpleasant experiences like melancholy from the death of one's beloved son while suffering from a chronic illness. The second (b) involves the suffering or pain brought about by the nature of impermanence of all phenomena. For instance, one can experience an exalted moment of joy and pleasure, but the potentiality and the nature of this momentarily "desirable" experience being subjected to change is suffering on a different level. The suffering of change is informed by the notion of impermanence or *anitya* (Sanskrit; Pali: *anicca*), as one of the three fundamental marks of existence, which maintains that all composite phenomena are subject to change. For instance, the pleasant experience of eating one's favorite ice cream could easily turn into a painful and unpleasant experience if s/he eats too much of it, or the desirable experience of basking in the afternoon sun could turn into a pain, a discomfort. At a doctrinal level, it means that all beings and things, having born or arisen, shall pass away or change. The fact that one's current "desirable" experience turns into a nuisance is something that even non-human animals undergo, but we assume that the awareness of the transient nature of a "desirable" experience is something that only humans can be cognizant of. (See Chapter 15, this volume.) Hence, they are referred to as "gross" and "subtle" impermanence (Garfield 2015: 40). The understanding of impermanence at a gross level involves realizing the changes over a certain period of time, whereas grasping impermanence at a subtle level involves having the awareness that everything changes at every moment. With the exception of having to realize the "subtle" impermanence, the first two forms of existential pain concern largely matters of everyday experience, and they are not "Buddhist truths" in the sense that they do not necessarily require robust philosophical argumentation or doctrinal ground, unlike the third (c) form of existential pain in Buddhism.

The third (c) form of existential pain concerns suffering arising out of human ignorance of the nature of reality, failure to understand the true nature of selflessness, impermanence, and dependent origination. It is a notion of existential pain from the perspective of Buddhist metaphysics, inextricably linked to and grounded on the notions of causal interdependence and no-self. We take ourselves (selfhood) to be entities existing independently and permanently because we are not cognizant of selflessness and interdependence of all things. Explicating the Tibetan philosopher Tsongkhapa's interpretation of *duhkha*, Jay Garfield explains that it is not mere ignorance, but the "positive superimposition of a characteristic on reality that it lacks" (Garfield 2015: 9). The positive superimpositions of characteristics onto reality that it lacks are our deluded perception of permanence of our phenomenal experiences and selfhood or ego, which are the main causes of our existential pain. When the Buddha declared that suffering could be eliminated, in one sense it meant the third form of existential pain, because like all beings the Buddha also endured all kinds of physical pains, including illness and death, and they are inevitable facts of existence. However, from the perspective of the theory of Karma, it meant all forms of existential pain, as we shall explain in the following section. Much of our psychological pain arises out of our ignorance, and only "enlightenment" or "awakening" to the true nature of reality and human existence could bring an end to this form of existential pain. The question of dealing with this subtler or higher form of existential pain requires the understanding of the fundamental Buddhist concepts like no-self, impermanence, and dependent origination.

3 The cause of suffering

The Buddhist analysis of existential pain suggests a hierarchical way of understanding and dealing with *duhkha* as a fundamental feature of existence. However, it is important to note that even mortality does not bring an end to one's existential pain. In this section, we will discuss the Buddha's Middle Path, which requires the understanding of concepts like no-self and dependent origination to explain the cause of existential pain and the human condition in Buddhist metaphysics. A brief discussion of the notion of karma is also important here because it helps us to contextualize and explain the causal theory of existential pain in Buddhism.

According to the Buddhist theory of *karma*, one's life process doesn't stop with the annihilation of the body (death) for the "mental continuum" or the individual stream of consciousness continues and takes a physical form elsewhere after death and keeps on taking on rebirth after rebirth until the individual achieves complete freedom or *nirvana* from this cyclic existence called *samsara* (Bhikkhu Bodhi 2005: 150). Without going into details of the Buddhist cosmological theory, Buddhism holds that there are six realms of rebirth (*bhavacakra* or the wheel of life: gods, humans, titans, ghosts, animals, and hell) where all beings take birth and rebirth governed by the law of karma. Keown uses an interesting analogy of karma functioning as the elevator in the building of Buddhist cosmology. Each floor designates different realms of existence, and it can go up or down (Keown 1996: 37). Karma, literally, means "action" and karmic actions are by definition moral actions, which means that they produce either good karma or bad karma. All karmically unproductive actions are neutral; they contribute nothing to one's spiritual or soteriological endeavors. The theory of karma functions like a metaphysical bank account of an individual's wholesome and unwholesome deeds, and depending on one's karmic currency, an individual being takes rebirth in different realms of rebirth or travels from one floor to another in Keown's Buddhist cosmology as the superstructure of a building (the topic of Buddhist ethics and moral prescription, or *sila*, is broadly addressed in the Noble Eightfold Path).

The second Noble Truth, the truth of the origin of suffering, is built on a theory of causality. The Buddha claimed his conception of causation or causal uniformity to be a "Middle Way" between the two extremes of *eternalism* and *annihilationism*, which attempts to find a mean between the former's claim of selfhood (*atman*) as unchanging and immutable, and the latter's complete denial of continuity altogether (Kalupahana 1992: 29). In the context of ancient Indian philosophical schools, the former refers to those who held the Brahmanical notion of *atman* and the latter to the materialists (the Charvaka/Lokayata) who completely rejected the notions of karma and rebirth. While it is clear from the theory of karma why the Buddha would reject the *annihilationist* stance, it is not obvious why he would reject *eternalism,* for he also propounds and posits a certain form of "continuity" across lives. This will be clear as we discuss the Buddhist conception of personal identity, and why his "middle path" is indeed a middle course of action between the two extremes. It is in his identification and elaboration of the second Noble Truth where the Buddha began to develop a systematic philosophical worldview that distinguished him from his contemporaries. While the Buddha claimed that "it is craving which leads to renewed existence, accompanied by delight and lust, seeking delight here and there; that is, craving for sensual pleases, craving for existence, craving for extermination" ("Setting in Motion of the Wheel of the Dhamma," in the Saṃyutta Nikāya, trans. Bhikkhu Bodhi 2000: see above), his analysis and explanation for the causes and conditions that give rise to existential pain propounds how our "primal ignorance" to the reality of our identity, impermanence, and dependent origination is the root cause and basis of craving, lust, jealousy, and all kinds of negative emotions.

The doctrine of *dependent origination* presents a detailed explication of the causal theory and describes the conditions that co-arise to cause existential pain and the continuation of *samsaric existence* – the condition of all sentient beings, it is believed, is to be caught in a continuous cycle of birth and death that arises from desire and attachment to a deluded view of the self and the nature of reality. The notion of dependent origination (*pratityasamutpada*) asserts that *existence* is in a constant flux or a series of interconnected phenomenal events, material and immaterial, without any real, permanent, and independent existence of their own, and it is best explained in the Twelve Links or the *Twelve Nidānas*, which most prominently appeared in the Pali *Nikāyas* as follows (quoted in Shulman 2008: 304):

> And what, monks, is dependent-origination? Dependent on (1) ignorance, monks, (2) mental dispositions. Dependent on mental dispositions, (3) consciousness. Dependent on consciousness, (4) name and form. Dependent on name and form, (5) the six bases (of the senses). Dependent on the six bases, (6) contact. Dependent on contact, (7) sensation. Dependent on sensation, (8) thirst. Dependent on thirst, (9) grasping. Dependent on grasping, (10) being. Dependent on being, (11) birth. Dependent on birth, (12) old age and death, sadness, pain, suffering, distress and misery arise. This is the origin of this whole mass of suffering. This, monks, I say is dependent-origination.

The Buddha is claimed to have said, "Whoever sees dependent origination sees the Dharma. Whoever sees the Dharma sees the Buddha," in *Majjhima Nikaya* (quoted in Sopa 1986: 105). The doctrine of the twelve links of dependent origination is the most central of all doctrines or theories in Buddhism, and in a sense, it is the hub where all Buddhist philosophical concepts or presuppositions come into position and play. For our purpose here, we will try to demonstrate how the twelve links of dependent origination present and explain the casual theory of existential pain. It begins by asserting that ignorance (*avidya*) is the root cause that triggers the samsaric existence. As indicated in the previous section, this ignorance is not mere "not knowing," but "not knowing" in the sense of misperception of ultimate reality, of the Four Noble Truths, and of transmigration and rebirth that gives rise to false views of reality and causes mental afflictions. Thus, ignorance is positioned at the root of all afflictions, and it leads to false thought-constructions or fabrication of the phenomenal world as perceived or misperceived through the six sense media. For instance, we misperceive the existence of an "I" or the reality of our perceptual world as permanent. Then contact (*sparsha*) happens between the sense organs (*shadayatana*), the sense objects (*nama-rupa*), and a moment of cognition or consciousness, and contact (tactile, visual, auditory, olfactory, gustatory, and mental) gives rise to "the capacity to utilize fluctuations of the object-field in terms of attractiveness, and neutrality" (Sopa 1986: 113). These fluctuations are sensations or feelings of pleasure, displeasure, or indifference produced through contact. Therefore, sensation or feeling (*vedana*) is based on contact such that different sensations of pleasant, unpleasant, or indifference are arisen. Sensation or feeling as the subject-side of the contact is taken to be the seat of karmic activity; craving or thirst (*trishna*) occurs here. It springs from the experiencing of feeling, which is caused and conditioned by karmic imprints from previous lives that come into their fruition fueling action and continuing the process of karmic production. Craving can take three forms: (a) sensual-craving, as in pursuing sensual desires; (b) becoming-craving, as attachment to one's own identity and experience; and (c) non-becoming-craving, as wishing to avoid or end one's own identity or experience (Thanissaro Bhikkhu 2008: 29). Grasping (*upadana*) is the process of appropriation and actualization of craving based on the five aggregates of form, feeling, perception, fabrication, and consciousness. This is where our desires are strengthened. For instance, through the experience of the phenomenal world that feeds sensations like craving, views of identity or "I-ness" are fabricated. Grasping sets in motion the process of becoming (*bhava*) as the coming into "existence" of craving and appropriation like a seed sprouting given all the necessary conditions like moisture and warmth. With becoming or *bhava* as the actualization and fruition of karmic seeds, it is the continuation and production of samsaric existence, and therefore, in a sense, becoming (*bhava*) and *samsara* are synonymous, though *becoming* is kind of an intermediate existence (Sopa 1986: 116). The eleventh link of dependent origination (*jati*) is the physical actualization of samsaric existence after a brief transition in *bardo* (intermediate state), and the last link of dependent origination is ageing and death, as the slow weakening of the five aggregates, the senses, and a unified consciousness in one body. The doctrine of dependent origination connects and presents the fundamental concepts in Buddhist metaphysics, including the theory of karma; and in particular, it explains how ignorance leads to craving and fabrication as the seed of existential suffering. Though it may demand more attention and elaboration, given the constraints of space and purpose here, we would like to discuss the doctrine of *no-self* in relation to its role dealing with existential pain in the following.

From the twelve links of dependent origination, we get a deeper understanding of how ignorance or misperception of reality leads to false constructions of reality and craving. The fabrication of an "I" or ego as an independent and permanent entity is the root cause of existential pain, the seat of karmic activity, which perpetuates an individual's cyclic existence in *samsara*. The teaching of no-self is an often misunderstood idea in Buddhism because it sounds as if Buddhists posit that there is no such thing as the self or person whatsoever, and therefore the ultimate end is *nirvana* understood as "extinction." Buddhists reject the ontological status of the self as the essence of a person – the part whose continued existence is essential for the person to exist (Siderits 2007: 32). The metaphysical theories of Buddhism maintain that all composite things are impermanent and all phenomena are empty of real, permanent, and independent existence (*svabhava*), including the false notion of self or "I." The Buddhist theory of personal identity as explicated in the doctrine of five *skandhas* claims that a person is an aggregate of five psychophysical elements. These are: (1) *rupa*: anything corporeal or physical; (2) feeling: sensations of feeling, pain, and indifference; (3) perception: those mental events whereby one grasps the sensible characteristics of a perceptible object like the color of a cap; (4) volition: mental forces responsible for bodily or mental activity; and (5) consciousness: the awareness of physical and mental states (Siderits 2007: 35–6). All of these *skandhas* are not only impermanent and subject to constant change, but also out of one's control. The most celebrated early Buddhist story explaining this concept is a conversation between the Greek King Malinda and the Buddhist monk Nagasena. Nagasena explains the doctrine of no-self with the analogy of a chariot (Siderits 2007: 50–4): the monk argues that there are no persons independent of the aggregates just as there are no chariots independent of their parts, and the names or words like "chariot" and "person" are only convenient designators. This logic of part–whole relationship and the idea that "chariot" is a convenient designator are crucial because they gesture toward the theory of two truths in Buddhism. Some philosophers maintain this theory of two truths to be the Buddha's most important philosophical contribution to ancient Indian philosophy, and the Buddhist philosopher Nagarjuna gave an exposition of and developed the theory profoundly in the second century (Thakchoe 2011). Although there is much debate among variants of theorists of the two truths, generally, the conventional truth refers to phenomenal truths or objects in our perceptual world as we experience and construct concepts and names like the chariot, and the ultimate truth rejects the ontological status of any object in the conventional or phenomenal world existing as an independent entity. Therefore, just as any object in the phenomenal world, a "person" is a conceptual fiction. It is indeed a convenient designator to fare in the conventional world but ultimately things are empty of independently existing essence. The realization and practice of this ontological attitude is key in Buddhism because such an attitude reduces our craving and attachment to the "self" that exists conventionally, and in turn mitigates our existential pain by realizing one of its main causes.

The centrality of understanding the concepts above in Buddhism is evident from the Noble Eightfold Path, which begins with "Right View" and "Right Intention" as the correct epistemic remedy for existential suffering. Right view entails the understanding of the Four Noble Truths, the three marks of existence, and the theory of karma and dependent origination. Most importantly, as suggested in our brief discussion of the theory of karma as the vehicle for *duhkha* or existential pain, in the twelve links of dependent origination we saw the connection that ignorance leads to craving which in turns causes karmic activity.

4 Conclusion

With the acceptance of *duhkha* as an inherent condition of existence, Buddhism offers methodical solutions to realistically reduce and ultimately eradicate existential suffering. The Noble Eightfold Path that involves what Flanagan calls the "threefold cord" offers an integrative approach that combines wisdom, morality, and meditation for alleviating existential pain (Flanagan 2011). Besides the deconstruction and debunking of the "self" in a philosophically gripping manner, there is an underlying pragmatism behind the notion of *anatman* in Buddhism. For instance, if there is no "self" in an ultimate sense, then there is no need for fear of death and there is little basis for clinging and ego. It is this realism that seems to make Buddhism an increasingly attractive and plausible worldview. As demonstrated, the issue of *duhkha* or existential pain is at the heart of Buddhist philosophy and across all Buddhist traditions, and it is the problem of existential pain that was the subject of the Buddha's rigorous philosophical and spiritual project. As a philosopher and physician, the Buddha investigated and diagnosed the causes of our existential pain and prescribed a set of practices that involves epistemic, ethical, and meditative training.

In light of the question whether pain plays a positive role in Buddhism, although it doesn't play a direct and positive role, the realization of the human condition as fundamentally *duhkha* and its arising from ignorance, attachment, and aversion is supposed to inspire a positive and more compassionate attitude to life. As some contemporary philosophers have wondered and contemplated upon, it is puzzling to think of how the *no-self* view of personhood engenders compassion and loving kindness for oneself or others (Flanagan 2011: 160). It is to ask the most fundamental question: what is the connection between the Buddhist metaphysic of the self and the ethic of compassion? An obvious Buddhist response to this would be to consider that subjective karmic imprints or impressions are believed to be stored and transmitted from one life to another, such that it encourages *right effort* to act and live a more compassionate life. This not only requires a metaphysical commitment to the law of karma, but also shows how the source of motivation for compassion is basically self-interest. A more sophisticated response to the question would require a deeper analysis of the ethic of compassion as understood in Buddhism. Compassion, as defined in classical Buddhist tradition, means "the heart that trembles in the face of suffering" (Feldman and Kuyken 2011: 144), and thus it is an orientation of the mind that recognizes the all-pervasive nature of suffering. The idea of compassion is constitutive of pain in the sense that it is a natural response to the recognition of existential pain. The realization of no-self or the fictional and impermanent nature of our existence generates a kind of compassion that is not directed to a particular individual or event but to existence itself in the face of the universality of pain in the world.

Related topics

Chapter 15: The lives of others: pain in non-human animals (Droege)
Chapter 23: Sacred pain: the use of self-inflicted pain in religion (Glucklich)

Further reading

Dīgha Nikāya: The Long Discourses of the Buddha: A Translation of the Dīgha Nikāya, trans. Maurice Walshe (Boston: Wisdom Publications, 1987).
Damien Keown, *Buddhist Ethics: A Very Short Introduction* (Oxford: Oxford University Press, 2005).
Walpola Rahula, *What the Buddha Taught* (New York: Grove Press, 1974).
Mark Siderits, "Buddha," in Edward N. Zalta (ed.), *The Stanford Encyclopedia of Philosophy* (Spring 2015 edition), <http://plato.stanford.edu/archives/spr2015/entries/buddha/>.

References

Bhikkhu Bodhi (trans.) (2000) *The Connected Discourses of the Buddha*. Boston: Wisdom Publications.
Bhikkhu Bodhi (trans. and ed.) (2005) *In the Buddha's Words: An Anthology of Discourses from the Pali Canon*. Boston: Wisdom Publications.
Feldman, C. and Kuyken, W. (2011) Compassion in the landscape of suffering. *Contemporary Buddhism* 12 (1): 143–155.
Flanagan, O.J. (2011) *Bodhisattva's Brain: Buddhism Naturalized*. Cambridge, MA: MIT Press.
Garfield, J.L. (2015) *Engaging Buddhism: Why It Matters to Philosophy*. Oxford: Oxford University Press.
Kalupahana, D.J. (1992) *A History of Buddhist Philosophy: Continuities and Discontinuities*. Honolulu: University of Hawaii Press.
Keown, D. (1996) *Buddhism: A Very Short Introduction*. Oxford: Oxford University Press.
Shulman, E. (2008) Early meanings of dependent origination. *Journal of Indian Philosophy* 36: 297–317.
Siderits, M. (2007) *Buddhism as Philosophy: An Introduction*. Indianapolis: Hackett Publishing Co.
Sopa, G.L. (1986) The special theory of pratityasamutpdda: the cycle of dependent origination. *Journal of the International Association of Buddhist Studies* 1(1): 105–118.
Strong, J.S. (1995) *The Experience of Buddhism: Sources and Interpretations*. Belmont, CA: Wadsworth Publishing Co.
Thakchoe, S. (2011) The theory of two truths in India. In E.N. Zalta (ed.), *The Stanford Encyclopedia of Philosophy* (Summer 2011 ed.). <http://plato.stanford.edu/archives/sum2011/entries/twotruths-india/>.
Thanissaro Bhikkhu (2008) *The Paradox of Becoming*. Access to Insight: Readings in Theravāda Buddhism. <http://www.accesstoinsight.org/lib/authors/thanissaro/paradoxofbecoming.pdf>.
Chögyam Trungpa (2009) *The Truth of Suffering and the Path of Liberation*. Boston: Shambhala.

25

PAIN AND THE DIVINE

Trent Dougherty

1 Introduction

This essay treats the following question: Can divine reality feel pain?[1] In so-called "Western religions" deriving from the Mediterranean, divine reality is generally considered to be an individual, personal being with a proper name such as "Elohim," "YHWH," "God,"[2] "Abba," or "Allah." In East Asian religions, divine reality is not generally conceived of as personal or even conscious. Thus the question hardly arises in religious traditions rooted in East Asia. In the personalist religions of the Abrahamic tradition, Judaism and Islam focus on God's transcendence in a way that Christianity – softened by the doctrine of the Incarnation – does not. Because Christianity holds that God became incarnate as a human, Christianity naturally raises our question more than do other traditions. After a brief survey of what various traditions have said, I will use as a focal lens recent work by Linda Zagzebski. In some bold new work, she defends a thesis that entails that the divine reality, taken to be the God of Christianity, experiences pain.

In Hinduism, one of the world's oldest religions, ultimate reality is inherently transcendent, despite immanent manifestation – in the form of polytheism – to common people. But of ultimate reality we are told that "it never feels pain, and never suffers injury" (Brihadaranyaka Upanishad 3.9.26). At the point of reaching Brahman, the self has transcended the realm of pleasure and pain (either by "absorption" into the One or by total annihilation or some other means).

Buddhism, as an outgrowth of Hinduism, seems to share this perspective. The first Noble Truth is that all life is suffering and the Eightfold Path to Enlightenment has as its destination Nirvana or the "unbinding" where all that troubles one – every form of desire – is gone. Of course, Buddhism is officially atheistic, so there is no divinity – either concrete or abstract – in the Buddhist ontology. Yet it is worth noting this agreement with Hinduism in order to treat the "divine" in the broadest possible sense.[3]

In Judaism, there is quite a split between the more anthropomorphic depictions of God in the Hebrew Scriptures, especially in the Pentateuch, and the main Jewish philosophers. In many places in the Hebrew Scriptures, God is portrayed as angry or jealous or in possession of other emotions, but perhaps the strongest statement comes in the description of God's frame of mind just before sending the Flood when assessing the wickedness of mankind.

"And the Lord was sorry that he had made humankind on the earth, and it grieved him to his heart" (Genesis 6:6, NRSV). This implication that God suffers emotionally at the hands of his creatures opens the door to the idea that God could feel pain. Indeed, if "pain" is taken widely enough – as I actually think it should – then this is just an *instance* of God feeling emotional pain. Later, we will narrow our scope to a stricter sense of "pain."

In stark contrast to the anthropomorphism of the Hebrew Scriptures are the words of Judaism's most illustrious philosopher, Maimonides. It is worth quoting him at length here.

> Whenever such evils are caused by us to any person, they originate in great anger, violent jealousy, or a desire for revenge. God is therefore called, because of these acts, "jealous," "revengeful," "wrathful," and "keeping anger" (Nah. i. 2), that is to say, He performs acts similar to those which, when performed by us, originate in certain psychical dispositions, in jealousy, desire for retaliation, revenge, or anger: they are in accordance with the guilt of those who are to be punished, and *not the result of any emotion: for He is above all defect!* The same is the case with all divine acts: though resembling those acts which emanate from our passions and psychical dispositions, *they are not due to anything superadded to His essence.*
>
> (Maimonides, trans. 1904: Guide for the Perplexed,
> 76–77, emphasis added)

In Judaism, there does not appear to be an official position with respect to where on the spectrum of anthropomorphism and abstraction one ought to be. Clearly enough, though, philosophical Judaism, as represented by Maimonides and the Maimonidean tradition developed by his followers such as Samuel Ibn Tibbon, has little place for God's feeling pain.

Christianity picks up this ambiguity for the most part, since it accepts the Hebrew Scriptures and developed out of Judaism. So the issue concerning the anthropomorphism of the Hebrew Scriptures recurs. There is a bit of anthropomorphism in the Gospels and Epistles, but far less.

Within the Christian theological tradition, one of the earliest clear statements by a fairly authoritative body is brief and to the point. "If anyone says that in the passion of the cross God felt pain, and not the body with the soul which the Son of God Christ had assumed he does not think rightly" (Council of Rome under Saint Damasus, CE 382, in Denzinger, *Enchiridion Symbolorum* 72).

The assumption here is that Jesus Christ was both human and divine, and he felt pain only in his humanity, or insofar as he was human, and not in his divinity, or not insofar as he was divine. This sentiment was expressed yet again over 200 years later in the Roman Council.

> Truly indeed we must believe and in every way profess that Our Lord Jesus Christ, God and Son of God, suffered the passion of the Cross *only according to the flesh;* in the Godhead however, he remained *impassible,* as the apostolic authority teaches and the doctrine of the Holy Fathers most clearly shows.
>
> (Roman Council, CE 860 and 863, under Saint Nicholas I,
> in Denzinger, Enchiridion Symbolorum 327)

We will discuss impassibility a bit at a couple of places below, but suffice it here to say that there is a strong tradition of affirming impassibility in God prior to the late twentieth century.

There is very little in Islam that treats the subject directly, but the very strong emphasis on God's transcendence and the influence of both late antique and medieval Judaism and

Christianity strongly suggest that God's feeling pain is very much not at home in Islamic theology.

In the next section, I consider a bold new view that is an apparent departure from this traditional view that God does not experience pain, at least *prima facie*. Others have argued against the doctrine of divine impassibility, but only Linda Zagzebski's recent work on omniscience both clearly entails that God feels pain, not just that God has negative emotions, and is grounded squarely in the theology of God's attributes. Therefore her work in that area will be the lens through which we focus on our question for the remainder of this chapter. First I will present an exposition of Zagzebski's theory. Then I will assess Zagzebski's arguments that God has the property of omnisubjectivity – arguments from omniscience and perfect empathy. Next, I consider some fairly obvious and traditional objections. Finally, I consider ways these objections could be circumvented.

2 On omnisubjectivity

I said at the outset that the question this chapter treated was whether divine reality felt pain. In the Christian tradition, there is much discussion of whether God "suffers," but almost invariably the question involves emotional suffering. I will focus on a theory which would have the direct implication that God felt "physical" pain, that is, that God hosted qualitatively identical phenomenal qualia (arguably non-physical things) as when, say, we stub a toe. That "physical" pain is indeed a particular quality of consciousness – one connected to our bodies in the right kind of way – is a thesis I shall not argue for here. (See Chapter 17, this volume, for discussion.) Few of the arguments against divine impassibility have any direct bearing on this thesis because they largely concern God having non-physical emotional responses to His creatures.

As we have seen, various traditions have had varying degrees of specificity with respect to the question of whether a divine being would or should be able to feel pain. The most developed treatment comes from within the Roman Catholic tradition of Christianity. This is not surprising, since that tradition is the most ambivalent to the question. On the one hand, God is conceived as being omnipotent and therefore able to avoid experiencing any suffering, including pain. But on the other hand, God is conceived as being omniscient and therefore would know what it is like to feel pain. Thus it is neither obviously ruled out nor obviously included. Furthermore, in the Christian tradition it is an imperative to balance the transcendent and the imminent in the divine due to the doctrine of the Incarnation and, thus, almost any Trinitarian Christian theism.

This ambiguity requires the adherent to explore the question in detail. This is just what Linda Zagzebski does in her seminal paper "Omnisubjectivity." In this section, I will explicate her view and present two arguments for it. I will also present rebutting arguments.

2.1 Setting it up

Zagzebski is very upfront about her proposal: "I propose that an omniscient being must have perfect total empathy with you and with all conscious beings. This is the property I call omnisubjectivity" (242).[4] Below, we will see what Zagzebski includes in an account of empathy. First, though, we'll sneak up on the issue a bit more to see its relevance to the present investigation.

To have omnisubjectivity is to exemplify "the property of consciously grasping with perfect accuracy and completeness the first-person perspective of every conscious being" (231).

More colloquially, it is "to know what it is like for conscious creatures to have their distinctive sensations and emotions, moods, and attitudes" (232). Clearly, then, if God is omnisubjective, then God feels pain. So, affirming omnisubjectivity is a very direct way to affirm that God feels pain. Since Zagzebski thinks omniscience entails omnisubjectivity, she'll see God's feeling pain as a heretofore little-noticed consequence of classical theism. (For more on contrasting the first- and third-person perspectives on pain, see Chapters 16 and 21, this volume.)

One reason she thinks omniscience entails omnisubjectivity is that she "take[s] for granted that if we could really 'get' what it is like to feel what another feels, see what she sees, and know what she knows from her own viewpoint, we would have a deeper and better kind of knowledge of her than if we merely know that she sees grey, feels frustrated, and knows she made a mess in the market" (232). This sounds sensible, and when combined with a perfect-being theology creates a *prima facie* expectation that God would have such a trait. But of course it is a *better* mode of knowledge only if it is a *possible* mode of knowledge. Otherwise, we'd have to say that perfect-being theology implies that God should be able to create a square circle. Thus, the key question is simply whether omnisubjectivity is logically possible. Zagzebski says little directly on behalf of its possibility as such (she does so indirectly, by arguing that God is omnisubjective and by providing a framework in which we might take ourselves to find it conceivable). Let's take a look at some of the details of Zagzebski's understanding in order to survey some of the issues that would have to be addressed in a full treatment.

For Zagzebski, the *reason* omniscience is supposed to entail omnisubjectivity is not because omnisubjectivity opens up another range of facts to be known. Indeed, it's not so much a form of knowledge at all that is at stake, but a form of *understanding*. Here, we should see omniscience not according to several common contemporary notions (Wierenga 2003; Freddoso 1984; Swinburne 1977; Hoffman and Rosenkrantz 2002) where, essentially, God knows the truth-value of every proposition. Rather, we should see omniscience as something like *ideal cognition* (Kvanvig 1990) or reroute the argument through ideal cognition. Ideal cognition requires of God not just unlimited breadth of knowledge, but unlimited depth of understanding.

Zagzebski's most specific claims regarding the requisite depth of understanding concern phenomenal qualia. "If any two qualia differ," she says, "God must be able to tell the difference between them. If the first person perspective on some state of affairs differs from the third person perspective on the same state of affairs, he must be able to distinguish them" (236). She further claims that "[t]he only way to distinguish qualia is to have them, and the only way to distinguish first and third person perspectives is to adopt those perspectives" (236). This is another discrimination claim, and so again is assuming an ideal-cognition notion of omniscience, since it requires not just knowing some fact, but the ability to make a fine discrimination that may or may not be a kind of knowledge. Let's grant the first claim about discrimination. What about the further claim about the "only way" to distinguish qualia? At first blush, this appears to be an unusual claim. For it's unclear why God couldn't just distinguish them by knowing which people are hosting them at which time. Furthermore, God could know the causal histories and consequences of the hosting of those qualia. *Prima facie*, this seems quite sufficient for God to distinguish between the qualia. At any rate, one wants to know why this would not be sufficient. It seems that, lurking alongside the ideal-cognition notion is the thesis that an ideal cognizer must know everything *in every way it can be known*. Knowing everything *in every way it can be known* entails knowing pain through feeling pain. And this property seems to go beyond omniscience to ideal cognition.

In the next section, in the course of discussing one of Zagzebski's arguments for the thesis that God is omnisubjective, I discuss the notion that there are multiple ways one and the same thing can be known.

2.2 The Argument from Omniscience

The first argument I will present in favor of the omnisubjectivity thesis is the broadest one I can glean from Zagzebski's text. It is, however, also the most loosely based on her actual words. Still, I think the argument is at least as strong and fits well with what she says.

The Argument from Omniscience

> Premise 1: God is omniscient.
> Premise 2: If God is omniscient, then he knows all the facts and knows them in all the ways they are known.
> Lemma: God knows all the facts in all the ways they are known. (From (1) and (2))
> Premise 3: One and the same fact is known in both third- and first-personal ways.
> Conclusion: God knows facts in both third- and first-personal ways.

Premise (1) can be taken as definitional. Premise (2) finds some motivation in perfect-being theology. For to know facts in all the ways they are known seems more perfect than not to do so. The question is what ways of knowing there are and what they come to. This makes premise (3) quite salient. One way to think about the matter is that there is a particular first-personal mode of presentation. We all know what it is like to come to learn that we are the subject of some action. Many times I grumble, "Who left the milk out again?!" only to realize later that it was me. When I say, "the person who got the milk out forgot to put it back" in this situation, the subject term "the person who got the milk out" refers to me. Thus, said sentence expresses the same proposition as "Trent forgot to put the milk back" since the subject phrase is a definite description which uniquely picks me out. Likewise for "I forgot to put the milk back" spoken by me, Trent. If we go with the coarse-grained theory that these sentences express the same proposition, we must admit that to bear the knowledge relation to that proposition via the modes of presentation captured in the different sentences makes for very different items of knowledge, since the propositions that are the relata are grasped by such different modes of presentation. They differ as much as *de re* and *de dicto* knowledge. This is not surprising, since we are up against the problem of *de se* knowledge. Zagzebski's suggestion is that God must know the facts via *each* mode of presentation to know them ideally.[5] *What it's like* to know what I express by "that same idiot left the milk out again" is very different from *what it's like* to know what I express by "I left the milk out again" even when I'm that idiot, when I *don't know* I'm the idiot. And this will be so regardless of the theory of propositions we hold. So if God must know each fact in each *way* it can be known, it appears he will have to adopt the first-person perspective on every proposition known by anyone.[6] And, as I discuss below, if God adopts the first-person perspective regarding a proposition concerning being in pain, then God feels pain.

Even if we accept the conclusion, it must be admitted, it is very hard to see what it would be for one being to adopt the first-person perspective of a distinct being. One initially thinks of the adopter essentially forgetting who they are, becoming absorbed in the perspective of the adoptee. But of course God could not forget he was God, so further explication of what it would even *be* to adopt the perspective of another would be a welcome addition to the picture. We will delve into this a bit more in the next section where we consider the argument from empathy.

2.3 The Argument from Empathy

In this section, I assess a more specific argument more directly anchored in Zagzebski's text. It finds its basis in the virtue of empathy. Since empathy is a virtue, a perfect being would be expected to display it perfectly. The argument is simple enough.

The Argument from Empathy

> Premise 1: God has perfect empathy.
> Premise 2: Perfect empathy entails taking the first-person perspective of others.
> Conclusion: God takes the first-person perspective of others.

This conclusion along with some plausible lemmas delivers the thesis that God feels pain. First we'll look at Zagzebski's account of human empathy. After that we will extend that account to divine empathy. This will set things up for evaluation of the key premise, premise (2).

Here are the key traits of human empathy, according to Zagzebski.

(i)   Empathy is a way of acquiring an emotion like that of another person.
(ii) When A empathizes with B, A thinks that the fact that B has a given emotion is a reason for her to have the same [or a very similar] emotion.
(iii) When A empathizes with B, A takes on the perspective of B.
(iv) When A empathizes with B, A is motivated from A's own perspective to assume the perspective of B.
(v)   An empathetic emotion is consciously representational. It loses its point once the target emotion disappears.

(238–240)

With respect to (i), I would have thought that empathy *just was* the ability to acquire an emotion in the right kind of way. But that's a small matter. It's important to consider how much follows from the acquisition of emotions. It's hard to believe that having the full perspective of another can be had just by having all their emotions. It is also controversial whether pain is an emotion, though I have defended the emotional view of pain.[7] However, on the assumption that pain is not an emotion, it is natural to extend the account of empathy to include acquiring the feelings of others, such as pain.

(ii) seems to me to overintellectualize empathy. Surely sometimes empathy is more intuitive and automatic than (ii) implies. Surely sometimes someone has empathy for another without thinking about reasons at all. But this is easily amended. Substitute for (ii), the following:

(ii★) When A empathizes with B, the fact that B has a given emotion motivates her to have the same (or a very similar) emotion.

(iii) is really too indeterminate to evaluate without an account of taking on a perspective. It will be easy for it to come out true on a loose reading. But on the closest specific reading in the neighborhood – that one literally takes on the first-person perspective of another – the question is, as I said above, what it would be for one being to adopt the first-person perspective of a distinct being.

I have little to say about (iv). Given that empathy is a virtue, it makes sense that it would be motivated from the virtuous perspective of the empathizing individual. But in her commentary on this item Zagzebski quotes from theorists whose ideas tend to work against the specific notion of perspective adopting Zagzebski seems to need for the strong reading of omnisubjectivity. For example, she quotes Goldman as saying that perspective adopting is "imaginatively assuming one or more of the other person's mental states." That does not seem to require literally acquiring the same first-person perspective as the object of empathy. Both Goldman and Oxley take perspective adopting to be "a kind of copy or simulation." It is unclear, to me at least, that copying or imagining or simulating really lets the empathizer know what it is like to be the object of empathy.[8] It is easy to see how it could get close, but it is hard to see how it could close the gap completely.

This leads quite naturally to the question whether this is a merely human limitation. Zagzebski says:

> If perfect empathy includes a complete and accurate representation of another person's emotions, perfect total empathy includes a complete and accurate representation of all of another person's conscious states. If A has perfect total empathy with B, then whenever B is in a conscious state C, A is conscious that B is in C and takes that fact to be a reason to acquire C herself. A acquires a state that is an accurate copy of C both in quality and in strength, and A is aware that her conscious state is a copy of C.
>
> *(241)*

Note that Zagzebski seems to be assuming that emotions are conscious states. This is not a universally shared view.[9] Furthermore, it's not perfectly clear to me whether, when she says that each person is in C, she is saying they are in type-identical states or whether they somehow indwell the same token state. I assume she means the former. Plausibly, type-identical phenomenal states are qualitatively indistinguishable. For this to entail the strong first-personal thesis, i.e., that one literally takes on the first-person perspective of another, the first-person perspective needs to be wholly accountable in qualitative terms.

For present purposes, however, what is relevant to our guiding question is not the strict first-personal claim but the qualitative duplicate claim. So we can weaken premise (2) for present purposes.

The Revised Argument from Empathy

Premise 1: God has perfect empathy.
Premise 2: Perfect empathy entails feeling the pain of others (understood thusly: hosting qualitatively type-identical phenomenal states).
Conclusion: God feels the pain of others.

This revised argument jettisons some of the baggage of the stronger argument but retains adequate strength to deliver the thesis that God feels pain. It would be good to briefly discuss plausible grounds for and objections to the premises of the Revised Argument from Empathy (RAE).[10]

Here is an argument for premise (1) of RAE:

Empathy Sub-argument (1)

Premise 1: God is a perfect being.
Premise 2: A perfect being has all virtues perfectly.[11]
Lemma: God has all virtues perfectly. ((1), (2))
Premise 3: Empathy is a virtue.
Conclusion: God has empathy perfectly. (Lemma and (3))

It is hard to disagree with any of the premises. They are all at least initially very plausible. The main problem that could arise would be if it were impossible for God to have certain virtues. For example, if one held to a strong enough doctrine of divine impassibility, then one may reject premise (2) of Empathy Sub-argument (1) simply on the grounds that the lemma is impossible.

Historically, the doctrine of divine impassibility has not primarily been that God does not *have* emotions or that God does not *experience* pleasure or pain, but, rather, that God is not *caused* (or, especially, caused *against his will*) to experience emotion, pain, or pleasure by creatures. So there are strong and moderate accounts of divine impassibility and corresponding arguments regarding God feeling pain.

Argument from Moderate Impassibility

Premise 1: God is perfect.
Premise 2: A perfect being cannot be caused to feel pain against his will.
Conclusion: God cannot be caused to feel pain against his will.

Argument from Strong Impassibility

Premise 1: God is a perfect being.
Premise 2: A perfect being can feel no pain.
Conclusion: God can feel no pain.

Clearly the Argument from Moderate Impassibility poses no threat to omnisubjectivity, for it is no part of that thesis that God's feeling pain is an effect caused against his will. The Argument from Strong Impassibility (ASI), on the other hand, does pose a threat, so we will briefly evaluate it, but it should be noted that the notion of impassibility at work in ASI is generally taken to be the minority position. The argument for premise (2) is intuitive and straightforward.

ASI Sub-argument

Premise 1: Feeling pain is a weakness(/vulnerability/liability).
Premise 2: All weakness (/vulnerability/liability) is imperfection.
Lemma: Feeling pain is an imperfection. ((1), (2))
Premise 3: A perfect being has no imperfections.
Conclusion: A perfect being can feel no pain. (Lemma and (3))

These are eminently sensible premises, so ASI presents a credible threat to the thesis that God feels pain. The main kind of reason plausibly advanced against premises (1) or (2) of ASI Sub-argument is that the ability to feel pain is the exercise of a power. We think animals are higher beings than plants because they have sentience and plants do not. Nociception is usually coincident with a form of sentience. More broadly, one simply might think that a being who can suffer along with creatures is a better, more perfect being than one who cannot (cf. Oord 2010). This latter move is liable to sound like wishful thinking or a confusion based on emotionalism to an advocate of the ASI Sub-argument, so there is likely to be a hard impasse here. It is clear that the literature needs more focused engagement by scholars representing the opposing perspectives on the notion of greatness involved and what would make feeling pain a great-making feature. Here is one line of question in particular that needs to be addressed. Does the notion of great-making that has the consequence that feeling pain is a great-making feature also have the consequence that feeling what it's like to hate on the basis of race is a great-making feature? If so, isn't that a reduction to absurdity?

3 Conclusion

If God is omnisubjective, then God feels pain. If God is omnisubjective, then God feels every kind of pain felt by any creature. So, in arguing for omnisubjectivity, Zagzebski is giving the most direct argument ever that God feels pain in the most detailed and robust sense heretofore known. I have outlined a research project for further study of this issue by raising a number of objections, pointing to unfinished business in the philosophy of language, and suggesting ways the view might be modified or otherwise motivated. A lot hangs on the possibility premise. Zagzebski avows "[i]t seems to me that it is possible that there is an omnisubjective being, at least, I know of no reason to think it is impossible" (242). I don't have any positive intuition that it is possible. I have a slight intuition that it is not, and I have expressed some honest skepticism about whether it is consistent with God's omnipotence and complete perfection. The ability to feel pain can present itself reasonably as both a perfection and an imperfection. Settling the matter is not easy. Clearly, further discussion of the possibility is warranted.

Related topics

Chapter 8: A neurobiological view of pain as a homeostatic emotion (Strigo and Craig)
Chapter 9: A view of pain based on sensations, meanings, and emotions (Price)
Chapter 16: Robot pain (Mandik)
Chapter 17: Pain and consciousness (Pereplyotchik)
Chapter 21: Can I see your pain? An evaluative model of pain perception (de Vignemont)

Notes

1 A related, but distinct question, is whether God *suffers* from experiencing pain. On some theories of pain, one can be in pain and not dislike it or desire for it to stop. I reject such theories (Dougherty 2014: ch. 2, §2), therefore, on my view, if God is in pain, God suffers. For the sake of space, this further question is not treated here.
2 In Christianity, "God" functions like a title term such as "President" or "Mom." In intimate cases, a title term functions also as a proper name. In this way, "God" functions like "Mommy."
3 For more on the role of pain and suffering in Buddhism, see Chapter 24, this volume.
4 All quotations in the section are from Zagzebski (2008) unless otherwise specified. She expands upon the notion in her 2013 book by the same name. Readers interested in finer details should consult that book.
5 And of course if the sentences express different facts, then it follows from the standard account of omniscience that God must know each of them.
6 One can envision an even stronger form of ideal-cognition theory according to which God must know every *possible* fact from every *possible* perspective, but that is too much to evaluate here. It may, however, serve as a basis for a *reductio* on the theory of omnisubjectivity.

7 Dougherty 2014: ch. 2, §2. For more on the idea that pain is an emotion, see Chapters 8 and 9, this volume.

8 The case could be different with imagining, if Jennifer Radden is correct that it is impossible to imagine pain without actually feeling pain. Thanks to Jennifer Corns for bringing this to my attention.

9 For more on the relation of pain and consciousness, see Chapter 17, this volume. Also, Robert Roberts thinks there can be unconscious emotions.

10 Zagzebski also offers an explanatory argument from the ability of omnisubjectivity to solve two puzzles of omniscience and to explain the property of actuality. I will not assess the strength of these indirect arguments here, as they would require us to go quite far afield.

11 To be just right, this premise would need to be further modified for arcane details, but it is easy to see how that process would go, and it is not relevant to present concerns.

References

Dougherty, T. (2014) *The Problem of Animal Pain: A Theodicy for All Creatures Great and Small*. London: Palgrave-Macmillan.

Freddoso, A. (1984) *The Existence and Nature of God*. South Bend, IN: University of Notre Dame Press.

Hoffman, J. and Rosenkrantz, G. (2002) *The Divine Attributes*. Oxford: Blackwell.

Kvanvig, J. (1990) Theism, reliabilism, and the cognitive ideal. In M. Beaty (ed.) *Philosophy and the Christian Faith*. Notre Dame: University of Notre Dame Press, pp. 71–91.

Maimonides, M. (1904) *Guide for the Perplexed*, trans. M. Friedländer. London: Routledge & Kegan Paul.

Oord, T.J. (2010) *The Nature of Love: A Theology*. Atlanta, GA: Chalice Press.

Swinburne, R. (1977) *The Coherence of Theism*. Oxford: Oxford University Press.

Wierenga, E. (2003) *The Nature of God: An Inquiry into Divine Attributes*. Ithaca, NY: Cornell University Press.

Zagzebski, L. (2008) Omnisubjectivity. In J. Kvanvig (ed.), *Oxford Studies in Philosophy of Religion*, vol. 1. Oxford: Oxford University Press, pp. 231–248.

26

THE PROBLEM OF PAIN IN THE PHILOSOPHY OF RELIGION

Steve Layman

The problem of pain is one aspect of the problem of evil. The problem of evil is generally considered the most important objection to traditional monotheism (the belief that there is exactly one God who is almighty, all-knowing, and perfectly good). "Evil" here refers to badness, as in "bad things happen to good people." And badness includes moral wrongdoing (e.g., assault and murder), loss (e.g., loss of health or loss of a loved one), and suffering. Suffering I take to be fairly intense and sustained pain, whether the pain is physical or mental in nature. So, we can speak of the "problem of pain" as one part of the problem of evil, the part that has to do with suffering in particular.[1]

By "physical pain" I mean the type of pain that has an apparent location in the body, e.g., a toothache or a sharp pain in the knee. By "mental pain" I refer to unpleasant experiences that do not have an apparent location in the body, e.g., feeling thoroughly miserable, feeling deeply depressed, feeling extremely anxious, and feeling very afraid. I emphasize that suffering is fairly intense and sustained pain. For example, a minor muscle ache is a form of pain but it would hardly count as suffering, and neither would a momentary pain even if it is a very sharp pain.

1 Rowe's formulation

A well-known formulation of the problem of evil by William Rowe accords suffering (and hence, pain) a central role (Rowe 1979: 336):

1 There exist instances of ... suffering which an omnipotent, omniscient being could have prevented without thereby losing some greater good or permitting some evil equally bad or worse.
2 An omniscient, wholly good being would prevent the occurrence of any ... suffering it could, unless it could not do so without thereby losing some greater good or permitting some evil equally bad or worse.
3 [So,] There does not exist an omnipotent, omniscient, wholly good being.

Why accept (2)? Consider an example. Suppose you have been seriously injured and a physician knows she could heal you in either of two ways: (a) simply by having you take one pill that has no harmful side effects or (b) by performing invasive surgery which would involve much post-operative pain over several months. A physician who opted for (b) in these circumstances would rightly be regarded as morally flawed – definitely not "wholly good." In the light of examples such as this, (2) seems very plausible.

Rowe's defense of premise (1) has become a focal point in philosophical discussions of the problem of evil:

> Suppose in some distant forest lightning strikes a dead tree, resulting in a forest fire. In the fire a fawn is trapped, horribly burned, and lies in terrible agony for several days before death relieves its suffering.
>
> *(Rowe 1979: 337)*

Clearly, an almighty God could prevent the fawn's suffering, e.g., by painlessly euthanizing the fawn. What greater good would be lost if God did that? Theists have struggled to locate plausible answers to such questions.

For present purposes, one thing is especially noteworthy about Rowe's example: it gets much of its force from our knowledge of what it feels like to be burned. Rowe is counting on his readers to understand that the fawn is undergoing an experience that is very unpleasant and hurtful.

2 Types of theistic responses

Theists may respond to the problem of pain in at least four basic ways. First, they can offer a theodicy, i.e., they can suggest reasons God has, or might have, for allowing suffering. We'll consider an illustrative theodicy momentarily.

Second, theists may offer the "overrider" response, i.e., they might simply admit that the suffering in the world counts as evidence against theism, but insist that this evidence against theism is overridden by other evidence that favors theism. Of course, this response is only as good as the evidence for theism, and many philosophers would deny that the evidence for theism is strong enough to play this role.

Third, many theists are so-called "skeptical theists," i.e., they call into question the assumption that we humans would be likely to know God's reasons for allowing suffering, assuming God has such reasons. We humans are perhaps a bit like a novice chess player who cannot fathom why a chess master has made a certain move. The novice would be foolish to reason thus: "I see no good reason for the chess master to move his rook *there*; hence, the chess master has no good reason to move his rook *there*." Similarly, because God is omniscient and the world is very complex, we would be foolish to infer that God has no good reasons for allowing suffering since we are unable to conceive of any such reasons. Skeptical theism is not without plausibility, but it comes at a cost. Traditional monotheism is a worldview and a worldview is supposed to help us make sense of our lives and of our place in the world. And while no worldview can explain everything, failing to explain some salient feature of our experience, such as suffering, is a serious deficit, especially if there are other worldviews that can explain such phenomena well. Thus, the most plausible versions of skeptical theism claim only that we should be skeptical about our ability to grasp God's reasons for allowing every instance of suffering and/or the total amount of suffering. These versions of skeptical theism can be combined with other responses to the problem of pain, e.g., with theodicies that offer explanations of much (but not all) suffering.

Finally, theists might offer the comparative response, i.e., they might argue that although theism does not explain every case or type of suffering, the main alternative views also have difficulty in accounting for the phenomena of suffering *in terms consistent with their philosophical underpinnings*; hence the problem of pain is not a good reason to reject theism in favor of the main alternative views. The comparative response is illustrated below in the case of philosophical naturalism.

3 The soul-making theodicy

John Hick's "soul-making" theodicy is perhaps the most promising theodicy on offer:

> God's purpose was not to construct a paradise whose inhabitants would experience a maximum of pleasure and a minimum of pain. [Instead] the world is ... a place of "soul making" ... in which free beings, grappling with the tasks and challenges of their existence ..., may become "children of God" and "heirs of eternal life."
>
> *(Hick 1990: 45–46)*

From this perspective, God has given us the power of making significant free choices. We can choose to help or harm one another. God could have made robots, without free will. But God wants us to freely choose the way of love – love of God and love of neighbor. Our freedom makes human life profoundly meaningful and provides the opportunity to develop virtues such as love, compassion, patience, and courage. God might have made a world in which suffering was excluded, but in such a world humans would arguably have lives of much less moral significance than in the actual world. While we may at times envy those who have relatively easy lives, we admire those who have faced serious hardship and suffering with courage, patience, and hope. Similarly, we admire and honor those who have sacrificed to help others who are suffering and in need. In short, a world with the many challenges and evils our world contains is one in which human beings can develop their best traits and capabilities.[2]

But theists generally claim that there won't be any suffering in heaven. So, why didn't God put us in heaven to begin with and skip this vale of suffering? From a theistic point of view, this question overlooks the great value of becoming a certain kind of person, a virtuous person. As Hasker notes:

> A courageous woman is different from a coward, even when no danger is present; the love of a person who has learned compassion and self-sacrifice has a distinctive quality even when no one is presently suffering. ... Heroes in many walks of life are often ... honored long after age and/or changed circumstances have made a repetition of their heroic achievements impossible ... . Such persons are valued for what they *are* and for what they *have done*, rather than for what they may yet do.
>
> *(Hasker 2004: 33)*

Furthermore, by giving us the opportunity to make moral and prudential choices in a setting involving hardship and trials, we are given a significant degree of choice regarding the sort of persons we will be. Beyond this, theists typically believe that a virtuous character is necessary for the sort of close relationship with God in which heaven consists. And many theists believe that the moral rigors of this earthly life prepare us for important spiritual tasks we'll be called upon to perform in the life after death.

But the soul-making theodicy seems to come up short in some cases. For example, it is surely inapplicable in the case of Rowe's fawn. And the suffering of children who die very young – too young to have had a chance to develop the virtues, does not seem to be explained by the soul-making theodicy. Is their suffering simply a means to the soul-making of others? Such a suggestion hardly seems compatible with the thesis that God is wholly good.

But the soul-making theodicy can and should include the idea that natural evil (i.e., the suffering caused by non-human factors such as diseases, earthquakes, and tornadoes) is caused by the operation of laws of nature. After all, an environment governed by laws of nature seems to be needed for soul-making because free action requires an environment that is predictable to a significant degree. Just consider a simple act such as walking across a room to give another person a loaf of bread. Such an act is taken on the assumption that the loaf of bread won't suddenly evaporate, that gravity won't fail, and that the recipient won't suddenly turn into a stone. Furthermore, the challenges and dangers of the natural world provide much of the stimulus for soul making.

But surely almighty God could create an environment governed by natural laws that do not produce devastating hurricanes, debilitating diseases, and so on? With this suggestion, however, the critic of theism wanders into highly speculative territory, for contemporary science tells us that our universe is "fine-tuned" for life. Extremely minor changes in the fundamental laws of nature would very likely produce a universe that would not support life. So, no one can say with confidence that God could create a physical universe that both supports life and is governed by laws of nature that do not produce natural evils.[3]

But almighty God can do miracles, so God can always intervene to prevent suffering (e.g., God could relocate Rowe's fawn so that it doesn't get burned). Yes, but as Hasker points out, God's "constant interference ... would negate the uniformity of natural order," which seems necessary for free action and soul making (Hasker 2004: 39). But a wholly good God is surely obligated to intervene in order to prevent the most intense instances of suffering, right? As Hasker points out, however, this assertion needs to be backed up by some plausible moral principle that distinguishes the natural evils God is obligated to prevent from those God is not obligated to prevent. And drawing up such a principle is no easy philosophical task (Hasker 2004: 39).

At this point it is also worth noting that reflections on the moral life may lead theists to question Rowe's second premise (which I here shorten slightly for the sake of convenience): *An omniscient, wholly good being would prevent the occurrence of any suffering it could, unless it could not do so without thereby losing some greater good.* Suppose a theist – let's call him Theo – who accepts Rowe's second premise is considering whether to inflict suffering on someone. Theo reasons as follows: "If the suffering is not necessary for a greater good, God will prevent me from inflicting it. But if I am successful in inflicting the suffering, then it is necessary for some greater good – a greater good that will be lost if the suffering does not occur." Hasker points out that this way of thinking about suffering undermines morality (Hasker 2004: 58–75). Virtuous acts would then often or even routinely be contrary to the greater good. And when we think about people inflicting suffering on others, we do not generally suppose that if the suffering is inflicted, it was necessary for some greater good. So, from this perspective, if God allows us to choose between good and evil, we ought to think that the evils are often gratuitous, i.e., not necessary for any greater good.[4]

The above discussion, though brief, illustrates three important things, it seems to me. First, it shows that the problem of pain raises many challenging questions for theism. Second, I believe it indicates that theists have reasonable answers to many of those questions. But third, it strongly suggests that theists have difficulty in producing a theodicy that explains all instances of suffering in a satisfying way. For example, it seems to me that the question, "why doesn't God intervene more often to prevent suffering?" is not given a fully satisfying answer.

4 The comparative response illustrated

At this point theists might have recourse to skeptical theism. Or they might offer the comparative response, that is, they might admit that theism lacks a fully adequate theodicy but argue that the main alternative views also have difficulty in accounting for the phenomena of suffering *in terms consistent with their philosophical underpinnings*; hence the problem of pain is not a good reason to reject theism in favor of the main alternative views. I will now illustrate the comparative response in the case of philosophical naturalism, which I take to be the chief contemporary rival of theism. Naturalism is the view that there is no God or anything like God (e.g., no angels or non-physical souls) and everything is physical. To clarify, the comparative response, as applied in the case of naturalism, is not an argument for the conclusion that naturalism is false; it is an argument for the conclusion that naturalism falters in accounting for the phenomena of suffering; hence, the phenomena of suffering do not provide a good reason to reject theism in favor of naturalism.

Before proceeding, it will be helpful to elaborate a bit on the phenomena of suffering. It is widely agreed that the phenomena of suffering commonly include at least the following:

(A) Certain subjective conscious experiences, for example, the hurtfulness of physical pain, the feeling of being miserable, the agony of anxiety, the dreadful feeling of depression, and the raw fear of more suffering to come.

(B) Suffering enters into a variety of causal relations. For example: (1) A person experiencing severe chronic pain may opt for suicide as a means of avoiding any further feelings of an extremely unwelcome sort. Here suffering seems to be among the causes of behavior. (2) The belief that others have been harmed or killed can cause suffering in the form of deep sadness, anxiety, or despair. Here a mental state (a belief) is apparently the cause of (or among the causes of) suffering. (3) After an earthquake, a family may sleep outside and suffer in the bitter cold because they fear that aftershocks will cause their house to collapse. Here suffering apparently results (in part) from the mental state of fear.

Just as theists falter in their attempt to explain why God would permit certain types of suffering, naturalists arguably falter in providing an adequate explanation of (A) and/or (B).[5] But for naturalists the problems arise because of weaknesses in their theories of the mind. To see this, we must examine a series of naturalistic theories of the mind. Of course, we cannot here examine every possible naturalistic theory, but perhaps enough can be said to highlight the challenging sorts of questions naturalism faces.

4.1 Epiphenomenalism

Epiphenomenalists hold that mental states are caused by physical states, but mental states themselves cause nothing. From this perspective, mental states are analogous to the shadows cast by a car as it moves down a road; the shadows are caused by the car's blocking the sun's rays but the shadows do not in turn have any causal effect on the car's motion. (Mental states do not cause physical states, such as brain states.) Nor is the shadow at a given moment caused by the shadow from the preceding moment; the shadows are caused by the car. (Mental states do not cause other mental states.)[6] Epiphenomenalists admit the reality of mental states, including the reality of subjective conscious experiences of pain. But by denying mental states any causal powers, epiphenomenalists must deny all of the phenomena included in (B) above. Relatively few naturalists endorse epiphenomenalism; the clash with common sense is simply too great.[7] It is hard to believe, for example, that pain does not cause victims of torture to scream or to feel fear. Nevertheless, as we shall see, some commonly held naturalistic theories of the mind seem to lead to ephiphenomenalism by implication.

4.2 Non-reductive physicalism

Non-reductive physicalism is a position favored by many philosophers, including many naturalists.[8] On this view, humans are entirely physical entities; they do *not* have non-physical souls. And mental states *supervene* on physical states, i.e., if one is in a mental state M, one is in that state by virtue of the fact that one is in a certain physical state P, and "anything that has P at any time necessarily has M at the same time" (Kim 2006: 198). But mental states are not wholly reducible to (and are not identical with) physical states (Kim 2005: 34). (By way of contrast, *reductive* physicalists hold that mental states are nothing over and above physical states.) Finally, mental states (or events) are causes; they can cause both physical states (or events) and mental states (or events) (Kim 2005: 35). For example, a decision (mental event) can cause my arm to rise (physical event). And the desire for food (a mental event) can cause the thought, "some pasta would taste good" (another mental event).

Jaegwon Kim has formulated an important objection to non-reductive physicalism, called the exclusion argument, which can be outlined as follows (Kim 2005: 194–197):

1   If a physical event has a cause, then it has a sufficient *physical* cause.
2   So, each brain-event (that has a cause) has a sufficient physical cause.
3   If a given brain event has a sufficient physical cause, it does not also have a mental cause.
4   So, mental events never cause brain events (and hence they never cause physical events, including bodily movements).

Premise (1), the "Closure Principle," is routinely assumed by scientists in all their research, including neuroscientists. And it is generally accepted by both non-reductive and reductive physicalists. Step (2) merely applies the Closure Principle to brain events. At this point it may be useful to construct a sort of picture to help us think about Kim's argument:

$$M_1 \qquad\qquad M_2 \qquad\qquad M_3$$
$$| \qquad\qquad\quad | \qquad\qquad\quad |$$
$$B_1 \quad\rightarrow\quad B_2 \quad\rightarrow\quad B_3$$

Suppose B_1, B_2, and B_3 are brain states and that M_1, M_2, and M_3 are mental states. The vertical lines tell us that the mental states supervene on the brain states. For example, M_1 supervenes on B_1 – if a person is in B_1, then he or she must be in M_1. The arrows tell us that B_1 is a sufficient cause for B_2 and that B_2 is a sufficient cause for B_3. (This is just a simplified way of picturing the point that brain states have sufficient *physical* causes.) The question, in essence, is this: if B_1 fully causes B_2, and B_2 fully causes B_3, what causal role do the mental states M_1, M_2, and M_3 play, if any? Step (3) gives Kim's answer: the mental states do not cause any brain states at all. How does Kim arrive at this answer? It is of course *logically possible* for an event to have two sufficient causes. For example, two assassins might strike a lethal blow at the same person and at the same moment. But given that B_1 is a sufficient cause of B_2, what distinctive causal role does M_1 play? It seems merely to ride piggyback on B_1, given that it supervenes on B_1.[9] Thus, non-reductive physicalism seems, by implication, to lead us to deny that there are mental causes of physical events – including actions.

An example may help to clarify Kim's point. Imagine that the functions of my smartphone supervene on the matter that constitutes it. I throw the phone at the window and the window breaks. Did my phone cause the breakage? It is natural to answer, "yes." But obviously, any physical object having the size, shape, weight, and solidity of my phone would also cause the window to break (if I threw it at the window). The information-processing functions of the smart phone make no distinctive causal contribution to the breaking of the window. They simply ride piggyback on the matter that constitutes the phone. Therefore, it seems we are speaking very loosely when we say the smart phone caused the breakage. The true causal account has nothing to do with the distinctively smartphone-ish aspects of the object. And Kim's point is that supervening mental states would similarly make no causal contribution to physical events in the brain.[10]

The exclusion argument also seems to force the non-reductive physicalist to deny that one mental state ever causes another mental state. For, given that mental states depend on physical (brain) states for their existence, causing a mental state requires causing the brain state it depends on. For example, in order to cause M_2, M_1 must cause B_2. Thus, mental–mental causation presupposes mental–physical causation. But as we have just seen, the exclusion argument rules out mental–physical causation. In short, the exclusion argument seems to show that non-reductive physicalism inadvertently leads to epiphenomenalism.[11]

4.3 Reductive physicalism

Reductive physicalists claim that mental states are wholly *reducible* to physical states, i.e., mental states are nothing over and above physical states. An example of reductive physicalism is the mind–brain identity theory, i.e., the view that mental states are identical to brain states. A standard objection to this theory is that it fails to account for subjective conscious experiences. No amount of information about the brain, neurons, dendrites, axons, and so on, tells us *what it is like* to feel a sharp pain or to smell ammonia. We might put the point this way: Suppose we could provide an extraterrestrial visitor with a complete set of biological facts about the human body, including all the neurobiological details about the workings of the human brain. If we confine ourselves to these physical facts, we leave out something important, namely, such subjective conscious experiences as the feeling of pain or the fear of falling.

A common reply is that the complete physical description does not leave out these subjective conscious experiences, it merely refers to them under a different (i.e., neurobiological) description. But here many philosophers agree with John Searle: a description of the world under third-person physical terms, such as scientists provide, is not a complete description of the world. What is left out is precisely the subjective, first-person, conscious phenomena, e.g., *what it is like* for a person to experience a dull ache or to feel dizzy (Searle 2004: 97–98). And Thomas Nagel is making the same point with his famous question, "what is it like to be a bat?" Imagine a researcher who can fully describe, in neurobiological terms, the workings of a bat's brain. Her account leaves out what it is like to experience the world in the way a bat does. And thus an interesting and important *feature of reality* has been omitted (Nagel 1974: 435–450). *Facts about first-person, conscious experiences are not metaphysically reducible to facts about neurobiology.*

Reductive functionalism is another form of reductive physicalism.[12] According to functionalists, a given mental state can be defined as an *internal state* of a person that serves as the causal link between inputs from the environment and outputs in the form of behaviors and other mental states. For example, pain can be defined as an internal state that serves as the causal link between tissue damage (e.g., a dog bite), behaviors (e.g., screaming, running away), and other mental states (e.g., being afraid or angry). Unfortunately, reductive functionalism faces a problem similar to that of the mind–brain identity theory. As Heil notes:

> Consider … the experience of a throbbing pain in my toe. Is this simply a matter of my being in a certain functional state (one that results in my believing that I have a pain in my toe, for instance, and disposes me to rub my toe)? If that were so, it would seem a simple matter to program a computing machine to be in a similar functional state. Yet it is odd to imagine that such a device might, solely because of the way we have programmed it, *feel pain*. What seems missing from the function-alist account is the *feeling* of pain. … And feelings, whatever they are, seem not to be functionally characterizable.
>
> (Heil 1993: 177)

Here the point is that the functionalist approach seems unable to capture "what it is like" to be in certain types of mental states. In short, functionalist analyses of certain mental states are deficient; and this seems especially clear in the case of subjective conscious experiences such as the *feeling* of pain, *the fear* of death, or the *feeling* of sadness. Thus, it appears that func-tionalism falters in accounting for the phenomena of suffering (especially the phenomena listed under (A) above).

Our examination of naturalistic theories of the mind is of course merely illustrative. But objections similar to those I've summarized have been raised against all the main naturalistic theories. Of course, many naturalists think that there are ways of getting around the problems I've summarized. So, they may think they face no serious problem of pain. But it is not as if there is a consensus among philosophers as to how physicalists can refute the well-known objections to their views. And notice that many theists also *think* that they have ways of getting around the problem of pain, e.g., many theists *think* they have an adequate theodicy. Many other theists *think* that a combination of (a) partially successful theodicies and (b) skeptical theism gives them an adequate response to the problem of pain. ("Given that we stand to God as a small child stands to an adult, we can hardly expect to understand *all* of God's reasons for allowing suffering.") So, do neither naturalists nor theists face a serious problem of pain? Or do both face a serious problem of pain? Advocates of the comparative approach claim that both do.

5 Theism and mental causation

Just at this point, however, naturalists may claim that theism, with its dualism of a non-physical God and a physical creation, and its historical tendency to back soul–body dualism, has severe difficulties in explaining mental causation (and hence difficulties in explaining phenomenon (B) above). And this is *in addition to* the more familiar problems in reconciling the existence of a good God with the facts about suffering. We cannot explore this claim in detail here, but let us note some factors that significantly complicate defending it.

1   It has often been argued that there is no conceivable way that a non-physical God (or non-physical soul) could interact causally with physical entities. So, such causal interac-tion cannot occur. But is it safe to assume that what we humans cannot conceive cannot occur? Well, prior to the rise of science, could humans *conceive* of the causal relation between a magnet and small bits of iron? No. Of course, prior to the rise of science, humans were *familiar* with the phenomenon of magnetism, but they had no

understanding whatsoever of the underlying mechanisms. Magnets were utterly myster-ious. Nevertheless, this fact clearly would *not* have provided a good reason to deny that magnets attract iron filings.

2   But theists and soul–body dualists face an energy-conservation objection, right? How can a non-physical God (or soul) cause an event in the physical world without violating the law of conservation of energy, i.e., that the total amount of energy in a causally isolated system remains constant? First, the universe is not a causally isolated system if God exists. Nor is it a causally isolated system if souls exert causal influence on the brain. Second, as Robin Collins has observed, the law of conservation of energy is based on the study of purely physical systems and thus it is not clear that the law applies to systems involving both physical causes and non-physical causes, such as God and the soul (Collins 2008: 33).

3   Theists may have resources for avoiding some of the problems of naturalistic theories of the mind. Theists can and should agree with physicalists that human mentality is depen-dent on brain activity; a blow to the head may cause a loss of consciousness and brain injury may permanently impair mental functioning. But the dependence relationship may not be as strong as physicalists claim (e.g., supervenience or identity), with physical events always "running the show." The brain might be more like a radio receiver: smash the receiver and the music stops, but the receiver is not, all by itself, the source of the music.

Given theism, God creates the physical world and sets in place those regularities we call laws of nature. Might God also be able to actualize the following sorts of relations between the mental and the physical?

- Some mental states or events are caused by a combination of both mental and physical states, neither of which are, by themselves, sufficient causes. For example, one thought – together with supporting brain activity – causes another thought.
- Some physical states or events are caused by a combination of both mental and physical states, neither of which are, by themselves, sufficient causes. For example, a decision (in combination with supporting neural activity) causes an action.

If such relationships are logically possible, God could presumably actualize them, and the causal connections of phenomenon (B) could be accounted for.

To sum up, the problem of pain is a very important objection to traditional theism. Theists try to respond in various ways. The soul-making theodicy seems to explain quite a bit of suffering, but not all of it. The overrider response is only as good as the positive evidence for the existence of a perfectly good God. Skeptical theism comes at a high cost unless it can be successfully combined with one of the other responses. Finally, via the comparative response, theists seek to put the problem of pain into perspective by arguing that rival metaphysical positions face significant problems of pain of their own.

Related topics

Notes

1 For the idea that pain itself involves presentations of badness, see Chapter 3, this volume.
2 I am here loosely paraphrasing Hick (1990: 46).
3 The main point of this paragraph is borrowed from Hasker (2004: 38).
4 Hasker observes that, from this perspective, any particular *instance* of evil is gratuitous, but the *class* of gratuitous evils cannot be empty.
5 For examples of naturalistic explanations of the phenomena highlighted in (B) see chapters in Section I of this volume, e.g. Chapters 2 and 4.
6 The shadow analogy is borrowed from Kim (2006: 179).
7 For a defense of epiphenomenalism, see Huxley (1874).
8 My characterization of non-reductive physicalism is borrowed from Kim (2006: 290–291), and (2005: 33–5). My formulation differs slightly from Kim's in that I use the term "states" whereas his formulation is in terms of property instantiations.
9 Throughout this paragraph I am paraphrasing Kim (2005: 48). And I have borrowed the phrase "ride piggyback" from him.
10 The smartphone example is borrowed from Jennifer Corns in email correspondence (23 November 2015), but the analysis of the example is mine and I must take responsibility for it.
11 For an expanded statement of the exclusion argument, see Kim (2005: 36–52). For an overview of attempts to respond to the exclusion argument, see Robb and Heil (2014).
12 There are multiple kinds of functionalism, see, e.g., Levin (2013). For a psychofunctionalist treatment of the qualitative features of pain, see, for instance, Chapters 15 and 18 of this volume.

Further reading

William Hasker, *The Emergent Self* (Ithaca, NY: Cornell University Press, 1999), criticizes physicalist theories of the mind and argues that the mind is an emergent individual with novel causal powers. Daniel Howard-Snyder, "The Argument from Inscrutable Evil," in Daniel Howard-Snyder (ed.), *The Evidential Argument from Evil* (Bloomington: Indiana University Press, 1996), 286–310, provides a defense of skeptical theism. C. Stephen Layman, *Letters to Doubting Thomas: A Case for the Existence of God* (Oxford: Oxford University Press, 2007), critically evaluates theistic and naturalistic perspectives on a range of issues, including religious experience, the fine-tuned universe, moral responsibility and free will, and evil. Alvin Plantinga, "Materialism and Christian Belief," in Peter van Inwagen and Dean Zimmerman (eds.), *Persons: Human and Divine* (Oxford: Oxford University Press, 2007), 99–141, provides a defense of substance dualism, including a critical discussion of Jaegwon Kim's famous pairing problem. Richard Swinburne, *Providence and the Problem of Evil* (Oxford: Oxford University Press, 1998), is an extended reflection on the problem of evil by one of the world's foremost philosophers of religion.

References

Collins, R. (2008) Modern physics and the energy-conservation objection to mind–body dualism. *American Philosophical Quarterly* 45(1): 31–42.
Hasker, W. (2004) *Providence, Evil, and the Openness of God.* New York: Routledge.
Heil, J. (1993) Philosophy of mind. In L. McHenry and F. Adams (eds), *Reflections on Philosophy: Introductory Essays.* New York: St. Martin's Press.
Hick, J. (1990) *Philosophy of Religion*, 4th ed. Englewood Cliffs, NJ.: Prentice Hall.
Huxley, T. (1874) On the hypothesis that animals are automata, and its history. *Fortnightly Review*, no. 22.
Kim, J. (2005) *Physicalism, or Something Near Enough.* Princeton: Princeton University Press.
Kim, J. (2006) *The Philosophy of Mind*, 2nd ed. Cambridge, MA: Westview Press.
Levin, J. (2013) Functionalism. In E.N. Zalta (ed.), *The Stanford Encyclopedia of Philosophy* (Fall 2013 ed.). <http://plato.stanford.edu/archives/fall2013/entries/functionalism/>.
Nagel, T. (1974) What is it like to be a bat? *Philosophical Review* 83(4): 435–450.
Robb. D. and Heil, J. (2014) Mental causation. In E.N. Zalta (ed.), *The Stanford Encyclopedia of Philosophy* (Spring 2014 ed.). <http://plato.stanford.edu/archives/spr2014/entries/mental-causation/>.
Rowe, W. (1979) The problem of evil and some varieties of atheism. *American Philosophical Quarterly* 16(4): 335–341.
Searle, J. (2004) *Mind: A Brief Introduction.* Oxford: Oxford University Press.

SECTION III

PRACTICAL IMPLICATIONS

Why does pain matter, practically?

PART III-I

Pain in ethics

27

BAD BY NATURE

An axiological theory of pain

Olivier Massin

This chapter defends an axiological theory of pain according to which pains are bodily episodes that are bad in some way. Section 1 introduces two standard assumptions about pain that the axiological theory constitutively rejects: (i) that pains are essentially tied to consciousness and (ii) that pains are not essentially tied to badness. Section 2 presents the axiological theory by contrast to these and provides a preliminary defense of it. Section 3 introduces the paradox of pain and argues that since the axiological theory takes the location of pain at face value, it needs to grapple with the privacy, self-intimacy and incorrigibility of pain. Sections 4, 5 and 6 explain how the axiological theory may deal with each of these.

Before starting, two methodological caveats are in order. First, the goal is here to understand *what pains are*: we want to spell out the *nature* of pains, that is, their *essence* or *real definition* (Fine 1994). Perhaps that nature is multifaceted: perhaps pains have several essential features. To express these, I shall use the following expressions interchangeably: "one essential feature of pain is to be *F*," "pains are essentially *F*," "part of the nature of pains is to be *F*," "what it is to be a pain is in part to be *F*."[1]

Second, the following purports to shed light on the nature of pain *from the stance of descriptive metaphysics*. One working assumption is therefore that at least part of the nature of pain is correctly captured by our pre-theoretical conceptions. Ordinary thinking about pain cannot be completely misguided (on pain of not being about pain), and may even prove subtler than expected.

1 Two dogmas about pain

Contemporary literature on pain tends to agree on two broad views about the nature of pain. The first may be called "Experience-Dependence":

Experience-Dependence: Part of the nature of pains is to be either experiences of bodily episodes, or experienced bodily episodes.[2]

That pains are by nature *experiences of bodily episodes* is a view endorsed in the the International Association for the Study of Pain's definition of pain, and constitutes the common denominator of a wide variety of theories of pain such as perceptualism (Armstrong 1993;

Pitcher 1970) evaluativism (Helm 2002; Cutter and Tye 2011; Bain 2013, Chapter 3, this volume) and recent adverbialist accounts (Aydede, Chapter 18, this volume).

The second way to essentially connect pains with experiences is to identify pain with *experienced bodily episodes*. Thus pains may be equated to *experienced physical bodily processes* (Smith et al. 2011), to *mind-dependent bodily sense-data* (Jackson 1977), or to *some experienced* sui generis *bodily pain-quality* on a par with pressures and temperatures. Note that even when reference is made to some physical episodes or qualities which, contrary to sense-data, may exist independently from experiences thereof, pains are not equated to such physical episodes or qualities *simpliciter*, but to such episodes or qualities *qua* experienced.

All in all, the first standard assumption about pain is that if we scrutinize the nature of pain, some experience will always be found, either because pain is itself an experience, or because pain is essentially the object of some experience. Experiences – or mental cognates: consciousness, feeling, perception … – necessarily figure in pain's *definiens*.

The second, perhaps even more widely shared, assumption about pain is that if we scrutinize the nature of pain, no value will ever be found. Pains are essentially non-axiological phenomena. Call that second standard assumption "Value-Independence":

Value-Independence: It is not part of the nature of pains to be bad.

It is not in the essence of pain to be value-laden. Pain's badness is not part of pain's nature. Value-Independence may be rephrased in the following way. Let us use "painfulness" as a topic-neutral term meant to capture the property, whatever it is, which makes a (bodily or mental) episode be a pain:

Painfulness: the property, whatever it is, in virtue of which an episode is a pain.

By stipulation, then, *pains are painful episodes*. In this terminology, Value-Independence amounts to saying that *painfulness is not a value*. Is Value-Independence really an orthodox assumption? Two objections may be raised against that proposal.

The first stresses that pains are widely held to be *necessarily* bad. This is true, but it is important to see that pains can be necessarily bad without being essentially bad. Compare with knowledge. Although knowledge is often held to be necessarily good, knowledge is scarcely ever defined in terms of its goodness. The same holds true of pain, following Value-Independence. When philosophers insist that pain is always bad, they do not want to suggest that "being bad" is part of the *definiens* of pain. In Fine's (2002: 271) terms, "[i]t is no part of what it is to be pain that it should be bad." Rather, the nature of pain is held to constitute the *supervenience basis* or *ground* of the badness of pain. It does not include that badness. This standard and often tacit assumption is clearly spelled out by Zangwill (2005: 127): "Pain necessitates (or suffices for) badness even though it is not part of pain's essence (or nature or being or identity) to be bad."

A second objection to the present claim that Value-Independence is orthodox is that *evaluativism*, one chief contemporary theory of pain, does analyze pains in term of values. Evaluativism (Helm 2002; Cutter and Tye 2011; Bain 2013, and Chapter 3, this volume) accounts for pains by appealing to experiences *representing some bodily episodes (disturbances, damages …) as being bad for us*.

It is true indeed that evaluativism uses value-terms in its *analysans* of pain. But, first, these value-terms lie within the scope of a non-factive psychological connective. "Experiencing *x* as bad" does not entail "*x*'s being bad." Hence, although pains, according to evaluativism, are essentially dependent on something *feeling bad*, they are not essentially dependent on anything *being bad*. Second, even when such evaluations are veridical, the value that is then actually exemplified is not a value *of pains*, but *of their object*, of what pains are about – typically, bodily damages (Bain 2013). (See also Chapter 30, this volume.)

Thus Value-Independence is in fact subscribed to even by evaluativists about pain. To claim that it is part of the nature of pain to represent its object as being bad is not to claim that it is part of the nature of pain to be bad. Representing bodily disturbances as bad constitutes, according to the standard evaluativist picture, the supervenience basis or ground of pain's badness. Pain's badness, here again, is a consequence, but not a part, of pain's nature.

On the whole, neither the view that pains are necessarily bad nor evaluativism contradicts Value-Independence. That Value-Independence represents the orthodox view is reflected in the division of labor within the field: psychologists, neuroscientists and philosophers of mind study the nature of pain; moral philosophers and value theorists try to shed light on its value.

By wrapping Experience-Dependence and Value-Independence together, one arrives at a fairly orthodox position about pains that could be called "Pain Psychologism":

> Pain Psychologism: It is in the nature of pains to be experiences or experienced, but it is not in the nature of pains to be bad.

2 The Axiological Theory of Pain

I believe that both Experience-Dependence and Value-Independence are mistaken: pains do not essentially depend on experiences, but they do essentially depend on value. Call this "anti-psychologism" about pain:

> Pain Anti-psychologism: It is neither in the nature of pains to be experiences nor to be experienced, but it is in the nature of pains to be bad.

To get to the version of Pain Anti-psychologism to be defended here, let us first zoom out so as to consider the broader class of *unpleasant or disagreeable sensations*, which includes pains, but also dizziness, tiredness, itches, prickles, nauseas, etc. (Corns 2014). Being painful, accordingly, is only one way of being disagreeable. Trivially, what all disagreeable sensations have in common is that they are disagreeable. Value-Independence holds that disagreeableness is a mental, non-axiological property. I believe, on the contrary, that what all these disagreeable bodily sensations have in common is that they are bad in some way. Disagreeableness is an axiological, non-mental property. More precisely:

> Axiological Theory of Disagreeable Sensations: x is a disagreeable sensation of S
> $=_{df} x$ is an episode in S's body which is finally, personally and *pro tanto* bad for S.

Disagreeableness is the final, personal, *pro tanto* and negative value of bodily episodes. Let me explain.

To say that pains and other disagreeable sensations are *finally* bad is to say that they are not instrumentally bad: pains are bad in themselves, independently of the value of their effects. Pain may well accrue some instrumental value as well, but such an instrumental value is typically positive.[3]

To say that pains or other disagreeable sensations are *personally* bad, by contrast to being bad *simpliciter*, is to say that their badness is related to the subject of the pain: a pain is bad *for* its subject, in a way it is not for others. Personal values should not be conflated with subjective values: some things may be bad for Julie (a poison, say) without her knowing or experiencing that they are bad for her (Rønnow-Rasmussen 2011). Note that the axiological theory is compatible with many different accounts of final personal values. Pain's badness may be taken to be a primitive non-natural property, analyzed in terms of fitting-attitudes (Rønnow-Rasmussen 2011), in terms of aptness to harm (Cutter and Tye 2011; see Zimmerman 2009 for a defense of the symmetrical view that personal goodness should be analyzed in terms of benefit), etc.

To say that pains or other disagreeable sensations are bad *pro tanto*, by contrast to being bad *in toto*, amounts to saying that pains are not necessarily bad *overall*. Perhaps pains are good or neutral on the whole, that is, all things considered – for instance because of their positive instrumental value. Likewise a medicine may be bad with respect to its taste, but good overall, because it saves life.

This way of characterizing the disvalue of pain and other disagreeable sensations is generally accepted (see, e.g., Goldstein 1989). But, as seen above, the standard take is that such final, personal *pro tanto* negative values are not essential to pain and other disagreeable sensations, but only necessary to them. In accordance with Pain Psychologism, disagreeableness is typically considered a non-axiological, mental property, which constitutes the supervenience basis of pain's disvalue. The Axiological Theory of Disagreeable Sensation maintains by contrast that disagreeableness *is* a negative value, so that being bad is part of what it is to be a disagreeable sensation.

To get an axiological account of *pains* from such an axiological account of disagreeable sensations, one simply needs to specify further the way in which bodily episodes are bad. Disagreeableness, as a personal final *pro tanto* disvalue of bodily episodes, is a thin value. Painfulness, I submit, is a thicker value, a value with more descriptive content. *Being painful is a way of being disagreeable, that is, a way of being finally personally bad.* As there are two main ways to get thick concepts from thin ones (see, e.g., Tappolet 2004; Elstein and Hurka 2009; Roberts 2011), there are two main ways to arrive at painfulness from disagreeableness. The first is to argue that what makes painfulness thicker than disagreeableness cannot be disentangled. Painfulness would be irreducibly thicker than disagreeableness: it would be a primitive thick value of the personal, *pro tanto* final kind. The second is to argue that the descriptive content of painfulness may be disentangled further (for instance, in terms of the kind of bodily episodes it accrues to – some possible candidates being bodily disturbances, damages, disorders, threats thereof, intense pressures, or extreme temperatures). I shall here remain neutral on this issue and will only assume that *painfulness is a thick value falling under the thinner value of disagreeableness.*

Axiological Theory of Pain: x is a pain of $S =_{df} x$ is an episode in S's body which is finally, personally and *pro tanto* bad in the relevant way for S.

In other words, a pain is a painful bodily episode, where *being painful* is understood as a thick value falling under the thin final personal *pro-tanto* value of *being disagreeable*.

The Axiological Theory of Pain (ATP) is a version of anti-psychologism about pain. The term "experience" does not figure in pain's *definiens*, but the term "badness" does. Using again "painfulness" as a topic-neutral term to denote the property, whatever it is, in virtue of which an episode is a pain, the contrast between the ATP and Pain Psychologism may be represented as follows:

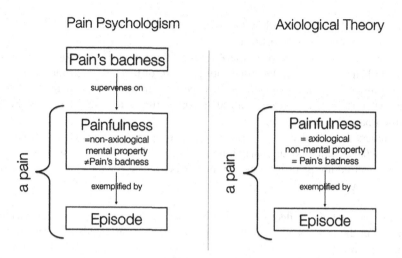

Figure 27.1

Although unorthodox, the view that algedonic properties such as pleasantness, unpleasantness, disagreableness or painfulness are value properties is not unprecedented. It has been embraced in various versions by Meinong (1972: 91, 95), Scheler (1973: 97, 105), Hartmann (1932: vol. 1, 131–132; vol. 2, 160), von Wright (1963: ch. 4), Goldstein (1989, 2000), Mendola (1990), Rachels (2000), Hewitt (2008) and Mulligan (2009). Here is von Wright:

> Most writers in the past regard pleasure as either some kind of sensation or as something between sensation and emotion. Moore, Broad, and the non-naturalists in general take it for granted that pleasantness is a "naturalistic" attribute of things and states and not an axiological term. This, I think, is a bad mistake.
>
> *(von Wright 1963: 63)*

Here are two initial motivations in favor of the ATP. The first is that in the standard psychologist picture, painfulness and pains' badness end up being phenomenologically redundant. The badness of a pain is not presented as an additional property, on top of its being a pain. Insofar as phenomenology is a good guide to the nature of pain, the distinction between the pain-making property of pains and the value of pain does not capture any genuine difference:

Premise 1: Our typical experiences of pains present us with pains as they are. (Experiences of pains are not systematically misleading.)

Premise 2: Our typical experiences of pains present us with painfulness – the property, whatever it is, in virtue of which pains are pains. (Pains are experienced as such, not as smells or sounds.)

Premise 3: Our typical experiences of pains present us with pains as being bad. Pains feel bad.

Premise 4: Our typical experiences of pains do not present us with the badness of pains as distinct from, and additional to, their painfulness. Pains are not experienced as being painful and, on top of that, bad.

Conclusion: Pains' badness is not distinct from painfulness.

A similar argument is put forward by Goldstein (2000) with respect to pleasure, to the effect that pleasure's goodness is essential to it.

The second motivation in favor of the ATP is that equating the essential property of pains with a value helps to solve the heterogeneity problem of pains – the problem of identifying what the multifarious kinds of bodily pains have in common: "what is the sensory resemblance between the intense freezing pain of an almost frozen foot and the diffuse hot pain of a sunburned back?" (Clark 2005).

If painfulness is construed as a non-axiological property or quality, this problem seems indeed intractable. But equating painfulness with a value paves the way for a plausible answer: what all bodily pains have in common is being bad for their subject. Clark puts his finger on that solution:

> For my part, when I reflect on these episodes of pain, the only common quality I can find in the feelings so designated seems to be that expressed by the general term "bad" or "aversive."
>
> *(Clark 2005)*

Clark does not endorse the ATP, however; for him, what all pains have in common is that their subject is disposed to avoid them. But it is telling that he naturally uses "bad" to capture the property common to all pains. As it happens, many answers to the heterogeneity problem – what all pains have in common is to be averted, to be worthy of being averted, to be disliked ... – echo well-known reductionist strategies with respect to values. A possible diagnosis is that such theories are presenting as a single account what is in fact the conjunction of two theories: an axiological theory of pain surreptitiously parceled with a reductionist theory of values.

In the rest of this chapter, I want to argue that on top of avoiding the phenomenological redundancy of pain's badness, and of providing a neat solution to the heterogeneity problem of pains, the ATP paves the way for a promising way of handling the vexing *paradox of pain*.

3 The ATP and the paradox of pain

Are pains in the mind or in the body? This question raises the famous paradox of pain – acutely described in Hill 2005, Chapter 5, this volume; Aydede 2009, 2013, Chapter 18, this volume; Hardcastle, Chapter 1, this volume. The three following features of pain suggest, initially, that pains should be in the mind:

Privacy: Only the subject of a pain can directly access it. If Julie has a pain, John cannot feel Julie's pain (at least not in the way Julie does; see de Vignemont's Chapter 21, this volume).

Self-Intimacy: Pains are necessarily felt or experienced. If Julie has a pain, Julie feels the pain she has (see Pereplyotchik's Chapter 17, this volume).

Incorrigibility: Feeling or experiencing a pain entails having a pain. If Julie feels that she has a pain, Julie has a pain (*see* Langland-Hassan's Chapter 20, this volume).

But a fourth feature of pains suggests that pains are not mental: namely, pains seem to be *located* in the body. Since mental episodes do not, from a descriptive standpoint, have bodily locations (although their reductive basis may have one in the brain), pain's bodily location runs afoul of the view that pains are mental. The paradox of pain is thus that the Privacy, Self-Intimacy and Incorrigibility of pains seem irreconcilable with their bodily location.

The standard way of handling the paradox is to give priority to the three mental aspects of pains – by endorsing Experience-Dependence – and to try to account, one way or another, for the phenomenon of pain location.

The ATP takes the opposite route: take pain's location at face value, and try to explain Privacy, Self-Intimacy and Incorrigibility in some other way. Rejecting Experience-Dependence on behalf of the location of pain is not an unprecedented move. Stumpf (1928) argues – tracing his view back to Malebranche – that pains are neither experiences nor emotions, but located qualities on a par with sounds and colors. As Bain (2007) usefully recalls, within analytic philosophy, the view that pains are objective conditions of the body has been endorsed or suggested by Cornman (1977), Graham and Stephens (1985) and Newton (1989). More recently, Reuter (2011) and Reuter et al. (2013) have argued on experimental grounds that in the folk conception, pain is an objective bodily condition rather than an experience or *sense-datum* (for discussion, see also Chapter 1). Hill (2005, Chapter 5, this volume) argues that at least one concept of pain is that of a bodily disturbance.

The ATP therefore belongs to the family of theories that equate pains with some objective bodily conditions rather than with mental states. But contrary to other objectivist theories of pain, the ATP equates pains with *value-laden* bodily conditions. Thanks to this, I shall now argue, the ATP is better suited than other objectivist theories to deal with the Privacy, Self-Intimacy and Incorrigibility of pains. More precisely, under the ATP:

- Privacy can be accounted for by relying on the axiological distinction between *personal and impersonal values*;
- Self-Intimacy can be accounted for by appealing to the metaphysical distinction between *modal and essential accounts of ontological dependence.*
- Incorrigibility can be explained away thanks to the psychological distinction between *pain and suffering.*

4 Tackling Privacy

According to the ATP, the value of pain is *personal*: Julie's pain is not bad *simpliciter* (as are moral values) but bad *for her*, in a way it is not bad for Paul. That pain's essential badness is personal is, I suggest, what explains pain's essential Privacy.

To get Privacy from personal badness, one needs to adopt a further but plausible claim about the epistemology of personal values: the only way to directly access the final badness of *x* for Julie is to *be* Julie. Paul can only *indirectly* access what is good for Julie, *by putting himself in Julie's shoes.* Julie has privileged access to what is good for her. Accessing what is good for her requires first empathizing with her (Rønnow-Rasmussen 2011: 60). On this assumption, and since on the ATP personal badness is essential to pains, pain's Privacy holds true of pain in virtue of its axiological constituent. In other words, because it is in the nature of pain to be personally bad, a pain can only be directly accessed by the person for whom it is bad.

It should be stressed that such a proposal by no means entails Experience-Dependence. As stressed above, that her pain is bad for Julie does not entail that Julie's pain is bad in her eyes, nor that she experiences her pain as bad. The ATP entails that pains are person-dependent, not that they are experience-dependent.

The following analogy may help shed light on the present proposal. Pains, as the ATP understands them, share many features with *reflections* – e.g., the reflection of the moon on the sea. Once personal values are recognized as essential ingredients of pains, pains accrue some metaphysical perspectivality and, consequently, some epistemological privacy, which closely resemble those of reflections.

Metaphysically, first, reflections are dependent on a viewpoint. This notwithstanding, reflections are independent of their being experienced. Reflections are not mere appearances in our mind, purely intentional objects. That reflections do not depend on our experiences of them is shown by the following facts: (i) experiences of reflections can be veridical or illusory, (ii) closing one's eyes does not destroy the reflection of the moon at the viewpoint one occupies, (iii) contrary to mind-dependent objects, reflections can be photographed,[4] (iv) reflections may cause warming and even fires. In the very same way that reflections are viewpoint-dependent but experience-independent, pains, thanks to their essential personal value, are subject-dependent but not experience-dependent.

Second, because of their metaphysical perspectivality, reflections are epistemologically private in the sense of being directly accessible only from the very point of view on which they essentially depend. Here again, the analogy with pains is quite strong. In the same way that the reflection of the moon at a viewpoint can only be directly seen from that viewpoint, the badness of a pain for a person can only be directly felt by that person. And in the same way that to access the moon's reflection from Julie's viewpoint one has to imagine oneself occupying Julie's viewpoint, to access Julie's pain one has to put oneself in her shoes. Thus pains – qua personally bad – like reflections, are private without being experience-dependent.

5 Tackling Self-Intimacy

Self-Intimacy, on the face of it, straightforwardly entails Experience-Dependence: if pains cannot exist without being experienced, then, trivially, pains depend on experience.

A first reaction, on behalf of the ATP, is simply to reject Self-Intimacy by defending the possibility of unfelt pains (see, e.g., Palmer 1975; see also Chapters 17 and 20, this volume). Although I sympathize with this line of thought, I am willing to grant Self-Intimacy so as to suggest that, under the ATP, it can be reconciled with Experience-Independence.

The starting idea is that the above argument from Self-Intimacy to Experience-Dependence relies on a flawed conception of ontological dependence (Fine 1995; Lowe 2001; Correia 2006). Suppose, as some old Catholic representations have it, that *God sees everything*. God being a necessary being, this entails that nothing can exist without being seen by God. Yet we do not want to conclude from this that everything is a sense-datum of God, that everything depends on God's seeing. The reason is, to paraphrase Fine (1995), that the *source* of the necessity in question does not lie in the dependent nature of the world, but in the necessary and omniscient nature of God. That *x* cannot exist without *y* does not yet establish that *x* ontologically depends on *y*. This impossibility has yet to flow from the nature of *x*.

This paves the way for the following account of Self-Intimacy, compatible with Experience-Independence. Pains are indeed necessarily felt, but the source of this necessity does not lie in pain's nature. Rather, it lies in the pain-tracking nature of consciousness. Consciousness is, with respect to one's pains, like God with respect to the world: it feels all of them. Thus, *the reason why there are no unfelt pains is not that pains are experience-dependent but that consciousness is pain-attracted.*

Why should it be so? Objectivist accounts of pain that accept Value-Independence have no clear answer available. If pains are on a par with sounds, smells, colors or other physical events, there is no reason why consciousness should track pains more than these.[5] If, on the other hand, pains are essentially bad for us, it is no wonder that pains attract consciousness. One of the essential functions of consciousness could be to monitor what is finally (dis) valuable for us.

This proposal faces however the following immediate objection: even if consciousness tracks by nature things that are bad for us, there is no guarantee that such things will lie within its field. Thus something finally bad for Julie may happen in her toe, but because of some nociceptive defect, Julie may fail to experience it. The ATP seems to entail that this finally bad episode would be an unfelt pain, thereby contradicting Self-Intimacy.

Self-Intimacy may however be rescued by restricting what counts as *Julie's body*. One may argue that if something bad for her is going on in Julie's toe, and that she cannot feel it, then this toe is not really *hers*. The parts of our body in which no algedonic sensations can be felt – such as the tips of our hairs, nails or teeth – are in one sense not ours: they do not belong to our *affective body* (de Vignemont and Massin 2015). If dysfunctions of the nociceptive systems modify the boundaries of the body that counts as ours, pain may be necessarily felt without being essentially felt.

6 Tackling Incorrigibility

I have argued that the ATP is compatible with – and even helps explain – Privacy and Self-Intimacy. My proposal for dealing with Incorrigibility – experiencing a pain entails having that pain – is different: I shall argue that Incorrigibility is false but that the ATP helps to disclose the grain of truth underlying it.

The case against Incorrigibility is relatively straightforward. Referred pains – where a pain is felt in another location than the one in which it really is – show that the felt location of a pain can be illusory (Hill 2005). Phantom limb pains – where a pain is felt in an amputated limb – show that experiences of pain can be hallucinatory. Although people suffering from phantom limb pains may well *be in pain*, in a sense to be elucidated soon, they still do not *have a pain*, as compellingly argued by Bain (2007). Pains can be mislocated, and even hallucinated. Incorrigibility, as it stands, should be rejected. (Cf. Chapter 20, this volume.)

If the case against Incorrigibility is so simple, why does Incorrigibility sound so compelling? The motivation underlying it seems to be that when Julie insists, sincerely, that she has an intense pain in her amputated limb, it will not do to reply to her that she's plain wrong. There is something she's right about. What is it?

The ATP points to the following answer. Bad things call for negative affective reactions: injustice calls for indignation; culpability calls for guilt; danger calls for fear, etc. Since pain, according to the ATP, is essentially bad, one is led to wonder: what is the appropriate affective reaction to pain? The answer, I submit, is *suffering*. Pains should be suffered. Enjoying a pain, or being indifferent to it, are incorrect affective responses to pain.

Although they are sometimes conflated or put under the same heading, pain and suffering are categorially distinct (a point urged by Scheler 1973: 105, 256–258, 333–338). Suffering – like fear, admiration, hate – is an emotion: an affective intentional state directed towards some (real or merely apparent) object or episode. Pains – like itches, tickles, nauseas – are non-intentional bodily episodes. Suffering is an attitude, pain is not. Pain is located, suffering is not. Pains are worthy of being suffered; suffering is our fitting affective reaction to pain. Although the distinction between pain and suffering becomes patent once pains are recognized as essentially bad, the ATP is not the only way to get to it. Feldman (2004) has championed the corresponding distinction between attitudinal and sensory pleasures;[6] Hill's distinction (Chapter 5, this volume) between *peripheral pain* and *central state pain* closely matches the distinction between pain and suffering;[7] and clinicians have long been aware that "[i]t is suffering, not pain, that brings patients into doctors' offices in hopes of finding relief" (Loeser 2000; see also Cassell 2004/1995).

With the pain/suffering distinction in hand, it becomes easy to account for the intuition underlying Incorrigibility. When Julie insists, sincerely, that she has an intense pain in her amputated limb, what she says is literally false. She has no pain in her limb, because she has no limb. *But* Julie is genuinely *suffering* from a hallucinatory pain. The plausibility of Incorrigibility relies on a conflation between pain and suffering. One may suffer a pain that one does not have, in the same way that one may fear a danger that one does not face. Suppose Julie hallucinates a tarantula over her head and insists that she is in real danger. She is not infallible about dangers for all that, quite the contrary. But she really is frightened by her hallucinatory perception. Likewise for her phantom limb "pains": she has no pain, but her pain hallucinations prompt genuine suffering. When we say, with an air of paradox, that Julie *is in pain* although she *has no pain*, what we mean is that Julie is genuinely suffering in reaction to a hallucination of pain.

Can we say more about the nature of suffering and its relation to pain? Suffering can be analyzed in terms of evaluative content, or suffering can be equated to some *sui generis* intentional mode. According to evaluative-content accounts of suffering, to suffer a (real or apparent) pain just is to experience/feel/perceive this pain as bad. According to intentional-mode accounts of suffering, to suffer a (real or apparent) pain is a *sui generis* affective attitude directed at the pain, an attitude we embrace in reaction to the pain being experienced as bad. Suffering being an emotion, this debate is an instance of the broader debate within emotions theory, between the so-called perceptualist accounts of emotions – which equate emotions to experiences of value (see, e.g., Tappolet 2000) – and the attitudinal account of emotions, which equates emotions to reactions to experiences of valuable things (see, e.g., Mulligan 2007; Deonna and Teroni 2012).

Without prejudging that complex issue, it may be noticed that pain asymbolia may provide a further reason to embrace the later, intentional-mode account of suffering. Pain asymbolics not only report feeling pain but, even more bafflingly, sometimes describe their pain as *hurting* and *painful* (see, e.g., Grahek 2007: 45; Bain 2014). Distinguishing the experience of the badness of a pain from the normal suffering reaction to it allows us to take these reports at face value. On that proposal asymbolics do experience their pain as bad, but fail to suffer it. *Feeling x as bad* and *suffering x* are distinct: the latter is the normal and correct reaction to the former. Subjects with phantom limb pains suffer from pains they feel, but do not have; patients with pain asymbolia fail to suffer from pains they have and feel.

In sum, equating pains with bodily episodes that are personally bad in a way allows us to (i) straightforwardly account for the location of pains, (ii) avoid the phenomenological redundancy between pain's badness and pain's painfulness, (iii) solve the heterogeneity problem for pains, (iv) explain the privacy of pain, (v) explain the self-intimacy of pain, and (vi) explain away the incorrigibility of pain.

Related topics

Acknowledgements

I am very grateful to Jennifer Corns and David Bain for invaluable comments on this chapter, as well as to the participants in the conference The Role of Phenomenal Consciousness, Glasgow, 24 October 2015. Thanks to Riccardo Braglia, CEO and Managing Director Helsinn Holding SA and the Fondazione Reginaldus (Lugano) for financial support of the work published here.

Notes

1 See Correia 2006 on such generic essentialist statements.
2 I shall eschew talk of consciousness to avoid vexing terminological issues, but the idea may be rephrased by saying that a pain either involves (i) the transitive consciousness of some bodily episode or (ii) a bodily episode of which one is transitively aware. For discussion see also Chapter 17, this volume.
3 The concept of final value is distinct from the concept of intrinsic value. An intrinsic value is a value that supervenes on the intrinsic properties of its bearers. A final value is a value that is not instrumental. Some final values may be extrinsic (Rabinowicz and Rønnow-Rasmussen 2000). This may be the case of disagreeableness: if disagreeableness is a personal value, it supervenes not only on the intrinsic properties of the bodily episodes it accrues to, but also on relations between such episodes and the subject to which that body belongs.
4 As Russell (1914) liked to recall in connection with closely similar examples, "The photograph cannot lie."
5 See Findlay 1961: 177, for a converging argument with respect to the motivational power of pains.
6 Two differences between the present view and that of Feldman are worth noting, though. First, Feldman (2004: 84) uses "disenjoying" instead of "suffering" to express the opposite of "enjoying." Second, while on the present proposal pains are *worthy* of being suffered (but not necessarily so), Feldman maintains that sensory pleasures are *necessarily* enjoyed. See Massin 2013 for an overview of different ways of drawing the sensory/attitudinal pleasures distinction.
7 Although I fully agree with Hill on the distinction, I disagree with him on two more superficial points. First, I disagree that the central affective state corresponds to our concept of *pain*. The concept of *suffering* is the one that captures such a negative mental state. Second and relatedly, I disagree with him that folk psychology fails to distinguish the two algesic concepts. For instance, we speak of "suffering pain" and consider it inappropriate (but not impossible or meaningless) to enjoy pain.

References

Armstrong, D.M. (1993) *A Materialist Theory of the Mind*. London/New York: Routledge.
Aydede, M. (2009) Is feeling pain the perception of something? *Journal of Philosophy* 106(10): 531–567.
Aydede, M. (2013) Pain. In E.N. Zalta (ed.), *The Stanford Encyclopedia of Philosophy* (Spring 2013 ed.). <http://plato.stanford.edu/archives/spr2013/entries/pain/>.
Bain, D. (2007) The location of pains. *Philosophical Papers* 36(2): 171–205.
Bain, D. (2013) What makes pains unpleasant? *Philosophical Studies* 166 (suppl. 1): S69–S89.
Bain, D. (2014) Pains that don't hurt. *Australasian Journal of Philosophy* 92: 305–320.
Cassell, E.J. (2004/1995) Pain and suffering. In S.G. Post (ed.), *Encyclopedia of Bioethics*, 3rd ed. London: Macmillan, pp. 1961–1968.
Clark, A. (2005) Painfulness is not a quale. In M. Aydede (ed.), *Pain: New Essays on Its Nature and the Methodology of Its Study*. Cambridge, MA: MIT Press, pp. 177–198.
Cornman, J.W. (1977) Might a tooth ache but there be no toothache? *Australasian Journal of Philosophy* 55: 27–40.
Corns, J. (2014) Unpleasantness, motivational oomph, and painfulness. *Mind & Language* 29: 238–254.

Correia, F. (2005) *Existential Dependence and Cognate Notions*. Munich: Philosophia.

Correia, F. (2006) Generic essence, objectual essence, and modality. *Noûs* 40(4): 753–766.

Cutter, B. and Tye, M. (2011) Tracking representationalism and the painfulness of pain. *Philosophical Issues* 2: 90–109.

Deonna, J.A. and Teroni, F. (2012) From justified emotions to justified evaluative judgements. *Dialogue* 51(1): 55–77.

de Vignemont, F. and Massin, O. (2015) Touch. In M. Matthen (ed.), *Oxford Handbook of Philosophy of Perception*. Oxford: Oxford University Press, pp. 294–311.

Elstein, D.Y. and Hurka, T. (2009) From thick to thin: two moral reduction plans. *Canadian Journal of Philosophy* 39(4): 515–535.

Feldman, F. (2004) *Pleasure and the Good Life: Concerning the Nature, Varieties, and Plausibility of Hedonism.* Oxford: Oxford University Press.

Findlay, J. (1961) *Values and Intentions*. London: Allen & Unwin.

Fine, K. (1994) Essence and modality. In J.E. Tomberlin (ed.), *Logic and Language*, special issue of *Philosophical Perspectives* 8: 1–16.

Fine, K. (1995) Ontological dependence. *Proceedings of the Aristotelian Society* 95: 269–290.

Fine, K. (2002) The varieties of necessity. T. Gendler and J. Hawthorne (eds.), *Conceivability and Possibility*. Oxford: Oxford University Press, pp. 253–281.

Goldstein, I. (1989) Pleasure and Pain: Unconditional, Intrinsic Values. *Philosophy and Phenomenological Research* 50: 255–276.

Goldstein, I. (2000) Intersubjective properties by which we specify pain, pleasure, and other kinds of mental states. *Philosophy* 75: 89–104.

Graham, G. and Stephens, G.L. (1985) Are qualia a pain in the neck for functionalists? *American Philosophical Quarterly* 22: 73–80.

Grahek, N. (2007) *Feeling Pain and Being in Pain*, 2nd ed. Cambridge, MA: MIT Press.

Hartmann, N. (1932) *Ethics*, trans. S. Coit. 3 vols. London: George Allen & Unwin; New York: Macmillan Co.

Helm, B. (2002) Felt evaluations: a theory of pleasure and pain. *American Philosophical Quarterly* 39: 13–30.

Hewitt, S. (2008) *Normative Qualia and a Robust Moral Realism*. PhD diss., New York University.

Hill, C.S. (2005) Ow! The paradox of pain. In M. Aydede (ed.), *Pain: New Essays on Its Nature and the Methodology of Its Study*, Cambridge, MA: MIT Press, pp. 75–98.

Jackson, F. (1977) *Perception: A Representative Theory*. Cambridge: Cambridge University Press.

Loeser, J.D. (2000) Pain and suffering. *Clinical Journal of Pain* 16(2): S2–S6.

Lowe, E. (2001) *The Possibility of Metaphysics: Substance, Identity, and Time*. New York: Oxford University Press.

Massin, O. (2013) The intentionality of pleasures and other feelings, a Brentanian approach. In D. Fisette and G. Fréchette (eds.), *Themes from Brentano*. Amsterdam: Rodopi, pp. 307–337.

Meinong, A. (1972) *On Emotional Presentation*, trans. M.-L. Schubert Kalsi. Evanston: Northwestern University Press.

Mendola, J. (1990) Objective value and subjective states. *Philosophy and Phenomenological Research* 50: 695–713.

Mulligan, K. (2007) Intentionality, knowledge and formal objects. *Disputatio* 2(23): 1–24.

Mulligan, K. (2009) *Emotion and Value*. Oxford: Oxford University Press.

Newton, N. (1989) On viewing pain as a secondary quality. *Noûs* 23(5): 569–598.

Palmer, D. (1975) Unfelt pains. *American Philosophical Quarterly* 12: 289–298.

Pitcher, G. (1970) Pain perception. *Philosophical Review* 79: 368.

Rabinowicz, W. and Rønnow-Rasmussen, T. (2000). A distinction in value: intrinsic and for its own sake. *Proceedings of the Aristotelian Society* 100(1): 33–51.

Rachels, S. (2000) Is unpleasantness intrinsic to unpleasant experiences? *Philosophical Studies* 99: 187–210.

Reuter, K. (2011) Distinguishing the appearance from the reality of pain. *Journal of Consciousness Studies* 18 (9–10): 94–109.

Reuter, K., Phillips, D., and Sytsma, J. (2013) Hallucinating pain. In J. Sytsma (ed.), *Advances in Experimental Philosophy of Mind*. London: Bloomsbury, pp. 75–100.

Roberts, D. (2011) Shapelessness and the thick. *Ethics* 121(3): 489–520.

Rønnow-Rasmussen, T. (2011) *Personal Value*. Oxford: Oxford University Press.

Russell, B. (1914) The relation of sense-data to physics. *Scientia* 16: 1–27.

Scheler, M. (1973) *Formalism in Ethics and Non-formal Ethics of Value*, trans. M. Frings and R.L. Funk. Evanston: Northwestern University Press.

Smith, B., Ceusters, W., Goldberg, L.J., and Ohrbach, R. (2011) Towards an ontology of pain. In *Proceedings of the Conference on Ontology and Analytical Metaphysics*. Tokyo: Keio University Press.

Stumpf, C. (1928) *Gefühl und Gefühlsempfindung*. Leipzig: Verlag von Johann Ambrosis Barth.

Tappolet, C. (2000) *Emotions et valeurs*. Paris: Presses Universitaires de France.

Tappolet, C. (2004). Through thick and thin: good and its determinates. *Dialectica* 58(2): 207–221.

von Wright, G. (1963) *The Varieties of Goodness*. London: Routledge & Kegan Paul.

Zangwill, N. (2005) Moore, morality, supervenience, essence, epistemology. *American Philosophical Quarterly* 42: 125–130.

Zimmerman, M. (2009) Understanding what's good for us. *Ethical Theory and Moral Practice* 12: 429–439.

28

PAIN AND TORTURE

Michael Davis

What is the relation between pain and torture? That's a hard question to answer – in part because, like most important words, "pain" has several senses, some competing and still in dispute, something that should be clear from the first section of this volume. There are three other reasons making it hard to answer the question with which I began. First, recent empirical studies suggest that not all "pain" is painful, that is, that some pain, even if intense, may not include any suffering (Corns 2014; see also Chapter 27, this volume). Yet, it seems no more than common sense that there is no torture without suffering. Second, insofar as pain is understood as a physical state, say, the firing of certain neurons, much that counts as torture may not be pain, for example, allowing a prisoner to shiver naked in a cold cell for weeks or months, with no place to sleep but a concrete floor. Third, there is etymology. The English word "pain" comes from the Latin *poena*, originally meaning legal punishment. Though that etymology does not tell us what "pain" means now, it does warn us that the word may have associations inappropriate for understanding torture (in part at least because much torture is illegal). Most (rough) synonyms for "pain," such as "hurt" or "agony," are free of such associations. I therefore propose to substitute one of those synonyms, "suffering," for "pain," hoping that the substitution clarifies my official subject without changing it.

"Torture" too has several senses. I shall focus on that sense explaining why we consider torture especially morally objectionable (that is, so morally objectionable that, like slavery, it can never be morally justified or only morally justified under the most pressing circumstances). That sense seems to me to be both central to our understanding of torture and the one most likely to be of interest to readers of this chapter.

This chapter has three parts: first, an explanation of why the standard legal definition of "torture" is inadequate for understanding what makes torture especially morally objectionable; second, an alternative to the legal definition designed to bring out what is especially morally objectionable about torture; and third, an explanation of why (and how) the most important competing definitions fail to do that.

1 Some inadequacies of the standard legal definition

On 10 December 1984, the United Nations General Assembly adopted the Convention against Torture and Other Cruel, Inhuman, or Degrading Treatment or Punishment. For the

334

purposes of that document (now endorsed by most countries), the term "torture" was defined as:

> any act by which severe pain or suffering, whether physical or mental, is intentionally inflicted on a person for such purposes as obtaining from him or a third person information or a confession, punishing him for an act he or a third person has committed or is suspected of having committed, or intimidating or coercing him or a third person, or for any reason based on discrimination of any kind, when such pain or suffering is inflicted by or at the instigation of or with the consent or acquiescence of a public official or other person acting in an official capacity. It does not include pain or suffering arising only from, inherent in or incidental to lawful sanctions.
>
> *(United Nations 1984)*

However useful this definition may be for some purposes (such as outlawing all official torture in signatory states), it does not help much with understanding torture as such. It leaves too much out. For example, an illegal organization, such as the mafia, seems (without official "consent or acquiescence") to be as capable of torture as any government. Even an individual (such as the Marquis de Sade) can torture. Torture is not even necessarily a relation among humans. Children sometimes torture insects. Cats seem to torture captured mice. Whoever or whatever does it, torture seems much the same, a relation between sentient beings (torturer and tortured) in which the one intentionally makes the other suffer. Any definition that is designed to capture what is especially morally objectionable about torture should acknowledge that (the centrality of sentience).

The term "torture" has its origin in the idea of "twisting" (as in "torque" and "tortuous"). Torture was originally tormenting the body until it twists uncontrollably. Though the modern literature on torture (like the UN Convention) distinguishes between "physical" and "mental" torture, all the examples of "mental torture" usually offered seem to be either physical in a straightforward sense or something other than torture (for example, intimidation). So, for example, keeping a prisoner awake until disoriented and incoherent seems to be physical torture. The means by which the prisoner is kept awake (loud noises, poking by a guard, and so on) are physical. The outcome is also physical. Sleep privation disrupts physical processes in body and brain (causing exhaustion, jumpiness, extreme depression, and other suffering associated with physical disease). Though there is generally little pain, and no scars or other physical marks, there is still much physical suffering – that is, a state of the body sufficiently unpleasant that a rational person would (normally) avoid it even at great cost. Even a dog or a rat can be made to suffer in that way – and what a dog or rat can suffer does not seem mental (as opposed to physical) in any *morally* significant sense.

The current distinction between "mental" and "physical" torture seems not to be philosophical (that is, a distinction arising from an attempt to understand torture). On virtually any philosophical account of the mental, the suffering torture produces must be mental (even when the suffering is located in some part of the body, for example, when I truthfully report that my crushed finger hurts). Indeed, we cannot even think of the (physical) torture of animals without attributing a mental state to them. Bodies without minds feel nothing. The distinction between "mental" and "physical" torture seems to be rhetorical rather than philosophical. Those defending torture seem to hope that torture that is "merely mental" (or "merely psychological") will seem less serious than the "physical" sort (hence the effort that the US government, for a time, put into making the distinction). So, for example, inducing "the misperception of suffocation" (say, by using a wet towel to cut off the interrogated's air supply) is often said to be mental (or psychological) torture – and so, a less severe form of torture than, say, burning the interrogated's chest with a red-hot poker (which scars the body) or beating him with a rubber hose (which leaves no outward marks however much it hurts).[1] The concealed assumption seems to be that mental suffering involves an intervening false belief that the torturer introduces ("the *misperception of suffocation*"). Physical torture does not require intervening beliefs (just sentience). Mental torture is then (so the argument runs) more like extortion or trickery than like physical torture. Since extortion and trickery do, on the whole, seem (though morally objectionable) less morally objectionable than physical torture, mental torture is (so the argument we are considering concludes) also less morally objectionable than physical torture.

One difficulty for this argument is that many of the common examples of "mental torture," such as the "*misperception of suffocation*" produced by a wet towel over the mouth and nose, have little or nothing to do with deception. Even if the interrogated is told that she will not suffocate during "waterboarding" (and she believes it), she will have the (misdescribed) "misperception of suffocation." Since her air supply is being cut off, she is in fact suffocating – and her body reacts accordingly in a largely automatic way. Even the terror she feels will be automatic. To call this reaction "mental" (or "psychological") makes it sound less automatic (and more human) than it in fact is. For that reason, I suggest limiting "mental" (and "psychological") to torture that ordinary animals, such as rats or dogs, cannot suffer. (Cf. Chapter 15, this volume.) There are, in fact, few plausible candidates for mental torture so understood.

For these reasons, I suggest we dismiss the distinction between physical and mental torture. Instead, we should agree, first, that all torture is mental insofar as it requires enough consciousness to suffer (cf. Chapter 17, this volume); and, second, that all torture is physical in that it (a) does not presuppose the intervention of conscious reason and (b) operates by mechanisms humans share with other animals. Torture is only one of many ways to mistreat a person. Threats, however cruel, are another. The two ways may occasionally overlap (as in repeatedly putting a gun to someone's head) but even then we can distinguish the torture from the threat (the repetition of the false executions producing the torture).

Torture often hurts a lot, but turning that statistical fact into a definition (as the UN Convention does *not*) opens the door to the paradoxical notion of "humane torture," another version of the mental/physical rhetoric. "Humane torture" is harsh treatment of the body causing extreme suffering but not much pain, for example, months of solitary confinement in a dark, damp, and unheated cell. Not only is there nothing humane about such treatment (except the absence of worse), but the suffering so generated, if intended, seems morally indistinguishable from what almost everyone classifies as torture, slow torture like the drop-drop-drop of the legendary "Chinese water torture," but torture nonetheless. The absence of anything that *hurts a lot* seems a technicality.

Torture can be undertaken for any of at least seven reasons. The UN Convention identifies four of these: (1) to obtain a confession ("judicial torture"), (2) to obtain information ("interrogational torture"), (3) to punish ("penal torture"), and (4) to intimidate or coerce the sufferer or others to act in certain ways ("deterrent" or "terrorist" torture). The Convention omits at least three other reasons to torture: (5) to destroy opponents without killing them (what we may call "disabling torture"); (6) to please the torturer or others ("recreational torture"); and (7) to honor a deity or the victim ("ritual torture"). Two of these omissions from the Convention are understandable. Recreational torture is something government is unlikely to engage in today, though individuals are, especially if a government declares the tortured beyond its protection. Ritual torture seems to belong to another time, say, to the time when the Huron or Iroquois of the eastern woodlands of North America were still powerful nations. (But see Chapter 23, this volume.) The other omission, disabling torture, is not so easy to understand. Governments today do seem to engage in such torture.

2 The alternative definition

What then makes torture (like slavery) especially morally objectionable? While torture is a form of what the UN Convention against Torture calls "cruel, inhuman, or degrading treatment," it seems to differ from other forms in the suffering it imposes (differing enough to be the only form the Convention absolutely forbids under all circumstances). Torture is (as the UN Convention says) *severe* suffering. But not all severe suffering is torture. Consider, for example, the suffering inflicted during a medical procedure (when, say, a surgeon today pops a dislocated shoulder back into place). Such suffering is plainly not something the Convention forbids – or indeed should forbid. There is also the suffering produced by caning, amputation, or other corporal punishments that most legal systems today disallow. However cruel, such punishment is not torture. The "executioner" (the official charged with executing the sentence) is not required to cause suffering, only to carry out a sentence, say, so many hard strokes of a cane upon the bare back. The suffering is (in the words of the Convention) "inherent in or incidental to lawful sanctions." The legislator may have chosen the punishment (in part) because it typically hurts, and the judge may have imposed it for the same reason. But those intentions are independent of the executioner's. In contrast, the torturer actually intends to cause the tortured to suffer (the suffering being either an end in itself or a means). So, for example, "drawing and quartering," though a punishment, was torture in this sense. The executioner was to carry out its various stages in such a way as to make the condemned suffer as much as possible.

While extreme suffering seems to be one morally significant feature of torture, part of what makes torture seem morally objectionable, it is not the only feature. Another is the vast inequality between tortured and torturer. In general, the tortured cannot stop the imposition of suffering, while the torturer has the power (in fact and perhaps even in law) to impose suffering of ever greater amounts almost indefinitely. I do not torture you when, in a street fight or wrestling match, I get you in a half nelson and force your arm upward until your distress makes you cry out and give up. I would, however, begin to torture you if, after you give up, I intentionally continued to force your arm upward.

The tortured's helplessness is of two kinds. First, there is physical helplessness. The tortured is often physically restrained, for example, tied to a chair or strapped to a table. Even when not physically restrained, the tortured may be weakened by lack of sleep, little or no food, or previous beatings. There are usually several torturers to one tortured. Second, there is generally an epistemic helplessness (or at least an extreme inequality in certain kinds of information). The torturers know much about the tortured. The tortured know little or nothing about those who torture them (generally, not even a name or badge number). The torturers have some idea how long the torture will last (even if only "as long as it takes" to get such-and-such). The tortured generally have no idea when the torture will end – or even what the torturers will do next. Torture is (or, at least, is supposed to be) more effective the more ignorance allows the tortured's fears to run wild.

It is nonetheless sometimes said in defense of interrogational or judicial torture that the duration of torture is under the tortured's control. There is some truth in this – but not much. When the torturer seeks information or a confession and the torture is still in its early stages, the tortured can (if he knows what is wanted) *decide* to give in (ending the torture). Indeed, in a well-regulated system of interrogational or judicial torture, the torture would begin, as it often did in early modern Europe, with the torturer showing the prisoner (the candidate for torture) "the instruments of torture," explaining the use of each. If the prisoner does not immediately confess or reveal what the torturer wants to know, the torture would begin, with great ceremony and relatively little suffering. The tortured would then be given another chance to reveal or confess. If he does not, the suffering would increase again. And so on. But if these appeals to reason fail, the torture would begin in earnest, its aim now not to extort information or confession but to achieve it by "breaking" the tortured.

The person subject to judicial or interrogational torture is "broken" when, and only when, he has become so distraught, so unable to bear any more suffering, that he can no longer resist any request the torturer might make. The tortured does not then even think about bargaining. He "pours out his guts." His conduct is no longer rational. He has lost self-control. He will say or do anything to end the torture. That, doubtless, is one reason why so much of what people say under torture is unreliable (Langbein 1977).

In principle, torture, all torture, is limited only by the tortured's endurance. The natural stopping point of torture is the tortured's death, the point at which he can no longer suffer. There is nothing in the concept of torture itself to limit it in any other way. The limit in judicial or interrogational torture arises from the reason justifying the torture, the prospect of extracting a confession or certain information. And, in practice, even judicial or interrogational torture has no *clear* limit. A torturer seldom, if ever, knows how much useful information the tortured has or how much the tortured must confess to have confessed "everything." Even someone seemingly broken may be holding a little back. How is the torturer to *know* unless he puts the tortured to the test? If more torture produces more information, the torturer learns that the tortured was holding back. If more torture produces nothing more, perhaps a little more torture will. The only time the torturer *knows* that he can force no more from the tortured is when the tortured has died. Until the tortured dies, the point at which the torture should stop is a matter of the torturer's judgment (or that of a superior). Torture is not an exact science.

Torture is typically voluntary only on one side. The torturer (or her superior) chooses whom to torture, how to torture, and when to stop the torture. The tortured seldom, if ever, have any such choice. What the tortured may choose is a course of action making torture likely or inevitable. For example, they choose to commit a crime, are caught, and refuse to confess in a country where the police routinely respond with torture. But many who are tortured do not choose even in this weak sense. They are tortured because, for example, they were caught in a sweep of "suspicious persons" or because they belong to some ethnic, religious, or other group the government wants to intimidate. They are simply "innocent bystanders." They lack even the attenuated power to choose not to be tortured further that the guilty told to confess have.

Torture is always presumptively *illegal*. Much torture is (without special legislation) aggravated battery of one sort or another, a serious crime (unless justified or excused), and so, many forms of torture are "violent" (in the sense of applying force against law or morality). But not all torture is violent (in this sense). Some tortures are not batteries (or, at least, not primarily batteries). They resemble non-violent crimes (or, at least, less violent crimes). If a suspect arrives at a detention center naked, failing to provide him with adequate clothing would be neglect (a non-violent crime). If he arrives clothed and sheds his clothing because a guard orders him to, his subsequent suffering from the cold in an unheated cell is not neglect but part of a positive criminal act including robbery (what right had the guards to take by force or threats the suspect's clothing without providing an adequate replacement?), assault (putting the suspect in reasonable fear of bodily injury to get him to undress), and aggravated kidnapping (holding him in the detention center against his will so that he can suffer severe privation). A legal system must explicitly, or by subterfuge, provide for torture if its agents are to torture with impunity. In even the most repressive state, lawful torture exists only as an exception to a general prohibition of battery, neglect, kidnapping, and similar crimes.

Whether resembling aggravated battery or another felony, torture seems substantially worse *morally* than the crime to which it otherwise corresponds. Perhaps part of what explains this difference in our moral assessment is the extreme inequality between (helpless) tortured and (powerful) torturer – making torture seem a kind of bullying. But more important to any explanation must be the way torture takes advantage of that inequality. Torture would be (conceptually) impossible if the tortured could physically protect themselves. It would be compromised, and perhaps much less effective, if the tortured were treated as having rights the torturer had to respect (say, on pain of later lawsuit or administrative penalty). Generally, torture goes on away from family, lawyer, and anyone else who might protect the tortured. Those who wish to torture someone first make him "disappear" (which is one reason that enlightened legal systems try to preserve communication between detainees and the outside world). For the torturer, the tortured must be no more than a living corpse (though, in interrogational or judicial torture, a dead man who can tell tales). The torturer imposes on the tortured what most of us think no human being should impose on another. Torture is therefore always humiliating. The especially humiliating forms of torture, including rough treatment of genitals and anus, are merely the extremes toward which the logic of torture pushes. To recognize any part of the body as beyond torment would offer the tortured some protection (and perhaps much reduce the torture's effectiveness).

Torture resembles punishment in at least four (related) ways. First, like torture, punishment would be a crime did the law not specifically provide otherwise. The death penalty resembles murder; imprisonment; kidnapping; and so on. Second, like torture, punishment (or rather the acts that constitute punishment) are all *prima facie* morally wrong. Third (and in consequence), punishment must have a positive defense (a plausible theory of punishment) to be morally acceptable. And, fourth, like torture, most punishments (death, imprisonment, caning, and so on) require that the convict be (more or less) helpless – handcuffed, under guard, or the like. Only reprimands, suspended sentences, and the like do not.

Punishment nonetheless differs from torture in at least four morally significant ways. First, punishment presupposes rationality. The insane, children, and other mental incompetents are generally exempt from (legal) punishment (and the morality of punishing them is at least controversial while their incompetence lasts). Torture as such requires only the ability to suffer. No theory of torture can plausibly define "torture" so that it is impossible to torture the insane, children, or any other mental incompetents so long as they can suffer. Second, punishment recognizes the convict as retaining certain rights (especially, the right to be treated as a human person). The concept of "mistreating the convict" is not empty in the way "mistreating the tortured" is. Third, punishment typically has a limit the convict knows as well as those who execute sentence. For example, even someone condemned to be drawn and quartered (typically) knows that he will not be caned or branded. Fourth, punishment (except for punishment that is also torture) does not seek the limit of what the convict can suffer (though it may in fact reach it). In that respect, punishment, unlike torture, does not take full advantage of its object's helplessness.

Torture can, of course, be domesticated in various ways. For example, most European legal systems that used torture to obtain confessions in criminal cases set conditions for how much torture (and what kinds) could be used. Torture could legally be used only to investigate relatively serious crimes. Even then a certain amount of evidence implicating a suspect was required before he could be lawfully tortured. More evidence was required for the more excruciating or debilitating tortures. The worst tortures were reserved for those suspected of the most serious crimes when the evidence was almost enough to convict even without a confession. Judges might be present both to put questions and to make sure the torturers did not overstep torture's legal limits. Yet, even domesticated in this way, torture still takes enough advantage of the tortured's helplessness to seem morally objectionable in a way that ordinary punishment does not. So, for example, though the torture of the Spanish Inquisition was domesticated in some such way as this, "the Spanish Inquisition" was nonetheless soon a byword for cruelty and remains so centuries after its abolition (Langbein 1977).

The tortured resemble medical patients in being relatively helpless. It is no surprise then that many devices of torture superficially resemble medical devices. The suffering torture inflicts is also sometimes not that different from what patients suffer. (Consider, for example, electric shock therapy or using a scalpel to peel away skin.) Yet, there is a fundamental difference between a physician, dentist, or other health-care professional and a torturer. The health-care professional should, and generally does, act in the interests of her patient (which is one reason why the health-care professions forbid members to serve torture in any way). Health-care professionals also now generally act with the patient's consent or the consent of someone acting in the patient's interest.[2] In principle, the torturer has no such professional interest in the tortured's welfare. And, in practice, the torturer is unlikely to care at all about it. The tortured is a mere means to someone else's end: a conviction, a bit of information, the torturer's gratification, or the like. The tortured is nothing more than a resource, something that can be misused or wasted but not mistreated.

To summarize: *torture is the intentional pushing of a sentient, helpless being to the limits of its ability to suffer, against that being's will and indifferent to its welfare.* Nothing in this conception of torture requires that the tortured be rational or even human. Nor does it require scars, crippling, or other long-term harm (physical or psychological) to result from the suffering. Torture occurs both when a being is intentionally made to suffer until it "breaks" and when the conduct in question, though reasonably designed to do that, fails (for example, when the tortured dies first or fails to break because he is "a brute"). Torture is a process which may include moments free of suffering. It is identifiable not by what is going on at any given moment but by the intentions of those who control the process. To treat humans in this way is always *prima facie* morally wrong and seldom, if ever, justified or excusable. It is morally worse than the moral wrongs it resembles insofar as it seeks to take full advantage of its subject's helplessness.[3]

3 Some unsatisfactory alternatives

There are at least three approaches to defining torture: the lexicographical, the agent-centered, and the victim-centered (as we may call them). The lexicographical is "scientific" insofar as it simply seeks to *report* (or systematize) usage. If successful, the lexicographical approach yields the concept of torture.[4] The trouble with the lexicographical approach is that we often need something sharper than the concept. Compare "money": The concept of money includes counterfeit money, play money, and currency withdrawn from use (such as the Italian lira or Confederate dollar), as well as pennies, dollar bills, bank checks, and commercial paper. When concerned with getting paid, I want "real money" ("real" signaling a certain conception of money narrower than the concept). What do I mean by "real money"? Of course, I intend to exclude counterfeit money, play money, and withdrawn currency. (I am no fool.) I might also (depending on my purpose) intend to exclude pennies (who wants to carry them around?), commercial paper (risky and hard to spend), and perhaps even checks (they sometimes "bounce"). In contrast, economists typically adopt another conception of money, one including checks and commercial paper, because checks and paper "really are money" (that is, something to be counted when trying to calculate the supply of money available for commerce).[5]

Much the same is true of any lexicographical definition of torture (for example, "severe mental anguish or physical pain"). It is such a definition that allows me to complain (without much exaggeration) that my dental hygienist tortures me every three months. But that complaint, though legitimate (since I do suffer a lot at her hands), uses "torture" in a sense distant from that which identifies torture as especially morally objectionable.[6] I do not consider my dental hygienist's conduct morally objectionable at all. Not only does she do only what I ask of her, she tries her best to avoid hurting me. Insofar as a lexicographical definition of "torture" simply reports usage without consideration of the use to which the word will be put, it is likely to be too general for a subject, such as what makes torture so morally objectionable, which requires more precision.

The other two approaches to defining "torture," the agent-centered and the victim-centered, are unlikely to yield a result too general in this way because they attempt to develop a conception that is morally useful (while not foreclosing the moral questions). The agent-centered approach seeks to develop a conception of torture by considering torture (primarily) from the *torturer's* perspective (emphasizing what the torturer intends). That is what I just did. That is also what the UN Convention did (though with a somewhat different end in view). In contrast, the victim-centered approach seeks to develop a conception of torture by considering torture (primarily) from the *victim's* perspective. (The parenthetical "primarily" is to remind us that both conceptions include both perspectives; the difference between the two, though important, is only in emphasis.)

David Sussman (2005) recently provided a good example of the victim-centered approach. Drawing (primarily) on the reports of torture victims, he defined torture as *a violent overwhelming of the victim's agency*. In most torture, the violence exploits "the victim's own participation" ("perverting" her agency), for example, by forcing her to answer questions. The victim is forced "into the position of colluding against [herself] through [her] own affects and emotions" (Sussman 2005: 4). But some "torture," what Sussman calls "ordeal," simply inflicts so much suffering that the "victim's will is ... turned into just a locus of suffering." For example, a soldier sentenced to a hundred lashes of the whip might break down, screaming uncontrollably, after the fortieth lash. While Sussman does distinguish ordeals from "torture proper" (because an ordeal does not ask for collusion), he nonetheless considers torture proper and mere ordeal to be alike in a fundamental way:

> Like interrogational torture [and, presumably, other forms of torture as well], ordeals involve not just an insult or injury to the victim's agency. Through the combination of captivity, restraint, and pain, the physical and social bases of rational agency are actively turned against such agency itself.[7]

Like torture, ordeals involve the violent destruction of moral autonomy (the perversion of rational agency by turning it against itself). Ordeals are, in this respect, morally objectionable in the special way that Sussman claims "torture proper" is.

Sussman's treatment of ordeals reveals one problem with the victim-centered approach, a departure from widely shared intuitions. Ordeals seem to be a moral category radically distinct from torture (though both do generally impose enough suffering to undermine moral autonomy at least temporarily). Ordeals include caning, branding, and other painful but (arguably) sometimes morally permissible rough treatment.[8] International law explicitly recognizes the difference between such rough treatment and torture. For example, the UN Convention against Torture excludes from its general prohibition of torture any "pain or suffering arising only from, inherent in or incidental to lawful sanctions," that is to say, Sussman's "ordeals" (for example, "a specific number of lashes"; Sussman 2005: 30).

Sussman's emphasis on moral autonomy (or "the bases of rational agency") suggests another problem with his approach to conceptualizing torture. What he presents is a phenomenology of torture from the perspective of a relatively sophisticated sufferer (the sort who might write an account like those on which the victim-centered approach typically relies). Sussman has nothing to say about the torture of animals, young children, the mentally infirm, or others who lack moral autonomy but who (apparently) can be tortured. Yet, torturing some non-autonomous beings, for example, infants or young children, seems to be at least as morally objectionable as torturing competent adults – an appearance any conception of torture should save or at least explain.

Underlying these two problems is a more fundamental one. Morality seems to be primarily about agency (what we should *do*) rather than about victimhood (what we *suffer*). What is fundamentally wrong with victim-centered analyses of torture – not only Sussman's but all of them – is precisely that they are victim-centered, that is, focused on what the victim suffers (or, at least, on what some victims – the morally autonomous – suffer), whether a disintegration of personality, sense of betrayal, loss of dignity, the suffering itself, or something else, rather than on the intention with which the victimizer (the torturer) acts (whether he succeeds or not).

In contrast, the agent-centered analysis above offers a clear distinction between torture and ordeals (however excruciating or debilitating the ordeal), a distinction that tracks not only legal documents such the UN Convention against Torture but common sense. Torture as such seeks to reach the limit of suffering that a helpless, unwilling being can endure – "breaking" him (if he does not die first). What Sussman identifies as "ordeal" is not torture in part at least because (according to the definition I offered) ordeals generally have a natural end before "breaking" (or death). For example, a sentence of so many strokes of the cane must end when that number of strokes is reached (however much or little the convict in fact suffers). Even a sentence of "caning to death" is not torture unless the caning is to be adjusted to maximize the suffering.[9] We must look (primarily) to the intentions of the torturer, not the effect on the tortured, to decide whether the suffering in question is torture – in the morally significant sense we are interested in when we condemn torture in terms more severe than those in which we condemn murder, kidnapping, robbery, battery, and the like (whether "torture proper" or something morally close, such as inhuman, cruel, or degrading treatment).

Related topics

Chapter 15: The lives of others: pain in non-human animals (Droege)
Chapter 17: Pain and consciousness (Pereplyotchik)
Chapter 23: Sacred pain: the use of self-inflicted pain (Glucklich)
Chapter 27: Bad by nature: an axiological theory of pain (Massin)

Notes

1 Consider this statement from an official French report done in 1955 (just after the Algerian war): "The water and the electricity methods, provided they are carefully used, are said to produce a shock which is

more psychological than physical and therefore do not constitute excessive cruelty." Quoted in Tindale 1996: 354. Note how "therefore" follows "more psychological than physical."

2 See, for example World Medical Association (2006): "[A physician shall] be dedicated to providing competent medical service in full professional and moral independence, with compassion and respect for human dignity … [and] respect the rights and preferences of patients, colleagues, and other health professionals."

3 Given this analysis, "torturing oneself" can only be torture by analogy or metaphor.

4 Dictionary definitions are sometimes lexicographical in this sense and sometimes something less, a mere list of various uses or senses.

5 I draw this distinction between concept and conception from Rawls (1971: 5).

6 This is one reason to reject the definition of torture in Kershnar (2012: 2–6): "imposing extreme suffering on [another]."

7 Sussman 2005: 33. The reference to "interrogational torture" here may suggest that interrogational torture is Sussman's subject throughout. While I think he has a tendency to write that way, especially near the article's end, his opening paragraphs make clear his subject is torture as such, for example: "In this article, I defend the intuition that there is something morally special about torture that distinguishes it from most other kinds of violence, cruelty, and degrading treatment" (Sussman 2005: 3).

8 For other victim-centered definitions that seem to have led their authors to make much the same mistake about ordeals, see Bedau 1987: 123–128, and Reiman 1985.

9 For a much longer explanation (and defense) of this analysis of torture, see Davis 2005 and 2007.

References

Bedau, H.A. (1987) *Death Is Different*. Boston: Northeastern University Press.

Corns, J. (2014) The inadequacy of unitary characterizations of pain. *Philosophical Studies* 169: 355–378.

Davis, M. (2005) The moral justifiability of torture and other cruel, inhuman, or degrading treatment. *International Journal of Applied Philosophy* 19(2): 161–178;

Davis, M. (2007) Torture and the inhumane. *Criminal Justice Ethics* 26(2): 29–43.

Kershnar, S. (2012) *For Torture: A Rights-Based Defense*. Lanham: Lexington Books.

Langbein, J.H. (1977) *Torture and the Law of Proof: Europe and England in the Ancien Regime*. Chicago: University of Chicago Press.

Rawls, J. (1971) *A Theory of Justice*. Cambridge, MA: Harvard University Press.

Reiman, J. (1985) Justice, civilization, and the death penalty: answering van den Haag. *Philosophy & Public Affairs* 14(2): 115–148.

Sussman, D. (2005) What's wrong with torture. *Philosophy & Public Affairs* 33(1): 1–33.

Tindale, C.W. (1996) The logic of torture. *Social Theory and Practice* 22(3): 349–374.

United Nations (1984) *The Convention against Torture and Other Cruel, Inhuman or Degrading Treatment or Punishment*, adopted and opened for signature, ratification and accession by General Assembly resolution 39/46, 10 December. Office the United Nations High Commissioner for Human Rights. <http://www.ohchr.org/EN/ProfessionalInterest/Pages/CAT.aspx>, accessed 11 February 2016.

World Medical Association (2006) *International Code of Medical Ethics*. World Medical Association. <http://www.wma.net/en/30publications/10policies/c8/>, accessed 12 March 2016.

29

PAIN AND EDUCATION

Avi I. Mintz

Parents and teachers inflict pain on the young in many ways. They frustrate a child's desire for immediate gratification by, say, refusing to purchase them a treat in the grocery store. Or they embarrass a student by identifying, for example, a computational error in math class. Or they punish a transgression by isolating or striking the child. Or perhaps they simply neglect the student's or child's call for attention. One may be inclined to say that "pain" is too strong a term for experiences like disappointment or frustration, and that we should reserve it for describing a more intense experience resulting in physical or psychological harm. (Cf. discussions of social pain in Chapters 7 and 13.) But such a definitional parameter should not be set casually because it might fail to acknowledge the very real intensity of children's reactions to parents' or teachers' actions; adults might dismissively classify something as benign but adolescents might feel it acutely – even an unpleasant "disappointment" can play a role in cognitive, moral, physical, or what is generally sometimes called "character" development. (See Chapter 30, this volume.) In this chapter, I shall call these negative experiences "pains of learning" or "educational pains," and I include under this umbrella such varied experiences as shame, embarrassment, confusion, anxiety, perplexity, frustration, and the experience accompanying bodily injuries.

1 Pains of learning in teaching and parenting

Too often the pain inflicted on children is taken to be either good or bad, something to be completely embraced or rejected. An influential debate in educational theory is illustrative: Progressive educational theorists in the early twentieth century – those who often claimed to be followers of John Dewey, the century's most influential educational philosopher – sought to liberate students' interests and intellect by promoting an education that included active movement, hands-on projects, and by connecting the curriculum to the students' lives outside of school (e.g., Dewey 1979/1915; Rugg and Shumaker 1928). These progressive educators viewed the strict disciplinary regime of "traditional classrooms" – those which featured students sitting silently in fixed rows of desks, drearily repeating some lesson they were coerced into memorizing – as oppressive and fear-inducing. Traditionalists sometimes justified students' boredom, fear, and anxiety as experiences that were good for their character, arguing that the ability to persevere for little reward in unpleasant circumstances is of great value in life. Progressive educators would quip that, in essence, the old, traditional education entailed the belief that it mattered not what children were taught, so long as they didn't like it. Isaac

Kandel, a long-time critic of child-centered progressive education, retorted that, for progressives, "it does not matter what a student studies, so long as he does like it" (Kandel 1943).

Such a dichotomy – whether students should enjoy their education or overcome their aversion to it – possesses so little nuance as to render it virtually useless; few scholars would defend the position that *all* learning should be enjoyable, or that students' enjoyment must be avoided in order to develop the right kind of character. Yet this kind of all-or-nothing thinking about pain and education persists. Parents of infants are confronted with, for example, advice to form nurturing, supportive attachments with their infants and toddlers by, among other things, feeding on demand and co-sleeping in order to minimize the babies' and toddlers' stress and anxiety.[1] Yet they are also presented with the opposite advice: to feed and put to sleep on a schedule, so that infants' and toddlers' pangs of hunger will encourage them to eat better when given the opportunity, and so that they will "self-soothe" (i.e., learn to cope with their distress) when left alone to sleep (e.g., Ferber 1985). While there are sophisticated arguments to be made on both sides of this debate, the public discourse tends to devolve into a choice between the need to shield versus the danger of shielding the young from unpleasant experiences.

In contemporary educational practice, a small minority of schools today keep alive the progressive vision that Isaac Kandel criticized, explicitly seeking to minimize the coercion and tedium involved in traditional schooling, offering instead the opportunity for students to pursue whatever they are inclined to do, whether that be music, literature, art, math, or video games.[2] At the other extreme, particularly in the United States, are the so-called "no-excuses" schools that have promoted rigid routines, uncompromising emphasis on academic success, and, sometimes, public shaming of students who score poorly on tests or who misbehave (e.g., Taylor 2015; Green 2014). Some educational theorists look at the more typical schools of today – not no-excuses schools nor the progressive schools but the kind of private and public schools that are the vast majority of schooling options – and argue that even they inflict "violence" upon students, causing "wounds" such as the anxiety caused by high stakes assessments, the spite that arises by schools' cultivation of competitiveness, and the diminished self that results from being controlled and coerced (Olson 2009; Harber 2004). Additionally, corporal punishment in classrooms is still common in most of the world (Pate and Gould 2012), as well as other forms of punishment such as confining students outside of class times (i.e., detention), assigning extra tasks, revoking students' privileges, or denying them access to their usual activities (e.g., suspending or expelling them).

Are the pains that occur in the course of schooling ever ethically or educationally warranted? An unsatisfactory response is to say simply that we ought to find a middle ground that is neither too indulgent of children's interests and whims nor too strict and punitive. While this position might hold some appeal in its broadest articulation, it provides little guidance in practice, nor is it particularly helpful as theory. What would that middle ground look like, for example, in one of the many countries in which teachers routinely paddle students? That they ought to paddle a misbehaving child neither too frequently nor too infrequently, neither too strongly nor too softly? The worthwhile question is whether paddling is itself an ethical means of fostering students' development in schools. More generally, is there a justifiable, pedagogically valuable role for particular pains of learning in teaching and parenting?

2 The case of corporal punishment as a pain of learning

Punishment, particularly corporal punishment, has long been the focus of debates about whether parents or teachers ought to inflict pain on their students. The issue, I would suggest, has led to the neglect of many other important kinds of pain relevant to education and child rearing. But since corporal punishment has received so much political, public, and scholarly attention, I first discuss some of the research on the topic and discuss some prominent philosophical responses to it. Thereafter, I turn to how educational pains unrelated to punishment might be, or might fail to be, pedagogically valuable.

Physical punishment for children's failures was routine a few generations ago and is still common in some schools and in many homes throughout the world, though its use varies dramatically by country. Japanese and American parents, for example, use corporal punishment far more frequently than European parents (Pate and Gould 2012: 63). In addition to differences among countries, use differs within countries. In Yemen corporal punishment is more than twice as likely to occur in rural homes as in urban homes (Pate and Gould 2012: 63). In the United States, corporal punishment is much more common in fundamentalist Christian homes (Flynn 1996; Pate and Gould 2012: 87). Indeed, American fundamentalist parenting has become a focus of public concern. A fundamentalist Christian parenting book, *To Train Up a Child* (Pearl and Pearl 1996), that advocated spanking and other disciplinary measures was targeted in a campaign calling for Amazon to stop selling it. Alarming media accounts have drawn attention to parenting practices in fundamentalist Christian communities. One family, for instance, that had sought to apply the disciplinary recommendations of *To Train Up a Child* murdered their adopted child in the process of "disciplining" her (Joyce 2013). Because fundamentalist culture emphasizes subordination so strongly (of wives to husbands, children to parents, all to god), beliefs about the value of corporal punishment accord with their values such that those parents would be less likely to be swayed by "permissive" arguments against its use.

The modern "children's rights" movement seeks to limit the use of corporal punishment, sometimes through legal challenges and sometimes via broader campaigns to encourage nation states to change their policies (Parker-Jenkins 1999). The Global Initiative to End All Corporal Punishment of Children, an advocacy group, reports that, as of this writing, 126 countries prohibit corporal punishment in schools and 72 permit it; 46 countries prevent corporal punishment in the home, while 152 permit it (GIECPC 2015). A prohibition against corporal punishment does not necessarily indicate an immediate elimination of its use (just as laws against tax fraud do not entail that no tax fraud occurs), but there is a correlation between prohibitions and the use of corporal punishment, and a prohibition may, over time, change a country's culture with respect to corporal punishment and result in decreased use.

The research on corporal punishment generally supports prohibiting it because, in addition to physical wounds, it may cause depression or increase aggression, among other things (e.g., Pate and Gould 2012). Some scholars, however, have pointed out that researchers have failed to demonstrate that the occasional use of mild forms of corporal punishment like spanking are indeed harmful (e.g., Larzelere and Baumrind 2010). Furthermore, some sociological research suggests the use of corporal punishment might be correlated with greater respect for parents (e.g., Lareau 2011). In addition, verbal discipline is often the fallback method for parents and teachers who do not use corporal punishment, and harsh verbal discipline has been shown to predict "adolescent conduct problems and depressive symptoms" (Baumrind et al. 2010: 161; Wang and Kenny 2014).

The fact that empirical studies have failed to find unambiguous harm from mild forms of parents' use of corporal punishment is only one complicating factor in determining whether it might be justified and ethical under certain circumstances. The second is the way that corporal punishment is employed across social groups. In the United States, black families and working-class and poor families are much more likely to employ it than are white, middle-class families (Flynn 1996; Lareau 2011). Some scholars and advocates in minority communities have raised concerns that many who call for eliminating corporal punishment are generally middle class and white and are promoting their own style of parenting in poor communities and communities of color. Parenting "remediation" programs that target these communities appear to some as an ethnocentric attempt to, what would be called in the not too distant past, civilize the savages (e.g., Brighouse and Swift 2013). Recently, the American football player Adrian Peterson unwittingly generated a rare public discourse about the relationship of race and parenting after he was indicted for beating his four-year-old son with a switch so severely that he required medical attention. While many in the media were quick to deplore Peterson's action, some argued that Peterson's critics were out of touch with Southern, African-American parenting norms. For example, former National Basketball Association player, Charles Barkley, stated that, if corporal punishment were to become illegal, "every black parent in my neighborhood in the South would be in trouble or in jail under those circumstances" (Sieczkowski 2014). In an era in which public policy is increasingly sensitive to cultural differences within a country, advocacy that appears ethnocentric and targets primarily the parenting practices of poor and marginalized communities, will raise ethical concerns – regardless of the validity of the advocates' argument (e.g., Brighouse and Swift 2013).

3 From corporal punishment to other educational pains

As I mentioned above, despite the fact that corporal punishment would be most people's primary association when asked about pain and education, corporal punishment is only one part of the terrain (and it is an area that, notwithstanding the caveats of some of the communities and scholars I described above, has seen a consensus against its use emerge). Arguably far more interesting and more important for parenting and teaching are other aspects of educational pain. While this essay is not the place to discuss at length the history of educational pain in philosophy, a brief digression on the topic will help elucidate some relevant conceptual distinctions. In the seventeenth century, John Locke argued that "*slavish discipline* makes a *slavish temper*" (Locke 1996/1693: §50, 34; Locke's emphasis). Locke worried that obedience because of "the fear of the rod" does not alter the underlying problematic inclination because the punishment (or fear thereof) only focuses the child's attention on his inability to satisfy the inclination (perhaps even inflaming it). Furthermore, the child should learn to obey reason, not the commands of others. Notably, Locke viewed using incentives like sugarplums to encourage virtuous behavior to be problematic as well. If a child acts virtuously to receive a treat, the child becomes acclimated to following the dictates of the appetites rather than following reason. To reason with children, Locke argued, is the surest path to developing a virtuous, rational adult. Despite his recognition of the problematic nature of harsh punishments and incentives that relate to the pleasures of the body, Locke did see a particular version of punishment and reward as essential to cultivating virtue. He advised that the great secret of education was getting children to internalize virtuous dispositions by praising or blaming their actions; the esteem or pain of shame experienced because of the child's desire to please a respected parent or tutor would form a virtuous character without recourse to the baser pleasures or pains of the body (Locke 1996/1693: § 52–58).

In the eighteenth century, in perhaps the most important work on parenting and education in the history of Western educational philosophy, Jean-Jacques Rousseau (1979/1762) argued that Locke did not go far enough. Praise or blame does not cultivate virtue. Rather, it subtly conveys that we should base our valuation of ourselves on what others think of us. He agreed with Locke that the way children are typically punished for misbehavior teaches primarily that a child must learn to do whatever the relevant authority demands of him. But rather than justify esteem or blame as Locke did, Rousseau sought to remove the authority from the child's horizon. Rousseau tells the story of a mischievous boy who, to cause a stir among the adults, broke the windows of his home. Rousseau did not scold him, nor did he reason with him (as Locke recommended).[3] He did not offer to repair the window or find other sleeping accommodations for the child. Any of those options would introduce punishment, subordination, and obedience into the equation, and therefore threaten the child's autonomy. Whenever possible, Rousseau counseled, a child should come to his own conclusions about the effects of his actions. To appreciate the folly of breaking a window, the child should sleep in a cold room.

Rousseau's argument that students should learn at their own pace and through their experiences (rather than via textbooks or lectures) was historically pivotal in opening the door to a re-examination of the aims and methods of education. But Rousseau, like Locke, is also helpful for understanding the difference between the pain involved in an authority punishing a child and other sorts of pains that are pedagogically productive. Rousseau argued that human flourishing required an ability to bear the ills of life – the inevitable loss of loved ones, the inevitable humiliations of failure, the inevitable illnesses and injuries. He thought that education had a role to play in cultivating our ability to deal with these pains; we should allow children to experience pains they can bear to help them acclimate to them (Mintz 2012).

Rousseau recognized that children and youth suffer because learning something involves an encounter with the limits of one's knowledge or a discovery of an unsatisfactory aspect of one's character or intellect. Confrontation with our ignorance or inadequacy is often unpleasant, but it is nevertheless necessary for learning and development. As the psychologist Fritz Oser has argued, an encounter with our mistakes and our inadequacies provides us with essential insight into how we might do something correctly, and this recognition of inadequacy or failure is sometimes painful (Oser 1996; Oser and Spychinger 2005; see also English 2013). For example, learning about injustices in our communities and in our world causes students to suffer at the suffering of others; learning about a historical injustice like genocide or contemporary injustices (the plight of the homeless) causes students emotional distress, but many argue that such experiences are a critical bridge to social justice (Nussbaum 1996; Mintz 2013).

In the remainder of this chapter, I focus on two main questions. First, how might we distinguish some of the necessary, valuable, or inevitable educational pains from others? Second, what conditions might teachers and parents create, such that their charges will respond productively to their educational pains?

4 Justifiable and productive educational pains

Despite the caveats about the potential for mild forms of corporal punishment to be ethical and developmentally valuable, corporal punishment per se, and punishment of all forms, introduces a variety of pains (e.g., shame, fear, anger, resentment) that might be detrimental to development and learning, particularly relative to other pains that might help achieve the same ends. Rousseau made the case that it is more educationally productive for the student to focus on her problem or activity rather than satisfying an authority, and that argument has found many supporters. John Dewey, like Rousseau, argued that children learn best when they encounter their own errors rather than have others point them out. Dewey was often criticized by his contemporaries for failing to understand that "discipline" is one of the primary aims of education. Dewey countered that there are two educationally relevant senses of discipline. On the one hand, "discipline" means punishing the child for failing to act as the authority desires. Discipline of this sort depends on "various kinds of physical, social, and personal pain" to control the child (Dewey 1976/1902: 207). In another sense, "discipline" is the by-product of sustained immersion in an activity in which one is interested. In this case it is the engagement in the activity – not the interest of avoiding "physical, social, and personal pain" – that cultivates discipline. One might best overcome inadequate carpentry abilities, for example, by continuously working with the wood, nails, and saws, eventually coming to master the skilled use of them. The child who attempts to build her first bird house experiences a relevant sort of pain in these activities, because she is regularly confronted with obstacles, frustrations, and distractions. Focused on the task at hand, one develops the "power to endure in an intelligently chosen course in face of distraction, confusion, and difficulty," a power Dewey identifies as "the essence of discipline" (Dewey 1916: 129).

This characterization of the two senses of discipline exaggerates and oversimplifies two matters. First, it seems to suggest that learning is ideally laissez-faire; that is, the teacher or parent should simply get out of the way and allow the student to teach herself through immersion in an activity, in a rich environment. Second, it seems to assume that children's interests will be sufficiently developed and robust to direct them to worthwhile activities. To respond to this latter point, it is certainly the case that interests are developed in many ways. Some adults who have a passion for playing a musical instrument, and continue to play because of intrinsic interest alone, were not interested when, as children, their parents or teachers required them to play; that is, interest may follow engagement with an activity, it does not always need to precede it. Furthermore, some would argue that there are some things that must be learned regardless of the student's interest because such topics serve the needs of the state, the family, or the child herself. Without wading into the voluminous debates about the centrality of students' interests, I suggest that, minimally, children's interests ought to be utilized in their education to whatever extent possible. When interest is absent, parents and teachers should creatively attempt to cultivate interest or endeavor to make the activity worthwhile for the student.

Regarding the authority's role in learning and development, there is likewise much scholarly debate. I would argue that a teacher or parent possesses expertise and experience that might assist the child in the activity, and there is no reason to withhold guidance and correction completely. Ideally, however, the correction and guidance will not impose upon the child sufficiently to transform the activity from one in which a goal is pursued to one in which the child simply follows or attempts to please the authority. Psychologists have suggested a helpful, related distinction. Students' struggle or failure is more pedagogically valuable in the midst of "task involvement" rather than "ego involvement" (Nicholls 1989). When children are pursuing an activity with a dominant focus on how they compare to others (which characterizes ego involvement) they are less likely to maximize their learning compared to when they are primarily interested in the task itself. This may seem obvious, but a child who spends her time assembling model airplanes because of her inherent interest in the task will probably, though not necessarily, become better at assembling models than the child who is primarily interested in, for example, assembling models faster than other children. The Rousseauean insight that a preoccupation with comparing oneself to others and with seeking approval from an authority may detract from learning is sound.

A classic study of extrinsic rewards found that children who were rewarded for solving a puzzle were less intrinsically motivated to engage in the task again at a later date than those who had not been extrinsically rewarded (Lepper and Greene 1975; Kohn 1999).

Nevertheless, ego involvement and extrinsic rewards can indeed be pedagogically effective. A professor who "grades on a curve," and makes high grades a scarce resource for which competition is fierce, may both increase the effort that her students put into the class and their willingness to tolerate frustration, anxiety, and other educational pains. But, at the same time, the ego involvement that grading on a curve encourages, and the extrinsic rewards of the grade, may ultimately undermine learning and development as the student's focus becomes divided between the material he is attempting to master, winning the professor's esteem, and comparing himself to his classmates. The educational pain of recognizing one's inadequacy or error is often unavoidable. But if students come to recognize the pain on their own, in the course of immersion in an activity, they may remain focused on what needs to be improved. When an authority corrects the student, or when the student is focused on how he compares to others or on obtaining an external reward, the pain of recognizing one's inadequacy or error is now compounded by additional educational pains that may not otherwise be present – the fear of reprimand, the fear of disappointing, the fear of *appearing* inadequate (as opposed to the fear that one is actually so). The more children and students can focus on the inquiry before them rather than on their relationships with authorities, the better.

Thus far, I have suggested that the pains of learning experienced through immersion in an activity are more justifiable and pedagogically productive than those that arise in the attempt to please or obey a relevant authority (though the latter may be justifiable and productive as well). Another issue that is of use in determining the value of certain pains of learning is task difficulty. Psychologists have found that if tasks are too easy, people are not inclined to pursue them. Yet tasks that are extremely difficult will be avoided as well. Ideally, tasks will have a moderate challenge – anything already mastered will be a bore, anything so far beyond one's current abilities will cause frustration and anxiety and breed helplessness. Thus educators must find tasks that are sufficiently difficult that a student will struggle to complete them, but that are not too far beyond current abilities (e.g., Shernoff et al. 2003).

5 Promoting productive responses to the pains of learning

The above analysis suggests that certain kinds of educational pains – those experienced through immersion in an intrinsically interesting task of moderate difficulty – are valuable and justifiable. But responses to pains vary widely. Why does one athlete get cut from a varsity high-school basketball team and never try out again, while someone like Michael Jordan uses the rejection to fuel an intense effort to improve? Why do some students fail a moderately difficult math course and decide to take no further math courses, while another retakes the course and plans to take others? There must be more to the matter, for example, than whether the math course was of moderate difficulty. Scholars studying academic achievement in schools found that a challenging curriculum alone did not lead to high student achievement. Rather, only when that challenging curriculum was accompanied by strong social support – the support of teachers, family, and a student's community who provide assistance and cultivate the confidence necessary for a student to persevere through frustration – did the standards yield the desired educational achievement (Lee et al. 1999). This lesson about the value of social support is particularly important considering how often educational reformers call for more rigorous standards. The frustration and struggle associated with a challenging curriculum may be an obstacle to further learning or a catalyst for it, depending on whether social support is present, among other things.

Furthermore, the struggle and frustration in the encounter with a challenging curriculum can be ameliorated when teachers offer explicit, concrete strategies and advice for success (e.g., Delpit 2006). Explicit discussion of strategies and social support are not, however, the same as guiding students though their work. Some teachers break math problems down into simple step-by-step procedures, thinking that "success breeds success" (Clifford 1990). Indeed, cross-cultural researchers in education have observed that Japanese teachers are much more likely than American, German, and teachers from many other countries, to present students with difficult problems and allow them to experience frustration and confusion. Japanese students are not only left to struggle with their failure, but Japanese teachers also seek to induce students' struggle and frustration by selecting problems that will likely cause them to err. In a math classroom, for example, a Japanese teacher might ask students to add fractions with different denominators knowing that most students will do so incorrectly, and will then have to struggle to figure out what went wrong (Stigler and Hiebert 1999). On the other hand, teachers in other countries are more likely to try to protect students from their confusion and frustration. American teachers, for example, are much more likely than Japanese teachers to tell students the procedure for correctly adding fractions before presenting them with a problem. They protect students from the pains of confusion and frustration while denying them an opportunity to grapple with the mathematical concept itself, something that improves students' understanding of the topic (Stigler and Hiebert 1999).

In addition to the importance of social support and explicitly providing students with the foundational competence such that they understand how they can achieve their goals (while avoiding leading students through their inquiry), a third factor might promote productive encounters with the pains of learning: equipping students with a better narrative of learning. A striking study found that middle schoolers' math scores could be raised by merely telling them on occasion over the course of a semester that success in mathematics was based on effort (not on innate ability) (Blackwell et al. 2007).[4] The lesson we might learn as parents and educators is the following: we ought to provide our students and our children with a narrative about learning in which their educational pains – failure, frustration, anxiety, and fear – are not indicators of innate deficits but are rather rungs on the ladder of educational success, a proper part of the educational journey.

6 Conclusion: why thinking about educational pain matters

Many young people routinely suffer in ways that society should help prevent – children are hungry, they are physically and emotionally abused, they are humiliated, and they are neglected. And in their homes and schools, they experience other pains such as self-doubt about their intellectual (or professional) potential. Because even self-doubt can be so painful some have argued that teachers should avoid criticism or correction that might harm self-esteem. The "self-esteem" movement in education that emerged in the 1990s in California explicitly argued for the educational value of affirmation (e.g., Mecca et al. 1989). Yet to shield a student from her own ignorance or ineffectiveness is anti-educational, and the implications of methods and aims of education devoted narrowly to enhancing students' self-esteem have been justly pilloried (e.g., Stout 2000; Smith 2002; Sykes 1995). But to posit simply that *all* educational pains are valuable is problematic as well. Certain educational pains are more justifiable and educationally productive than others. Parents and teachers must take care about which ones children will experience, and they must lay the foundation for children to have productive responses to the pains of learning.

Related topics

Chapter 7: Neuromatrix theory of pain (Roy and Wager)
Chapter 13: Psychogenic pain: old and new (Sullivan)
Chapter 30: Pain and justified evaluative belief (Cowan)

Notes

1 The defenders of "attachment theory" are probably the best example of contemporary advocates for reducing children's stress and anxiety. See, for example, Attachment Parenting International's website, AttachmentParenting.org.
2 Sudbury Valley School, for example, has about twenty schools in the United States and another dozen or so in Europe, Israel, Japan, and Brazil. These schools in many ways resemble A.S. Neill's Summerhill School as children spend their days planning and administering their own activities, choosing what to study (or not to study), and generally managing their days as they see fit (Neill 1992). For a discussion of the Democratic School of Hadera in Israel, see Hecht 2011.
3 Rousseau believed that young children were not yet capable of sophisticated reasoning. The children who were reasoned with, as Locke had advised, really just offered performances of reasoning to satisfy and impress adults. Rousseau, who valued authenticity, would prefer children to respond bluntly and directly (Rousseau 1979/1762: 89–90). Rousseau believed that the children who reasoned with adults were merely performing for accolades.
4 The psychologist Carol Dweck has conducted highly influential work on praise, distinguishing praise of effort from less developmentally valuable praise of ability. She found that ability praise made students *more* inclined to avoid their mistakes and failures rather than overcome them (Cimpian et al. 2007; Dweck 1999; Kamins and Dweck 1999).

References

Baumrind, D., Larzelere, R.E., and Owens, E.B. (2010) Effects of preschool parents' power assertive patterns and practices on adolescent development. *Parenting: Science and Practice* 10: 157–201.

Blackwell, L.S., Trzesniewski, K.H., and Dweck, C.S. (2007) Implicit theories of intelligence predict achievement across an adolescent transition: a longitudinal study and an intervention. *Child Development* 78: 246–263.

Brighouse, H. and Smith, A. (2013) Forum reply. In J.J. Heckman (ed.), *Giving Kids a Fair Chance*. Cambridge, MA: MIT Press, pp. 107–112.

Cimpian, A., Arce, H.-M.C., Markman, E.M., and Dweck, C.S. (2007) Subtle linguistic cues affect children's motivation. *Psychological Science* 18: 314–316.

Clifford, M.M. (1990) Students need challenge, not easy success. *Educational Leadership* 48: 22–26.

Delpit, L.D. (2006) *Other People's Children: Cultural Conflict in the Classroom*. New York: New Press.

Dewey, J. (1916) *Democracy and Education: An Introduction to the Philosophy of Education*. New York: Free Press.

Dewey, J. (1976/1902) The child and the curriculum. In *The Middle Works, 1899–1924*, vol. 2, ed. J.A. Boydston. Carbondale: Southern Illinois University Press.

Dewey, J. (1979/1915) *Schools of To-morrow*. In *The Middle Works, 1899–1924*, vol. 8, ed. J.A. Boydston. Carbondale: Southern Illinois University Press.

Dweck, C.S. (1999) Caution – praise can be dangerous. *American Educator* 23: 4–9.

English, A.R. (2013) *Discontinuity in Learning: Dewey, Herbart and Education as Transformation*. Cambridge: Cambridge University Press.

Ferber, R. (1985) *Solve Your Child's Sleep Problems*. New York: Simon & Schuster.

Flynn, C.P. (1996) Normative support for corporal punishment: attitudes, correlates, and implications. *Aggression and Violent Behavior* 1: 47–55.

GIECPC (Global Initiative to End All Corporal Punishment of Children) (2015) *Global Progress towards Prohibiting All Corporal Punishment*. GIECPC. <http://www.endcorporalpunishment.org/progress/>.

Green, E. (2014) *Building a Better Teacher: How Teaching Works (and How to Teach it to Everyone)*. New York: W.W. Norton & Co.

Harber, C. (2004) *Schooling as Violence: How Schools Harm Pupils and Societies*. London: RoutledgeFalmer.

Hecht, Y. (2011) *Democratic Education: A Story of a Beginning*. Washington, DC: Bravura Books.

Joyce, K. (2013) Hana's story: an adoptee's tragic fate, and how it could happen again. *Slate.com*. <http://www.slate.com/articles/double_x/doublex/2013/11/hana_williams_the_tragic_death_of_an_ethiopian_adoptee_and_how_it_could.html>.

Kamins, M.L. and Dweck, C.S. (1999) Person versus process praise and criticism: implications for contingent self-worth and coping. *Developmental Psychology* 35: 835–847.

Kandel, I.L. (1943) *The Cult of Uncertainty*. New York: Macmillan.

Kohn, A. (1999) *Punished by Rewards: The Trouble with Gold Stars, Incentive Plans, A's, Praise, and Other Bribes*. Boston: Houghton Mifflin Co.

Lareau, A. (2011) *Unequal Childhoods: Class, Race, and Family Life*, 2nd ed. Berkeley: University of California Press.

Larzelere, R.E. and Baumrind, D. (2010) Are spanking injunctions scientifically supported? *Law & Contemporary Problems* 73: 57–87.

Lee, V.E., Smith, J.B., Perry, T.E., and Smylie, M.A. (1999) Social support, academic press, and student achievement: a view from the middle grades in Chicago. In *Improving Chicago's Schools: A Report of the Chicago Annenberg Research Project*. Chicago: Consortium on Chicago School Research.

Lepper, M.R. and Greene, D. (1975) Turning play into work: effects of adult surveillance and extrinsic rewards on children's intrinsic motivation. *Journal of Personality and Social Psychology* 31: 479–486.

Locke, J. (1996/1693) *Some Thoughts concerning Education: and, Of the Conduct of the Understanding*, ed. R.W. Grant and N. Tarcov. Indianapolis: Hackett Publishing Co.

Mecca, A.M., Smelser, N.J., and Vasconcellos, J. (1989) *The Social Importance of Self-Esteem*. Berkeley: University of California Press.

Mintz, A.I. (2012) The happy and suffering student? Rousseau's *Emile* and the path not taken in progressive educational thought. *Educational Theory* 62: 249–265.

Mintz, A.I. (2013) Helping by hurting: the paradox of suffering in social justice education. *Theory and Research in Education* 11: 215–230.

Neill, A.S. (1992) *Summerhill School: A New View of Childhood*. New York: St. Martin's Griffin.

Nicholls, J.G. (1989) *The Competitive Ethos and Democratic Education*. Cambridge, MA: Harvard University Press.

Nussbaum, M. (1996) Compassion: the basic social emotion. *Social Philosophy and Policy* 13(1): 27–58.

Olson, K. (2009) *Wounded by School: Recapturing the Joy in Learning and Standing Up to Old School Culture*. New York: Teachers College Press.

Oser, F.K. (1996) Learning from negative morality. *Journal of Moral Education* 25: 67–74.

Oser, F.K. and Spychinger, M. (2005) *Lernen ist schmerzhaft: Zur Theorie des negativen Wissens und zur Praxis der Fehlerkultur*. Weinheim: Beltz.

Parker-Jenkins, M. (1999) *Sparing the Rod: Schools, Discipline and Children's Rights*. Stoke-on-Trent: Trentham Books.

Pate, M. and Gould, L.A. (2012) *Corporal Punishment around the World*. Santa Barbara, CA: Praeger.

Pearl, M. and Pearl, D. (1996) *To Train Up a Child*. Pleasantville: No Greater Joy Industries.

Rousseau, J.J. (1979/1762) *Emile: or, On Education*, trans. A. Bloom. New York: Basic Books.

Rugg, H. and Shumaker, A. (1928). *The Child-Centered School: An Appraisal of the New Education*. New York: World Book Co.

Shernoff, D.J., Csikszentmihalyi, M., Schneider, B., and Shernoff, E.S. (2003) Student engagement in high school classrooms from the perspective of flow theory. *School Psychology Quarterly* 18: 158–176.

Sieczkowski, C. (2014) Charles Barkley defends Adrian Peterson, says "every black parent in the South" hits their kids. *Huffington Post*. <http://www.huffingtonpost.com/2014/09/15/charles-barkley-adrian-peterson_n_5822258.html>.

Smith, R. (2002) Self-esteem: the kindly apocalypse. *Journal of Philosophy of Education* 36: 87–100.

Stigler, J.W. and Hiebert, J. (1999) *The Teaching Gap: Best Ideas from the World's Teachers for Improving Education in the Classroom*. New York: Free Press.

Stout, M. (2000) *The Feel-Good Curriculum: The Dumbing-Down of America's Kids in the Name of Self-Esteem*. Cambridge, MA: Perseus Books.

Sykes, C.J. (1995) *Dumbing Down Our Kids: Why America's Children Feel Good about Themselves but Can't Read, Write, or Add*. New York: St. Martin's Press.

Taylor, K. (2015) At Success Academy Charter Schools, high scores and polarizing tactics. *New York Times*, 6 April.

Wang, M.-T. and Kenny, S. (2014) Longitudinal links between fathers' and mothers' harsh verbal discipline and adolescents' conduct problems and depressive symptoms. *Child Development* 85: 908–923.

30

PAIN AND JUSTIFIED EVALUATIVE BELIEF

Robert Cowan

I believe that I am sitting at a computer and that birds are singing outside. Not only do I believe these things, I seem justified (in the sense associated with evidence or probability of truth) in doing so. Further, my beliefs seem justified independently of their standing in relations of inferential support to other beliefs of mine, i.e., the justification is "immediate."

A natural account of how these beliefs are immediately justified appeals to the fact that I perceive (or seem to perceive) the computer and the birds. Indeed, it is commonly thought that perceptual experiences are a source of immediate justification for beliefs about the world.[1]

Consider now another class of beliefs of mine: I believe that the pain in my foot is bad, and that there are moral reasons against intentionally causing pain in other sentient creatures. Unlike the previous cases, which are empirical beliefs, these are commonly categorized as evaluative beliefs, i.e., roughly, beliefs about the (dis)value of the world. These beliefs also seem immediately justified. But unlike the empirical cases, it is less obvious how they are justified. For one thing, it might be a stretch to claim that we can perceive via the five canonical sensory modalities that something is bad or wrong. As a sign of the difficulties here, note that some philosophers (see, e.g., Price 1991/1758) have been led to posit a non-sensory faculty of rational intuition in order to account for evaluative justification. But many doubt the existence of such a thing.

Although there are other potential candidate sources – e.g., desire, emotion – in this chapter, I consider an alternative and under-discussed account of evaluative justification which appeals to conscious painful pains (hereafter, simply "pains"). On this view, pains are not only the objects of some justified evaluative beliefs, but are also a source of immediate justification. Call this the "Pain View."

Note two initial attractions of the view. First, by contrast with rational intuition, very few doubt the existence of pains (but see Chapter 1, this volume). Second, pains are widely thought to be "intrinsically" motivational (see, for instance, discussion in Chapters 3 and 4, this volume). This coheres with the common view that evaluative beliefs are intimately linked to motivation, e.g., if I sincerely believe that causing pain is wrong then I'll be in some way motivated to refrain from doing so.

My primary aim is to assess the Pain View. I first introduce a contemporary theory of pain – "Evaluativism" (see Bain 2013, and Chapter 3, this volume; Cutter and Tye 2011;

354

Helm 2002) – according to which pains are (roughly) perceptual experiences of the badness of bodily damage. I focus exclusively on this view partly due to space constraints but also because Evaluativism is naturally associated with the Pain View: if pains are perceptual then perhaps they have the same epistemology as other perceptual phenomena, i.e., they can immediately justify. I then introduce two theories of immediate justification which ground two versions of the Pain View. I then assess whether, on the assumption of Evaluativism, pains can immediately justify evaluative beliefs, and if so, of what kind. Finally, I briefly discuss the idea that a distinctive "moral" pain could immediately justify evaluative beliefs.

1 Pain Evaluativism

I once burnt my finger on a stove while attempting to cook spaghetti Bolognese. My finger was red and swollen, and it really hurt. Both of these things – my damaged finger and my pain – were in some sense bad.[2] I'll refer to the former (associated with the damage in my finger) as "bodily-badness" and the latter (associated with the painful experience) as "experiential-badness." Note also that I was rationally motivated (but see Cohen and Fulkerson 2014 for doubts about this) to do something about my finger and experience: to run my finger under cold water, to apply antiseptic, and (eventually) to take some paracetamol.

As a paradigmatic pain episode, theories of pain are supposed to account for it. One theory that has enjoyed recent popularity, and will constitute my focus, is:

> Evaluativism: S undergoes a (painful) pain just in case S undergoes a somatosensory experience that represents a bodily disturbance of a certain sort, and that same experience additionally represents the disturbance as bad-for-S.

There are various ways of making this more precise. For now I'm going to assume that the representational content of pain is: *there is a bodily disturbance, d, at location, l, and d is bad-for-me* (Cutter and Tye 2011: 97). In Section 5 I'll consider alternatives.

From this general characterization, we can see that Evaluativists think that the evaluative content of a pain is concerned with bodily-badness, e.g., in the case of the spaghetti my pain represented (roughly) the disturbance in my finger as bad-for-me. This evaluative layer of content apparently explains why I was rationally motivated to do something about the disturbance in my finger: roughly, it was because I was in a state representing the disturbance as bad (Bain 2013). Related to this, Evaluativists think that the evaluative content of pain partially constitutes (and explains) the *painfulness* of pain, i.e., the nasty, yucky feeling that we experience. Indeed, Evaluativists think that the representation of bodily-badness is what is lacking in cases of non-painful pains, e.g., asymbolics, morphine patients, etc.

Although Evaluativism is a theory of pain, proponents also have views about the badness associated with pain.

While Evaluativists agree that bodily-badness is represented in pain, there isn't consensus regarding its nature. Cutter and Tye (2011) assume an objectivist view according to which bodily-badness is *aptness to impede proper functioning of the organism*, but Helm (2002) thinks that subjects need to *care* about their functioning in order for an impediment to that functioning to be bad.

Evaluativists also differ regarding the nature and existence of what I called experiential-badness, i.e., the badness associated with the painful feeling. For example, Bain (2013) thinks that the representation of bodily-badness is itself experientially-bad (not simply painful), while Cutter and Tye (2014) seem to deny the existence of experiential-badness (at least of an intrinsic sort). Bain (2014) also adds the assumption that a necessary and perhaps constitutive condition of the representation of bodily-badness (and hence, of experiential-badness) is that the subject *cares* about their own body. Such bodily care is apparently lacking in asymbolics.

Finally, Evaluativists tend to characterize both bodily and experiential-badness as *bad-for-the-subject* (Bain 2013: Cutter and Tye 2011). In value theory this is commonly understood as prudential disvalue, of the sort which detracts from the subject's welfare.

2 Two epistemologies

I now introduce two theories of immediate perceptual justification.[3] The first of these claims that experiences can confer immediate justification because of their special phenomenology:

> Presentationalism: a perceptual experience, *e*, can confer (defeasible) immediate justification for believing that *p* iff the experience has presentational phenomenology with respect to *p*.

To understand this, compare looking at a red ball with simply thinking about one. In the former case, but not the latter, you are apparently *presented* with the ball and its redness. Due to this your experience (but not your thought) of the ball can confer immediate justification for believing that there is a red ball in front of you.

In more detail: an experience with presentational content with respect to *p* – such as the red ball experience – will involve it seeming to the subject that *p*, the subject being passive in the face of the experience, and the seeming not being "held" for some further reason. I'm assuming that presentational phenomenology is conscious (see Chapter 17, this volume, for more on the relationship between pain and consciousness).

Note, however, that some Presentationalists require more for presentational phenomenology. To understand this, consider the view that experiences can represent the backside of objects, e.g., a tomato, when we observe their front side. While some Presentationalists would accept that this sort of experience has presentational phenomenology (e.g., it seems to you that there is a backside, etc.), others deny it. One reason for doubt is that there is (arguably) a sense in which you aren't (and don't seem to be) *perceptually aware* of the backside of objects even if they are represented in experience. Perhaps such awareness is crucial for presentation (see Chudnoff 2013).

The second view about immediate perceptual justification is:

> Reliablism: a perceptual judgment that *p* (i.e., a judgment that *p* formed in response to a perceptual experience) is immediately justified (defeasibly) iff the judgment that *p* is produced by a reliable process.

A reliable process with respect to *p* is one which outputs a favorable ratio of true : false judgments that *p*. That is what distinguishes forming a belief about a red ball in response to visual experience from forming a belief about the existence of a red ball on the basis of thinking about it. The former judgment, but not the latter, is produced by a reliable process.

Unlike Presentationalism, which requires (at least) that an experience makes it seem to one that *p* in order for a perceptual judgment that *p* to be immediately justified, Reliabilists do not require that an experience makes it seem to a subject that *p*. The content *p* need not show up in the representational contents of experience. What matters is whether forming a judgment that p in response to an experience of a particular sort is a reliable process.

As is well known, Reliabilists must provide (*inter alia*) some principled account of process individuation. To illustrate: when I make the experiential judgment that there is a red ball in front of me, was the process *being formed in response to a visual experience*, or *being formed in response to this token experience*, or something in between? Which of these we adopt will make a difference to the verdicts that Reliabilists give as to whether particular perceptual judgments are justified or not.

We now have all of the necessary theory on the table. Two versions of the Pain View can be developed: a Presentationalist theory according to which pain has presentational phenomenology with respect to evaluative content, and a Reliabilist view according to which forming evaluative judgments in response to pains is a reliable process. Given the general characterization of Evaluativism, and the assumption of its truth, I now assess the prospects for both versions of the Pain View.

3 Pain Presentationalism

Can pains immediately justify beliefs about bodily-badness, i.e., beliefs with content *there is a bodily disturbance, d, at location, l, and d is bad for me*? According to Presentationalism, this requires that pain has presentational phenomenology with respect to bodily-badness. Does it?

Before answering this, note that Evaluativists – specifically, those who think representing bodily-badness partially constitutes/explains experiential-badness – may have independent reasons for being attracted to defending the idea that pains have something like presentational phenomenology. Proponents face the challenge (the "messenger shooting objection") that representing something as bad, e.g., believing that leaving the EU is bad-for-me, needn't itself be bad for a subject. So why is pain different? One answer is that pain presents (bodily-) badness, rather than merely representing it. Being presented with badness can, itself, be bad for you (see Bain Chapter 3, this volume).

On a permissive view, I see little reason to deny that pains have presentational phenomenology with respect to bodily-badness. If Evaluativism is true, then a pain will be something that subjects are passive in the face of, not based on further reasons, and will involve it seeming to the subject that *there is a bodily disturbance, d, at location, l, and d is bad for me*.

If, however, we require more for presentational phenomenology, e.g., something analogous to perceptual awareness (see above), I'm less clear about whether pains can immediately justify evaluative beliefs. Consider this: if bodily-badness turns out to be aptness to impede proper functioning (as Evaluativists seem to think) then there is a sense in which we aren't aware of that when in pain. It might be objected that we could be aware of this feature in experience, but just not under that description. But more would need to be said before we had clear reasons for thinking that there is more robust presentational phenomenology with respect to bodily-badness. This is compounded by a more general worry that, when in pain, the only badness that we are "aware" of is what I have called "experiential-badness, " i.e., the nasty feeling of painfulness. We aren't obviously aware of bodily-badness. (Cf. Chapter 27, this volume.)

Can pains immediately justify beliefs about experiential-badness, i.e., beliefs with content *there is a painful pain, P, and P is bad for me*? According to Presentationalism, this requires that pain has presentational phenomenology with respect to experiential-badness. Does it?

Given the standard formulation of Evaluativism, the answer is "no," since experiential-badness is not (re)presented in pain. For there to be a positive answer, Evaluativism would need to be amended such that pains were (in some sense) *self-presenting*, i.e., they present their own experiential-badness.

In this context it is worth noting John McDowell's (1994, 1998) view that (roughly), when I am in pain, my pain presents itself to me. However, as Bain (2009) has argued, on McDowell's view, pains are not only self-presenting, but are also self-verifying, since they constitute their own subject matter, i.e., a pain, *P*, is accurate just in case one is undergoing pain, *P*. This is a problem because there are apparently no other precedents for this combination of features in our mental economy. If that's right, then it might preclude developing Evaluativism along these lines. Hence the Pain View would be false with respect to beliefs about experiential-badness.

4 Pain Reliabilism

Are judgments about bodily-badness in response to pain produced by a reliable process? In order to enable a clear assessment I need to take a stand on process individuation. I'll assume (warily) that the process is *being formed in response to a pain experience*, and (for now) that the relevant outputs are judgments with content *there is damage at location, l, that is bad for me*. Is that process reliable?[4]

Here are two reasons to think not.

First, as Jennifer Corns (2014) points out, there are a large number of cases where ordinary subjects undergo pains but where there is no bodily damage, and hence no bodily-badness.[5] These include paradigmatic cases of sensory pains like headaches, migraines, lower-back pain, chronic pain, referred pain, and pain after healing. She notes that "the poor correlation between pain and tissue damage is now widely accepted by pain scientists and clinicians" (Corns 2014: 371). (See also Chapter 6, this volume.)

Second, if bodily-badness comes in degrees (see Cutter and Tye 2011; Chapter 2, this volume), e.g., a minor cut is *less* bad than a gaping wound, and if judgments about bodily-badness are about degrees of badness, then there is even more scope for extensive mismatch between the intensity of pain and the badness of the damage (I'm assuming that judgments about bodily-badness are connected to the degree of painfulness of pain). Again, Corns points out that "the same type of tissue damage (typed by cause and severity) undergone by differ-ent people, and even by the same person at different times is commonly known to involve different affect" (Corns 2014: 373). She suggests that perhaps most pains will turn out to be illusory with respect to bodily-badness.

If these points are correct, then pains may not be able to result in immediately justified judgments about bodily-badness, due to their being insufficiently reliable.

Against this, it might be objected that subjects can train themselves to avoid forming eva-luative judgments in cases where pains misrepresent. If that's right, then perhaps forming beliefs about bodily-badness in response to pains can be reliable. Nothing I've said rules out this possibility. I'm not claiming that subjects couldn't form immediately justified evaluative beliefs in response to pain, just that it's a good deal less obvious than in the case of, e.g., shape judgments in response to vision.

Another objection is that subjects may form beliefs in response to pains that have a more coarse-grained content, e.g., *there is something wrong/bad with me*. Given that this avoids a commitment to the existence of bad bodily damage at a particular location, this content could be veridical in many of the supposed "problem" cases that Corns identifies. For example, in cases of lower-back pain, it may be true that something is going badly with the subject's body/functioning, such that forming judgments in response to this sort of experi-ence would be a reliable process. Note, however, that this wouldn't obviously avoid problems concerning the reliability of judgments concerning degrees of badness. Perhaps, though, pain judgments have an evaluative content that is compatible with a whole host of non-zero degrees of badness.

On this picture, subjects could form immediately justified beliefs that *there is something wrong/bad with me* in response to pains. Perhaps this judgment (and indeed the pain) could serve as a prompt to engage in activities which might identify harmful damage to the body, e.g., seeking medical attention. In this way pains and pain judgments would have a similar epistemic function to that claimed by Michael Brady (2013) to be possessed by emotions, i.e., they can serve as starting points for search activities to understand why and if their contents are true.

Are judgments in response to pain about experiential-badness produced by a reliable process? Although the standard statement of Evaluativism denies that experiential-badness is represented in pain, this doesn't, by itself, entail that a Reliablist Pain View is false. This is because Reliabilists don't require that a content, *p*, show up in the contents of an experience in order for a belief that *p* formed in response to that experience to be immediately justified. All that matters is that the belief is produced by a reliable process.

Given this it might seem that there is little reason to deny that forming beliefs about experiential-badness, e.g., *this pain feels bad*, in response to pain could be a reliable process. Subjects are typically assumed to be quite reliable with respect to this sort of content. Although that seems right, more needs to be said about how subjects can come to be reliable. Is this an innate capacity we have? Or does it require learning, e.g., the adoption of prior evaluative beliefs about the experiential-badness of pain? The answers to these questions may have an epistemological upshot. For example, if we require prior evaluative beliefs in order to be reliable, this raises questions about whether the justification is immediate.

5 What evaluative content?

So far I have been mostly assuming – as Evaluativists do – that pains have the following sort of content (simplified for ease of expression):

(A)   There is bodily damage that is bad-for-me.

However, it seems that there are other potential candidates. Here is a non-exhaustive list of alternatives:

(B)   There is bodily damage that is bad.
(C)   My bodily damage is bad-for-me.
(D)   My bodily damage is bad.

(A)/(C) differ from (B)/(D) regarding the kind of badness that is represented. In (A)/(C) the kind of badness is *badness-for-the-subject* while in (B)/(D) it is *badness simpliciter*. The former is relative to a particular subject, and is associated with prudential badness. The latter is not relativized to a particular subject, i.e., it is subject neutral. This is allegedly successfully referred to when someone says "the Holocaust was bad for everyone who suffered in it, but it was also a bad event over-and-above the suffering of those individuals."

(A)/(B) also differ from (C)/(D) regarding whether the bodily damage represented is proprietary or not. In (A)/(B) the damage is non-proprietary, i.e., it is not represented as belonging to the subject, while in (C)/(D) it is.

Which of these is the content of pain is important for at least two reasons.

First, it is significant for Presentationalists vis-à-vis what sorts of contents pains might immediately justify (it's not as crucial for Reliabilists since they don't require that pain has content, *p*, in order for a judgment that *p* (formed in response to pain) to be immediately justified).[6]

Second, it has importance for moral philosophy. If pain has content (B) then subjects of pain would, in a sense, be committed to the disvalue of bodily damage wherever they encounter it, e.g., in other people. Pain would represent to the subject that a particular instance of bodily damage is bad, not simply *their* bodily damage, or simply *bad-for-them* (contrast this with content (C) – if pain has this content then it seems that pain only commits them to the disvalue (for them) of *their* bodily damage). If (B) is pain's content then this may make it more plausible that it could play a role in justifying moral beliefs such as intentionally causing bodily damage in other beings is *pro tanto* wrong. It might also open up an avenue for responding to certain kinds of egoism, i.e., (roughly) the view that we only have reason to do what is in our own interests. If (B) is the content of pain then even egoists – who are sometimes subjects of pain – might be presented in pain with reasons both to refrain from causing and reasons to alleviate bodily damage wherever they find it (this requires the plausible assumption that when one is presented with badness, one is presented with reasons).[7]

How might we determine which of (A)–(D) is correct?

One method is to argue by elimination. For example, we could dispense with (C)/(D) if it could be shown that subjects can have pains in the absence of representing bodily parts as *theirs*. In this context the work of Frederique de Vignemont (2015) is potentially significant. She argues that in cases of Alien Limb, i.e., where subjects do not identify limbs as belonging to *them*, subjects can nevertheless have pain experiences (thus, according to Evaluativism, (re) presenting bodily-badness). One way of interpreting this is that such cases demonstrate that pains do not have proprietary content – i.e. they don't involve the (re)presentation of *my* bodily damage.[8] Thus, we could eliminate (C)/(D) as possible specifications of pain's content.

Against this, it might be suggested that perhaps Alien Limb subject's pain experiences do (re)present body parts as theirs, but they resist this when they make judgments. Or maybe we can't assume that Alien Limb subjects have the same sort of pains as "normal" subjects. Much more would need to be said.

If, however, an argument based on Alien Limb cases could be made to work, we would be left with either (A) or (B) as the remaining candidates.

Here is a line of argument present in the literature which allegedly supports (A) over (B) (in Cutter and Tye 2011, who take it from Pautz 2010). Imagine two agents Mild and Severe, who are part of two distinct groups that have evolved differently such that bodily damage, *d*, is very apt to impede for Severe vis-à-vis her functioning but is significantly less so for Mild. Now suppose that Mild and Severe are conjoined, and that they are each subject to the same token instance of bodily damage, *d*, at the point where they are joined. Cutter and Tye assume that Mild would undergo a mild case of pain, while Severe would undergo a very painful pain, since they would be representing different degrees of badness. If their pains were representing badness *simpliciter* then this would seem to entail that one or both of Mild and Severe are misrepresenting the badness of *d*. But apparently that is counterintuitive. On this basis, Cutter and Tye suggest that both subjects must be representing *badness-for-them* (as per (A)), as only this is consistent with neither of Mild and Severe misrepresenting the badness of *d*.

One way of responding to this is to call into question the evolutionary story Cutter and Tye tell about the role and content of pain. Another option is to account for the lack of misrepresentation by positing contents (C) or (D) (but note my discussion of Alien Limb cases).

However, even if the Mild/Severe example is (perhaps in conjunction with the Alien Limb cases) successful in providing us with reasons to think that (A) is pain's content, that doesn't entail that no pains have content (B). Perhaps having particular sorts of concepts and beliefs can non-trivially affect – i.e., via "cognitive penetration" – the content of pains, such that it could come to have a content along the lines of (B) (see Chapter 22, this volume). For example, perhaps we are able to take up an impersonal stance on bodily-badness when we undergo pains, and this influences its content (see Nagel 1986 for a related discussion). However, even if that is possible, note that pain wouldn't be playing a fundamental role in revealing the badness *simpliciter* of bodily damage. Instead it would be pain plus whatever mental item(s) cognitively penetrate the pain. This could have implications for whether pains themselves could play epistemically and morally significant roles of the sort outlined above. For example, it wouldn't be true that by simply undergoing a pain one is in a sense committed to the badness *simpliciter* of bodily damage. Instead, it would require that they take up a particular (optional) stance on their pains.

6 Moral pain

At least since Plato, philosophers have thought that something like a pain could be a source of justified evaluative beliefs.[9]

The most striking example of this can be found in the Moral Sense Theory of Frances Hutcheson (1991/1725). On Hutcheson's view approbation (a pleasure) and disapprobation (a pain) are ways of sensing the moral qualities of people's motives and actions. Note that Hutcheson had quite a permissive view of what a sense is: "a determination of the mind, to receive any idea from the presence of an object which occurs to us, independent on our will" (Hutcheson 1991/1725: 264–265).

Aside from having a different kind of object (motives), these kinds of pains and pleasures are distinct from the pains I have so far been discussing in that they exhibit an independence of the subject's concern for their own interests (recall what some Evaluativists say about the connection between pain and care). As Hutcheson wrote: "some actions have to men an *immediate goodness* ... by a *superior sense,* which I call a *moral one,* we *approve* the actions of others ... a like perception we have in reflecting on such actions of our own, without any view of natural advantage from them" (Hutcheson 1991/1725: 264–265). It is from disapprobation that we get our concepts of moral badness, wrongness, etc. It also appears to underlie moral judgments about the badness of intentions and actions.

If we were to (anachronistically) combine Hutcheson's Moral Sense Theory with an Evaluativist account of moral disapprobation we would (roughly) get the following:

> Moral Pain Evaluativism: *S* undergoes a moral pain just in case *S* is in an experiential state which represents a subject's (perhaps *S*'s) motive as bad (independently of *S*'s self-interest).

Unfortunately, space constraints preclude anything like a full discussion of whether a Pain View about moral pain is plausible. I'll say a little about the epistemology of moral pain before finally considering objections to its existence.

Briefly, could moral pains have presentational phenomenology with respect to the moral badness of intentions? On a permissive account the answer may appear to be "yes." If, however, we have a more robust view of what is required for presentational phenomenology, e.g., requiring something akin to perceptual awareness, then it may be doubtful that such presentational phenomenology is present in cases where we consider the motives of others, since we don't seem to be "aware" of other people's motives.[10] Rather than respond to that challenge, a proponent of Presentationalism about moral pain might claim that it is nevertheless plausible that moral pains with respect to our own motives possess presentational phenomenology, and can thus be a source of immediate justification for evaluative beliefs. However, I think Presentationalists will then need to address a challenge from C.D. Broad (2016/1944: 149), which goes roughly like this: the pain-like phenomenology we allegedly experience when considering the motives of others is the same (or very similar) to that experienced when we consider our own. If there is no presentational phenomenology in the former case, then that provides us with reason to think it is also lacking in the latter case. Perhaps, then, Presentationalists need to defend the view that we can be presented with the badness of other people's motives.

Could judgments about the moral badness of intentions and actions, formed in response to moral pains, be reliable? Hutcheson seemed to think that our moral sense was reliable because it was designed by God. But contemporary Reliabilists will likely want to avoid this sort of appeal. In any case, regarding the motives of others, we might worry about whether we could be reliable about their moral qualities in the absence of true beliefs that the agents had the motives in question. But that might mean that one's moral pain-based judgments are only mediately justified because the process that produces them would only be conditionally reliable, i.e., only reliable given the input of true beliefs about intentions. Perhaps, though, such judgments could nevertheless be independent of the subject possessing justification for believing other evaluative propositions, hence they could still be (with respect to evaluative propositions) epistemically fundamental evaluative judgments. Note that such worries may not arise with respect to judgments about our own motives, e.g., perhaps we are directly aware of (or acquainted with) our own motives. However, in order to fully address questions about reliability – and indeed to fully address questions about presentational phenomenology – we would need to know more about what moral badness consists in. For example, if it turns out that moral badness is a dispositional property which manifests itself in the experience of moral pains (perhaps in "normally functioning" subjects), that might increase the plausibility of the claim that judgments about moral badness formed on the basis of moral pains could be reliable. But that is of course a substantial question in value theory.

I end by briefly considering a couple of objections to the existence of moral pain.

One might object to the characterization of disapprobation as pain. It might be thought that pain is intimately connected with damage, and that there is no damage implicated in cases of morally bad intentions. In response: although there is not obviously any bodily damage involved, there is a sense in which a morally bad motive is one which is (or is apt to) damage one's social relations with other moral agents (note that this would involve complicating the characterization of Moral Pain Evaluativism). Moral pain could thus be the registering of the badness of this damage.

A more fundamental objection is that there is no such thing as a distinctive moral pain, i.e., it's a mysterious posit like rational intuition. Although it is uncontroversial that there are moral emotions, e.g., guilt, indignation etc., emotions and pains are distinct kinds of entity. One response to this challenge is that at least some negative emotions, e.g., guilt, are themselves usefully categorized as kinds of pain (but see Corns 2015 for reasons to reject this). Another is to argue that moral "pain" is better thought of as an instance of moral displeasure rather than pain per se (Hutcheson himself employed the language of "(dis)pleasure"), and that this is the affective component of some moral emotions. If that's right, and the affective component of moral emotions were the bearer of representational content (see Goldie 2000), then moral displeasure could play a crucial epistemic role vis-à-vis the justification (perhaps the immediate justification) of evaluative beliefs. (See related discussion of social pain and other negative experiences as pains in Chapters 7, 13, and 29.)

However, as is the case with the Pain View about "standard" pains, much work needs to be done – e.g., concerning the nature of presentational phenomenology, the nature of badness, etc. – in order to make a Pain View about moral pain acceptable.

Related topics

Chapter 1: A brief and potted overview on the philosophical theories of pain (Hardcastle)
Chapter 3: Evaluativist accounts of pain's unpleasantness (Bain)
Chapter 4: Imperativism (Klein)
Chapter 6: Advances in the neuroscience of pain (Apkarian)
Chapter 7: Neuromatrix theory of pain (Roy and Wager)
Chapter 13: Psychogenic pain: old and new (Sullivan)
Chapter 17: Pain and consciousness (Pereplyotchik)
Chapter 22: Pain and cognitive penetrability (Jacobson)
Chapter 27: Bad by nature: an axiological theory of pain (Massin)
Chapter 29: Pain and education (Mintz)

Acknowledgements

Many thanks to Jennifer Corns for helpful discussion and comments on earlier drafts of this chapter.

Notes

1 Immediate justification is commonly assumed to be defeasible. For example, even if my perceptual experience immediately justifies the belief that there is a computer, this could be undercut if I become aware I am hallucinating. I'm also assuming throughout that perceptual experiences are non-factive.
2 The badness is commonly thought to be *pro tanto* rather than all-things-considered because bodily damage or a pain experience could have good consequences overall, e.g., it might prompt the sufferer to be more careful in future.
3 The distinction between these two theories is highlighted in Chudnoff 2013.
4 Given that many think that something like reliability is a necessary condition for knowledge, the discussion in this section is of general relevance to the question of whether pains are a source of immediate knowledge.
5 Corns argues against perceptualist views of pain, of which Evaluativism is a type. I'm granting that pains could be perceptual, but am instead casting doubt on the reliability of judgments formed in response to them, e.g., perhaps ordinary agents are seldom in the optimal conditions in which pain reliably tracks damage and badness.
6 On the assumption of Reliabilism, it could be the case that judgments formed in response to pains with all of contents (A)–(D) could be immediately justified. Much work would, of course, need to be done to make this plausible.
7 Another way of putting all of this: if (B) is the content of pain, then pain could play a role vis-à-vis justification about bodily-badness, as Mill seemed to think desire could play vis-à-vis justification about the goodness of happiness. See his *Utilitarianism*.
8 This is not how de Vignemont argues. She regards Alien Limb cases as putting pressure on the view that care for one's body is a necessary condition for undergoing a painful pain experience.
9 Something like a pain – the feeling of respect for law – figures in Kant's moral philosophy. See his *Groundwork*. However, it doesn't appear to play an *epistemic* role. At best it plays a motivational role.
10 These points wouldn't obviously apply with respect to the consideration of hypothetical cases.

Robert Cowan

References

Bain, D. (2009) McDowell and the presentation of pains. *Philosophical Topics* 37(1): 1–24.
Bain, D. (2013) What makes pains unpleasant? *Philosophical Studies* 166 (suppl. 1): S69–S89.
Bain, D. (2014) Pains that don't hurt. *Australasian Journal of Philosophy* 92(2): 1–16.
Brady, M.S. (2013) *Emotional Insight: The Epistemic Role of Emotional Experience.* Oxford: Oxford University Press.
Broad, C.D. (2016/1944) Some reflections on moral-sense theories in ethics. In B. Colburn (ed.), *Methods of Ethics.* Proceedings of the Aristotelian Society Virtual Issue 3. London: Aristotelian Society, pp. 138–166.
Chudnoff, E. (2013) *Intuition.* Oxford: Oxford University Press.
Cohen, J. and Fulkerson, M. (2014) Affect, rationalization, and motivation. *Review of Philosophy and Psychology* 5(1): 103–118.
Corns, J. (2014) The inadequacy of unitary characterizations of pain. *Philosophical Studies* 169(3): 355–378.
Corns, J. (2015) The social pain posit. *Australasian Journal of Philosophy* 93(3): 561–582.
Cutter, B. and Tye, M. (2011) Tracking representationalism and the painfulness of pain. *Philosophical Issues* 21(1): 90–109.
Cutter, B. and Tye, M. (2014) Pains and reasons: why it is rational to kill the messenger. *Philosophical Quarterly* 64(256): 423–433.
de Vignemont, F. (2015) Pain and bodily care: whose body matters? *Australasian Journal of Philosophy* 93(3): 542–560.
Goldie, P. (2000) *The Emotions: A Philosophical Exploration.* Oxford: Oxford University Press.
Helm, B.W. (2002) Felt evaluations: a theory of pleasure and pain. *American Philosophical Quarterly* 39(1): 13–30.
Hutcheson, F. (1991/1725) *An Inquiry concerning Moral Good and Evil.* In D.D. Raphael (ed.), *British Moralists 1650–1800*, vol. 1. Indianapolis: Hackett Publishing Co.
McDowell, J. (1994) *Mind and World.* Cambridge, MA: Harvard University Press.
McDowell, J. (1998) *Mind, Value, and Reality.* Cambridge, MA: Harvard University Press.
Nagel, T. (1986) *The View From Nowhere.* Oxford: Oxford University Press.
Pautz, A. (2010) A simple view of consciousness. In R. Koons and G. Bealer (ed.), *The Waning of Materialism.* Oxford: Oxford University Press.
Price, R. (1991/1758) *A Review of the Principal Questions and Difficulties in Morals.* In D.D. Raphael (ed.), *British Moralists 1650–1800*, vol. 2. Indianapolis: Hackett Publishing Co.

PART III-II

Pain in medicine

31

AN INTRODUCTION TO THE IASP'S DEFINITION OF PAIN

Andrew Wright

A quick trawl through this volume will confirm that the International Association for the Study of Pain's (IASP's) definition of pain is *the* go-to definition for those with an interest in pain. However, philosophers who approach the IASP's definition ("the definition") hoping to gain a quick and easy insight into the way scientists view pain are likely to be disappointed by its opacity. This chapter is intended to provide an introduction to the motivations that lay behind the development of the definition, to its history, its utility and its meaning. I want to stress that this chapter is an introduction; it is not intended to provide a thorough analysis of the definition. As such, I do not fully explore some of the issues that arise. For example, questions of whether pain is necessarily unpleasant, and whether our identification of experiences as pain is infallible (see Chapter 20, this volume). Additionally, some issues of detail that are relevant to the definition are beyond the scope of this chapter and are omitted. For example, the distinctions between "tissue damage," "potential tissue damage" and "undamaged tissue," and the relationship between tissue damage and pain (for contrasting perspectives on these distinctions and relations, see Chapters 5–10, this volume).

This chapter is divided into five sections. The first is a brief introduction to the history and motivations that prompted the development of the IASP's Taxonomy of Pain Terms. The fact that the definition is a constituent of a taxonomy raises the question of whether the definition is an adequate taxonomic tool. I use the process of evaluating whether the definition is taxonomically appropriate as a means of unraveling the intended meaning of the definition. I explain the evaluative process in the second section and conduct the evaluation in the subsequent sections titled "Clarity" and "Narrow Scope, Broad Scope and Brevity." My conclusion is that the definition is not adequate for taxonomic purposes. In the final section, I speculate on the competing aims that might explain this inadequacy.

1 The need for a taxonomy

The IASP was founded in 1973 and its first taxonomy of pain terms was published in 1979. John Bonica, who can be described as *the* motivating force behind the development of this taxonomy (Jones 2010), "considered the development and implementation of a universally accepted taxonomy on pain one of the most urgent and most important objectives of IASP"

(Jones 2010: 22). He memorably described the commonplace inconsistent use of key terms as the "tower of Babel conditions" (IASP 1979: 247) that prevailed at the time. The IASP's Taxonomy was intended to provide a "minimum standard vocabulary for members of *different disciplines* who work in the field of pain" (IASP 1979: 249, my emphasis). However, in apparent contradiction, the editorial that introduced the 1986 taxonomy "emphasized something that was implicit in the previous definitions ... the terms [in the taxonomy] have been developed for use in *clinical practice* rather than for experimental work, physiology or anatomical purposes" (IASP 1986: S216, my emphasis). It is difficult to discern this implication in Bonica's (1979) introduction.

How should these comments be interpreted? Despite appearances to the contrary there is, in my view, no tension here. A significant proportion of the terms in the taxonomy define subtly distinct *pain conditions* like "allodynia," "hyperalgesia" and "neuralgia." These distinctions are critical for differential diagnosis and communication between clinicians, so relevance for clinical practice may well have motivated the inclusion of many terms. Indeed, Bonica's reference to "tower of Babel conditions" may refer to the inconsistent use of terms that label pain conditions rather than an inconsistent use of the term "pain." In my view, and I explain my thinking in the concluding section, the scientific community uses "pain" consistently because the ordinary concept of pain underpins the use of "pain" in almost all theoretical, experimental and clinical contexts. Additionally, the idea that *taxonomic* definitions might be formulated in a fashion that is appropriate for clinicians but inappropriate for workers from other disciplines makes little sense. The demand of taxonomy is always one of classification, and the requirements imposed by classification are always the same whether or not the terms being defined are most relevant for clinicians.

The structure of the taxonomy is straightforward. All the terms other than "pain," which is the first entry, are arranged alphabetically. The majority of these definitions are supported by a note which is intended to have a broadly explanatory function. In line with Bonica's tenet that the taxonomy is not "'fixed' for all time and cannot be modified as we acquire new knowledge" (IASP 1979: 247), the taxonomy has been regularly reviewed and expanded: from nineteen entries in 1979 to thirty-one entries in 2014, and most entries have been revised.

The definition and its note are:

Pain – "An unpleasant sensory and emotional experience associated with actual or potential tissue damage, or described in terms of such damage" (IASP 2014).

Note – "The inability to communicate verbally does not negate the possibility that an individual is experiencing pain and is in need of appropriate pain-relieving treatment. Pain is always subjective. Each individual learns the application of the word through experiences related to injury in early life. Biologists recognize that those stimuli that cause pain are liable to damage tissue. Accordingly, pain is that experience we associate with actual or potential tissue damage. It is unquestionably a sensation in a part or parts of the body, but it is also always unpleasant and therefore also an emotional experience. Experiences which resemble pain but are not unpleasant, e.g., pricking, should not be called pain. Unpleasant abnormal experiences (dysesthesias) may also be pain but are not necessarily so because, subjectively, they may not have the usual sensory qualities of pain. Many people report pain in the absence of tissue damage or any likely pathophysiological cause; usually this happens for psychological reasons. There is usually no way to distinguish their experience from that due to tissue damage if we take the subjective report. If they regard their experience as pain and if they report it in the same way as pain caused by tissue damage, it should be accepted as pain. This definition avoids tying pain to the stimulus. Activity induced in the nociceptors and nociceptive pathways by a noxious stimulus is not pain, which is always a psychological state, even though we may well appreciate that pain most often has a proximate physical cause" (IASP 2014).

"Pain" is one of the few definitions that has escaped revision, though its supporting note (henceforth "the note") has been subjected to revision in the form of the addition of the first sentence. I take this revision to be a response to criticism by K.J.S. Anand and Kenneth Craig, which I briefly discuss in the penultimate section of this chapter. Other alterations have been insignificant.[1] Crucially for the evaluation I undertake in coming sections, the note not only concerns both explanation and usage, it also subserves an *essential* taxonomic function.

The explanation for the longevity of the definition is that the IASP believes that the "existing definition of 'pain' has proven very useful and is an appropriate one" (Loeser and Treede 2008: 473).[2] It is not entirely clear what Loeser and Treede's distinction between utility and appropriateness is intended to convey in the context of taxonomy. Roughly, a definition is taxonomically appropriate (henceforth "t-appropriate") if it picks out all and only tokens of X. Taxonomic utility ("t-utility") and t-appropriateness cannot come apart, because a definition has utility as a means of picking out all and only tokens of X iff it is t-appropriate. It may be that Loeser and Treede (and by extension the IASP as an organization)[3] take "utility" to convey clinical value in abstraction from t-utility, there being no obstacle to the independence of clinical utility and t-appropriateness. However, as "pain" is advertised as a constituent of a taxonomy, the utility (rather than the t-utility) of the definition will not influence my assessment of the definition as a taxonomic tool. Additionally, there is no need for specific evaluation of the t-utility of the definition because t-utility depends on t-appropriateness. So an evaluation of the t-appropriateness of the definition is the main focus of this chapter.

2 Taxonomic appropriateness

Taxonomic definitions are expressed in terms of features that are intended to distinguish all and only tokens of the class being defined (call these "taxonomic features"). Taxonomy often concerns the taxonomic features of things that already fall under an informal classification. In the case of pain, we have a good idea of what should fall under the formal (taxonomic) class because the ordinary concept PAIN constitutes an informal class. So the key test of the t-appropriateness of the definition is that it neither classifies pains as non-pains nor non-pains as pains. However, this does not mean that the taxonomic process is just an endorsement of informal classification.

Consider an informal class of things – R. All tokens of R have the features *f* and *g*, but some things (*NRs*) that are not informally classified as *Rs* also have *f* and *g*. So *f* and *g* are not ideal for the purpose of conferring taxonomic respectability on R. A lack of taxonomically ideal features suggests that the informal class is linked by custom (i.e., that R is an arbitrary classification). What if the informal class lacks unique features? Should tokens of *NR* fall under the formal classification (*TR*), or should another feature – *h*, which links only the majority of *Rs* – determine the formal classification (thereby some *Rs* would not fall under *TR*)? These taxonomic uncertainties have a significant bearing on the definition and note, and they are important considerations in my evaluation.

A definition is *accurate* if it picks out all and only *Xs*. In terms of the criteria I introduce below, a definition is accurate if it satisfies both Narrow and Broad Scope. Although accuracy is the key test, it is not the only test of t-appropriateness; all definitions should also have the twin virtues of clarity and brevity. In this context, "clarity" means that the taxonomic features of a definition should be obvious. If the taxonomic features of a definition are opaque then it will not be clear whether some candidates qualify as *X* or not. "Brevity" is not so easily pinned down. I take it a definition which includes taxonomically irrelevant information can be improved. Also, a definition would not be t-appropriate if non-taxonomic information obscures the taxonomic features of that definition, i.e., wordiness may contribute to opacity.

Overall then, the IASP's definition of pain would be ideally t-appropriate if it satisfied the following four criteria:

Clarity: The taxonomic features of the definition should be obvious.

Narrow Scope: The definition should not classify pains as non-pains.

Broad Scope: The definition should not classify non-pains as pains.

Brevity: The taxonomic features of the definition should be formulated economically and the formulation should exclude taxonomically irrelevant information.

This is a not strict test. In practice, there is some wiggle room. If the taxonomic features of the definition are obvious then it would be unreasonable to conclude that the definition is not t-appropriate when its only failing is a little wordiness. There is also some flexibility in Narrow and Broad Scope because it is controversial whether certain organisms have the capacity to experience pain (see, for instance, Chapters 15 and 16, this volume) and whether certain experiences are pains – I call these (putative) experiences p-pains. For some commentators a failure to exclude some or all p-pains would represent a contravention of Broad Scope. For others the exclusion of p-pains would contravene Narrow Scope. The question of whether some or all p-pains are pains has no bearing on my evaluation, but I take it that the definition should not exclude any p-pains from classification as pain without good reason (and if there were good reason there would be no controversy, i.e., they would not qualify as p-pains). To do otherwise would be arbitrary. I take the avoidance of arbitrariness to be tacitly implied by Narrow Scope. By contrast, there is no good reason to weaken a strict understanding of Clarity; if the taxonomic features of the definition are not clear then the definition is not t-appropriate.

To recap, given that the definition is a constituent of the IASP's Taxonomy, I assume that Loeser and Treede's claim that the definition "has proven very useful and is an appropriate one" refers to t–utility and t-appropriateness. As the former depends on the latter, an evaluation of t-appropriateness amounts to an evaluation of t-utility. The function of a taxonomic definition of pain is to express clearly and succinctly the features that pick out all and only pains. Failure to do so would provide a very good reason to reject Loeser and Treede's claim.

As Narrow and Broad Scope cannot be evaluated unless the taxonomic features of the definition are clear, I begin by evaluating Clarity. It will soon be obvious that the note is *required* for taxonomic purposes. For this reason I evaluate the clarity of three versions of the definition: the definition itself; the conjunction of the definition and the relevant parts of the note (the "conjunction"); and an interpretation of the IASP's intentions which is derived from the conjunction (expressed under "Def" in the following section). As the opacity of the conjunction is such that it cannot be evaluated against Narrow Scope, Broad Scope and Brevity without interpretation (as in Def), I evaluate only the definition and Def against these criteria.

3 Clarity

According to the IASP something is a pain iff it is either:

i   An unpleasant sensory and emotional experience associated with actual or potential tissue damage; or
ii An unpleasant sensory and emotional experience which is described in terms of actual or potential tissue damage.

Both disjuncts are opaque. Considered in isolation from the note the nature of the association between the experience and tissue damage is a mystery. (For discussion of the puzzles that this relationship can raise, see, e.g., Chapters 1, 5 and 18, this volume.) It is also implausible that the requirement for description in (ii) was meant to be interpreted literally because, as we shall see, it has absurd consequences. I begin with the former.

There is only one reference to an association in the note – "pain is that experience we *associate* with actual or potential tissue damage" (IASP 2014, my emphasis). This is because "[e]ach individual learns the application of the word [pain] through experiences related to injury in early life" and "[b]iologists recognize that those stimuli that cause pain are liable to damage tissue" (IASP 2014). This is not very illuminating. Is pain associated with tissue damage because we (the folk) have learned this association, or is pain associated with tissue damage because biologists recognize a causal relationship between tissue damage and pain? If the association is learned then *all* of the experiences that fall under (ii) would be picked out by (i). This is inconsistent with the contingency of (i). By contrast, the phrase "liable to damage tissue" reflects the contingent relationship between token pains and their usual cause. So I take the association in (i) to be a causal relationship between pathology and pain. This understanding is supported by the emphasis in the note on the contingency of this relationship.

In this light, (ii) represents the IASP's solution to the problem of characterizing pains that lack a pathological cause. On a literal reading, "described in terms of actual or potential tissue damage" seems to exclude straightforward pain reports like "my knee hurts" because they do not refer to tissue damage. But as the relevant parts of the note are cashed out in terms of "report," the requirement in (ii) should be interpreted loosely to include these reports. Strictly speaking, the definition is obscure because the note is *needed* to understand that (ii) is intended to include pain reports. However, even though this understanding diffuses the problem slightly, a requirement for report is also too demanding.

Consider Joe and his reticent friend Jean who are the subjects of qualitatively identical unpleasant sensory and emotional experiences that are not caused by actual or potential tissue damage (i.e., their experiences are not pains by (i)). Joe reports his experience as a pain, so his experience is a pain by (ii). But Jean is silent, so her qualitatively identical experience is not a pain. This is plainly absurd. Furthermore, an interpretation of (ii) in terms of a requirement for report contradicts what I take to be an avowal by the IASP, expressed in the first sentence of the note, not to exclude the (putative) experiences of organisms *because* they lack the ability to communicate verbally. (Cf. Chapters 15 and 20, this volume.)

References to report and the addition of the opening sentence to the note clarify the IASP's *intent*. They do not clarify the *definition*. The note cannot alter the fact that the requirement for description is a taxonomic feature of (ii). References to "report" in the note suggest that this requirement should not be interpreted literally, but then the first sentence of the note is a declaration that a requirement for report should not be a taxonomic feature of (ii) either.

This is all very confusing. For the moment, I will put the difficult matter of formulating (ii) in a way that reflects the IASP's intention to one side as I want to introduce a taxonomic feature of the note that has an impact on the disjunctive nature of the definition.

Dysesthesias are unpleasant sensory and emotional experiences that are usually caused by nerve damage (Fields 1999) so they qualify as pains under (i). This is a taxonomic problem because the subjects of some dysesthesias say that their experiences do not feel like pain (Fields 1999). The IASP solves this problem by using the note to explicitly exclude dysesthesias that lack the "usual sensory qualities" of pain from classification as pain.[4]

The use of "usual" in this context is perplexing because it suggests that pains are either characterized by usual or unusual qualities. Nothing in the note offers a solution to the thorny problem of distinguishing the experiences that would not be pains because they lack the usual sensory qualities of pain (e.g., some dysesthesias) from the experiences that would be pains even though they lack the usual sensory qualities of pain. For this reason I assume that the IASP means "particular sensory qualities" where "particular" means the qualities that subjects recognize as pain. So some dysesthesias are not pains, because they lack this particularity.

Problematically for the disjunctive nature of the definition, there is no non-arbitrary reason why this reason for specifically excluding dysesthesias should not generalize to all pains. In effect this makes the first disjunct redundant. To see the problem, consider a version of the conjunction:

Def: Something is a pain iff it is either:

(i*)   An unpleasant sensory and emotional experience with particular sensory qualities which has a pathological cause; or

(ii*) An unpleasant sensory and emotional experience that could in principle be identified as pain by its subject because it has particular sensory qualities which normally have a pathological cause.

This version requires a little unpacking. I prefer the more general term "pathological cause" to the "pathophysiological cause" mentioned in the note because the latter seems to exclude anatomical pathology. The plural "particular sensory qualities" is intended to convey the widely held view that pain (conceived as a type) is characterized by different sensory qualities and not that a token pain is constituted by more than one sensory quality. More importantly, (i*) is explicit about the association between the experience and tissue damage. Also, (ii*) employs an in-principle clause to eliminate the absurdity mentioned above in a way that is consistent with the IASP's intention not to exclude the (putative) experiences of organisms because they lack the capacity for self-report. This clause is focused on the subject of the experience: *if* the subject had the ability to learn "the application of the word [pain] through experiences related to injury in early life" (IASP 2014), then that subject would learn to identify the appropriate experiences as pain.

To restate the problem mentioned above, the requirement that pains have the particular sensory qualities of pain generalizes to both disjuncts. With this in place, all the experiences that fall under (i*) also fall under (ii*). Consequently (i*) is taxonomically redundant and the disjunctive structure of the definition is meaningless.

The universal applicability of (ii*) is not an indication that (i) and (ii) are intended to have different functions. If it were otherwise (ii) would be the obvious candidate for the taxonomic disjunct as it corresponds with (ii★). And, given the statement that "the terms [in the taxonomy] have been developed for use in clinical practice" (IASP 1986: S216), presumably (i) would be intended to have a clinical function. This understanding of the functions of (i) and (ii) is implausible for three reasons.

First, even though (ii★) is derived from (ii) and the note, it is incredible that (ii) is intended to have universal scope, because it requires description. Second, the either/or structure of the definition is inconsistent with the claim that (i) and (ii) have different functions. Third, the clinical utility of (i) is questionable. Certainly, the information that some pains lack a pathological cause would be a useful reminder to clinicians not to disregard reports of pain in the absence of pathology. However, even if the association in (i) were explicit (as in (i★)) this information cannot be inferred from (i) because (i) is consistent with the view that all pains have a pathological cause. The either/or structure of the definition is needed to see the contingency of (i). The IASP would not present important clinical information in such an obscure manner.

The conclusion that the definition and the conjunction contravene Clarity cannot be avoided. Although the note provides some insight into the association in (i) and the description in (ii), it also confuses because the note contradicts some taxonomic features of the definition. In effect, assuming the authority of the note, the definition does not accurately represent the IASP's intentions. Strictly speaking, Def is not under scrutiny here as it represents a significant revision of the IASP's formulations of both definition and note. Nevertheless, I consider the t-appropriateness of Def in this and subsequent sections of this chapter because I see it as a representation of the IASP's intent. As far as Clarity is concerned Def has a significant and fatal flaw: its disjunctive structure. Although clarity would be improved by eliminating (i★), I will not evaluate the t-appropriateness of (ii★) because it is too removed from its origins in the conjunction.

4 Narrow Scope, Broad Scope and Brevity

In the first section of this chapter, I mention that criticism by K.J.S. Anand and Kenneth Craig was (almost certainly) the catalyst for the only substantial alteration to the note: the addition of the sentence beginning, "The inability to communicate verbally ..." Their claim was that "[i]n its present form ... the definition of pain challenges our understanding of pain because *it does not apply* to living organisms that are incapable of self-report" (Anand and Craig 1996: 3, my emphasis). They were concerned that knowledge of the IASP's definition might lead some clinicians to deny treatment to neonates and very young children on the basis that they cannot experience pain.[5] (For discussion see Chapter 36, this volume.) Surprisingly, none of those who defended the definition seem to have noticed that Anand and Craig's claim is false.[6] By (i) an organism is in pain if it is the subject of an unpleasant sensory and emotional experience associated with a cut (say) so there is no *requirement* for self-report in the definition. However, the definition does exclude some of the p-pains of organisms incapable of self-report.

By (ii), an experience that is excluded by (i) is a pain iff it is an unpleasant sensory and emotional experience described in terms of actual or potential tissue damage. So (ii) excludes some p-pains *because* their subjects are incapable of self-report. In the preceding section I argued that (ii) is too demanding because it excludes all experiences that would be classified as pain but for the fact that their subjects do not report them for *whatever* reason. Although revision of (ii) in accord with the opening sentence of the note (as in (ii★)) would address this problem, the possibility of revision does not alter the wording and hence the failing of the definition.

Thus far, I have not mentioned that being unpleasant is a requirement of both disjuncts so it is a necessary condition on pain. This is potentially problematic because subjects with pain asymbolia, and some of those who have either been treated with morphine or had lobotomies, identify experiences as pain, yet report that their experiences are not unpleasant. These experiences, which do not qualify as pain because they are not unpleasant, present an interesting counterpoint to dysesthesias. The IASP excludes dysesthesias from classification as pain because they lack the particular sensory qualities of pain, so by the IASP's own lights having these qualities seems a good reason not to exclude these affectively neutral experiences from classification as pain. Unless the IASP has a good reason for making unpleasantness a necessary condition on pain, these affectively neutral experiences should have the status of p-pains if not pains. Perhaps the failure to provide a reason for making unpleasantness a necessary condition is an omission rather than an arbitrary decision. If this is right then it would be unreasonable to conclude that this omission is taxonomically fatal, and so Def would escape the charge that it contravenes Narrow Scope. If it is not just an omission then the charge sticks. Either way the definition contravenes Narrow Scope because (ii) requires self-report.

The use of the note to exclude some dysesthesias amounts to an admission by the IASP that the definition is too broad in scope. However, the question of whether the definition *is* too broad in scope is moot. The reason the IASP gives for the exclusion of some dysesthesias is that they lack the "usual sensory qualities of pain." This phrase may be intended to convey the reason that pains are characterized by *unique* sensory qualities, but recognition does not imply that pains *are* characterized by such qualities. It may be that the experiences we identify as pain are a motley collection of sensory qualities linked by nothing more than a learned ability to identify them as pain. Accordingly, in Def, I take it that the qualities are usual (in my terms they are "particular") in the sense that their subjects recognize them as pain. So the IASP's exclusion of dysesthesias appears to be based on the assumption that a subject's identification of an experience as a pain or a non-pain is infallible. Dysesthesias provide reason to doubt this assumption.

This problem presses because some itches are pains by (i); i.e., they are unpleasant sensory and emotional experiences that are causally related to histamine release associated with tissue damage. However, as *all* the experiences we label as "itches" are united by the urge to scratch (Hall 2008) we have good reason to accept that itches form a formal (taxonomic) class distinct from pain. The trouble is that if there is no good reason to accept the requirement for particular sensory qualities then some itches (some non-pains) would qualify as pain. Whether or not the IASP has a good reason for imposing this requirement, the definition contravenes Broad Scope because it fails to exclude either some itches (if the relevant dysesthesias are p-pains) or both some itches and dysesthesias. Of course, Def is consistent with Broad Scope if the IASP has a good reason, but if it does not have a good reason then the requirement for particular sensory qualities is illegitimate.

It is clear from this evaluation that parts of the note were formulated to subserve an essential taxonomic function. Putting aside other criticisms, it can be said that the taxonomic inappropriateness of the definition is an intrinsic consequence of this strategy. So, even though the wording of the definition is admirably succinct, the definition is not intended to express all the taxonomic features that pick out all and only pains. Considered together the taxonomically relevant parts of both the definition and note contravene Brevity for the simple reason that Def is more succinct than these relevant parts. Unfortunately, Def also contravenes Brevity because (ii*) picks out all the experiences that fall under (i*). The upshot is that the taxonomically redundant disjunct (i*) obscures the taxonomic features of Def.

5 Concluding remarks – the utility of the definition

The definition, the conjunction and my interpretation of the conjunction (Def) are not t-appropriate. Indeed, they miss their taxonomic target by a mile. Why? As the first entry in the IASP's Taxonomy the definition is intended to have taxonomic utility, but it is also intended to have clinical utility. In attempting to achieve both ends the IASP has fallen well short of the standard for t-appropriateness. My hunch is that the definition has endured because its t-utility is of little or no relevance to most clinicians and pain scientists. In this section, I explain why a taxonomic definition has little utility for clinicians and pain scientists, and I speculate on the thinking that underpins the wording of the definition and note.

Although John Bonica stated that the inconsistent use of terms motivated the development of the taxonomy as a whole, I doubt that it motivated the definition of pain. The experiences that fall under the ordinary concept of pain are the focal point of pain science because researchers investigate and clinicians assess and treat these experiences. For this reason the use of a definition that does not align with the ordinary concept of pain would have limited value and in many settings it might hamper communication. In this light, the IASP's reference to the "usual sensory qualities of pain" and the recommendation to accept pain reports as evidence of pain can be seen as an attempt to embrace the ordinary concept. The exclusion of experiences that subjects do not recognize as pain and experiences that are not unpleasant is consistent with this conjecture; the idea of a pain that does not feel like a pain is at odds with the ordinary concept, and affectively neutral pains seem beyond the realm of everyday experience. (Cf. Chapter 1, this volume.)

In view of the scientific importance of the ordinary concept there has been and is little pressure on the IASP to formulate a taxonomically appropriate definition. My guess is that greater pressure was exerted by the fact that some clinicians have used the absence of (relevant) pathology as a reason to deny that patients are in pain or for dismissing some pains as insignificant. This conjecture explains the basic disjunctive structure of the definition; the category pain is exhausted by (a) pains that have a pathological cause, and (b) pains that lack a pathological cause. The IASP's laudable commitment to the promotion of medical research and the provision of adequate treatment motivated its desire to solve the taxonomic problem posed by (b) in a manner which was intended to have both taxonomic and clinical utility. Although its solution, expressed in (ii), is a startlingly inappropriate taxonomic tool, its inadequacy has not been noticed because t-utility is of little practical importance to the scientific community as a whole.

This explanation is consistent with the IASP's decision not to reformulate the definition to exclude some dysesthesias. The use of the note to exclude dysesthesias is evidence of the IASP's desire for both taxonomic and clinical utility. A relatively small proportion of abnormal sensations seems an insufficient reason to reformulate an otherwise taxonomically adequate definition that the IASP would claim carries a clear clinical message in the content of its disjuncts.[7] The IASP has simply not considered the taxonomic significance of this strategy. The use of the note to introduce the requirement for the "usual sensory qualities" represents an acknowledgement that the scope of the definition is too broad and it raises doubts about the coherence of the disjunctive structure of the definition.

This account explains why the IASP's definition is taxonomically inappropriate. The importance of clinical utility explains the IASP's desire to formulate a taxonomic definition that has clinical utility. The inappropriateness of the definition as a taxonomic tool reflects this blurred focus. The irrelevance of t-utility for most workers in the field of pain, explains why the definition has escaped significant negative criticism. In this light my assumption that Loeser and Treede's claim that the "existing definition of 'pain' has proven very useful" (Loeser and Treede 2008: 473) refers to t-utility may be mistaken; they may be expressing the IASP's view that the definition is *clinically* useful.

Overall, I see the process of formulating the definition and the reviews that have been conducted since 1979 as missed opportunities. The note is the appropriate vehicle for justifying taxonomic features and for taxonomically irrelevant but clinically important information; a taxonomic definition is not. If the IASP's Taxonomy Committee had observed this distinction then perhaps it would have produced a definition that clearly picks out all and only pains. The message that emerges from this chapter is that philosophers should be very wary of any conclusions they might draw from cursory consideration of the IASP's definition of pain and its explanatory note.

Related topics

Chapter 1: A brief and potted overview on the philosophical theories of pain (Hardcastle)
Chapter 5: Fault lines in familiar concepts of pain (Hill)
Chapter 6: Advances in the neuroscience of pain (Apkarian)
Chapter 7: Neuromatrix theory of pain (Roy and Wager)
Chapter 8: A neurobiological view of pain as a homeostatic emotion (Strigo and Craig)
Chapter 9: A view of pain based on sensations, meanings, and emotions (Price)
Chapter 10: Pathophysiological mechanisms of chronic pain (Thacker and Moseley)
Chapter 15: The lives of others: pain in non-human animals (Droege)
Chapter 16: Robot pain (Mandik)
Chapter 18: Pain: perception or introspection? (Aydede)
Chapter 20: Pain and incorrigibility (Langland-Hassan)
Chapter 36: Fetal pain and the law: abortion laws and their relationship to ideas about pain (Derbyshire)

Notes

1　There have been two other changes to the note: the phrase "but are not unpleasant" has been moved without any change to the meaning of the sentence in which it appears; and the latest version states "[t]here is *usually* no way to distinguish their experience from that due to tissue damage if we take the subjective report" (IASP 2014; my emphasis), which is more equivocal than the 1979 formulation which omits the word "usually."

2　This quotation comes from a report of a meeting of the IASP's Taskforce on Taxonomy in November 2007. The recommendations of the taskforce were reviewed by the entire editorial board of the IASP's journal *Pain* (Loeser and Treede 2008) so I take the quotation as an endorsement by the IASP more broadly.

3　See the preceding footnote.

4　There is a tension between the exclusion of *some* dysesthesias because they lack the usual sensory qualities of pain and the definition of dysesthesia as "[a]n unpleasant abnormal sensation, whether spontaneous or evoked" (IASP 2014). If some dysesthesias may be pains (as explicitly stated in the note) then these dysesthesias would have the usual sensory qualities of pain. So how could these experiences fall under a characterization as abnormal sensations? I leave this question open.

5　The clinical importance of ensuring adequate pain treatment should not be underestimated. Not only does pain have the capacity to cause suffering, there is also evidence that untreated acute pain predisposes subjects to chronic pain (Hanley et al. 2007; Møiniche et al. 2002).

6　In particular, see comments on Anand and Craig's (1996) editorial by Stuart Derbyshire, Harold Merskey and Patrick Wall in *Pain* 67, pp. 209–211.

7　Almost certainly, the similar problem posed by some itches was not identified.

References

Anand, K. and Craig, K. (1996) New perspectives on the definition of pain. *Pain* 67: 3–6.

Bonica, J. (1979) The need of a taxonomy. *Pain* 6: 247–248.

Fields, H. (1999) Pain: an unpleasant topic. *Pain* 6 (suppl.): S61–S69.

Hall, R.J. (2008) If it itches, scratch! *Australasian Journal of Philosophy* 86(4): 525–535.

Hanley, M., Jensen, M.P., Smith, D.G., Ehde, D.M., Edwards, W.T., and Robinson, L.R. (2007) Pre-amputation pain and acute pain predict chronic pain after lower extremity amputation. *Journal of Pain* 8 (2): 102–109.

IASP (International Association for the Study of Pain) (1979) Pain terms: a list with definitions and notes on usage. *Pain* 6: 249–252.

IASP (International Association for the Study of Pain) (1986) Pain terms: a current list with definitions and notes on usage. *Pain* 3 (suppl.): S216–S221.

IASP (International Association for the Study of Pain) (2014) *IASP Pain Terminology.* <http://www.iasp-pain.org/Taxonomy>, accessed 31 December 2015.

Jones, L.E. (2010) *First Steps: The Early Years of IASP 1973–1984.* Seattle: IASP Press.

Loeser, J. and Treede, R. (2008) The Kyoto Protocol of IASP basic pain terminology. *Pain* 137: 473–477.

Møiniche, S., Kehlet, H., and Berg, J. (2002) A qualitative and systematic review of preemptive analgesia for postoperative pain relief. *Anesthesiology* 96: 725–741.

32

PHILOSOPHY AND "PLACEBO" ANALGESIA

Daniel E. Moerman

1 Pain is in the brain

It is important to distinguish between injury, nociception, and pain. Injury occurs in the finger when you hit it with a hammer. The nociception system conveys to the brain the information about the injury. The pain, however, is not in the finger (though it seems to be, hence complicating phenomenological accounts), rather it's in the brain (cf. Chapters 5 and 27). The best example of this is found in the situation known as phantom limb pain. Occasionally when a person loses a limb, an arm, or leg for example, she might feel the leg still there. And it might hurt, even terribly. Sometimes, the lost limb feels as if it is badly contorted, wrapped around her own neck. For an interesting case and review see (Bunch et al. 2015). The recognition of this implausible phenomenon helps us understand what is unfortunately called the "placebo effect"; I will return to the issue of the name later.

2 Placebos and pain

It has been widely recognized for many years that intense pain can respond to an injection of sterile saline or a few pills (preferably large multicolored capsules), that is, inert treatment; this is referred to as "placebo analgesia." The simple fact of placebo analgesia is often greeted with great suspicion. "Everyone knows" that pain is the result of injury or real physical illness, and therefore it will require real medicine for effective treatment. Such "knowledge" is at least in part a consequence of the highly mechanistic understanding of human physiology which is generally part of contemporary medicine. As one student of the subject suggests, "[i]n the mechanistic tradition that still underlies much of modern biomedicine, believing in the power of a placebo to erase pain is as irrational as filling the gas tank of your car with Earl Grey tea" (Morris 1997: 187). Irrational or not, contemporary research has laid out very clearly the neurobiology of placebo analgesia (Benedetti and Amanzio 1997). And the oddness here is diminished by the recognition that, as I've noted, pain is in the brain.

3 Active and inert treatments: what is the difference?

In what follows I will on occasion contrast "active treatments" and "inert treatments." Examples of active treatments might include morphine for pain, aspirin for a headache, or alcohol as an anti-infective agent, deep-brain stimulation for Parkinson's, and cortisol for immunosuppression. For a classic list, see the World Health Organization's Model Lists of Essential Medicines (WHO 2015).

Examples of inactive treatments are those which ordinarily "we in the know" understand to be mimics of the active treatments lacking that which we understand to *be* active, so a syringe of saline water rather than morphine, or a tablet of starch made to mimic an aspirin tablet, etc. These inactive treatments are often termed "placebos," a term which I prefer to avoid, but with which I have no argument. The history of the term is complex and interesting, and often gotten wrong. For what I consider to be the correct interpretation of the evolution of the term see (Moerman 2002: 10–11).

The dilemma here is that, as already noted, these "placebo treatments" (legitimate term) are sometimes quite effective (active, if you will) and have what are called "placebo effects." But I would argue that this usage betrays a very faulty logic. If the thing is inert (sterile saline), then it can't have any effect. If it *is* effective, it can't be due to the placebo. However, other sorts of things can affect the sick or inflamed. The confidence of the physician, the color of the pills, the shape and decor of the physician's office; many other things can support that inert treatment, things which I prefer to call "meaning" in Polanyi's sense (Polanyi 1966; Polanyi and Prosch 1975). In what follows, I will attempt to flesh out this argument, and make it plausible. And meaningful.

4 The classic experiment

The classic experiment which led to much recent research in this area was done in the late 1970s, following the earlier recognition that humans had endogenous opioids in their brains, first established in 1974 and 1975 (Hughes et al. 1975). A handful of peptides called endorphins (from "endogenous morphine") were identified, ironically enough, through medical research on addiction. It seemed that these peptides could actually moderate pain.[1] Subsequently, working with young people who were having wisdom teeth removed, Levine and colleagues gave their patients various drugs to treat the post-operative pain. Drugs were given double-blind through an intravenous drip so that no one knew who was getting what. Most patients were given placebo as their first pain treatment about two hours after the surgery. Then, an hour later, they were given another treatment, either a second placebo or the opiate antagonist naloxone.[2] Although there were no differences in the pain reported by the two groups at the time of the second treatment, another hour later the patients who received naloxone reported significantly more pain than those who got a second placebo. *Naloxone had reversed placebo analgesia* (Levine et al. 1978). This was a brilliant experiment, but it had flaws,[3] and it occasioned a negative response for years (at this writing, the paper has been cited 1,032 times according to Google Scholar). This was not a perfect experiment; a lot went on which I haven't described, and the paper was very controversial. But, eighteen years later, Fabrizio Benedetti said of this paper that it marked the date that "the biology of placebo was born" (Benedetti 1996). It is now generally recognized that this was the first study to show convincingly that inert treatment could stimulate the production of endogenous opiates in the brain. In a personal communication about this study, Howard Fields, one of the authors, told me "[t]he first time we did this and did not have morphine as a possibility, there was no placebo effect. Once we truly blinded it, so that nobody really knew what they were getting [or giving], we started seeing robust effects from saline infusions." When the clinicians knew there was no possibility of morphine, there were no "placebo effects." When morphine was possible (even if very improbable) there were robust effects from saline infusions. For a direct test of this issue, which showed the same thing but much more clearly, see a wonderful paper by Gracely (Gracely et al. 1985).

Benedetti, in effect, repeated Levine's study years later addressing all the critiques of the original study with a much larger pool of subjects. The conclusions were the same – naloxone blocked placebo-induced analgesia. In addition, he showed that a drug called proglumide enhanced the effect of injection of inert saline. It is an even more masterful study than the one it replicated (Benedetti 1996).

More recently, very ingenious fMRI studies of placebo analgesia have shown more precisely where and how these changes are occurring. One study showed that "placebo analgesia was related to decreased brain activity in pain-sensitive brain regions, including the thalamus, insula, and anterior cingulate cortex, and was associated with increased activity during anticipation of pain in the prefrontal cortex, providing evidence that placebos alter the experience of pain" (Wager et al. 2004: 1162). It is important to note that the brain changes noted with placebo treatment are essentially the same as those that occur with treatment with opiates (Wager et al. 2004). And it is also the case that the prefrontal cortex is the area generally associated with abstract thought and thought analysis, where you make sense of things, where you create meaning (Miller and Cohen 2001).

5 Beyond pain

It is also the case that although the plurality of research has been done on pain, similar recent work has focused on other conditions including depression, anxiety, Parkinson's disease, and many more. There are similar findings. Inert treatments mimic the neurological activity of effective active treatments. In some cases, the frequency of effective inert treatments is nearly the same as that of effective active treatments. Notably, this is the case in depression where, it has been argued, while there are modest statistical differences between drug and control groups in trials, "the clinical relevance of the differences has not been established" (Moncrieff and Kirsch 2015).

It is worth noting that this is a very popular area of study. Thousands of studies are published every decade, and the number of publications is almost always up; see Table 32.1, which shows the number of responses in Google Scholar to the query "placebo effect research" by decade from 1940 to the present.

Table 32.1 Google Scholar citations, by decade, for the search "placebo effects research"

Decade	Google Scholar "placebo effect research"	Factor change from previous decade
1940–49	437	—
1950–59	2,500	5.7
1960–69	7,450	2.9
1970–79	16,400	2.3
1980–89	25,500	1.5
1990–99	21,800	0.8
2000–9	179,000	8.2
2010–present	233,000	1.3

Source: Google Scholar, <https://scholar.google.com>, accessed September 2014.

6 Colorful pills

Consider a simple case, colorful pills. There is ample evidence to conclude that inert pills of different colors have different effects and that colors can enhance, or reduce, the effect of active treatments. Throughout the "Western world," red, yellow, and orange pills tend to be stimulants, or uppers (red is "hot"), while blue and green pills tend to be tranquilizers, or downers (blue is "cool") (de Craen et al. 1996). There is however some interesting variation in this pattern. In Italy, a few studies have shown that while part of this pattern is true for women – blue placebos are effective sleeping pills – it is not so for Italian men, for whom blue placebos act as stimulants, inhibiting sleep (Cattaneo et al. 1970; Lucchelli et al. 1978). A native Italian colleague suggested the following hypothesis: blue is the color of the Virgin Mary, a comforting figure for many Italian women (Google "Virgin Mary" images); on the other hand, the Italian national football team is the Azzurri, or "Blue" (Google "Azzurri" images) which for many Italian men is a figure of intense excitement, vigor, and valor (and, too often, catastrophe), hardly sleep inducing; fans chant in unison "Forza Azzurri" which can be translated to the English phrase "Go Blue," which anyone from Michigan will recognize. So, we might conclude that the blue placebo has different significance for men than for women (in Italy), that it shows a different sign, or, in my preferred terms, it "means" different things to men and women.

I argue that these variations in space, time, and gender in the effectiveness of placebos is a measure of how their meanings vary in time and space. Moreover, I would argue that this is a key to understanding what is happening when a person responds to an inert pill. It's not the pill that creates the response; the pill is, after all, inert. And that's what "inert" means. No one would be tempted to call these "inert responses," since that is certainly an oxymoron. But it does make sense to see them as a species of "meaning response."

7 Open–hidden experiments

A final example of the meaning response in medicine: Benedetti has done a series of experiments (Benedetti et al. 2003) reversing the terms of the standard experiment with placebos. He arranged with hospitalized post-surgical patients to do this experiment, where patients could be given their standard post-surgical analgesia surreptitiously through an intravenous line. Half the patients were attended by a clinician when the analgesia was administered, the "open administration group," while the other half were not attended by a physician, the "hidden administration group."

> The open administration was performed at the bedside by a doctor, who told the patients that the medication was a potent painkiller, according to routine clinical practice. In other words, the patients were informed that their pain was going to subside within a few minutes. By contrast, the hidden administration was given by the preprogrammed machine without any doctor or nurse in the room, so that the patients were totally unaware that a painkilling medication was being given.
>
> Thus, the main difference between open and hidden injections was the knowledge that a medication was being given, and an engagement with another human being. Both the open and the hidden groups rated their pain by themselves in a pain diary at 30 and 60 minutes after morphine infusion, on the basis of a numerical rating scale ranging from 0 = *no pain* to 10 = *unbearable pain* .... After the injection of morphine, the pain decrease in the open condition was larger than in the hidden

condition at both 30 min, $t(40) = -3.322$, $p = .002$, and 60 min, $t(40) = -4.766$, $p = .001$. Thus, the hidden administration of morphine was less effective than the open one.

(Benedetti et al. 2003)

He repeated variations of this experiment with other illnesses (Parkinson's disease, state anxiety, beta blockade) and physiological conditions (muscarinic antagonism), and in all of them, open administration of drug or other treatment was more effective than hidden administration.

What shall we call the difference between the open and hidden administration of treatment? All the patients received standard medical treatments – morphine, subthalamic brain stimulation, atropine, etc. – of known effectiveness. The drugs were always effective. Most important, in this study *there were no placebos*. Unless we are prepared to call doctors placebos, which is utterly ridiculous;[4] for a discussion of the idea of psychotherapy being placebo, see Kirsch et al. (2015) and Moerman (2002: ch. 7, 89–99, and Chapter 12, this volume). This is from the conclusions to Benedetti's paper:

> It is probably wrong to call placebo effect the difference between open and hidden treatments, since no placebos are given. *Meaning response is perhaps more appropriate ...* in order to make it clear that the crucial factor is not so much the treatment per se but rather the meaning around the medical treatment. In other words, placebo effects also occur without the administration of any placebo. Therefore, it might be time to limit the use of the term placebo effect to those situations in which inert (dummy) medical treatments are given ... However, it is worth noting that even if a placebo is given, there is no such thing as a placebo effect, since this term deflects our gaze from what is really important (the meaning and the meaning-induced expectations) and aims it at what is not (the inert pills and, in general, the inert medical treatments).
>
> *(Benedetti et al. 2003, emphasis mine)*

A number of other scholars have argued that meaning is central to the "placebo effect." Among them are Howard Brody (Brody and Brody 2000), Ted Kaptchuk (2011), and, from a somewhat different perspective, David Newman (2009).

8 Factors causing the placebo effect meaning response to vary: genes and/or gender

There is very little evidence for genetic differences among people regarding their ability to respond to meaning in a medical context. There is some.

Researchers in Ted Kaptchuk's group at Harvard have identified a genetic polymorphism that shows that people with different alleles of a gene (Catechol-O-methyltransferase val158met – or COMT) respond differently to the same placebo treatment of Irritable Bowel Syndrome. The gene is involved in the process by which the body makes dopamine and is involved in processes associated with meaning response such as reward, pain, memory, and learning (Hall et al. 2012; Hall and Kaptchuk 2013).

Finally, Luana Colloca and colleagues have recently shown that observational learning can also induce analgesic effects (Colloca and Benedetti 2009). Moreover vasopressin, a hormone released by the hypothalamus, can enhance the placebo effect in women, but not men

(Colloca et al. 2016). This hormone has quite different effects on men and women; to oversimplify, they argue that it might encourage women to tend-and-friend while it encourages men to fight-or-flight. The former state leaves people more ready to listen and hear while the latter encourages them to ignore, or even dehumanize, the other. In this way people seem to sort themselves into in-group behavioral dynamics. These results complement and resemble clinical findings observed in the open–hidden studies (Benedetti et al. 2003; Colloca et al. 2004) in which social interactions induce pain relief. Despite the fact that the underlying psychosocial mechanisms are distinct, the outcomes observed in experimental and clinical settings are comparable in magnitude to those in the open–hidden studies. The outcomes are at least similar.

9 Some philosophical considerations

Many philosophical considerations of the placebo effect address ethical issues: what happens when a physician lies to a patient and instead of giving him a real drug, she gives him an inert substitute? But most of the situations we have seen show that this is an irrelevant non-issue. Having the physician on hand to advise the patient on what his morphine will do (and thereby enhancing its effectiveness) is hardly some sort of chicanery, and not unethical. Indeed, we might prefer to argue that it is unethical to deprive the patient of the clinician's presence by replacing her with a more efficient, cost-saving robot computer. Neither would deliberately avoiding blue sleeping tablets for Italian men seem to me unethical. *Al contrario.*

Other philosophical approaches to placebo phenomena are varied; most concern mechanisms. They regularly grant the significance of meaning, but wonder how meaning becomes action. For many investigators, a key to understanding the issue involves what some call "conditioning," and others call "learning." One of the first to do this was Robert Ader who worked with rats (Ader and Cohen 1975), and later humans in whom he claimed to have conditioned autoimmune processes (Giang et al. 1996). Kirsch has also written and studied conditioning and placebo effects (Montgomery and Kirsch 1997); he has also proposed expectancy as an approach to placebo (Kirsch 1999). Finally, Luana Colloca and Franklin Miller have proposed a fascinating semiotic approach to the placebo effect (Miller and Colloca 2010).

In both conditioning and expectancy arguments, the individual must have experience with effective drugs or other experiences (like a mother's caresses and caring when her infant is soothed) that the "placebo" can interact with. That is, the conditioned response depends on an unconditioned (e.g., real) one. Insofar as this might be the case, the very common argument that "all medicine was the placebo effect until the invention of penicillin" (see, e.g., Shapiro and Shapiro 1997) is clearly nonsense. You can't have conditioned responses without unconditioned ones. That view also ignores the wide presence throughout the premodern world of highly effective plant medicines, including many still in use today: digitalis from the lovely plant foxglove (*Digitalis* spp.), opium from poppies (*Papaver somniferum*), curare from *Strychnos toxifera*, and aspirin, a minor modification of the more toxic salicylates from a number of plants, including willows (*Salix* spp., after which the salicylates were named) and meadowsweet (*Spirea* spp., after which aspirin is named). Certainly there were inert medications utilized throughout antiquity and beyond which acted as placebos, but only because people could learn about the powers of medicines, and be affected positively by other unrelated objects and experiences after learning from conditioning stimuli.

Other more recent philosophical approaches to meaning responses include interesting work by Jordi Vallverdú who focuses on how emotion can engage different physiological functions without having active pharmaceuticals involved (Vallverdú 2013). Similarly, André

LeBlanc approaches the emotional dimensions of meaning responses from the perspective of "full correspondence," pursuing the notion of "feeling what happens" (LeBlanc 2014). Mark Sullivan considers "psychogenic pain" in his consideration of how trauma and pain are related (Chapter 13, this volume).

Giulio Ongaro draws on enactivism to broaden and deepen the concept of meaning as the working axis of the "placebo effect." He writes:

> "Placebo effect," then, is simply a pharmacocentric misnomer. In enactivist terms, we can better think of it as a response to a milieu that holds meaning for the individual, remembering that anything is meaningful to the extent that it relates to the organism's norm at the particular condition the individual finds himself in. To be more precise, we can say that the placebo effect is a meaning response with a positive valence, while the nocebo effect is a meaning response with a negative valence.
>
> *(Ongaro 2013: 13)*

10 Discussion

Even in this brief chapter, it should be apparent that "placebo phenomena" are extremely broad and varied, far broader and more varied than I have indicated here. There has been only limited research on the role of placebos and the cannabinoid receptor site system, for example; a start is shown in recent work by Benedetti who (with colleagues) showed that some elements of placebo analgesia are mediated not by the opioid system, but by the cannabinoid system. They suggest that "the endocannabinoid system has a pivotal role in placebo analgesia in some circumstances when the opioid system is not involved" (Benedetti et al. 2011: 1228, abstract). More mysteries to solve.

At the same time as there is stunning scholarship on the anatomy and physiology of the placebo effect, I'd argue that the literature on ethical dimensions of the issue are often premodern. In a very influential paper published in *Scientific American* in 1974,[5] philosopher Sissela Bok phrased the problem this way. Writing in the wake of the emergence of the double-blind trial as the "gold standard" of medical evidence, Bok argued that deceptive practices, like giving patients inert drugs that they thought were active treatments, were deeply unethical, a form of lying that would be "corrosive of medical authority": "Honesty may not be the highest social value; at exceptional times, when survival is at stake, it may have to be set aside. To permit a widespread practice of deception, however, is to set the stage for abuses and growing mistrust." She concludes her article by citing Augustine writing about official sanction for white lies, saying "little by little and bit by bit this will grow and by gradual accessions will slowly increase until it becomes such a mass of wicked lies that it will be utterly impossible to find any means of resisting such a plague grown to huge proportions through small additions" (Bok 1974: 23). A few years later, a scholar as accomplished as Howard Brody (PhD in philosophy; dissertation on the placebo effect; MD) could write a paper titled "The Lie that Heals: The Ethics of Giving Placebos" in the *Annals of Internal Medicine* (Brody 1982). These attitudes persist; I can attest to this as I personally have been excoriated in the Internet blogosphere for holding different views, that meaning responses can be (or simply cannot avoid being) an integral part of medicine.

How different this is than the body of work by Bruce Barrett in Madison, Wisconsin. A long series of studies culminated in this one (Rakel et al. 2011) in which 719 patients with a new-onset common cold (a viral infection) were randomized into three groups. One group received treatment but no patient–clinician interaction, one group received "standard" interaction, and one received "enhanced interaction"; in the latter group, the clinicians used a set of practices characterized by "the mnemonic PEECE: (P) Positive prognosis, (E) Empathy, (E) Empowerment, (C) Connection and (E) Education." That is, they paid attention to their patients, they called them at home to find out how they were doing, etc. Patients rated clinician empathy with a standard scale; interleukin-8 and neutrophil counts (which measure the intensity of a viral infection) were obtained for nasal wash at baseline and forty-eight hours later. The two ratings of empathy and cold intensity were closely but inversely related. Those in the enhanced-care group experienced statistically significantly reduced cold severity and duration (Rakel et al. 2011). I don't see any lies here, neither do I see anything "corrosive of medical authority." I do see people enhancing patients' understandings of both their illnesses and their treatments. I see them manipulating meaning in a way that was beneficial to the patients.

Finally, some have argued that the problem with a concept like the "meaning response" is broader than that range of phenomena called the "placebo effect" (Jennifer Corns, personal communication). The literal physical anguish and joy of "a teenage girl in love" is clearly a "meaning response," and not a "placebo effect." The terror we might feel while watching a horror movie like *Psycho* or *The Cabinet of Dr. Caligari* is a meaning response in reaction to light flickering on a wall; there is nothing there at all, yet we scream together. The intense satisfaction after a wonderful dinner after a busy day of, say, hiking, and that mellow glow that accompanies the port in front of the fire afterwards, are partly a consequence of the stimulation of μ-opioid receptor sites in the gut (Holzer 2009), but surely the meanings of the meal, both those of its content and its structure (Douglas 1972), are clearly meaning responses, and not placebo effects. But I don't see that this is a problem, indeed it is an advantage, because we can each experience meaning responses in non-medical contexts to enhance our appreciation of them in the more serious world of hospitals, life, and death.

Related topics

Chapter 5: Fault lines in familiar concepts of pain (Hill)
Chapter 12: Biospsychosocial models of pain (Hadjistavropoulos)
Chapter 13: Psychogenic pain: old and new (Sullivan)
Chapter 27: Bad by nature: an axiological theory of pain (Massin)

Acknowledgements

Special thanks to Jennifer Corns for interesting discussions about these issues. Thanks also to Luana Colloca for helpful discussion of issues of gender and vasopressin, and other dimensions of this chapter. Giulio Ongaro and I had a very helpful discussion of enactivism. Lola Romanucci-Ross, my native Italian colleague, has always been helpful to me, including here. For Cynthia.

Notes

1 Controversy ensued when people realized that the humans could produce substances to which they could become addicted.
2 Naloxone, an opiate antagonist, blocks the receptor sites in the brain to which opiates bind. The metaphor is that it's like an uncut door key which can slide into the lock, but not unlock it, at the same time preventing the real key from sliding into the lock.
3 The study was small; it had a complicated design, more complicated than I have described. The authors' conclusions were plausible, and in the end correct, but could easily be challenged at the time; for example, see Gracely et al. 1983.

4 Physicians are hardly inert: they are living breathing people, often people we (their patients) have known for decades, who have delivered our babies, mended our broken arms, alleviated our migraines. Even if this particular doctor is not one we have known before, she often knows one of our favorite doctors (best is when our old favorite was a professor of this new person). Our psychiatrists may have known us longer than do our children, and know things about us that the kids will never know (I dearly hope). Doctors are not inert.

5 Google Scholar lists sixty-four publications citing this paper between 1 January and 1 November 2015, fifty-one years after it was published.

References

Ader, R. and Cohen, N. (1975) Behaviorally conditioned immunosuppression. *Psychosomatic Medicine* 37: 333–340.

Benedetti, F. (1996) The opposite effects of the opiate antagonist naloxone and the cholecystokinin antagonist proglumide on placebo analgesia. *Pain* 64: 535–543.

Benedetti, F. and Amanzio, M. (1997) The neurobiology of placebo analgesia: from endogenous opioids to cholecystokinin. *Progress Neurobiology* 52: 109–125.

Benedetti, F., Maggi, G., Lopiano, L., Lanotte, M., Rainero, I., Vighetti, S., and Pollo, A. (2003) Open versus hidden medical treatments: the patient's knowledge about a therapy affects the therapy outcome. *Prevention & Treatment* 6(1). doi:10.1037/1522-3736.6.1.61a.

Benedetti, F., Amanzio, M., Rosato, R., and Blanchard, C. (2011) Nonopioid placebo analgesia is mediated by CB1 cannabinoid receptors. *Nature Medicine* 17: 1228–1230.

Bok, S. (1974) The ethics of giving placebos. *Scientific American* 231: 17–23.

Brody, H. (1982) The lie that heals: the ethics of giving placebos. *Annals of Internal Medicine* 97: 112–118.

Brody, H. and Brody, D. (2000) Three perspectives on the placebo response: expectancy, conditioning, and meaning. *Advances in Mind–Body Medicine* 16(3): 216–232.

Bunch, J.R., Goldstein, H.V., and Hurley, R.W. (2015) Complete coverage of phantom limb and stump pain with constant current SCSI aystem: a case report and review of the literature. *Pain Practice* 15: E20–E26.

Cattaneo, A.D., Lucchilli, P.E., and Filippucci, G. (1970) Sedative effects of placebo treatment. *European Journal of Clinical Pharmacology* 3: 43–45.

Colloca, L. and Benedetti, F. (2009) Placebo analgesia induced by social observational learning. *Pain* 144: 28–34.

Colloca, L., Lopiano, L., Lanotte, M., and Benedetti, F. (2004) Overt versus covert treatment for pain, anxiety, and Parkinson's disease. *Lancet Neurology* 3: 679–684.

Colloca, L., Pine, D.S., Ernst, M., Miller, F.G., and Grillon, C. (2016). Vasopressin boosts placebo analgesic effects in women: a randomized trial. *Biological Psychiatry* 79(10): 794–802. doi:10.1016/j. biopsych.2015.07.019.

de Craen, A.J., Roos, P.J., de Vries, A.L., and Kleijnen, J. (1996) Effect of colour of drugs: systematic review of perceived effect of drugs and of their effectiveness. *British Medical Journal* 313: 1624–1626.

Douglas, M. (1972) Deciphering a meal. *Daedalus* 101: 61–81.

Giang, D.W., Goodman, A.D., Schiffer, R.B., Mattson, D.H., Petrie, M., Cohen, N., and Ader, R. (1996) Conditioning of cyclophosphamide-induced leukopenia in humans. *Journal of Neuropsychiatry and Clinical Neuroscience* 8: 194–201.

Gracely, R.H., Dubner, R., Wolskee, P.J., and Deeter, W.R. (1983) Placebo and naloxone can alter post-surgical pain by separate mechanisms. *Nature* 306: 264–265.

Gracely, R. H., Dubner, R., Deeter, W.R., and Wolskee, P.J. (1985) Clinicians' expectations influence placebo analgesia. *Lancet* 1(8419): 43.

Hall, K.T. and Kaptchuk, T.J. (2013) Genetic biomarkers of placebo response: what could it mean for future trial design? *Clinical Investigation* 3: 311–314.

Hall, K.T., Lembo, A.J., Kirsch, I., Ziogas, D.C., Douaiher, J., Jensen, K.B., Conboy, L.A., Kelley, J.M., Kokkotou, E., and Kaptchuk, T.J. (2012) Catechol-O-methyltransferase val158met polymorphism predicts placebo effect in irritable bowel syndrome. *PloS One* 7: e48135.

Holzer, P. (2009) Opioid receptors in the gastrointestinal tract. *Regulatory Peptides* 155: 11–17.

Hughes, J., Smith, T.-W., Kosterlitz, H.-W., Fothergill, L.A., Morgan, B.-A., and Morris, H. (1975) Identification of two related pentapeptides from the brain with potent opiate agonist activity. *Nature* 258: 577–580.

Kaptchuk, T.J. (2011) Placebo studies and ritual theory: a comparative analysis of Navajo, acupuncture and biomedical healing. *Philosophical Transactions of the Royal Society B: Biological Sciences* 366: 1849–1858.

Kirsch, I. (1999) *How Expectancies Shape Experience*. Washington, DC: American Psychological Association.

Kirsch, I., Wampold, B., and Kelley, J.M. (2015) Controlling for the placebo effect in psychotherapy: noble quest or tilting at windmills. *Psychology of Consciousness: Theory, Research, and Practice*. doi:10.1037/cns0000065.

LeBlanc, A. (2014) "Feeling what happens": full correspondence and the placebo effect. *Journal of Mind and Behavior* 35(3): 167–184.

Levine, J.D., Gordon, N.C., and Fields, H.L. (1978) The mechanism of placebo analgesia. *Lancet* 2(8091): 654–657.

Lucchelli, P.E., Cattaneo, A.D., and Zattoni, J. (1978) Effect of capsule colour and order of administration of hypnotic treatments. *European Journal of Clinical Pharmacology* 13: 153–155.

Miller, E.K. and Cohen, J.D. (2001) An integrative theory of prefrontal cortex function. *Annual Review of Neuroscience* 24: 167–202.

Miller, F.G. and Colloca, L. (2010) Semiotics and the placebo effect. *Perspectives in Biology and Medicine* 53: 509–516.

Moerman, D.E. (2002) *Meaning, Medicine, and the "Placebo Effect."* Cambridge/New York: Cambridge University Press.

Moncrieff, J. and Kirsch, I. (2015) Empirically derived criteria cast doubt on the clinical significance of antidepressant-placebo differences. *Contemporary Clinical Trials* 43: 60–62.

Montgomery, G. and Kirsch, I. (1997) Classical conditioning and the placebo effect. *Pain* 72(1–2): 107–113.

Morris, D.B. (1997) Placebo, pain, and belief: a biocultural model. In A. Harrington (ed.), *The Placebo Effect: An Interdisciplinary Exploration*. Cambridge, MA: Harvard University Press, pp. 187–120.

Newman, D.H. (2009) *Hippocrates' Shadow*. New York: Simon & Schuster.

Ongaro, G. (2013) *Enactivism and the Placebo Effect*. MSc diss., University of Edinburgh.

Polanyi, M. (1966) *The Tacit Dimension*. Garden City, NY: Anchor Books/Doubleday & Co.

Polanyi, M. and Prosch, H. (1975) *Meaning*. Chicago: University of Chicago Press.

Rakel, D., Barrett, B., Zhang, Z., Hoeft, T., Chewning, B., Marchand, L., and Scheder, J. (2011) Perception of empathy in the therapeutic encounter: effects on the common cold. *Patient Education and Counseling* 85(3): 390–397. doi:10.1016/j.pec.2011.01.009.

Shapiro, A.K. and Shapiro, E. (eds.) (1997) *The Powerful Placebo from Ancient Priest to Modern Physician*, Baltimore: Johns Hopkins University Press.

Vallverdú, J. (2013) The meaning of meaning: new approaches to emotions and machines. *Aditi Journal of Computer Science* 11: 25–38.

Wager, T., Rilling, J., Smith, E., Sokolik, A., Casey, K., Davidson, R., Kosslyn, S., Rose, R., and Cohen, J. (2004) Placebo-induced changes in fMRI in the anticipation and experience of pain. *Science* 303: 1162–1167.

WHO(World Health Organization) (2015) *WHO Model Lists of Essential Medicines*. WHO. <http://www.who.int/medicines/publications/essentialmedicines/en/>, accessed 2 January 2016.

33

PAIN MANAGEMENT

Carolyn Berryman, Mark Catley and Lorimer Moseley

1 Introduction

Identifying the underlying etiologies and mechanisms of many pain states is a major clinical and research challenge. Pain, nociception and pathology do not share a straightforward, isomorphic relationship and our inability to understand the underlying etiology can color our attitudes towards the symptoms. Despite this, clinical management requires a framework within which consistent, evidence-based, soundly reasoned, effective, feasible and cost-effective management strategies can be delivered.

Effective pain management depends on a diverse and deep knowledge set because pain is a highly complex multifactorial experience. Several concepts are fundamental here. First, contemporary perspectives in the pain sciences consider that pain is a protective experience rather than a "damage-marker" or some other measure of the state of the tissues. (Cf. chapters in Section I of this volume, e.g., Chapters 2, 4, 8 and 9.) Neither the actual state of the tissues nor the amount of activity in nociceptive fibers determines the emergence of pain (Wall and McMahon 1986). Pain emerges when real or apparent threat is sensed and a response is activated (McMahon et al. 2013). Second, pain exists entirely within consciousness, which differentiates it from nociception, which is the detection, transformation, transmission and processing of a potentially dangerous stimulus or event, and from other protective physiological responses (see Butler and Moseley 2013; Moseley and Butler 2015a, 2015b; cf. Chapter 17, this volume.) Third, the multifactorial nature of pain is best considered within a biopsychosocial framework (see Chapter 12, this volume). That is, pain involves a complex and variable interaction of biological (for example genetic profile, neurotransmitter profile, real-time biological status of the body), psychological (for example mood, personality, thoughts and beliefs) and social (for example cultural, familial, socioeconomic) factors and needs to be considered in context.

This chapter outlines pain management from a clinical perspective. The chapter explores what components contribute to the delivery of optimal pain management and how we currently measure whether we have met that goal. A wide range of pain management strategies are subsequently presented, culminating in the ultimate aim of management: self-management.

2 What is the aim of pain management?

The general aim of pain management is to identify in context and address – using pharmacological, psychological (cognitive and behavioral), physical, cortical, virtual and/or self-management strategies – modifiable causes or contributions to the patient's loss of well-being. Pain relief is the most obvious, but not the only, therapeutic goal. Management also aims to restore physical and psychosocial function to sufficient levels to enable meaningful engagement in activities of daily living, to prevent recurrent injury, and to minimize ongoing health-care and medication utilization (Gatchel et al. 2014). Meeting patients' expectations about outcomes and assessing and providing evidence-based information about their condition aims to facilitate acceptance and empower self-management (Moseley and Butler 2015b; Pincus and McCracken 2013).

The clinician is encouraged to look beyond local tissue sources of nociception and consider the severity and impact of the pain, the multimodal nature of the experience, the contributing factors and comorbidities such as depression, hypertension, diabetes and cardiovascular disease (Barnett et al. 2012; Haanpää et al. 2010). Indeed, chronic pain of high severity has been associated with increased all-cause mortality and in particular mortality due to cardiovascular disease (Torrance et al. 2010). Because there are tight restrictions imposed on time and resources in clinical practice, and pain is complex and multimodal in nature, the assessment and management of pain can be very challenging (Mills et al. 2016).

3 Delivering optimal pain management

That pain be considered the fifth vital sign, as proposed by the American Pain Society (Campbell 1996), invites mandatory consideration of pain in all clinical interactions. This invitation, to raise pain to the level of essential information, was spawned by concern for the under-treatment of pain. The initiative encouraged health-care professionals to actively listen and respond to their patients' pain rating, often leading to the prescription of opioids when other pharmaceutical interventions such as paracetamol failed (Sullivan and Ballantyne 2016; Campbell 2016). Most clinical guidelines endorse this invitation (SIGN 2013; NICE 2013, 2014; Schlug et al. 2015) and also call for a comprehensive, multidimensional, and robust clinical assessment of the pain state.

Because living with pain may be associated with a deterioration in quality of life, social withdrawal, loss of work capacity, cognitive impairment, altered mood, depression and cardiovascular disease, early access to care is critical (Torrance et al. 2010; Breivik et al. 2006). Of course, delivery of optimal pain management at the appropriate time relies on the capacity of the system to deliver it, and the quality of the care itself. Current systems of pain care delivery worldwide are arguably lagging behind societal needs and provide fragmented and inconsistent access to services of variable quality (PainAustralia 2010; Dubois and Follett 2014).

Indeed, wholehearted commitment to health professional pain education at tertiary level and beyond is yet to be given in most training institutions, despite recommendations from the International Association for the Study of Pain and open access to its standardized curricula for pain education for health professionals (see IASP 2012). In general, undergraduate pain education occurs in a piecemeal fashion, swallowed up in other topics, and is not given stand-alone time or resources (Morone and Weiner 2013; Briggs et al. 2011). The issue is compounded by a lack of experienced pain education faculty and as a result, many clinicians emerge from training deficient in the skills necessary to optimally assess and manage pain

(Morselli et al. 2010; Ripamonti et al. 2012). One way forward taken by Australia is the instantiation of a national framework for the assessment and management of pain, which formalizes resource allocation towards training, development and distribution of the necessary capacity for timely management of pain (PainAustralia 2010).

4 Measuring outcomes

Pain intensity remains the primary outcome measure of most clinical encounters and is usually recorded as a rating out of 10 where 10 is the worst pain the patient could imagine (Morone and Weiner 2013). Pain intensity has long been criticized for being a one-dimensional measure of a multidimensional problem and findings suggest that other outcome measures or a combination of outcome measures such as functional capacity, emotional well-being, sleep quality and life enjoyment might better represent the effectiveness of a given management strategy (Lazaridou and Edwards 2016). The Fibromyalgia Impact Questionnaire, for example, is often used in clinical and academic settings to quantify the functional impact of the disease (Burckhardt et al. 1991). Choosing a clinically relevant measure with good psychometric properties is a difficult task that may be facilitated by an evidence website such as the International Centre for Allied Health Evidence, which provides access to at least sixty-two benchmarked outcome measures for pain conditions and includes an outcomes calculator (iCAHE 2014).

5 Screening tools

Theoretically, screening tools that identify patients at risk of poor prognosis should help finite resources be directed to those patients who will most benefit. For example, the STarT Back tool (Murphy et al. 2016) stratifies the risk of chronic low-back pain after an acute episode into low, medium and high, and suggests treatments for each risk level. The Örebro Musculoskeletal Pain Screening Questionnaire aims to identify people at risk of developing ongoing pain due to psychosocial factors, assessing five risk categories and providing guidance for cut-off scores (Johnston 2009). Other tools might screen for neuropathic pain components, for example the Leeds Assessment of Neuropathic Symptoms and Signs (Bennett 2001), the Neuropathic Pain Questionnaire, PainDETECT and ID Pain (Haanpää et al. 2009); or for contributing mood states, such as the Depression, Anxiety Stress Scale. These tools are yet to be perfected and as yet none are established as gold-standard screening tools, but work to this end is under way (Rhon and Fritz 2015; Traeger et al. 2015). Some examples of tools in current use are presented in Table 33.1.

6 Pharmacological strategies

The World Health Organization cancer pain ladder for adults (WHO 2015) provides guidelines for both the method of delivery and the type of drugs to deliver depending on pain severity. Recommendations from the first rung of the ladder include drugs that are commonly prescribed and also commonly used without prescription across many health-care settings, including the management of non-cancer pain. For example, in mild, acute and chronic pain states the ladder recommends use of: paracetamol, non-steroidal anti-inflammatory tablets or creams and weak opioids (Breivik 2012). Further up the ladder the more fragile the relationship between pain and recommendations becomes. For example, in chronic low-back pain there is low- to moderate-quality evidence for the short-term efficacy

Table 33.1 A selection of clinically useful screening tools

Screening tool	Availability	Measure	Suitability
STarT Back	Freely available at Keele University (2016)	9-item index stratifies 3 levels of risk of transition of acute to chronic pain	Back pain only
Brief Pain Inventory	Freely available from multiple Internet sites	9-item self-report questionnaire that reports pain severity and pain interference during activities of everyday life	Useful in many presentations including cancer
Leeds Assessment of Neuropathic Symptoms and Signs	Full text and scale available at ResearchGate (Bennett 2001)	Objective (2 tasks) and subjective (5 questions) analysis of sensory disturbance	Identifying patients in whom neuropathic signs and symptoms contribute to the pain state
Neuropathic Pain Questionnaire	(Krause and Backonja 2003)	12-item questionnaire, 10 sensory items and 2 affective items	Identifying patients in whom neuropathic signs and symptoms contribute to the pain state
Depression Anxiety and Stress Scale	Free to download, fee for manual from University of New South Wales (UNSW 2014)	42-item self-report scale for evaluating 3 negative emotional states – depression, anxiety and stress	Useful in many presentations

of prescription opioids (recommendations from the second rung), and a comprehensive assessment of the potential risk of side effects prior to use is necessary. There is no evidence for the effectiveness of opioids in long-term use for chronic non-cancer pain (Chaparro et al. 2013), but they remain the mainstay for the control of cancer pain (WHO 2015).

Guidelines for the treatment of neuropathic pain (NICE 2013) also recommend para-cetamol as a first-rung drug, often in conjunction with topical preparations such as lidocaine, tricyclic antidepressants, gabapentinoids and selective noradrenergic re-uptake inhibitors (Haanpää 2012; NICE 2013; Finnerup et al. 2015). Strong opioids and tramadol for neuro-pathic pain are worth considering when there is insufficient pain relief. Critically, contention exists about the effectiveness, risk and cost of any pharmacological approaches to chronic pain because of the complexity and uncertainty of the mechanisms underlying the pain presenta-tion. (See, in this volume, Chapter 10, for more on chronic pain mechanisms, and Chapter 35, for more on controlled pain-relieving substances.)

7 Psychological strategies

Fundamental to the notion that pain is a protective experience, rather than a marker of true tissue damage, is that anything that threatens the person in pain will increase the likelihood and intensity of pain. Critically, these threatening influences occur outside of awareness, although some correlates of threat are often noticeable, for example stress, anxiety and fear (Zeidan et al. 2012). Psychological strategies that target threatening cognitive and behavioral contributors to pain play a major role in any pain management program. For more information on cognitive-behavioral therapy and acceptance and commitment, and meditation strategies see Chapters 11 and 12, this volume.

8 Therapeutic neuroscience education

"Explain Pain" (EP) refers to the delivery of education about the biological mechanisms that underpin pain (Moseley and Butler 2015b). The skilled clinician shifts the patient's understanding of pain from that of a marker of injury to that of a marker of the perceived need to protect body tissue. Heuristics, such as "hurt does not equal harm," help to embed the new message, but practical examples using tales of phantom limb pain, where there is pain but no tissue damage, and heroic sporting feats such as kicking the winning goal with a broken ankle are used to challenge current concepts of the meaning of pain. Grounded in conceptual change theory – that is, the explanation of the processes by which a person's current concepts of an entity interact with and change to a new set of concepts that are incompatible with the original (Posner et al. 1982) – EP is differentiated from earlier components of cognitive-behavioral therapy by focusing on the patient's knowledge and knowledge framework about pain (for a full review and discussion of the components see Moseley and Butler 2015b). EP is delivered clinically in one-on-one or group sessions (Moseley 2004) and is thought to effect a cognitive modulation of pain. Positive shifts in the understanding of pain, behavioral changes, participation in rehabilitation and diminished catastrophization have also been shown in randomized controlled trials (Moseley et al. 2004; Moseley 2002).

9 Operant learning theory: graded activity and pacing

At the heart of operant learning theory is the belief that pain behaviors are a major component of the pain presentation, and that their expression is subject to reinforcement. That is, positive and negative reinforcement of behavior is thought to lead to strengthening and weakening of the behavior respectively (Fordyce 1982; Gatzounis et al. 2012). For example, demonstration of protective and communicative behaviors such as guarding and vocalization is thought to become more frequent when positive reinforcement is given, such as expressions of sympathy from a spouse (Newton-John 2002). Similarly, weakening of the behavior is expected following negative reinforcement. Success with operant learning theory is predicated on a good behavioral analysis. Patterns of behavior, the context in which they take place and postures or activities associated with increased or decreased pain are noted through interview, diary keeping, activity-recording technology and direct or indirect observation. Realistic goals are set with mutual consent and then strategies such as graded activity, pacing activity, and time-contingent medication dosing are used to reach the goals (see Gatzounis et al. 2012 for a full review). Graded activity refers to the patient performing exercises to quota (75–90 percent of exercise tolerance) with an ongoing adjustment of the quota as improvement occurs. Pacing refers to breaking down activity into smaller chunks and using breaks in between. The aim is that rest will become contingent on the time or part of activity completed, and extinguish contingency on the negative reinforcement of pain. A similar framework exists for time-contingent medication. Surprisingly, despite frequent use, operant conditioning alone seems no more effective than usual care for decreasing pain, increasing function, or attaining earlier return to work in people with chronic low-back pain (van der Giessen et al. 2012).

10 Hypnosis

Hypnosis can relieve pain in subgroups of chronic pain patients with flow-over effects into take-home self-management skills (Jensen and Patterson 2014). Mood states such as anxiety and depression can also be modified by hypnosis, in addition to suggestions that may be made to improve activity levels, increase active coping skills and improve the quality of sleep (Jensen 2011; Jensen et al. 2011). Mechanisms of relaxation, distraction and focused attention have been postulated to underpin the effects of hypnosis (Jensen and Patterson 2014).

11 Physical, complementary and alternative medicine strategies

Complementary and alternative medicines include, but are not limited to, spinal manipulation or cracking, mobilization, acupuncture, massage, homeopathy, herbalism, exercise, electrotherapy, cryotherapy and aromatherapy (Mills et al. 2016). The vast majority of published literature attributes the effects of these interventions to cognitive factors associated with expectations and the therapeutic process, rather than tissue or peripheral nervous system modulation (see Chapter 32, this volume, and Moerman 2002; Moerman and Jonas 2002; Moseley 2008). Poor- to moderate-grade evidence supports manipulation and massage over placebo or no treatment for pain relief and improved function in the short term in acute or subacute spinal pain. Small health gains (mostly decrease in pain severity) have been consistently reported for acupuncture in people with chronic low-back pain (Furlan et al. 2010; SIGN 2013), but whether or not it depends on the needles being inserted is open to debate. There is no evidence to support the efficacy of homeopathy and, because the proposed mechanisms of action (memory of water for substances with which it has previously been in contact; BHA 2016) are unscientific, its medical use has been challenged on ethical grounds (Zawiła-Niedźwiecki and Olender 2016).

General exercise is known to have a positive effect on people with chronic pain (Liddle et al. 2004), although much of the supporting evidence is low quality. The discussion centers on the difference between being physically active, which is no talisman against the deleterious effects of a largely inactive life, as besets many individuals with chronic pain, and exercise, which is deemed a subset of physical activity that is planned and focuses on improved physical fitness. Exercise governed by indicators such as the breathlessness scale and heart-rate quota is an important component in full recovery from a pain state (Bement and Sluka 2016). The numerous benefits of therapist-prescribed exercise include pain modulation, improved flexibility, strength and better coordination. Although not widely acknowledged or explored, it is plausible that exercise also trains the neural component of movement; that is, it not only improves neuromuscular processes in the periphery, but it is thought to train cortical motor programs as well (Wallwork et al. 2015).

Transcutaneous electrical nerve stimulation (TENS) emerged as a viable modality for pain management after publication of the gate control theory of pain (Melzack and Wall 1965). TENS is conventionally used at high (greater than 50 hertz) or low (acupuncture mimic, less than 10 hertz) frequencies, for periods at a time. The TENS machine is of wearable and portable size, the frequency may be modulated to prevent habituation, and the electrodes are self-adhesive. Pain relief is thought to be in response to stimulation of the large-diameter nerve fibers, the same ones that one would normally self-stimulate by rubbing the site of immediate injury and thus, by the gate control theory, inhibit noxious afferent impulses. The evidence in support of TENS use is mixed: a recent meta-analysis reported level-I and -II evidence for effective pain relief in people with chronic lower-back pain when TENS was used for a period of less than five weeks (Jauregui et al. 2016), while a comprehensive, but older, Cochrane review reported inconsistent evidence for any benefit (Khadilkar et al. 2005).

Enthusiasm for using heat or cold therapy (wraps, packs or electrotherapy generated) for pain modulation is based primarily on empirical experience. Indeed a recent review of its use in acute musculoskeletal pain states and delayed-onset muscle soreness found limited evidence of short-term effectiveness for either modality (Malanga et al. 2015). Electrotherapy agents that may produce thermal effects, such as short-wave diathermy units (electro-magnetically generated heat that is discharged through the tissues because they act as the capacitor) and ultrasound (which operates as a form of mechanical energy applied directly over the painful area, coupled to the skin with an aqueous gel, and a low depth of penetration), also have a limited evidence base (Harris and Susman 2002). Laser therapy for painful conditions has become a popular intervention based on the significant antinociceptive effects reported in animal studies (Chen et al. 2008; Hsieh et al. 2015), but human studies have so far failed to provide sufficient evidence of benefit (Glazov et al. 2016).

12 Training the brain

Recent developments have seen the emergence of strategies that aim to reinstate normal representation of the body in the brain. For example, the somatosensory homunculus, shown to be distorted in chronic pain (Flor et al. 1997), can be re-established using training with sensory stimuli (pinprick) (Flor et al. 2006). Motor patterns have also been shown to be distorted in association with several pain conditions including chronic neuropathic pain (Lefaucheur et al. 2006). Graded motor imagery, which presents movement patterns to the brain through recognition of photographs or diagrams and a left/right judgement task progressing in a stepwise fashion to explicit movement, has randomized control trial support (Bowering et al. 2013; Parsons 2001).

13 Surgical interventions and imaging

The effectiveness of invasive techniques, such as injecting anesthetic or steroid into a purported painful joint, or blocking or damaging the nerve to a purported painful part, for pain relief and improved function, seems to depend on the accurate selection of patients. Using a range of diagnostic criteria, multiple systematic reviews that consider the evidence for various invasive techniques show moderate evidence for the long-term effectiveness of damaging the nerves that supply painful areas in people with chronic back or neck pain, as well as injecting lidocaine into the space around the spinal cord for people with spinal stenosis (Manchikanti et al. 2016b). There is mixed or minimal evidence for other interventions, including implantable devices that release drugs into the space around the spinal cord, or electrical devices that stimulate spinal cord neurons at an analgesic frequency or analgesic or steroidal injections into the purported painful joint (Manchikanti et al. 2015, 2013, 2016a).

Yet, despite fragile support, there has been a rapid and very large increase in some of these interventions. For example, joint injections have increased 293 percent overall between 2000 and 2013 in a Fee-for-Service Medicare population in the United States (Manchikanti et al. 2015). This raises the possibility that some management strategies may be driven by factors other than evidence-informed patient and clinician decision-making. The routine use of X-rays, that cannot and do not image pain, in the majority of pain states (Pransky et al. 2010) is perhaps also an example of the consequences of a litigious society where evidence-based decision-making is disrupted in favor of ruling out distant possibilities of sinister underlying pathology. As clinicians we need to be accountable to our motives and offer management strategies that have the greatest likelihood of success based on our knowledge of the evidence and our clinical evaluation of the presenting patient.

14 Self-management and virtual strategies

The overarching aim of most interventions for pain is to achieve a state where self-management is possible (Mackey et al. 2016). Development of self-management skills may involve competency and compliance with a home exercise and/or psychological program, access to online resources, access to health-care professionals via Telecare or the Internet, or self-help support groups. The recent flourish of applications for monitoring progress, activity and pain levels throughout the day adds another dimension to the ability to capture and share information between patient and clinician and thus promote self-management. Future options for home management may also include the ability to address brain images of the body by exercising in a virtual world, provided by a pair of goggles, or working through virtual exercises delivered to electronic devices (Harvie et al. 2015, 2016).

Related topics

Chapter 2: Pain and representation (Cutter)
Chapter 4: Imperativism (Klein)
Chapter 8: A neurobiological view of pain as a homeostatic emotion (Strigo and Craig)
Chapter 9: A view of pain based on sensations, meanings, and emotions (Price)
Chapter 10: Pathophysiological mechanisms of chronic pain (Thacker and Moseley)
Chapter 11: Psychological models of pain (Williams)
Chapter 12: Biopsychosocial models of pain (Hadjistavropoulos)
Chapter 17: Pain and consciousness (Pereplyotchik)
Chapter 32: Pain and "placebo" analgesia (Moerman)
Chapter 35: Pain and controlled pain-relieving substances (Aggarwal and Pettus)

References

Barnett, K., Mercer, S., Norbury, M., Watt, G., Wyke, S., and Guthrie, B. (2012) Epidemiology of multimorbidity and implications for health care, research, and medical education: a cross-sectional study. *Lancet Neurology* 380: 37–43.

Bement, M. and Sluka, K. (2016) Exercise-induced hypoalgesia: an evidence-based review. In K. Sluka (ed.), *Mechanisms and Management of Pain for the Physical Therapist*. Philadelphia: Wolters Kluwer.

Bennett, M. (2001) The LANSS pain scale: the Leeds assessment of neuropathic symptoms and signs. *Pain* 92: 147–157.

BHA (British Homeopathic Association) (2016) *How does homeopathy work?* BHA. <http://www.britishhomeopathic.org/how-does-homeopathy-work/>.

Bowering, K.J., O'Connell, N.E., Tabor, A., Catley, M.J., Leake, H.B., Moseley, G.L., and Stanton, T.R. (2013) The effects of graded motor imagery and its components on chronic pain: a systematic review and meta-analysis. *Journal of Pain* 14: 3–13.

Breivik, H. (2012) A major challenge for a generous welfare system: a heavy socio-economic burden of chronic pain conditions in Sweden – and how to meet this challenge. *European Journal of Pain* (London, UK) 16: 167.

Breivik, H., Collett, B., Ventafridda, V., Cohen, R., and Gallacher, D. (2006) Survey of chronic pain in Europe: prevalence, impact on daily life, and treatment. *European Journal of Pain* (London, UK) 10: 287–333.

Briggs, E., Carr, E., and Whittaker, M. (2011) Survey of undergraduate pain curricula for healthcare professionals in the United Kingdom. *European Journal of Pain* (London, UK) 15: 789–795.

Burckhardt, C., Clark, S., and Bennett, R. (1991) The fibromyalgia impact questionnaire: development and validation. *Journal of Rheumatology* 18: 728–733.

Butler, D. and Moseley, G.L. (2013) *Explain Pain*. Adelaide, Australia: Noigroup Publications.

Campbell, J.N. (1996) APS 1995 Presidential address. *Pain Forum* 5: 85–88.

Campbell, J.N. (2016) The fifth vital sign revisited. *Pain* 157: 3–4.

Chaparro, L., Furlan, A., Deshpande, A., Malais-Gagnon, A., Atlas, S., and Turk, D. (2013) Opioids compared to placebo or other treatments for chronic low-back pain (review). *Cochrane Database of Systematic Reviews*, no. 8: CD004959. doi:10.1002/14651858.CD004959.pub4.

Chen, K.H., Hong, C.Z., Kuo, F.C., Hsu, H.C., and Hsieh, Y.L. (2008) Electrophysiologic effects of a therapeutic laser on myofascial trigger spots of rabbit skeletal muscles. *American Journal of Physical Medicine & Rehabilitation* 87: 1006–1014.

Dubois, M. and Follett, K. (2014) Pain medicine: the case for an independent medical specialty and training programmes. *Academic Medicine* 89: 863–868.

Finnerup, N.B., Attal, N., Haroutounian, S., McNicol, E., Baron, R., Dworkin, R.H., Gilron, I., Haanpää, M., Hansson, P., Jensen, T.S., Kamerman, P.R., Lund, K., Moore, A., Raja, S.N., Rice, A.S., Rowbotham, M., Sena, E., Siddall, P., Smith, B.H., and Wallace, M. (2015) Pharmacotherapy for neuropathic pain in adults: a systematic review and meta-analysis. *Lancet Neurology* 14: 162–173.

Flor, H., Braun, C., Elbert, T., and Birbaumer, N. (1997) Extensive reorganisation of primary somatosensory cortex in chronic back pain patients. *Neuroscience Letters* 224: 5–8.

Flor, H., Nikolajsen, L., and Jensen, T. (2006) Phantom limb pain: a case of maladaptive CNS Plasticity? *Nature Neuroscience* 7: 873–881.

Fordyce, W.E. (1982) A behavioural perspective on chronic pain. *British Journal of Clinical Psychology* 21 (pt. 4): 313–320.

Furlan, A., Yazdi, F., Tsertsvadze, A., Gross, A., van Tulder, M., Santaguida, L., Cherkin, D., Gagnier, J., Ammendolia, C., Ansari, M., Posterman, T., Dryden, T., Doucette, S., Skidmore, B., Daniel, R., Tsouros, S., Weeks, L., and Galipeau, J. (2010) *Complementary and Alternative Therapies for Back Pain II: Evidence Report/Technology Assessment, No. 194*. Prepared by the University of Ottawa Evidence-Based Practice Center under Contract No. 290–2007-20059-I (EPCIII). AHRQ Publication No. 10(11)-E007. Rockville, MD: Agency for Healthcare Reseach and Quality.

Gatchel, R., McGeary, D., McGeary, C., and Lippe, B. (2014) Interdisciplinary chronic pain management past, present and future. *American Psychologist* 69: 119–130.

Gatzounis, R., Schrooten, M.G., Crombez, G., and Vlaeyen, J.W. (2012) Operant learning theory in pain and chronic pain rehabilitation. *Current Pain and Headache Reports* 16: 117–126.

Glazov, G., Yelland, M., and Emery, J. (2016) Low-level laser therapy for chronic non-specific low back pain: a meta-analysis of randomised controlled trials. *Acupuncture in Medicine*. doi:10.1136/acupmed-2015-011036.

Haanpää, M. (2012) The assessment of neuropathic pain patients. *Pain Management* 3: 59–65.

Haanpää, M.L., Backonja, M.-M., Bennett, M.I., Bouhassira, D., Cruccu, G., Hansson, P.T., Jensen, T.S., Kauppila, T., Rice, A.S.C., Smith, B.H., Treede, R.-D., and Baron, R. (2009) Assessment of neuropathic pain in primary care. *American Journal of Medicine* 122: S13–S21.

Haanpää, M., Gourlay, G., Kent, J., Miakowski, C., Raja, S., Schmader, K., and Wells, C. (2010) Treatment considerations for patients with neuropathic pain and other medical comorbidities. *Mayo Clinic Proceedings* 85: S15 S25.

Harris, G. and Susman, J. (2002) Managing musculoskeletal complaints with rehabilitation therapy: summary of the Philadelphia Panel evidence-based clinical practice guidelines on musculoskeletal rehabilitation interventions. *Journal of Family Practice* 51: 1042–1046.

Harvie, D.S., Broecker, M., Smith, R.T., Meulders, A., Madden, V.J., and Moseley, G.L. (2015) Bogus visual feedback alters onset of movement-evoked pain in people with neck pain. *Psychological Science* 26: 385–392.

Harvie, D.S., Hillier, S., Madden, V.J., Smith, R.T., Broecker, M., Meulders, A., and Moseley, G.L. (2016) Neck pain and proprioception revisited using the Proprioception Incongruence Detection Test. *Physical Therapy* 96: 671–678.

Hsieh, Y.L., Hong, C.Z., Chou, L.W., Yang, S.A., and Yang, C.C. (2015) Fluence-dependent effects of low-level laser therapy in myofascial trigger spots on modulation of biochemicals associated with pain in a rabbit model. *Lasers in Medical Science* 30: 209–216.

IASP (International Association for the Study of Pain) (2012) *IASP Curricula*. Updated 2012. <http://www.iasp-pain.org/Education/CurriculaList.aspx?navItemNumber=647>.

iCAHE (International Centre for Allied Health Evidence) (2014) *iCAHE Outcome Calculators*, University of South Australia. <http://www.unisa.edu.au/Research/Sansom-Institute-for-Health-Research/Research/Allied-Health-Evidence/Resources/OC/>.

Jauregui, J.J., Cherian, J.J., Gwam, C.U., Chughtai, M., Mistry, J.B., Elmallah, R.K., Harwin, S.F., Bhave, A., and Mont, M.A. (2016) A meta-analysis of transcutaneous electrical nerve stimulation for chronic low back pain. *Surgical Technology International* 28: 296–302.

Jensen, M. (2011) Psychosocial approaches to pain management: An organizational framework. *Pain* 152: 717–725.

Jensen, M. and Patterson, D. (2014) Hypnotic approaches for chronic pain management. *American Psychologist* 69: 167–177.

Jensen, M., Ehde, D., Gertz, K., Stoelb, B., Dillworth, T., At, H., and Kraft, G. (2011) Effects of self-hypnosis training and cognitive restructuring on daily pain intensity and catastrophizing in individuals with multiple sclerosis and chronic pain. *International Journal of Clinical and Experimental Hypnosis* 59: 43–63.

Johnston, V. (2009) Örebro Musculoskeletal Pain Screening Questionnaire. *Australian Journal of Physiotherapy* 55: 141.

Keele University (2016) *STarT Back*. Keele University. <http://www.keele.ac.uk/sbst/>.

Khadilkar, A., Milne, S., Brosseau, L., Robinson, V., Saginur, M., Shea, B., Tugwell, P., and Wells, G. (2005) Transcutaneous electrical nerve stimulation (TENS) for chronic low-back pain. *Cochrane Database of Systematic Review*, no. 2: Cd003008.

Krause, S.J. and Backonja, M.M. (2003) Development of a neuropathic pain questionnaire. *Clinical Journal of Pain* 19: 306–314.

Lazaridou, A. and Edwards, R. (2016) Getting personal: the role of individual patient preferences and characteristics in shaping pain treatment outcomes. *Pain* 157: 1–2.

Lefaucheur, J., Drouot, X., Meanrd-Lefaucheur, I., Keravel, Y., and Nguyen, J. (2006) Motor cortex rTMS restores defective intracortical inhibition in chronic neuropathic pain. *Neurology* 67: 1568–1574.

Liddle, S., Baxter, G., and Gracey, J. (2004) Exercise and chronic low back pain. What works? *Pain* 107: 176–190.

Mackey, L.M., Doody, C., Werner, E.L., and Fullen, B. (2016) Self-management skills in chronic disease management: what role does health literacy have? *Medical Decision Making* 36(6): 741–759.

McMahon, S., Koltzenburg, M., Tracey, I., and Turk, D. (2013) *Wall and Melzack's Textbook of Pain*, 6th ed. Amsterdam: Elsevier.

Malanga, G.A., Yan, N., and Stark, J. (2015) Mechanisms and efficacy of heat and cold therapies for musculoskeletal injury. *Postgraduate Medicine* 127: 57–65.

Manchikanti, L., Abdi, S., Atluri, S., Benyamin, R.M., Boswell, M.V., Buenaventura, R.M., Bryce, D.A., Burks, P.A., Caraway, D.L., Calodney, A.K., Cash, K.A., Christo, P.J., Cohen, S.P., Colson, J., Conn, A., Cordner, H., Coubarous, S., Datta, S., Deer, T.R., Diwan, S., Falco, F.J., Fellows, B., Geffert, S., Grider, J.S., Gupta, S., Hameed, H., Hameed, M., Hansen, H., Helm, S., 2nd, Janata, J.W., Justiz, R., Kaye, A.D., Lee, M., Manchikanti, K.N., McManus, C.D., Onyewu, O., Parr, A.T., Patel, V.B., Racz, G.B., Sehgal, N., Sharma, M.L., Simopoulos, T.T., Singh, V., Smith, H.S., Snook, L.T., Swicegood, J. R., Vallejo, R., Ward, S.P., Wargo, B.W., Zhu, J., and Hirsch, J.A. (2013) An update of comprehensive evidence-based guidelines for interventional techniques in chronic spinal pain II: Guidance and recommendations. *Pain Physician* 16: S49–S283.

Manchikanti, L., Kaye, A.D., Boswell, M.V., Bakshi, S., Gharibo, C.G., Grami, V., Grider, J.S., Gupta, S., Jha, S.S., Mann, D.P., Nampiaparampil, D.E., Sharma, M.L., Shroyer, L.N., Singh, V., Soin, A., Vallejo, R., Wargo, B.W., and Hirsch, J.A. (2015) A systematic review and best evidence synthesis of the effectiveness of therapeutic facet joint interventions in managing chronic spinal pain. *Pain Physician* 18: E535–E582.

Manchikanti, L., Hirsch, J.A., Kaye, A.D., and Boswell, M. V. (2016a) Cervical zygapophysial (facet) joint pain: effectiveness of interventional management strategies. *Postgraduate Medicine* 128: 54–68.

Manchikanti, L., Knezevic, N.N., Boswell, M.V., Kaye, A.D., and Hirsch, J.A. (2016b) Epidural Injections for Lumbar Radiculopathy and Spinal Stenosis: a comparative systematic review and meta-analysis. *Pain Physician* 19: E365–E410.

Melzack, R. and Wall, P. (1965) Pain mechanisms: a new theory. *Science Education* 150: 971–978.

Mills, S., Torrance, N., and Smith, B. (2016) Identification and management of chronic pain in primary care: a review. *Current Psychiatric Reports* 18: 22–31.

Moerman, D. (2002) *Meaning, Medicine and the "Placebo Effect."* Cambridge: Cambridge University Press.

Moerman, D.E. and Jonas, W.B. (2002) Deconstructing the placebo effect and finding the meaning response. *Annals of Internal Medicine* 136: 471–476.

Morone, N.E. and Weiner, D.K. (2013) Pain as the fifth vital sign: exposing the vital need for pain education. *Clinical Therapeutics* 35: 1728–1732.

Morselli, M., Bandieri, E., Zanin, R., Buonaccorso, L., D'Amico, R., Forghieri, F., Pietramaggiori, A., Potenza, L., Berti, A., Cacciapaglia, G., Molitierno, A., Galli, L., Artioli, F., Ripamonti, C., Bruera, E., Torelli, G., and Luppi, M. (2010) Pain and emotional distress in leukemia patients at diagnosis. *Leukemia Research* 34: E67–E68.

Moseley, G.L. (2002) Combined physiotherapy and education is effective for chronic low back pain: a randomised controlled trial. *Australian Journal of Physiotherapy* 48: 297–302.

Moseley, G.L. (2004) Evidence for a direct relationship between cognitive and physical change during an education intervention in people with chronic low back pain. *European Journal of Pain* (London, UK) 8: 39–45.

Moseley, G.L. (2008) Placebo effect: reconceptualising placebo. *British Medical Journal* 336: 1086.

Moseley, G. and Butler, D.S. (2015a) *The Explain Pain Handbook: Protectometer.* Adelaide, Australia: Noigroup Publications.

Moseley, G.L. and Butler, D.S. (2015b) Fifteen years of explaining pain – the past, present and future. *Journal of Pain* 16: 807–813.

Moseley, G.L., Nicholas, M.K., and Hodges, P.W. (2004) A randomized controlled trial of intensive neurophysiology education in chronic. *Clinical Journal of Pain* 20: 324–330.

Murphy, S.E., Blake, C., Power, C.K., and Fullen, B.M. (2016) Comparison of a stratified group intervention (STarT Back) with usual group care in patients with low back pain: a non-randomised controlled trial. *Spine* 41(8): 645–652.

Newton-John, T.R.O. (2002) Solicitousness and chronic pain: a critical review. *Pain Reviews* 9: 7–27.

NICE (National Institute for Health and Care Excellence) (2013) *Neuropathic Pain in Adults: Pharmacological Management in Non-specialist Settings.* London: NICE.

NICE (National Institute for Health and Care Excellence) (2014) *Osteoarthritis: Care and Management.* London: NICE.

PainAustralia (2010) *National Pain Strategy.* Melbourne: PainAustralia.

Parsons, L.M. (2001) Integrating cognitive psychology, neurology and neuroimaging. *Acta Psychologica* 107: 155–181.

Pincus, T. and McCracken, L. (2013) Psychological factors and treatment opportunities in low back pain. *Best Practice & Research: Clinical Rheumatology* 27: 625–635.

Posner, G., Strike, K., Hewson, P., and Gertzog, W. (1982) Accommodation of a scientific conception: towards a theory of conceptual change. *Science Education* 66: 211–227.

Pransky, G., Buchbinder, R., and Hayden, J. (2010) Contemporary low back pain research – an implication for practice. *Best Practice & Research: Clinical Rheumatology* 24: 291–298.

Rhon, D. and Fritz, J. (2015) COMParative Early Treatment Effectiveness between physical therapy and usual care for low back pain (COMPETE): study protocol for a randomized controlled trial. *Trials* 16: 423.

Ripamonti, C., Santini, D., Maranzano, E., Berti, M., and Roila, F. (2012) Management of cancer pain: ESMO clinical practice guidelines. *Annals of Oncology* 23: vii139–vii154.

Schlug, S., Palmer, G., Scott, D., Halliwell, R., and Trinca, J. (2015) *Acute Pain Management: Scientific Evidence,* 4th ed. Melbourne: Australian and New Zealand College of Anaesthetists, Faculty of Pain Medicine.

SIGN (Scottish Intercollegiate Guidelines Network) (2013) *Management of Chronic Pain.* Edinburgh: SIGN.

Sullivan, M.D., and Ballantyne, J.C. (2016) Must we reduce pain intensity to treat chronic pain? *Pain* 157: 65–69.

Torrance, N., Elliott, A., Lee, A., and Smith, B. (2010) Severe chronic pain is associated with increased 10 year mortality: a cohort record linkage study. *European Journal of Pain* (London, UK) 14: 380–386.

Traeger, A., Henschke, N., Hubscher, M., Williams, C.M., Kamper, S.J., Maher, C.G., Moseley, G.L., and McAuley, J.H. (2015) Development and validation of a screening tool to predict the risk of chronic low back pain in patients presenting with acute low back pain: a study protocol. *BMJ Open* 5: e007916.

UNSW (University of New South Wales) *DASS: Depression, Anxiety, Stress Scales. Psychology.* UNSW. Updated 10 November 2014. <http://www2.psy.unsw.edu.au/dass/>.

van der Giessen, R.N., Speksnijder, C.M., and Helders, P.J. (2012) The effectiveness of graded activity in patients with non-specific low-back pain: a systematic review. *Disability and Rehabilitation,* 34: 1070–1076.

Wall, P.D. and McMahon, S.B. (1986) The relationship of perceived pain to afferent nerve impulses. *Trends in Neurosciences* 9: 254–255.

Wallwork, S.B., Bellan, V., Catley, M.J., and Moseley, G.L. (2015) Neural representations and the cortical body matrix: implications for sports medicine and future directions. *British Journal of Sports Medicine.* doi:10.1136/bjsports-2015-095356.

WHO (World Health Organization) (2015) *Cancer Pain Relief.* Geneva: WHO.

Zawiła-Niedźwiecki, J. and Olender, J. (2016) A not-so-gentle refutation of the defence of homeopathy. *Journal of Bioethical Inquiry* 13: 21–25.

Zeidan, F., Grant, J., Brown, C., McHaffie, J., and Coghill, R. (2012) Mindfulness meditation-related pain relief: evidence for unique brain mechanisms in the regulation of pain. *Neuroscience Letters* 520: 165–173.

PART III-III

Pain in law

34

PAIN AND THE LAW

Ben A. Rich

1 Introduction

This chapter will consider how pain, and the related yet conceptually distinct phenomenon of suffering, are addressed in the law. The focus will be civil rather than criminal law, and predominantly the sub-domain of civil law known as torts. A tort is a civil wrong in which the injured party may be compensated with an award in damages. The examples and illustrations will be drawn largely from the Anglo-American sources with which the author is most familiar. I will begin with an analysis of the term "pain and suffering" as it is commonly used in tort law. This will be necessarily brief, and perhaps singularly unsatisfying from a philosophical perspective, because of the largely unreflective approach the law has taken to what many scholars consider a deeply profound and significant dimension of the human experience. Next, I will discuss the critical role of pain and suffering as the basis for "non-economic damages" in tort litigation through a concise overview of the vigorous ongoing debate among legal scholars as to whether the award of such damages comports with the role of tort law in the legal system.

Thereafter I will examine another controversial topic – the role of law in setting the parameters for prescribing opioid analgesics to treat chronic non-cancer pain. Chapter 35 of this volume provides a detailed discussion of the nature and utilization of these medications. The United States has been the locus of high-profile legal cases, particularly disciplinary proceedings by medical licensing boards and litigation (both civil and criminal) arising out of both alleged over- and under-prescribing of pain medications, as well as policy initiatives. The concluding section will focus on the role of the law in end of life care. The pursuit of a peaceful death by patients with a terminal condition has generated significant case and statutory law in many Western nations. I will focus on seminal cases which highlight competing considerations.

I direct the reader to other chapters of this volume for related topics. Fetal pain, which has found its way into many recent anti-abortion provisions of state law in the United States, is considered in Chapter 36 of this volume. Chapter 28, on pain and torture, relates to recent challenges in the United States to the use of lethal injection on the grounds that when not undertaken by medical professionals there is a high risk of severe pain and distress constituting cruel and unusual punishment in violation of the Eighth Amendment to the Constitution. Once again in 2015 the US Supreme Court ruled against challengers of a lethal injection protocol.[1]

2 "Pain and suffering" in the law of torts – semantics over substance

[P]hilosophy might learn from tort law the difference between practical reality and philosophical frivolity.

Bernard Williams, Philosophical Foundations of
Tort Law *(Williams 1995)*

One commentator on pain and suffering damages in American tort law observed: "The response of the legal system to the doctrinal and factual complexity of pain and suffering has been to make this element of damages procedurally simple but analytically impenetrable" (Leebron 1989: 265). To explicate this distinction, consider first the procedural simplicity aspect. The relevant California Civil Jury Instruction is typical, stating that non-economic damages include: "past and future physical pain/mental suffering/loss of enjoyment of life/ disfigurement/physical impairment/inconvenience/grief/anxiety/humiliation/emotional distress." The instruction goes on to state: "No fixed standard exists for deciding the amount of these damages. You must use your judgment to decide a reasonable amount based on the evidence and your common sense."[2] Confirming the generic and non-analytic nature of such damages, one California appellate court decision on point notes:

> In general, courts have not attempted to draw distinctions between the elements of "pain" on the one hand and "suffering" on the other; rather, the unitary concept of "pain and suffering" has served as a convenient label under which a plaintiff may recover not only for physical pain but for fright, nervousness, grief, anxiety, worry, mortification, shock, humiliation, indignity, embarrassment, apprehension, terror or ordeal. Admittedly these terms refer to subjective states, representing a detriment which can be translated into monetary loss only with great difficulty.[3]

I will consider this "difficulty" further in the next section. Legal discourse in both academic journals and court decisions adopts a distinction, which permeates lay discourse as well, between "physical pain" and "mental suffering." A distinction touched on at various points throughout the volume. For purposes of this chapter, suffice it to say that the law (case, statutory, or legal theory) has not undertaken a fine-grained analysis of the distinction between pain and suffering in the experiencing subject. One must move outside of the law, most notably into the extensive writing of physician Eric Cassell, for an authoritative discussion of the distinct yet intricately interrelated aspects of pain and suffering (Cassell 2004).

In the absence of any legal analysis of the distinction between pain and suffering, common law jurisprudence has afforded the trier of fact (judges or juries) considerable latitude in calculating damages for non-pecuniary loss. This latitude only increases concerns about the responsible discharge of this duty (Diamond 1993). Similarly, there are no uniform criteria for reviewing courts to utilize. Some apply an abuse of discretion standard, while others hold that overturning an award requires a determination that the magnitude of the verdict shocks the judicial conscience (Schnapper 1989).

Assessing the appropriateness or inappropriateness of non-economic damage awards is further complicated by the fact-specific nature of each case. The non-economic component of the award can be substantial yet justifiable, and may include elements in addition to pain and suffering such as loss of consortium (companionship) and emotional distress. Compensating for the non-economic losses suffered by victims of negligence requires jurors to exercise their fallible human judgment in order to convert injury into a monetary amount (Kritzer 2014: 980). The resulting vagaries in damage awards have prompted calls for reform.

Professor Joseph H. King Jr. is a prominent critic who argues that "pain and suffering damages and the policy goals of modern tort law are conceptually and operationally incompatible" (King 2004: 166). The ostensible goal of damage awards in personal injury cases is to return the plaintiff, to the greatest extent possible, to the position s/he would have been in prior to the incident/accident attributed to the culpable act or omission of the defendant. King and other commentators insist that it is an illusion that monetary damages can be rationally calculated so as to correspond with the non-economic effects of pain and suffering; therefore only economic damages for the medical expenses of treatment for the plaintiff's distress and to offset loss of earning capacity are consistent with the objectives of tort law.

In a similar critique, a US federal circuit court of appeals judge characterized damage awards for pain and suffering as "the irrational centerpiece of the tort system" which undermines its integrity by contravening two essential values of the rule of law, i.e., rationality and predictability (Niemeyer 2004). He compares the problem to that raised by punitive damage awards, which are not intended to compensate the plaintiff, but rather to punish the defendant and deter others from similar conduct. These too are untethered from any standards of acceptability. Consequently, he urges legislatures to impose constraints to insure that pain and suffering damages may only be awarded for the purpose and to the extent that they address the impact pain and suffering have or may be anticipated to have in the future on the patient's life.

Another commentator, however, argues that damage awards for pain and suffering are not markedly different from many other varieties of non-economic damages countenanced by the law. Intentional torts such as assault and false imprisonment are the earliest causes of action allowing monetary awards to compensate for intangible loss (Rabin 2006). Others include criminal conversation and alienation of affections actions by spouses whose marital relations have been compromised by someone's wrongful actions, and libel and slander claims alleging that written or oral statements damaged the reputation of the plaintiff. In all of these a court may award the victim money for a harm that has no precise monetary equivalent. Therefore, if pain-and-suffering damage awards seriously undermine the integrity of the tort system, so too do awards for many other non-monetary injuries. I note too that Chapter 11 (on psychological models of pain) and Chapter 21 (on seeing the pain of others) discuss the nature of the challenges courts face in assessing another person's experience of pain and reasonably compensating them for it.

3 The politics of pain management: opioid analgesics for chronic non-cancer pain

And do you have a picture of the pain?

Phil Ochs, "Crucifixion Lyrics"[4]

Statutory and regulatory law in the United States, among others, is the product of the political process. In the United States examples include federal statutes such as the Controlled Substances Act (CSA), discussed more extensively below, and state laws such as so-called "intractable pain statutes" (recognizing the legitimacy of opioid prescribing for otherwise unrelievable pain conditions). The politicization of pain relief varies markedly depending on its origins, nature, and ramifications. Pain medicine has traditionally divided pain into three general types: acute, chronic non-cancer, and cancer or pain associated with life-threatening or terminal illness (Turk and Okifuji 2010). Until recently, because neither acute nor end of life pain management through opioid analgesia generated much political controversy, they were largely left to the health professions to manage unconstrained by oppressive regulatory oversight. The exceptions regarding pain at the end of life, i.e., palliative sedation and lethal prescriptions, will be addressed in the next section of this chapter. The same, however, has not been true of chronic pain.

The credibility of complaints of pain is a significant factor. Victims of traumatic injury or patients who have had major surgery present vivid and tangible evidence of the cause and severity of their pain. Moreover, with recovery and healing their need for high doses of strong pain medications can reasonably be anticipated to decline in a matter of days, at most weeks. Patients with advanced cancer or other terminal conditions often experience distressing symptoms requiring pharmacological management. The imminence of the patient's death also mitigates concerns about addiction or drug-seeking behaviors.

Chronic pain is by definition pain that has persisted for at least three months and may continue indefinitely (NIH 2011). Some medical professionals argue that chronic pain should be considered a disease entity unto itself rather than a persistent symptom of some other underlying condition (Tracey and Bushnell 2009). Moreover, it is not unusual for chronic pain to be present in the absence of any visible pathology. A more extensive discussion of chronic pain is provided in Chapter 10 of this volume.

Much of the law governing pain relief, both internationally and in individual countries, is focused on "controlled substances" – narcotics with an abuse potential but also effective in pain management. The Single Convention on Narcotic Drugs of 1961 (Single Convention) established basic requirements for development of national laws and regulations to address the worldwide problem of drug abuse and diversion (United Nations 1977). Most nations are now parties to the Single Convention, thereby ostensibly acknowledging the need for laws affecting the use of narcotics to recognize their legitimate role in patient care while at the same time seeking to prevent their abuse, diversion, or trafficking. The International Narcotics Control Board (INCB) was established as the United Nations affiliate agency providing oversight over the implementation of the Single Convention by signatory nations. A series of INCB reports has noted that laws and regulations relating to opioid analgesics continue to impose severe and burdensome restrictions on both their availability and appropriate use (INCB 2014).

The United States has provided an instructive example of the persistent tensions created by legal regimes intended to permit the legitimate use of narcotics while preventing or punishing their illegitimate use. The federal CSA (Controlled Substances Act) is the primary drug control legislation at the national level.[5] The CSA was a primary component of the Comprehensive Drug Abuse Prevention and Control Act of 1970, which was in turn the capstone of a series of federal drug control statutes dating back to 1914.[6] The CSA establishes five classification "schedules" for controlled substances ranging from Schedule I (high abuse potential and no currently recognized medical benefit, e.g., heroin, LSD, marijuana), to Schedules II and III, recognized medical benefits but significant abuse potential, to Schedules IV and V with recognized medical benefits and significantly lower abuse potential. The "scheduling" of medications is not fixed. In 2014, hydrocodone combination products were changed from Schedule III to Schedule II based on a conclusion that their abuse potential was more like those drugs currently in Schedule II.[7] There has also been increased pressure on the Drug Enforcement Administration (DEA) to recognize that marijuana has been demonstrated to provide medical benefit to certain patients (Bostwick 2012).

The DEA is the agency charged with enforcing the CSA. While the DEA readily disclaims either the legal authority or the intent to regulate the practice of medicine, among the most consistently cited barriers to pain management is physician fear of regulatory scrutiny by federal and state agencies (Rich 2000). This perception of regulatory scrutiny was enhanced by state laws in the United States and many European countries requiring multiple-copy prescription forms (MCPFs) for stronger analgesics such as morphine and fentanyl. One copy of the prescription went to some regulatory agency. Physicians uncomfortable with this level of scrutiny routinely prescribed weaker analgesics which did not require the special form. MCPF requirements have been abandoned in most of the US and some western European countries but are still prevalent in other countries (Cherny et al. 2010).

In the 1990s the laws and regulatory policies concerning opioid analgesia, especially for chronic pain, underwent a genuine transformation. Recognizing physicians' concerns about treating pain aggressively with opioids, many states enacted Intractable Pain Treatment Acts (IPTAs) which purported to provide immunity from regulatory sanctions for physicians who prescribed opioids to chronic pain patients. These statutes introduced many uncertainties, including the very definition of intractable pain (Joranson 1997). Moreover, such laws imposed no affirmative obligation on physicians to provide appropriate pain management. What ultimately improved the management of pain, particularly in the United States, was the recognition by the medical profession, prompted in part by litigation, that failure to adequately treat pain constituted substandard medical practice.

In 1991 a North Carolina jury awarded millions of dollars in damages in a lawsuit alleging under-treatment of the pain by a nursing home of an elderly man dying of cancer.[8] Ten years later, a California jury awarded over a million dollars in damages to the family of another elderly man dying from cancer, finding that the under-treatment of his pain by a physician constituted elder abuse.[9] In the ten-year period between these two cases, the Oregon Board of Medical Examiners became the first such board to take disciplinary action against a physician for repeated instances of inadequate pain management.[10] The Medical Board of California took a similar action several years later in response to a complaint by the family of an elderly nursing home patient dying of mesothelioma.[11] The clinical details of these cases are beyond the scope of this chapter and are described in detail elsewhere (Rich 2002).

In the United States, the consciousness raising about the role of pain management in quality patient care also included the Joint Commission for the Accreditation of Health Care Organizations (now the "Joint Commission") and the Federation of State Medical Licensing Boards, both of which issued policies and standards emphasizing the duty of health-care institutions and professionals respectively to promptly and effectively assess and manage pain. For a discussion of pain management, see Chapter 33 of this volume.

In contradistinction to these initiatives, US federal prosecutors zealously prosecuted physicians for allegedly violating the CSA by prescribing controlled substances in a manner that was not for a "legitimate medical purpose" or in the "course of professional practice," the magic words distinguishing legitimate from illegitimate prescribing. In such cases, prosecutors attempt to prove that the physician's conduct, usually involving a large number of patients or criminal investigators posing as patients, deviated so far from acceptable medical practice that it was, quite literally, outside the bounds of medical practice altogether. Jurors in such prosecutions are urged to view the defendant physician as nothing more than a drug dealer in a white coat with a medical degree.

The problem, which prosecutors and their expert witnesses exacerbate, is that in many such cases there is no simple, straightforward dichotomy between acceptable pain management and distributing drugs by prescription outside the bounds of medical practice. Rather, there is a qualitative range from exemplary practice, to acceptable practice, to substandard care (medical malpractice), to practice perhaps warranting suspension or even revocation of one's license to practice medicine – all of which are civil matters, and conviction for a crime.

Analogously, a patient may die as a result of medical error, but only in cases in which the physician's conduct amounted to reckless or intentional disregard of patient safety would a criminal prosecution ever be pursued, as opposed to a civil malpractice claim or disciplinary action by a medical board. Utilizing alleged violations of the CSA in an effort to imprison physicians for many years has even, in egregious cases, brought major professional organizations to the practitioner's defense in an effort to reinforce the distinction between substandard practice and criminal conduct.[12]

The "trapped between a rock and a hard place" metaphor characterized the prevailing perception of many physicians in the decade of the 1990s. This dilemma continues as the rate of prescription drug abuse and overdose deaths exponentially increased in the first decade of the twenty-first century. Major pharmaceutical companies were targeted for their role in promoting newly developed extended-release opioids as safe and effective therapies for chronic pain. The paradigm case was the highly profitable extended-release opioid Oxycontin manufactured by PurduePharma. In early 2007, the company and three of its top executives pleaded guilty to criminal charges of misleading physicians, regulators, and the general public on matters concerning the abuse potential of the drug and agreed to pay over $600 million in fines.

One legal response to the prescription drug abuse epidemic has been state prescription drug monitoring programs. These electronic databases allow physicians to determine what prescriptions for controlled substances their patients have received, when, and from whom. Patients seeking such medications from multiple physicians raise concerns about drug abuse or diversion. Most medical guidelines for prescribing controlled substances advise physicians to require their patients to take only controlled substances s/he prescribes, only as directed, and to fill prescriptions at a single pharmacy.[13]

4 Law and the pursuit of a peaceful death

He might have been resigned to die, but I suspect he wanted to die without added terrors, quietly, in a sort of peaceful trance.
Joseph Conrad, Lord Jim *(Conrad 1989/1900: 108)*

Laws related to care of terminally ill patients differ markedly among nations, ranging from relatively liberal approaches in the Netherlands, Belgium, and Switzerland to very restrictive laws often reflecting the dominance of particular religious traditions, such as Roman Catholicism or Islam. A comprehensive overview of this field, even focused on a single country, is beyond the scope of this chapter. It is also important to note that in some jurisdictions, for example Canada and the United States, a flurry of recent activity indicates the state of flux characterizing this area at the confluence of law, ethics, and medicine.

Historically, Anglo-American jurisprudence has reflected a philosophical bright line between the relief of pain and suffering (morally obligatory) and the deliberate causing or hastening of a patient's death (morally prohibited). Based upon this distinction, sedation to unconsciousness for refractory distress is permitted, whereas until recently provision of a lethal medication constituted a violation not only of professional standards but also the criminal law (Quill et al. 1997). Similarly, withholding or withdrawing life-sustaining interventions has been viewed by many as simply allowing for a natural death, whereas providing medication with the expectation that it will cause the patient's death constitutes assisted suicide or euthanasia even when provided at the request of a decisionally capable, terminally ill patient. For purposes of the discussion in this section I will use the term "aid in dying" (AID), which reflects an emerging consensus view among many health professional organizations that the term "assisted suicide" inappropriately stigmatizes both patients who utilize a lethal prescription and the physicians who prescribe it.[14] Note that Chapter 37 of this volume adopts the "assisted death" terminology in its discussion of the relationship between pain and the utilization of this end of life option.

The United States Supreme Court attached great significance to such distinctions when, in 1997, it unanimously ruled that the US Constitution recognizes no right to lethal medication for terminally ill patients. Nevertheless, the ruling left each state to determine whether or not to permit this end of life option.[15] The states of Oregon, Washington, Vermont, and California have enacted laws permitting physicians to write a lethal prescription for a terminally ill, decisionally capable patient who requests one, while Montana permits this practice by virtue of a decision by its Supreme Court. A similar finding by a trial court in New Mexico is currently on appeal by the state to its highest court. The Montana court decision stands in stark contrast to the Supreme Court decisions in *Glucksberg* and *Quill*, reflecting an emerging view that these long-held distinctions do not stand up to scrupulous analysis of causation and intent as these concepts have been applied in other areas of the law.[16]

Laws permitting terminally ill patients access to lethal prescriptions by willing physicians tend to be grounded from a legal perspective on the liberty interests of individuals to control what happens to their own body, and from an ethical perspective the correlative right to respect for individual autonomy. As well-entrenched as these principles may be in Anglo-American jurisprudence, courts have not hesitated to recognize the legitimacy of certain constraints upon them arising out of governmental interests. These interests were invariably invoked during the formative period of the so-called "right to die" litigation in the United States in the last quarter of the twentieth century. In seminal cases such as that of Nancy Cruzan, decided by the Supreme Court in 1990, the court, as many others had before in state court rulings, stated that whenever a patient or surrogate's right to refuse treatment was asserted, it must be balanced with four "countervailing interests of the state": (1) preserving life, (2) preventing suicide, (3) protecting the interests of innocent third parties (i.e., minor children), and (4) upholding the ethical integrity of the medical profession.[17]

In the decades since these interests were initially elucidated, US courts have increasingly found that the liberty interests of the individual take precedence over the authority of the state to dictate precisely whether, how, and when a patient dies. The doctrine of double effect (DDE), which originated in the medieval Roman Catholic theology of Thomas Aquinas, has been invoked by courts in their efforts to maintain a distinction between on the one hand relieving pain and suffering or allowing the discontinuation of life support and AID on the other. DDE purports to be a device by which one can determine the moral acceptability of engaging in an action which has both a good and a bad outcome, both of which can be ascertained in advance. Four conditions must be met:

1   The action itself must be morally good or at least morally neutral.
2   Only the good consequence may be intended, although the bad consequence will be foreseeable.
3   The good consequence must not be brought about by means of the bad consequence.
4   The good and bad consequence must be proportionate in their significance, i.e., a morally trivial benefit may not be achieved by means of a morally grave harm (McIntyre 2014).

In their embrace of DDE, courts have failed to acknowledge that the second element of DDE runs counter to a basic legal principle concerning intent. The criminal law in particular, but negligence law as well to a certain extent, operates on a presumption that every competent adult intends or at least can be held accountable for the natural and probable consequences of his or her actions, i.e., those which are foreseeable. By postulating a moral distinction between what one intends and what one merely foresees, DDE diverges from the law of intent in a significant way which the courts have failed to acknowledge.

Another confounding factor which DDE and the legal cases invoking it fail to address is that there are two persons involved in decisions to withhold or withdraw treatment or pursue AID by medical means – the physician and the patient. Many legal decisions appear to presume, without carefully examined evidence on a case-by-case basis, that a physician's intent in discontinuing life support is to respect the patient's autonomy or to unburden the patient of interventions which no longer remediate the underlying condition. In contrast, courts tend to presume that when a physician provides a lethal medication, s/he necessarily intends the patient's death rather than to respect the patient's wishes to assert control over the dying process (Rich 2007). Such presumptions take a simplistic view of intent, and in their narrow focus on the mental state of the physician appear to reduce the patient to a cipher whose intent is of no moral consequence (Quill 1993). This critique is particularly pertinent when the accepted paradigm for patient care is one of shared decision-making, in which patients and physicians are engaged in a medical joint venture (Rich 2001: 59–60).

Often invoking DDE, opponents of AID offer sedation to unconsciousness (palliative sedation) as the morally acceptable alternative in cases of refractory distress. In the *Glucksberg* and *Quill* decisions the court specifically noted this alternative to a lethal prescription was constrained by no legal barriers. Patients who have been plaintiffs in cases challenging laws criminalizing AID, including not only the Montana case previously noted but also a recent decision by the Supreme Court of Canada, argue that from their perspective dying in a chemically induced coma is not only undignified, but subjects their family and loved ones to a prolonged, distressing, and unwarranted death bed vigil.[18]

It is important to recognize the insights that have been gained from over eighteen years of data collection under the Oregon Death with Dignity Act (ODWDA). One of these key insights, with significant implications for Chapter 37 of this volume, is that intractable pain or refractory suffering are far down the list of most often cited reasons for pursuing this end of life option. Concerns about loss of autonomy, dignity, and the capacity to engage in activities that give life meaning and purpose are the prime motivating factors for those who have sought a lethal prescription.[19]

When considering legal issues associated with AID, courts are confronted with two distinct types of argument by those who maintain that current public policy does not countenance this option and never should. One is of the deontological variety, most pithily expressed in the exhortation "doctors must not kill!" (Gaylin 1998). Advocates of this position often reach far back to the Hippocratic Oath's pledge to "give no deadly drug" as authority for a categorical prohibition on any form of AID. Counter-arguments take many forms, from challenges to this interpretation of the Oath, or its relevance to twenty-first-century medical practice, to the legalistic variety which maintain that traditional distinctions between "killing" and "allowing to die" fail to acknowledge that when a physician discontinues life-sustaining measures s/he is causally connected to the patient's death in a more direct and immediate way than when writing a prescription for a lethal dose of medication which the patient may or may not ever take. This was precisely the point made by the Montana Supreme Court in the *Baxter* case.

The other type of argument is consequentialist in nature, raising concerns about slippery slopes and undue risks posed to vulnerable populations such as the economically disadvantaged or the physically disabled. At least in the United States, while these arguments might have had persuasive potential prior to the implementation of the ODWDA, data from the Oregon experience strongly suggest that there has been no slippage in the limits of the legislation, and it has posed no threat to any vulnerable groups. The absence of any data suggesting abuses or other harms resulting from the law prompted organizations such as the American Public Health Association and the American College of Legal Medicine to formally support such laws (Tucker 2009).

Recently there has been increased discussion as to whether access to lethal medication should be limited to patients with a terminal illness. In the Netherlands, Belgium, and Switzerland physicians can provide such assistance to patients with non-terminal conditions, including mental illness. The language of the recent Canadian high court decision, noted earlier, affords this option to patients with a "grievous and irremediable medical condition" with no requirement of terminality and no specific exclusion of psychiatric conditions. An extensive analysis of this ethically charged issue is beyond the scope of this chapter. However, there is a critical distinction between the existence of a diagnosed mental illness, including clinical depression, and a lack of decisional capacity. Most mental health professionals acknowledge that many psychiatric conditions do not necessarily preclude decisional capacity (Appelbaum 2007). Proponents of expanding access to AID to those with a non-terminal condition argue that willing physicians should not be precluded from assisting patients with a serious and incurable medical condition to end their lives so long as it is an informed and authentic choice and reasonable alternatives have been explored (Schuklenk and van de Vathorst 2015). Underlying this argument is the proposition that mental suffering from a psychiatric disorder can be as great as from a terminal condition. However, opponents of AID under any circumstances are likely to characterize any efforts to expand access as a clear instance of the slippery slope phenomenon.

Related topics

Chapter 10: Pathophysiological mechanisms of chronic pain (Thacker and Moseley)
Chapter 11: Psychological models of pain (Williams)
Chapter 21: Can I see your pain? An evaluative model of pain perception (de Vignemont)
Chapter 28: Pain and torture (Davis)
Chapter 33: Pain management (Berryman, Catley, and Moseley)
Chapter 35: Pain and controlled pain-relieving substances (Aggarwal and Pettus)
Chapter 36: Fetal pain and the law: abortion laws and their relationship to ideas about pain (Derbyshire)
Chapter 37: Pain, mental suffering, and physician-assisted death (Weinstock)

Notes

1 Glossip v. Gross, United States Supreme Court, No. 14–7955 (June 29, 2015), Opinions, Supreme Court of the United States, <http://www.supremecourt.gov/opinions/14pdf/14-7955_aplc.pdf>, accessed 23 July 2015.
2 California Civil Jury Instructions 3905A, Physical Pain, Mental Suffering, and Emotional Distress (Noneconomic Damage) – 2003, Justia, <https://www.justia.com/trials-litigation/docs/caci/3900/3905a.html>, accessed 14 June 2015.
3 Capelouto v. Kaiser Foundation Hospitals, 500 P. 2d 880 (1972).
4 Phil Ochs, "Crucifixion Lyrics," from *Live in Lansing* (1973), Lyrics, Universal Music Publishing Group, <http://www.metrolyrics.com/crucifixion-lyrics-phil-ochs.html>, accessed 22 June 2015.

5 Controlled Substances Act, Pub. L. No. 91–513, 84 Stat. 1242 (1970).
6 Comprehensive Drug Abuse Prevention and Control Act of 1970, United States House of Representatives, H.R. No. 91-1444 (September 10, 1970).
7 "Controlled Substances Schedule," United States Department of Justice Drug Enforcement Administration Office of Diversion Control, <http://www.deadiversion.usdoj.gov/schedules/>, accessed 18 July 2015.
8 Estate of Henry James v. Hillhaven Corp., No. 89 CVS 64 (N.C. Super. Ct. January 15, 1991).
9 Bergman v. Chin, No. H205732–1 (Sup. Ct. Alameda County, CA 1999).
10 "Stipulated Order in the Matter of Paul A. Bilder, M.D.," Oregon Board of Medical Examiners, September 1999.
11 "In the Matter of the Accusation against Eugene B. Whitney, M.D.," Medical Board of California, Decision, December 2003.
12 United States v. Hurwitz, 459 F. 3d 463 (4th Cir. 2006).
13 "State Prescription Drug Monitoring Programs," United States Department of Justice Drug Enforcement Administration Office of Diversion Control, <http://www.deadiversion.usdoj.gov/faq/rx_monitor.htm>, accessed 20 July 2015.
14 "Patients' Rights to Self-Determination at the End of Life," American Public Health Association, Policy No. 20086, 28 October 2008, <https://www.apha.org/policies-and-advocacy/public-health-policy-statements/policy-database/2014/07/29/13/28/patients-rights-to-self-determination-at-the-end-of-life>, accessed 28 December 2015.
15 Washington v. Glucksberg, 521 U.S. 702 (1997); Vacco v. Quill, 521 U.S. 793 (1997).
16 Baxter v. Montana, 224 P. 3d 1211, MT (2009).
17 Cruzan v. Director, Missouri Department of Health, 497 U.S. 261 (1990).
18 Carter v. Canada (Attorney General), 2015 SCC 5, 1 S.C.R. 333.
19 Oregon Department of Health Services, 2015 summary of the Oregon Death with Dignity Act, 2014, <https://public.health.oregon.gov/ProviderPartnerResources/EvaluationResearch/DeathwithDignityAct/Documents/year17.pdf>, accessed 23 July 2015.

References

Appelbaum, P.S. (2007) Assessment of patients' competence to consent to treatment. *New England Journal of Medicine* 357: 1834–1840.
Bostwick, J.M. (2012) Blurred boundaries: the therapeutics and politics of medical marijuana. *Mayo Clinic Proceedings* 87: 172–186.
Cassell, E.J. (2004) *The Nature of Suffering and the Goals of Medicine*, 2nd ed. New York: Oxford University Press.
Cherny, N.I., Baselga, J., de Conno, F., and Radbruch, L. (2010) Formulary availability and regulatory barriers to accessibility of opioids for cancer pain in Europe: a report from the ESMO/EAPC Opioid Policy Initiative. *Annals of Oncology* 21: 615–626.
Conrad, J. (1989/1900) *Lord Jim*. London: Penguin Books.
Diamond, S.S. (1993) What jurors think: expectations and reactions of citizens who serve as jurors. In R.E. Litan (ed.), *Verdict: Assessing the Civil Jury System*. Washington, DC: Brookings Institution, pp. 282–305.
Gaylin, W., Kass, L.R., Pellegrino, E.D., and Siegler, M. (1998) Doctors must not kill. *JAMA* 259: 2139–2140.
INCB (International Narcotics Control Board) (2014) *Report of the International Narcotics Control Board for 2014*. New York: United Nations. <https://www.incb.org/incb/en/publications/annual-reports/annual-report-2014.html>, accessed 18 July 2015.
Joranson, D.E. (1997) State intractable pain policy: current status. *APS Bulletin* 7: 7–9.
King, J.H., Jr. (2004) Pain and suffering, noneconomic damages, and the goals of tort law. *Southern Methodist University Law Review* 57: 163–209.
Kritzer, H.M., Liu, G., and Vidmar, N. (2014) An exploration of "noneconomic" damages in civil jury awards. *William & Mary Law Review* 55: 971–1027.
Leebron, D.W. (1989) Final moments: damages for pain and suffering prior to death. *New York University Law Review* 64: 256–357.
McIntyre, A. (2014) Doctrine of double effect. In E.N. Zalta (ed.), *The Stanford Encyclopedia of Philosophy* (Winter 2014 ed.). <http://plato.stanford.edu/archives/win2014/entries/double-effect/>, accessed 21 July 2015.

Niemeyer, P.V. (2004) Awards for pain and suffering: the irrational centerpiece of our tort system. *Virginia Law Review* 90: 1401–1421.

NIH (National Institutes of Health) (2011) Chronic pain: symptoms, diagnosis and treatment. *MedlinePlus* 6: 5–6. <https://medlineplus.gov/magazine/issues/spring11/articles/spring11pg5-6.html>.

Quill, T.E. (1993) The ambiguity of clinical intentions. *New England Journal of Medicine* 329: 1039–1040.

Quill, T.E., Lo, B., and Brock, D.W. (1997) Palliative options of last resort: a comparison of voluntarily stopping eating and drinking, terminal sedation, physician-assisted suicide, and voluntary active euthanasia. *JAMA* 278: 2099–2104.

Rabin, R.L. (2006) Pain and suffering and beyond: some thoughts on recovery for intangible loss. *DePaul Law Review* 55: 359–377.

Rich, B.A. (2000) An ethical analysis of the barriers to effective pain management. *Cambridge Quarterly of Healthcare Ethics* 9: 54–70.

Rich, B.A. (2001) *Strange Bedfellows: How Medical Jurisprudence Has Influenced Medical Ethics and Medical Practice.* New York: Kluwer Academic/Plenum Publishers.

Rich, B.A. (2002) Moral conundrums in the courtroom: reflections on a decade in the culture of pain. *Cambridge Quarterly of Healthcare Ethics* 11: 180–190.

Rich, B.A. (2007) Causation and intent: persistent conundrums in end of life care. *Cambridge Quarterly of Healthcare Ethics* 16: 63–73.

Schnapper, E. (1989) Judges against juries – appellate review of federal civil jury verdicts. *Wisconsin Law Review* 1989(2): 237–353.

Schuklenk, U. and van de Vathorst, S. (2015) Treatment-resistant major depressive disorder and assisted dying. *Journal of Medical Ethics* 41: 577–583.

Tracey, I. and Bushnell, M.C. (2009) How neuroimaging studies have challenged us to rethink: is chronic pain a disease? *Journal of Pain* 10: 1113–1120.

Tucker, K.L. (2009) At the very end of life: the emergence of policy supporting aid in dying among mainstream medical and health policy associations. *Harvard Health Policy Review* 10: 45–47.

Turk, D.C. and Okifuji, A. (2010) Pain terms and taxonomies of pain. In S.M. Fishman, J.C. Ballantyne, and J.P. Rathmell (eds.), *Bonica's Management of Pain*, 4th ed. Philadelphia: Wolters Kluwer/Lippincott Williams & Wilkins, pp. 13–23.

United Nations (1977) *Single Convention on Narcotic Drugs, 1961, as Amended by the 1972 Protocol Amending the Single Convention on Narcotic Drugs, 1961.* New York: United Nations.

Williams, B. (1995) Afterword: what has philosophy to learn from tort law? In D.G. Owen (ed.), *Philosophical Foundations of Tort Law*. Oxford: Clarendon Press, pp. 487–497.

35

PAIN AND CONTROLLED PAIN-RELIEVING SUBSTANCES

Sunil Kumar Aggarwal and Katherine Pettus

Pain relieving substances that pharmacologically reduce neurological transmission of pain signals are one vital toolset in the management and treatment of moderate to severe pain. (See, in this volume, Chapter 33, on pain management, and Chapters 11 and 12 on psychological models of pain, and the biopsychosocial model in particular.) International treaties regulate the cultivation, manufacture, distribution, and consumption of many plants, plant-based medicines, and pharmaceutical preparations that constitute these substances, many of which have been known since time immemorial to relieve moderate to severe pain.

These treaties, drafted and ratified during the mid-twentieth century (post-Second World War period), identify some plants and preparations that contain their active ingredients, as "narcotic drugs" and "psychotropic substances" (United Nations 1972/1961, 1971, 1988). The Single Convention on Narcotic Drugs (United Nations 1972/1961), considered the "cornerstone" treaty, "recognises that the medical use of narcotic drugs continues to be indispensable for the relief of pain and suffering, and that adequate provision must be made to ensure the availability of narcotic drugs for such purposes," yet contains only narrowly drafted provisions allowing appropriately trained and licensed professionals to manufacture, distribute, and prescribe some of these substances. The Single Convention contains no binding operational paragraphs obliging states parties to make controlled substances available to their citizens, yet allows parties to apply "measures of control more strict or severe" than those provided for in the Convention, in order to accomplish the treaty's supply-control objectives, if they deem such severe measures appropriate (art. 39).

Classifying (legally produced and distributed) medicines as "narcotic drugs" and "psychotropic substances," and attaching criminal justice consequences to "unauthorised" production, distribution, or consumption, of *both* controlled medicines and illicitly produced and marketed "street drugs," creates a fundamental tension that circumscribes professionals' willingness to prescribe even essential medicines such as morphine for the control of pain. To this day, the legal tensions, combined with the public and professional association of morphine with addiction, also circumscribes patients' and families' willingness to (respectively) consume and administer morphine to palliate symptoms and relieve pain. This tension presents as a public health crisis in many countries, being what experts have dubbed "the global

414

pandemic of untreated pain" (ESMO 2013). This epithet references the fact that in more than 150 UN member states, home to more than 5.5 billion of the world's people, medications stronger than aspirin or paracetamol (acetaminophen) are unavailable to relieve severe pain due to end-stage chronic and malignant diseases, HIV/AIDS, burns, trauma, surgery, and other conditions (Krakauer et al. 2010).

The pandemic can best be understood in the context of the multiple relationships, and the lack thereof, which have configured social and professional attitudes toward controlled substances for more than a century since the colonial powers began to draft the first drug control instruments in 1912 (UNODC 2008). Granting that "there are no good or bad drugs; there are only good and bad relationships with drugs" (Weil and Rosen 2004), the contemporary global movement to reconfigure the relationships between society and controlled substances entails transforming multiple social relationships with, *inter alia*, pleasure, pain, law, governance institutions, and suffering/mortality. We describe those ongoing, minimally coordinated, multiple transformations, as a paradigm shift (Kuhn 1970).

Since the global context, including the state of the science of pain relief and substance use, in which the post-war era treaties were drafted and ratified, has changed dramatically since that period, the entire spectrum of civil society concerned with drug policy is encouraging governments to adjust accordingly, and to work together to produce a more appropriate legal and normative framework. Most recently, the World Health Assembly passed a resolution calling on states to integrate palliative care into their health-care systems, to make controlled medicines available as necessary (WHO 2014), and some member states have called on the Commission on Narcotic Drugs (CND 2015) to align global drug policy with the Sustainable Development Goals (SDGs) (see OESA 2015). A UN Special Session on the World Drug Problem was held in April 2016, and this issue of improving access to controlled medicines was high on the agenda, as even CND member states are joining civil society to call for coordinated action and new governance approaches.

This chapter excavates some of the deeply rooted negativity surrounding the use of controlled pain-relieving substances, and discusses strategies that advocacy communities are taking to support more rational and ethical relationships with these often proscribed, rather than effectively *prescribed*, medicines. We argue that developments in the disciplines of medicine and public health, including pain treatment, palliative care, and addiction sciences, combined with the growth of civil society networks and the globalization of communications, are driving what we identify as a paradigm shift in this aspect of drug control policy.

The extent to which unduly restrictive domestic regulations formulated under the old paradigm, which proscribes many legitimate clinical relationships with controlled medicines, has added to the quantum of human suffering raises important philosophical and ethical questions. Currently, the unacceptability, unaffordability, inaccessibility, and unavailability of controlled medicines in many parts of the world effectively prevents pharmacists, physicians, or nurses from either learning about, recommending, or researching pain-relieving substances for patients who could potentially benefit from their rational use. We claim that it is ethically unacceptable to perpetuate ignorance about the medical utilization of such substances, when there is a traditional, as well as unconsolidated contemporary body of knowledge and praxis regarding pain relief. Finally, we consider whether stipulating a right to pain relief might influence governance practice to facilitate processes that would make controlled pain-relieving substances more available to patients who need them.

1 Background

Humans and animals have experienced unrelieved pain and distress since the beginning of our life on earth. Most indigenous societies have known how to relieve pain and symptoms by cultivating or gathering plants and preparing the medicines to relieve them (see Chapter 32, this volume). Morphine is derived from opium, which was deemed "God's own medicine" by William Osler, the widely recognized "Father of Modern Medicine." The opium poppy, in stone carving, adorns the marble ceilings of a central chamber sanctuary building of the Aesclepian healing cult's temple ruins in Epidauros, Greece (Askitopoulou 2002). This is a place so important to the practice of Western medicine that our words "therapy" and "clinic" and our symbol of medicine – a snake intertwined on a staff – all ultimately derive from the language and practices of this healing cult, which sprang up in the last third of the fifth century BCE in rural Greece.

Societies and countries at ground zero of the global pandemic of untreated pain have all but lost their traditional relationships with plant-based medicines that relieve severe pain, as national laws forbid the cultivation of their sources, and preparations derived therefrom. Unbeknownst to many state parties, cultivation for such purposes is not illegal under the drug control treaties, though. Their laws and regulations erroneously either ban, or strictly police, traditional relationships with pain-relieving plants, and closely oversee modern health providers' relationships with their powerful contemporary pharmaceutical descendants such as morphine. Moral panic – "the process of arousing social concern over an issue – usually the work of moral entrepreneurs and the mass media" (Scott and Marshall 2009: 489) – around drugs, has had a very long half-life, and until very recently has configured the health-law systems of even advanced democracies, generating multiple negative externalities, only one of which is the pandemic of untreated pain. The original, missionary driven (Tyrrell 2010; Nadelmann 1990) supply-control paradigm, which construed habitual or non-medical use of "narcotic drugs and psychotropic substances," theologically, as "evil" (Lines 2015), has been at the root of the moral panic that originally fueled the pandemic of untreated pain.

2 The legal framework of the pandemic

Let us identify the pain-relieving substances in question. International law, beginning with the Single Convention on Narcotic Drugs (United Nations 1972/1961) organizes opioid analgesics used for the relief of moderate to severe pain ("drugs") into "schedules," which detail how and by whom these substances should be made available (which relationships are legitimate for medical consumption, if indeed they should be available at all). (See Chapter 34, this volume.) The drug control treaties assign the WHO, through its Expert Committee on Drug Dependence, to this scheduling task. The principle opioid analgesics are: morphine, diacetylmorphine (heroin), hydromorphone, oxycodone, fentanyl, and methadone. All except heroin are included in the WHO Model List of Essential Medicines. Unprocessed opium is still actively used in medicine in preparations known as paregoric and deodorized tincture of opium. Regarding non-opioids, one essential medication for both anesthesia and pain relief is ketamine, which some countries have chosen to control under domestic law, and which China has repeatedly, and unsuccessfully, petitioned to bring under international control, because of reported non-medical use in the region. Additionally, benzodiazepines such as lorazepam and diazepam, anxiolytics that help treat anxiety in burn patients and related types of patients in pain, synergistically improve the efficacy of opioid analgesics.

The current international framework does not recognize the efficacy of non-opioid analgesic substances, such as cannabis and cannabinoid-based medicines derived from it, despite growing modern acceptance of this traditional plant medicine. Although the drug control treaties do leave room for medicinal uses of controlled substances, and some countries, in the last ten to twenty years, have begun to experiment with medical cannabis access systems for pain and other conditions, the majority of countries ban any and all access, even for medical use. The use of psychedelics such as psilocybin and LSD (lysergic acid diethylamide) for pain relief, which has been suggested in early data for intractable conditions such as cluster headaches, and the use of these and other members of the psychedelic class for psychiatric conditions such as PTSD (post-traumatic stress disorder), existential distress in terminal illness, and drug dependence (Tupper et al. 2015), is entirely unrecognized and uncodified in the current legal framework.

Contrary to popular linguistic usage, no pain-relieving substances (even cannabis and heroin) are actually "illegal." Logically, no substance, or object *in itself*, can be "illegal." A plant, a synthetic substance, or medicine, or preparation, cannot be criminalized, ticketed, sent to prison, or executed. Of course crops can be, and are, destroyed, and police seize and impound caches of so-called illicit drugs, but what the law defines as "illegal," is the behavior of the farmer who produces and distributes opium poppies without a license, or a pharmacist who dispenses morphine without a prescription. In other words, the law has banned or circumscribed particular relationships between farmers, chemists, distributors, and patients and substances it deems harmful, calling addiction "evil." Scientific developments and evidence advanced by civil society are calling that dominant paradigm into question, or at least imprecating it with greater nuance.

A confluence of several related factors, associated with the national and transnational development of civil society, has precipitated the call by palliative care and human rights advocates for governments to rectify the crisis/pandemic of untreated pain. First, modern pharmaceutical science, pain, and palliative medicine professionals and anesthesiologists have developed and refined clinical, legitimate, means to relieve severe pain; second, the International Narcotics Control Board has annually tracked and released data on UN member states' consumption of controlled medicines, such that academic groups and civil society can analyze it; and third, human rights experts have identified severe unrelieved pain as violations of both the right to the highest attainable standard of health, and the right to be free from cruel and degrading treatment.

The actual inaccessibility, unaffordability, and unavailability of controlled medicines in most parts of the world is similarly produced by a multitude of factors, which present differently in each country and community. Backed by states, the pharmaceutical industry has monopolized the raw materials, and profited from the marketing of many pain-relieving substances. Affordability depends largely on government subsidies, and since demand for cheap unpatented medicines such as morphine is low where the regulatory environment is unduly restrictive, industry has either exited the market entirely or marked up prices to account for uncertainty. In 2011, ninety-two percent of the world's medical supply of morphine was consumed by 17 percent of the global population, namely high-income countries; and low- and middle-income countries, which account for 83 percent of the global population, consumed only 8 percent (United Nations 2014).

National controls required by international law need not in themselves pose a problem for member states once providers and regulators are trained to safely handle, prescribe, and administer opioids (as appropriate to task). The problem, as noted above, is that few are appropriately trained and licensed. With regard to controlled substances such as cannabis, for which little legal relationship has been possible until recently, these laws do, of course, pose a problem for providers and patients wishing to access it for medical purposes such as the treatment of pain, epilepsy, HIV and cancer palliation, PTSD, etc.

3 Ideological roots of the contemporary pandemic

Between the eighteenth and twentieth centuries, Western colonial powers constructed substances such as opium, coca, and cannabis used by many societies for millennia for medical, ceremonial, and recreational purposes, first as legal, profitable commodities, and then as "evil," addictive "narcotic drugs" whose cultivation, manufacture, trade, and consumption societies must closely regulate and monitor "for the health and welfare of mankind." Later, psychedelic substances – both naturally derived and semi-synthetic, such as psilocybin, LSD, and dimethyltryptamine – psychostimulants, anxiolytics, and other classes, were similarly obfuscated and vilified as "psychotropic substances" and subjected to control. It is hardly surprising that, just as the imperial lineage of relationships with those substances (particulary opium, the biotic source of morphine) and their legal 'subjects' who traditionally produced and consumed them were distorted and exploitative, subsequent societies' social, legal, and clinical (disciplinary) relationships with those substances should likewise be distorted and exploitative.

The modern legacy of that imperial lineage, which originally thrived on Chinese market demand for opium, and Great Britain's insatiable desire for the revenues therefrom, is (unsurprisingly) characterized by the (mimetic) fear of addiction that pervades even the clinical culture surrounding opioid analgesics such as morphine. The cultural obsession with addiction undermines medical confidence in the appropriate use of morphine, and has saturated contemporary public opinion such that the ethical practice of pain relief is virtually unknown in most countries. While fear of addiction might have been a rational response to a vacuum of scientific knowledge about the substances in question when the dominant elites were negotiating the drug control treaties during the first half of the twentieth century, more sophisticated contemporary discourses and practices that distinguish between tolerance, dependence, and problematic use are now filling that epistemological vacuum.

Paradigm shifts, as philosopher Thomas Kuhn (1970) noted, occur when new evidence and practices challenge the dominant worldview, altering affected subjects/actors/participants' perceptions and customs with education and collective development. The current drug control paradigm is starting to shift as the anomalies proliferate under the gaze of modern, evidence-based practice advanced by global civil society. The fault lines emerging between the former and emerging paradigms create multiple political and discursive policy spaces for the development of more ethical, social, clinical, juridical, and political practices, all of which can bring public health into more fruitful alignment with the newly approved SDGs. The development of pain and palliative medicine and addiction science in recent decades exemplifies the way scientific progress can precipitate shifts from foundational, non–evidence-based assumptions, such as those underlying drug control policy, to more rational approaches, currently being called for by both civil society and UN member states.

The policy perspective informing the emerging paradigm views the rational response to problematic substance use ("addiction," or "the world drug problem") as integrating harm reduction, evidence-based treatment, and palliative care into public health systems. The framers of the drug control treaties did not have those policy options at hand, because they were ideologically driven, because the science we have at hand today simply was not there, and because there was no meaningful civil society engagement in drug policy. Lacking those tools, the framers' default option was to designate criminal and administrative law as the blunt instrument to arbitrate both medical and non-medical relationships with the substances they wished to control, thereby consolidating social fear and moral panic associated with the stigma of "addiction."

What well-governed, modern liberal societies might construct as reasonable – to endorse rational government policies that make pain-relieving substances available to clinicians and patients, even if those substances can have psychoactive active effects on some people – simply has not been an option until very recently, and only in a handful of states. In the vast majority, substances consumed by *outsider* social groups continue to be restricted, proscribed, and contrabanded (Helmer 1975). "*Faux* health science" logics of *euphoria pathologization, asocial addictionology*, and *pharmacologicalism* underpin official explanations, past and current, of selective substance prohibition and restriction by health-administrative governmental bureaucracies. The foregoing are not neologisms; they name particular prohibitionist ideologies at play which we will describe in greater detail below.

Let us begin with the origin and logic of *euphoria pathologization*. With regards to the clinical treatment of moderate to severe pain, the dominant paradigm tends to err on the side of believing that some pain-relieving substances may do the job "too well." A compulsion in the body politic to limit or proscribe pain-relieving substances, due to concern that they might either be used by those not in pain, for "idle pleasure," or to replace the experience of pain with "an excess" of pleasure, can certainly be characterized as a Puritanical compulsion to limit certain embodied experiences, though this impulse is certainly not unique in history. A movement known as progressivism, which was very much tied to Euro-American Christian Protestant groups, was highly successful in the late nineteenth and early decades of the twentieth century in inserting this compulsion into national law in various countries and colonial empires as well as emerging international compacts.

The impulse to limit "excess pleasure," even if it means limiting the potential of pain relief in society, is based in ignorance and an impoverished worldview that underappreciates what philosopher Richard Shusterman (1999) called somaesthetics: "the critical, meliorative study of the experience and the use of one's body as a locus of sensory-aesthetic appreciation and creative self-fashioning." The abandonment of somaesthetics not only leads to lost opportunities for study and exploration in spiritual studies, psychology, and health sciences, it also limits pain relief. This is because the lack of social recognition and appreciation of an aesthetic value, or more specifically, a somaesthetic value, to the use of some pleasurable substances has allowed a Puritanical impulse to restrict the range of substances readily available for pain relief. In the modern framing, rejection of the value of pleasure, elation, or sensory-aesthetic appreciation is seen in the pathological view taken with use of the term "euphoria," which implies a kind of artificial, transient, shallow, and manufactured state of being that serves no laudable social or individual purpose and is best avoided at all cost.

The second paradigmatic ideology is *asocial addictionology*. This is a view of addiction that essentially individualizes and chemically determines the disorder rather than understanding it as a by-product of, or adaptation to, an impoverished social environment and a lack of psychosocial integration – a position which has garnered strong evidence and scholarly support (Alexander 2008). When laws are built only out of an individualized or asocial addictionology, dissuading the individual addict or "potential addict" from making close contact with his or her preferred substance becomes the fundamental ordering mission of law, and punishing individuals through criminal sanction who facilitate ingestion of such substances or who possess the substances for the purposes of later consumption is intended to "interrupt addictive behaviors" and dissuade others from taking them up. Increasing restriction or frank absolute prohibition of substances is clearly the eventual outcome of such laws, given our current international drug control laws, and if they happen to stifle the use of such substances for the relief of pain – so be it, as that is essentially seen as an "acceptable social sacrifice" for the greater good of curbing and preventing further substance addiction. A social addictionology would instead recognize the value in treating addiction as more a disorder of social bonding, and a legal framework designed to manage and prevent addiction with this understanding would place primary emphasis on helping problematic users connect to needed health and social services and would take up the more fundamental task of working to restructure society so that investment is made in early childhood support, education, and other essential areas that would help to reduce the number of vulnerable individuals who would feel isolated, socially disconnected, or psychologically traumatized as victims of violence or structural violence. In this rendering, laws would be geared more towards rehabilitating and preventing potential social circumstances that foster addiction and not exclusively tunnel vision focused on the availability of particular substances.

This leads to the final ideology, which has fostered overcontrol of pain relieving substances to the point of inaccessibility. This is *pharmacologicalism*, a term coined by psychopharmacologist Richard DeGrandpre to describe the ideological "foundation for the moral ordering of drugs," whereby drugs are seen to be inherently good or evil, independent of context (DeGrandpre 2006). Understanding this pervasive bias requires serious consideration of the role of social factors in influencing the outcomes of all substance or drug use. The role of social factors in influencing drug effects is fundamental, especially for psychoactive substance use. DeGrandpre summarizes many lines of evidence that support this and states that "there are times when it appears that the drug context, with all its layers of meaning, is at least as efficacious in producing druglike effects. This is demonstrated not only in laboratory investigations but also in the rituals of drug taking itself" (DeGrandpre 2006: 19). The implications of this perspective yield such a radical critique of our conventional views that a block quotation from DeGrandpre's *The Cult of Pharmacology* (DeGrandpre 2006: 27) will be helpful. He explains:

> The idea that a drug has an essence that the user inevitably consumes along with the drug itself is part of a system of "pharmacologicalism." Technically speaking, pharmacologicalism, like racism, is an ideological system rooted in a set of assumptions that, although false and exaggerated, govern a whole range of perceptions, understandings, and actions. A key supposition of pharmacologicalism is that pharmacological potentialities contained within a drug's chemical structure determine drug outcomes in the body, the brain, and behavior. Accordingly, nonpharmacological factors play little role, whether in the realm of the mind or of the world of society and culture. In this highly reductionist system drugs have moral attributes that stem not from social and psychological forces but rather from the sphere of molecules. As a result, pharmacologicalism dictates that the moral status of a drug exists as a purely scientific question that can be documented and classified once and for all, not as a societal one that must be considered and reconsidered across time and place. Society, culture, and history can be ignored. ... Pharmacologicalism thus provided a scientific foundation for the moral ordering of drugs, which then allowed for a disparate, compartmentalized treatment of them as angels (Ritalin) or demons (cocaine).

The dominance of the pharmacologicalistic ideology helps to give a molecular chemical scientific underpinning to the legal arrangement by which some substances are touted and widely available (e.g, tobacco, alcohol, caffeine, sugar, cacao) and others are stigmatized and illicit. DeGrandpre's example of psychostimulant Ritalin (methylphenidate) versus the coca-leaf-derived cocaine is apropos because in blinded experiments, human subjects are unable to distinguish one drug from the other, and in brain imaging, the two drugs produce nearly identical results (he cites work by Nora Volkow, the current director of the US National Institute on Drug Abuse). Yet, Ritalin is widely used even in children to treat attention deficit disorder and cocaine is bathed in an aura of dangerousness and illicitude. Cocaine, it is important to note, *is* legally allowed for scientific and medical use; it is used as a topical anesthetic and has been used for this purpose in otorhinolaryngological surgeries, though certainly use is extremely limited due to factors discussed (Harper and Jones 2006).

To take another example of a stigmatized drug, heroin, also known as diamorphine or diacetylmorphine, is a semi-synthetic opioid produced by a single chemical modification to morphine, which is itself extracted from the sap of the unripened opium poppy. Heroin is legal to use medically as a pain-relieving and palliative substance in the United Kingdom and for opioid dependence syndrome in Canada and several European countries, but it is absolutely banned in most of the rest of the world, even though UK care providers report excellent results with this substance for both pain relief and palliation of breathlessness (Saunders and Platt 2003: 724–725), and even though the body promptly converts heroin into morphine when it is administered (Halbsguth et al. 2008). Moreover, morphine, use of which is treated differently under law, is far more widely available in some countries, yet extremely restricted and widely unavailable in many others (United Nations 2014).

An ideology that relies on the perceived properties of the *substances* to classify their position on the spectrum of legitimate to forbidden relationships misses the social, cultural, and historical *contexts* within which people's relationships with the substances are embedded. Policymakers will only succeed in managing those relationships to optimize public health outcomes when they stop reifying the substances, consider those multiple contexts of their use, and depathologize euphoria and acknowledge somaesthetics. And they can only do that authentically, with full information, when the "affected populations" (patients and health-care workers, problematic and non-problematic users, etc.) themselves are involved in the policymaking process.

4 A right to pain relief and palliative care

From the perspective of someone who is experiencing severe pain, all that matters is whether pain relief is within or out of reach. National laws, customs, and regulations, can either barricade or facilitate that reach. A stipulated right to palliative care and pain relief could bridge some of the gaps described above and stimulate the strengthening of public health infrastructure required by the (aspirational) right to the highest attainable standard of health. A right to pain relief and palliative care is desirable for ethical and political reasons, and can be construed as obligatory within the developing body of human rights law, which includes both the rights to health and to be free from cruel and degrading treatment. Experts interpret the failure to provide palliative care and essential pain medicines as a violation of international human rights law (Nowak and Hunt 2008; UNGA 2013).

The severe untreated pain and symptoms associated with serious illness destroy a person's dignity, protection of which is the core principle of human rights law. Described in political terms, the pain and symptom relief palliative care provides restores a suffering (even a dying) person's agency, the connection between a person and the world which risks being severed by severe pain and distress. (See Chapter 37, this volume.) When societies see morphine as a medicine "only for the dying," they misunderstand its power to restore agency to those who are in severe pain, although they might not be terminal or actively dying. Agency extends to spiritual and loving attitudes, as much as to the ability to be productive, which the patient may or may not have lost, depending on whether her pain and symptoms are controlled. A view of, and valuing of, agency as only productive in economic terms underlies the policy indifference towards morphine and other controlled medicines as pain-relieving substances. Something that is "only for the dying," whose agency is of no value anyway, is, tautologically, useless. This is yet another example of how ideological fixation on the *substance* displaces the value of multiple other available *relationships* not yet considered. The property of people in their own persons is internally connected with the claim recently made in the *Lancet* (Lancet 2015) that the right to health, and we would add the right to pain relief and palliative care, is a "necessary component of resilient human security."

Such a right, whose respect, protection, and fulfillment by governments would be monitored by civil society and informed electorates, would accord all seriously ill people – from the neonate to frail elderly – the protection and honor they deserve in a decent society. Optimally, it would also strengthen the relationships between people in diverse countries through knowledge-sharing and other projects. These relationships between peoples would be based in the solidarity and accompaniment that "lends a voice to suffering" as "the condition of all truth," in Theodor Adorno's (1983: 17–18) immortal words. We have suggested that the science and philosophy of pain that attends to the voice of suffering can support this emerging paradigm and generate more ethical practices in medicine and global health.

5 Conclusion

Solving the global pandemic of untreated pain calls for a new global and national governance paradigm that supports healthy relationships with pain-relieving substances whose use in many UN member states is currently effectively proscribed, or irrationally regulated, through fear of "diversion and abuse." A governance model built on evidence-based policy, and that incentivizes multisectoral collaboration rather than competition between implicated ministries, exemplifies this paradigm. While representative democracy is certainly not the only available polity to operationalize such a governance system, the accountability built into well-functioning constitutional systems with independent judiciaries, and regulatory oversight of health-care systems, ensures (at least *de jure*) that health-care providers in those countries are able to treat patients' pain and symptoms appropriately.

Accountability procedures and "quality improvement" indicators guide the implementation of clinical guidelines and *de facto* best practices. Conversely, in the locus of the pandemic, states still in the process of building or consolidating such accountability structures have yet to prioritize the appropriate training of human resources to handle and prescribe controlled medicines in accordance with international legal standards and guidelines (Gilson et al. 2012). Since citizens in countries with weak health-care systems and civil society structures are not in a position to hold policymakers and health systems accountable for this inability, the international pain and palliative care community can intervene on their behalf to advocate for health system strengthening, a right to palliative care and pain relief, training of human resources, and so on. The policy goals are to bridge clinical and regulatory knowledge gaps, and build robust accountability systems that allow health-care providers to use controlled substances safely and effectively to reverse the global pandemic.

Related topics

Chapter 11: Psychological models of pain (Williams)
Chapter 12: Biopsychosocial models of pain (Hadjistavropoulos)
Chapter 32: Pain and "placebo" analgesia (Moerman)
Chapter 33: Pain management (Berryman, Catley, and Moseley)
Chapter 34: Pain and the law (Rich)
Chapter 37: Pain, mental suffering, and physician-assisted death (Weinstock)

Further reading

Michel Foucault, *The Government of Self and Others: Lectures at the Collège de France 1982–1983* (New York: Palgrave Macmillan, 2010). (For further reading on governmentality.)

Eugen Wolters, "Our Language Shapes Our Reality, New Study Suggests," *Critical-Theory.com*, 2013, <http://www.critical-theory.com/language-shapes-reality-study-reveals/>. (For more about how truth regimes operate.)

Willem van de Ven, *The Social Reality of Truth: Foucault, Searle and the Role of Truth within Social Reality*, MMA thesis in philosophy, Tilburg University, 2012. (For more on the role of truth regimes in the social construction of reality.)

Office of the United Nations High Commissioner for Human Rights, *Right to Pain Relief: 5.5 Billion People Have No Access to Treatment, Warn UN Experts – World Hospice and Palliative Care Day – Saturday 10 October 2015*, <http://www.ohchr.org/EN/NewsEvents/Pages/DisplayNews.aspx?NewsID=16590&LangID=E>.

UN General Assembly, *International Covenant on Economic, Social, and Cultural Rights*, 16 December 1966, United Nations, Treaty Series, vol. 993, p. 3, <http://www.refworld.org/docid/3ae6b36c0.html>.

References

Adorno, T. (1983) *Negative Dialectics*, trans. E.B. Ashton. New York: Continuum.

Alexander, B. (2008) *The Globalisation of Addiction*. Oxford: Oxford University Press.

Askitopoulou, H., Konsolaki, E., Ramoutsaki, I., and Anastassaki, M. (2002) Surgical cures under sleep induction in the Asclepieion of Epidauros. In J.C. Diz (ed.), *The History of Anaesthesia: Proceedings of the Fifth International Symposium on the History of Anaesthesia*. Amsterdam: Elsevier, pp. 11–18.

CDN (Commission on Narcotic Drugs). (2015) CND Intersessional – 15th October 2015. *CND Blog*. http://cndblog.org/2015/10/cnd-intersessional-15th-october-2015/, accessed 23 October 2015.

DeGrandpre, R. (2006) *The Cult of Pharmacology*. Durham, NC: Duke University Press.

ESMO (European Society for Medical Oncology) (2013) ESMO press release: untreated cancer pain a "scandal of global proportions," survey shows. <http://www.esmo.org/Press-Office/Press-Releases/ESMO-Press-Release-Untreated-Cancer-Pain-a-Scandal-of-Global-Proportions-Survey-Shows>, accessed 23 October 2015.

Gilson, A., Maurer, M., LeBaron, V., Ryan, K., and Cleary, J. (2012) Multivariate analysis of countries' government and health-care system influences on opioid availability for cancer pain relief and palliative care: more than a function of human development. *Palliative Medicine* 27(2): 105–114.

Halbsguth, U., Rentsch, K., Eich-Höchli, D., Diterich, I., and Fattinger, K. (2008) Oral diacetylmorphine (heroin) yields greater morphine bioavailability than oral morphine: bioavailability related to dosage and prior opioid exposure. *British Journal of Clinical Pharmacology* 66(6): 781–791.

Harper, S. and Jones, N. (2006) Cocaine: what role does it have in current ENT practice? A review of the current literature. *Journal of Laryngology & Otology* 120(10): 808–811.

Helmer, J. (1975) *Drugs and Minority Oppression*. New York: Seabury Press.

Krakauer, E., Wenk, R., Buitrago, R., Jenkins, P., and Scholten, P. (2010) Opioid inaccessibility and its human consequences: reports from the field. *Journal of Pain and Palliative Care Pharmacotherapy* 24(3): 239–243.

Kuhn, T. (1970) *The Structure of Scientific Revolutions*. Chicago: University of Chicago Press.

Lancet (2015) Don't forget health when you talk about human rights. *Lancet* 385(9967): 481.

Lines, R. (2015) "Deliver us from evil"? – the Single Convention on narcotic drugs, 50 years on. *International Journal on Human Rights and Drug Policy* 1: 3–13. <http://www.hr-dp.org/files/2013/12/12/Human_Rights_and_Drugs_Vol_1_-_Editorial.pdf>, accessed 24 October 2015.

Nadelmann, E. (1990) Global prohibition regimes: the evolution of norms in international society. *International Organization* 44(4): 479–526.

Nowak, M. and Hunt, P. (2008) Special Rapporteur on the question of Torture and the Right of everyone to the highest attainable standard of physical and mental health. Letter to Mr D. Best, Vice-Chairperson of the Commission on Narcotic Drugs, 10 December 2008.

OESA (Office of Economic and Social Affairs, United Nations) (2015) *Sustainable Development Topics.* <https://sustainabledevelopment.un.org/topics>, accessed 23 October 2015.

Saunders, C. and Platt, M. (2003) Pain and impending death. In R. Melzack and P.D. Wall (eds,), *Handbook of Pain Management.* Edinburgh: Churchill Livingstone, pp. 721–726.

Scott, J. and Marshall, G. (2005) *A Dictionary of Sociology.* Oxford: Oxford University Press.

Shusterman, R. (1999) Somaesthetics: a disciplinary proposal. *Journal of Aesthetics and Art Criticism* 57(3): 299–313.

Tupper, K., Wood, E., Yensen, R., and Johnson, M. (2015) Psychedelic medicine: a re-emerging therapeutic paradigm. *Canadian Medical Association Journal* 187(14): 1054–1059.

Tyrrell, I. (2010) *Reforming the World: The Creation of America's Moral Empire.* Princeton: Princeton University Press.

United Nations (1971) *Convention on Psychotropic Substances.* Signed at Vienna on 21 February 1971.

United Nations (1988) *United Nations Convention against Illicit Traffic in Narcotic Drugs and Psychotropic Substances.* Signed at Vienna on 20 December 1988.

United Nations (2014) *World Drug Report 2014.* Office on Drugs and Crime, United Nations, No. E.14.XI.7.

United Nations (1972/1961) *Single Convention on Narcotic Drugs, as amended by the Protocol amending the Single Convention on Narcotic Drugs, 1961.* Signed in Geneva on 25 March 1972.

UNGA (UN General Assembly) (2013) *Report of the Special Rapporteur on Torture and Other Cruel, Inhuman or Degrading Treatment or Punishment, Juan E. Méndez.* Office of the United Nations High Commissioner for Human Rights. <http://www.ohchr.org/Documents/HRBodies/HRCouncil/RegularSession/Session22/A.HRC.22.53_English.pdf>.

UNODC (United Nations Office on Drugs and Crime) (2008) *One Hundred Years of Drug Control.* <https://www.unodc.org/documents/data-and-analysis/Studies/100_Years_of_Drug_Control.pdf>.

Weil, A. and Rosen, W. (2004) *From Chocolate to Morphine: Everything You Need to Know about Mind-Altering Drugs.* Boston: Houghton Mifflin Co.

WHO (World Health Organization) (2014) *Strengthening of Palliative Care as a Component of Comprehensive Care throughout the Life Course.* World Health Assembly Resolution 67.19 (24 May 2014). <http://apps.who.int/gb/ebwha/pdf_files/WHA67/A67_R19-en.pdf?ua=1>, accessed 24 October 2015.

36

FETAL PAIN AND THE LAW

Abortion laws and their relationship to ideas about pain and fetal pain

Stuart W.G. Derbyshire

1 Early abortion laws

Prior to the nineteenth century, abortion largely remained outside the purview of the law (Spivack 2008). In the Middle Ages, detecting pregnancy was not straightforward: women did not gain weight in early pregnancy, and baggy clothes often hid weight gain in later pregnancy. Menstruation could stop for many reasons and was not reliably connected to the onset of pregnancy. In many cases, pregnancy became clearly known only when the pregnant woman felt her fetus move.

Even then pregnancy remained uncertain, fraught and not something benign. Pregnancy threatened the woman's life, and the risk of deformity and stillbirth were high. Only successful birth removed the pregnancy as a source of threat and revealed the infant as a recognizable person. Consequently, medieval courts did not view the ending of pregnancy as the ending of a human life.

Advances in the understanding of pregnancy and the emergence of medicine as a professional career in the nineteenth century contributed to changes in the attitudes towards abortion. In both the United Kingdom and the United States, newly emerging medical associations worked to create distinctions between the proper and improper practices of medicine, with abortion considered improper. Physicians further developed their technical authority with increasingly sophisticated descriptions of female physiology, which they related to the natural function of women as child bearers. Here, physicians conformed to a more general nineteenth-century belief that motherhood was natural and so the interruption of pregnancy was a violation of natural intent, and a selfish refusal by women to perform their marital duty (Leslie 2010).

Consequently, in the United Kingdom, the 1861 Offences against the Person Act provided for life in prison for unlawfully procuring a miscarriage at any stage of gestation. In the United States, the 1873 Comstock Law did not directly ban abortion, but the procurement of contraception or abortifacient devices by the US Postal Service carried a prison sentence of up to five years. By the end of the nineteenth century, most US states had laws banning abortion. Notably, however, the motivations to restrict abortion were not based on moral concern for the fetus, but on concern to enhance the medical profession and protect women's natural roles as wives and mothers.

2 Early twentieth century

After the First World War the average UK household declined from six to four children (Brookes 1988). This decline triggered state concern about the family. The 1918 Maternity and Child Welfare Act established local authority and child-welfare committees, and enabled the authorities to provide salaried midwives, health visitors, infant-welfare centers, day nurseries, and food supplements for needy infants and mothers. Concerns about the health of infants inevitably spilt over into concerns about the pregnant woman and her fetus, and imbued fetal life with a new significance.

Concerns about the fetus were also encouraged by campaigns to increase the use of contraception. Campaigners drew a distinction between abortion, which was used by the poor to kill the fetus, and contraception, which prevented pregnancy and was a morally superior form of birth control. Birth control was more fitting with middle-class concerns for planning, and for the poor to be thrifty.

By the early 1930s, contraception was becoming a private decision, left to individual conscience, while abortion was being marginalized as a desperate form of birth control (Leslie 2010). The legal landscape was also shifting. Middle-class women who used contraception could afford an abortion, induced by a medical practitioner, when contraception failed. In addition to the improved safety, they received protection from prosecution because their doctor could argue that the abortion was a necessary treatment. Working-class women obtaining an "amateur" abortion, in contrast, were unable to claim the procedure as "medical." Widespread use of amateur abortion by working-class women created conflict with the law and medicine, and generated momentum to examine the question of therapeutic abortion both legally and medically (Brookes 1988).

In 1938, the British gynaecologist, Aleck Bourne, tested a desperate case by performing an abortion upon a fourteen-year-old girl who had been raped (BMJ 1938a). The judge in the subsequent trial ruled that Bourne had performed the abortion to protect the life of the mother who would have otherwise become a "mental wreck" had the pregnancy continued (BMJ 1938b). Thus the Bourne case set an important precedent in establishing that abortion to protect the life of the woman could include considerations of psychiatric health.

3 Later twentieth-century UK law reform

Following the Second World War, medical concern over therapeutic abortion continued. Reports of associations between maternal rubella and congenital infant defects began to emerge before the war, and in 1946 the *Lancet* noted that abortion had been recently recommended in the US to "prevent the birth of a defective child" following the pregnant woman's exposure to rubella (Lancet 1946). Although discussed, widespread legal support for abortion to prevent fetal abnormality was not forthcoming, leading the *British Medical Journal* to moot the possibility that abortion might be procured on psychiatric grounds by demonstrating that the mother had great anxiety at the thought of having an abnormal child (Jeffcoate 1960).

In 1959, the Distillers Company announced the introduction of a new sedative, "Distaval," now better known as thalidomide. Thalidomide was recommended to help pregnant women sleep and prevent morning sickness. Tragically, thalidomide caused terrible fetal abnormalities. The thalidomide disaster generated public outrage, with several well-publicized cases of women strenuously pursuing an abortion. Sherri Finkbine, for example, flew to Sweden from the United States to get an abortion (Hindell and Simms 1971). Distillers withdrew thalidomide in 1961, but a measles epidemic in 1962 maintained fears regarding the birth of disabled infants.

Following the thalidomide tragedy, the number of therapeutic abortions carried out by the British National Health Service rose sixfold, but no doctor was prosecuted (Hindell and Simms 1971). Subsequently, British medical bodies did not fully support legal changes. In 1966, the British Medical Association (BMA) advised that there was a body of medical opinion viewing the law as not needing amendment because the law covered all the accepted medical indications for therapeutic abortion (BMJ 1966a; Gleeson 2007). The Royal College of Obstetricians and Gynaecologists (RCOG) also opposed the need for abortion law reform on similar grounds and added that abortion posed "considerable" dangers, even to the healthy woman (BMJ 1966b). RCOG was openly skeptical of figures from Scandinavia, Eastern Europe, Russia and Japan that demonstrated low levels of mortality and indicated abortion to be safer than continuing pregnancy. Both the BMA and RCOG expressed suspicion of parliamentary efforts to interfere in medical matters. They maintained that abortion was to be decided by medical professionals and not by parliament or women.

Nevertheless, concerns remained among the profession about doctors' liability should a judge or jury narrowly interpret the *Bourne* ruling (BMJ 1966a; Gleeson 2007). There was also widespread public support for abortion to prevent fetal abnormality. An influential 1962 poll by the Abortion Law Reform Association (ALRA) indicated that 91 percent of British women supported legal termination in the event of fetal abnormality (Pyn 1973). ALRA spearheaded the UK law reform campaign and was successful in recruiting prominent doctors to its cause. ALRA also gradually persuaded the BMA to support reform, which was critical in securing the introduction of the 1967 Abortion Act (UK).

The 1967 Act legalized abortion up to twenty-eight weeks gestation if two doctors agreed that its continuance would pose a greater threat to the physical or mental health of the woman than if the pregnancy were terminated. The 1967 Act, therefore, did not meet the desire of ALRA for abortion to be provided at the request of the pregnant woman. Instead, abortion remained a question to be decided by the medical profession, as the BMA and RCOG desired. In practice, however, once it became apparent that RCOG was wrong, and abortion was revealed to be an exceptionally safe procedure, the requirement that the woman be provided with the better option for her health made it difficult to refuse an early abortion.

4 Later twentieth-century US law reform

Legalization in the United States followed a different course. Following the Second World War, the UK Parliament successfully introduced a national health plan making health care free for all citizens. President Truman pursued similar reform in the US, but the American Medical Association (AMA) mobilized against reform. In 1961, the AMA opposed Kennedy's efforts to introduce health insurance for the elderly. In 1965, the AMA tried, but failed, to block the introduction of Medicaid. Distracted by efforts to maintain a fee-for-service medical system, the AMA paid little attention to the abortion issue (Halfmann 2011). Instead, legal reformers and social campaigners drove the liberalization of abortion in America.

In 1967, the National Organization for Women (NOW) adopted a *Bill of Rights*, which included the demand that women be able "to control their own reproductive lives by removing from penal codes the laws limiting access to contraceptive information and devices and laws governing abortion." NOW lobbied states for abortion reform and filed lawsuits when those efforts failed. Unlike ALRA in the UK, NOW did not bring the AMA into their effort for reform.

Altering state legislation through political pressure gradually yielded reforms in state abortion laws. By 1970 a majority of US states still banned abortion in most circumstances, but fourteen states allowed abortions in limited cases associated with rape, incest or extreme physical risks to the health of the woman. Alaska, Hawaii and Washington, DC, allowed abortion to protect the health of the woman, including psychological and physical well-being as a part of health. Hawaii also allowed abortion on request, but access was restricted to Hawaiian residents. A landmark change occurred in New York in April 1970 when the New York State Legislature narrowly passed a law to vastly liberalize access to abortion in New York State. Previously, the law permitted abortion only to save the life of the pregnant woman. The new law permitted abortion, on request, during the first twenty-four weeks of pregnancy, and there was no residency requirement. During the first year of legal abortion in New York State, over 100,000 non-residents travelled to New York for an abortion (Harris et al. 1973).

Buoyed by this success, legal reformers looked increasingly towards the state and federal courts to protect access to abortion as a part of constitutional law. This effort succeeded in 1973 with the landmark ruling of the Supreme Court in *Roe v. Wade*. *Roe* made all statutes preventing access to abortion before twelve weeks unconstitutional. Between twelve and twenty-four weeks a balance was to be struck between the duties to the woman and recognition of the increasingly valued status of the fetus. After twenty-four weeks, the court ruled that states could regulate abortion to protect fetal life. This latter ruling was associated with the increasing viability of the fetus to survive outside the womb as a pregnancy proceeds. Twenty-four weeks was considered by the court to be the point of viability.

The late 1960s through the 1970s was a period of international abortion reform. Australia, Austria, Canada, Denmark, Finland, France, Greece, Hungary, Italy, New Zealand, Norway, Singapore and Sweden either legalized abortion for the first time or introduced substantial legal reforms (Cook and Dickens 1978). These new laws mobilized opposition to abortion and increased vocal concern about the fetus, a concern that was less present, or muted, prior to reform (Brookes 1988). The United States, however, was perhaps the most unique case in that reform was mediated through the judiciary, without much engagement of the medical professions or elected political representatives. The Supreme Court ruling was based on the woman's constitutional right to privacy.

Arguably, the court introduced a policy that was more liberal than that supported by public opinion (Beck 2015; Halfmann 2011). Certainly the policy clashed with many state legislatures and *Roe* ushered in a period of legal argument and contest over abortion that continues today. Since at least 2003, that argument has included the issue of fetal pain.

5 Fetal pain science

Discussion about the possibility of fetal pain began in earnest in 1994 when a team of surgeons described a hormonal stress response in the fetus during an injection (Giannakoulopoulos et al. 1994). The team behind the report was pioneering newly invasive *in utero* procedures and had observed the fetus recoiling when needled. This led them, and their pregnant patients, to moot the possibility of fetal pain.

Without language or other effective means to assess any felt, subjective, experience, the team measured objective markers that are consistent with pain, including the release of cortisol and β-endorphins. Cortisol and β-endorphin levels were higher after needling direct into the hepatic vein, which is innervated with sensory nerves, compared with the placenta, which is not. Subsequently, it has been demonstrated that the increased cortisol response is blunted if the fetus is pretreated with fentanyl (Fisk et al. 2001).

The suggestion that the fetus can feel pain was met with immediate skepticism and the original report itself stated that, "a hormonal stress response cannot be equated with pain" (Derbyshire 1994; Giannakoulopoulos et al. 1994). Several researchers subsequently questioned whether the fetus has sufficient neural development for pain prior to twenty-four weeks gestation (Derbyshire 2006; Fitzgerald 2005; Lee et al. 2005; RCOG 2010) and whether the fetus ever has sufficient conceptual development for pain (Derbyshire and Raja 2011).

In 2003, President Bush passed the Partial-Birth Abortion Ban Act. The Act was challenged in New York, California and Nebraska and overturned. During each state trial, however, Dr. Kanwaljeet ("Sunny") Anand testified as an expert witness that the fetus would feel pain during abortion procedures after twenty weeks gestation and probably earlier. Anand argued that the brainstem is sufficient for pain experience, which is functional from around eighteen weeks gestation (Giannakoulopoulos et al. 1994). Anand also pointed to evidence that the brainstem can process sensory information and that anencephalic children, with profound to total loss of cortical tissue, are awake and respond to noxious stimuli (Oberlander et al. 2002; Tuber et al. 1980). Thus Anand challenged the general consensus, discussed later, that the cortex is necessary for pain.

During the 1980s, Anand revolutionized the use of anesthesia during pediatric surgery (Anand et al. 1987). At that time, infants undergoing surgery rarely received anesthesia because it was believed that the risks of anesthesia were too great. Anand and colleagues, however, demonstrated considerable clinical benefits from infant anesthesia, including improved survival.

Anand and Hickey (1987) claimed that the improved outcomes were due to infant pain relief, and they speculated that the fetus might also be pain-capable. Subsequently, Anand and Craig (1996) called for the IASP definition of pain to be revised by removing the references to language and subjectivity (see Chapter 31 of this volume for further critical discussion of the IASP definition). Removing such references, they argued, would enable recognition of fetal pain.

The arguments that Anand raises encompass neuroscience and the nature of what it is to feel. These issues are not easy to resolve. (See in this volume, for instance, Chapters 6–9 and 17.) Being more tangible, and more available to direct, empirical measurement, most discussion has focused on the neuroscience. Certainly, it makes sense to ask what are the necessary neural structures for pain experience and when they develop. Although the relationship between the structure of the nervous system and subjective experience is far from being understood, most neuroscientists agree that some relationship is necessary. According to this broadly accepted view, prior to the development of the necessary neural structures, it can be agreed that pain is not possible.

6 The neural structures necessary for pain

Pain during surgery requires a functional peripheral nervous system that can detect noxious stimuli. The receptors in skin and the internal organs that respond to noxious stimuli are known as nociceptors. Nociceptor activity follows tissue damage and is intimately involved in the pain from tissue damage. Blocking nociceptors with local anesthetic prevents pain during tissue damage and people born without nociceptors, due to a rare genetic defect, never experience pain from tissue damage (Cox et al. 2006). Thus, prior to the development of nociceptors, fetal pain during an abortion is improbable.

To rapidly detect noxious stimuli and effectively signal the threat of tissue damage or otherwise alert the organism to a need to protect (see Chapters 4 and 8 of this volume), nociceptors sit in the outer surface of the skin. Nerve terminals and fibers deep in the skin begin to develop from around six weeks' gestation and they extend out towards the periphery from around ten weeks. The receptors closest to the surface of the skin are likely to be immature nociceptors, although their presence is only certain from seventeen weeks' gestation (Terenghi et al. 1993).

In the context of abortion, the absence of nociceptors prior to at least ten weeks' gestation effectively eliminates fetal pain as a concern in the first trimester. Fetal pain might still be claimed based on the disturbance of a homeostatic state, or activation of receptors wholly or partly dissociated from tissue damage, but the author is only aware of one attempt to argue that fetuses feel pain in the first trimester. That attempt is through the website of Doctors on Fetal Pain, and focuses on nociception.

Although there is broad agreement that nociceptors are necessary for pain from tissue damage, there is far less agreement regarding the necessary components of the central nervous system to process signals arriving from the periphery. The existence of reflexive recoil from needling, and associated hormonal stress response at eighteen weeks, demonstrate that nociceptive fibers have penetrated the spinal cord and are relaying to the thalamus by eighteen weeks (Giannakoulopoulos et al. 1994). Anand and others accept nociceptive activity reaching the thalamus at eighteen weeks as the minimal necessary requirement for pain experience (Anand 2007; Lowery et al. 2007; Merker 2007). This acceptance is based on the proposal that spinal–thalamic–brainstem loops are sufficient to generate an experience of pain.

Many neuroscientists, however, believe that the cortex is also necessary for an experience of pain (Lee et al. 2005; RCOG 2010; and see Chapter 7 of this volume). The cortex is the outer layer of the brain, generally associated with higher-order thinking, and often considered to be necessary for subjective awareness, including the awareness of pain (Apkarian et al. 2005; Derbyshire 2006; Tracey and Mantyh 2007). Signals from nociceptors do not reach the cortex until around twenty-four weeks' gestation (Hevner 2000; Kostović and Jovanov-Milosević 2006; Ulfig et al. 2000).

After twenty-four weeks, argument as to whether fetal pain is possible hinge on the subjectivity of pain, rather than on the neuroscience (Derbyshire and Raja 2011). Pain involves a language of distress, and includes signals for help, that extend beyond the stand-alone brain to incorporate a community of minds that the fetus will only become a part of after being born (Sullivan and Derbyshire 2015).

Elsewhere, a distinction has been drawn between being in pain and *knowing that* I am in pain (Tallis 2005; see also Chapter 20, this volume). Both an older infant and a fetus might be said to feel pain, but only the older infant can experience *that they are in pain* and explicitly share their condition with others as an acknowledged fact of being in pain (Derbyshire and Raja 2011). This distinction is similar to that drawn between pain as a subjective experience and pain as a bodily state, which is discussed elsewhere (Corns 2014; and see Chapters 5 and 27, this volume). It might be accepted that the fetus is capable of a bodily pain without explicit recognition, or subjective feeling, of pain. Such a bodily pain might be readily supported by thalamic–brainstem loops as Anand and others maintain (Anand 2007; Devor et al. 2015; Merker 2007), whereas the cortex might be necessary for a pain that is explicitly felt.

Whether pain as a mere expression of a bodily state, without a subjective component, carries no, or less, moral compulsion than pain as a sensation with an aversive, subjective, content is contentious (Derbyshire 1999; Derbyshire and Raja, 2011; Brugger 2012). The potential immorality of inflicting pain on the fetus during abortion is critical to the ongoing efforts to change abortion laws to prevent fetal pain.

7 Fetal pain laws in the US

The countries where abortion remains legal after eighteen weeks, albeit under highly variable conditions and restrictions, include Britain, China, Canada, Germany, India, Japan, Poland, Russia, Singapore, South Africa, Spain, Sweden, The Netherlands and Vietnam (CRR 2013). It is in these countries, therefore, that policy on abortion might become more restrictive following debate over the possibility of fetal pain. To the author's knowledge, however, only the UK and the US have attempted to restrict abortion based on the possibility of fetal pain.

Following the Partial-Birth Abortion Ban Act trials of 2003, the Bush administration submitted the Unborn Child Pain Awareness Act in 2005, which was subsequently debated in Congress in 2006. Although the Act secured a majority in Congress it did not secure the two-third majority necessary to pass as a law and so the Act lapsed.

Subsequent to the failed Unborn Child Pain Awareness Act, multiple US states began to deliberate their own fetal pain legislation. Nebraska went first, signing into law the Pain-Capable Unborn Child Protection Act in April 2010. The Nebraska law states, "[a]t least by twenty weeks after fertilization there is substantial evidence that an unborn child has the physical structures necessary to experience pain." And it goes on to state, "it is the purpose of the State of Nebraska to assert a compelling state interest in protecting the lives of unborn children from the stage at which substantial medical evidence indicates that they are capable of feeling pain." The following year, Alabama, Idaho, Kansas and Oklahoma filed their own, largely identical, fetal pain laws, being joined by Georgia and Louisiana in 2012, Arkansas, North Dakota and Texas in 2013, West Virginia in 2015 and Wisconsin in 2016. Currently, twelve US states have legislation restricting abortion to a twenty-week time limit based on fetal pain, and at least a further thirteen states have deliberated the possibility (Calhoun 2012).

These state laws are a direct challenge to the constitutional principle, established by *Roe*, that abortion remains the choice of the woman prior to viability, established at twenty-four weeks. It is therefore likely that the issue of fetal pain will arrive at the Supreme Court because the fetal pain laws prohibit abortion four weeks earlier than *Roe*. The Supreme Court will need to decide if the state rulings can be accommodated within the constitution.

Any discussion of fetal pain laws by the Supreme Court will follow many past discussions and amendments of the original *Roe* ruling. Past cases include *Harris v. McRae*, 1976 (allowing bans on the use of Medicaid for abortion); *Belloti v. Baird*, 1981 (allowing pregnant minors to seek an abortion without parental notification); *Webster v. Reproductive Health Services*, 1989 (upholding bans on the use of public employees and facilities to perform abortions); and *Planned Parenthood v. Casey*, 1992 (allowing state involvement before the end of the first trimester, enforced waiting periods, pre-abortion counseling, and parental consent laws). Following these rulings came the partial-birth abortion arguments, described earlier, which opened the way to the current fetal pain bills and an expected further clash in the Supreme Court. Thus, legal arguments over fetal pain in the US are part of a procession of legal arguments stretching back to *Roe*.

8 Fetal pain laws in the UK

In contrast the to the busy history of abortion law in the United States, the 1967 Abortion Act, UK, has only been amended once. In 1990, the Human Fertilisation and Embryology Act introduced a time limit of twenty-four weeks for almost all abortions except those on grounds of fetal anomaly, from which any limit was removed. In all other respects, the 1967 Act remains as it was. In 2007, the UK House of Commons Science and Technology Committee (House of Commons 2007) was tasked to review the 1967 Act. As part of their review, the Committee examined the issue of fetal pain and concluded that there is good evidence that the fetus launches a physiological reaction to noxious stimuli but no good evidence for pain being consciously felt (see Chapter 17 of the current volume for further discussion of pain as a conscious experience). The report concluded without recommending any change to the 1967 (amended 1990) Abortion Act (UK).

Two members of the Committee, however, were concerned that the main Committee report ignored important evidence regarding fetal pain and development. One of the members, Nadine Dorries, subsequently tabled an amendment to the proposed Human Fertilisation and Embryology Bill in May 2008 to include a reduction in the upper limit of abortion from twenty-four weeks to twenty weeks. The amendment was defeated by 332 votes to 190. A separate twenty-two-week limit amendment was defeated by 304 votes to 233 on the same evening.

One consequence of the Committee report was to trigger the UK Department of Health to request the RCOG (Royal College of Obstetrics and Gynaecology) to update the 1997 RCOG Working Party report on fetal awareness. The updated report was published in 2010 and contained the following summary statement:

> In reviewing the neuroanatomical and physiological evidence in the fetus, it was apparent that connections from the periphery to the cortex are not intact before 24 weeks of gestation and, as most neuroscientists believe that the cortex is necessary for pain perception, it can be concluded that the fetus cannot experience pain in any sense prior to this gestation.
>
> *(RCOG 2010)*

Thus the RCOG report upheld the central finding of the original Science and Technology Committee report and maintained support for the 1967 Abortion Act as amended in 1990. Since 2008, no further parliamentary efforts have been made to alter abortion law in the UK.

9 Can science resolve the issue of abortion?

Ever since *Roe*, abortion has been a highly contested issue in the US, but the issue has been much less contested in the UK and other countries. Several commentators have noted that the introduction of abortion as a concession to psychiatric health concerns, and to resolve the problem of fetal abnormality, left the control of abortion in medical hands (Halfmann 2011; Leslie 2010). The difficult political issues associated with abortion, such as bodily sovereignty, gender roles and the role of motherhood, as well as incendiary moral and emotional questions associated with guilt, promiscuity, sexuality and blame were thereby subsumed under the relatively neutral language of "mental health" and the seemingly esteemed, reasonable and unarguable science from the men and women of medicine.

In the US, in contrast, abortion was introduced as the consequence of the right to make private and personal decisions free from interference from the state or other body, including medical associations. Thus, American physicians did not act as the gatekeeper of abortion to decide "appropriate" cases for abortion. Consequently, bitter arguments over the rights of the woman versus the rights of the fetus and the nature and meaning of abortion have continued.

On the surface, it might seem that fetal pain ought to be a more prominent issue in the UK where abortion is an issue of medical authority. Pain is a medical issue and might be expected, therefore, to generate more angst in the UK than in the US. In the US, however, fetal pain is wrapped into the ongoing legal arguments and battles over autonomy and the rights of the woman versus the fetus. In the UK, in contrast, the argument over fetal pain is wrapped into a scientific/medical argument about the fetus, which was adequately resolved by the consensual scientific/medical authority manifested in the 2010 RCOG report.

The resolution of the fetal pain issue in the UK, and its continuance in the US, therefore, is not because the UK is "more scientific" and has resolved the scientific issue of fetal pain while the US has not. The resolution of the fetal pain issue in the UK, and the ongoing argument in the US, are a consequence of particular histories and local politics. Even if all the issues of gestational science were to be resolved, including the unknowns of fetal pain, the legal and political arguments about abortion would continue because it is the meaning of scientific facts that matters. And meaning is negotiable.

If the fetus has an inchoate mental life, rendering it pain-incapable, that does not mean the fetus becomes expendable. Similarly, if the fetus has a form of minimal mental existence, making it pain-capable, that does not mean the fetus becomes inviolable. Metaphysical questions regarding the meaning of personhood and the rights and wrongs of terminating fetal life are not resolved by deciding if and when the fetus becomes pain-capable. In both the UK and the USA, therefore, the efforts to resolve the moral question of abortion through the scientific issues relating to fetal pain cannot succeed.

In both countries, the development of the fetus, which is an issue for science, is being used to try and infer the moral and legal rights of the fetus, which is a distinctively non-scientific question (Robertson 2015). Science may provide a description or explanation of natural events, but does not deliver justifications for action. In 1966, the RCOG argued against the legalization of abortion by exaggerating the dangers associated with abortion. To an extent, the RCOG tried to evade the difficult moral and social issues posed by abortion in favor of the seemingly more concrete, and indisputable, empirical facts of safety. But even if abortion is dangerous, we can still allow women to expose themselves to danger.

Similarly, even if it is accepted that the fetus cannot feel pain during abortion, it does not follow that abortion is morally acceptable. To demand that abortion be accepted on the basis that a fetus feels no pain confuses facts with morality. The facts of fetal pain are highly contested, but even if fetal pain were resolved, that resolution would not render abortion moral or immoral. We may decide that the pain of the fetus is morally sufficient to override the legality of abortion in all circumstances, or only in some circumstances, or in no circumstances at all. We may decide that the potential for pain in the fetus requires an alteration in the procedure, such as including an analgesic, or we may decide no changes are necessary. What society does about unwanted pregnancies remains a moral, political and social question that cannot be resolved by deciding the pain-capability of the fetus.

Related topics

Chapter 4: Imperativism (Klein)
Chapter 5: Fault lines in familiar concepts of pain (Hill)

Chapter 6: Advances in the neuroscience of pain (Apkarian)

Chapter 7: Neuromatrix theory of pain (Roy and Wager)

Chapter 8: A neurobiological view of pain as a homeostatic emotion (Strigo and Craig)

Chapter 9: A view of pain based on sensations, meanings, and emotions (Price)

Chapter 17: Pain and consciousness (Pereplyotchik)

Chapter 20: Pain and incorrigibility (Langland-Hassan)

Chapter 27: Bad by nature: an axiological theory of pain (Massin)

Chapter 31: An introduction to the IASP's definition of pain (Wright)

References

Anand, K.J.S. (2007) Consciousness, cortical function, and pain perception in non-verbal humans. *Behavioral & Brain Sciences* 30: 82–83.

Anand, K.J.S. and Hickey, P.R. (1987) Pain and its effects in the human neonate and fetus. *New England Journal of Medicine* 317: 1321–1329.

Anand, K.J.S. and Craig, K.D. (1996) New perspectives on the definition of pain. *Pain* 67: 3–6.

Anand, K.J.S., Sippel, W.G., and Aynsley-Green, A. (1987) Randomised trial of fentanyl anasthesia in preterm babies undergoing surgery: effects on the stress response. *Lancet* 1: 243–248.

Apkarian, A.V., Bushnell, M.C., Treede, R.-D., and Zubieta, J.-K. (2005) Human brain mechanisms of pain perception and regulation in health and disease. *European Journal of Pain* (London, UK) 9: 463–484.

Beck, R. (2015) Twenty-week abortion statutes: Four arguments. *Hastings Constitutional Law Quarterly* 43: 187–240.

BMJ (1938a) The trial of Mr. Bourne. *British Medical Journal* (23 July): 185.

BMJ (1938b) Therapeutic abortion and the law. *British Medical Journal* (30 July): 225–227.

BMJ (1966a) Therapeutic abortion: report by B.M.A. Special Committee. *British Medical Journal* (2 July): 40–44.

BMJ (1966b) Legalized abortion: report of the Council of the RCOG. *British Medical Journal* (2 April): 850–854.

Brookes, B. (1988) *Abortion in England 1900–1967*. Beckenham: Croom Helm.

Brugger, E.C. (2012) The problem of fetal pain and abortion: Toward an ethical consensus for appropriate behavior. *Kennedy Institute of Ethics Journal* 22: 263–287.

Calhoun, L.J. (2012) The painless truth: challenging fetal pain-based abortion bans. *Tulane Law Review* 87: 141.

Cook, R.J. and Dickens, B.M. (1978) A decade of international change in abortion law: 1967–1977. *American Journal of Public Health* 68: 637–644.

Corns, J. (2014) The inadequacy of unitary characterizations of pain. *Philosophical Studies* 169: 355–378.

Cox, J.J., Reimann, F., and Nicholas, A.K., Thornton, G., Roberts, E., Springell, K., Karbani, G., Jafri, H., Mannan, J., Raashid, Y., Al-Gazali, L., Hamamy, H., Valente, E.M., Gorman, S., Williams, R., McHale, D.P., Wood, J.N., Gribble, F.M., and Woods, C.G. (2006) An SCN9A channelopathy causes congenital inability to experience pain. *Nature* 444: 894–898.

CRR (Center for Reproductive Rights) (2013) *The World's Abortion Laws Map*, 2013 update. <http://www.reproductiverights.org/sites/crr.civicactions.net/files/documents/AbortionMap_Factsheet_2013.pdf>, accessed 23 January 2016.

Derbyshire, S.W.G. (1994) Fetal stress responses. *Lancet* 344: 615.

Derbyshire, S.W.G. (1999) The IASP definition captures the essence of pain experience. *Pain Forum* 8: 106–109.

Derbyshire, S.W.G. (2006) Can fetuses feel pain? *British Medical Journal* 332: 909–912.

Derbyshire, S.W.G. and Raja, A. (2011) On the development of painful experience. *Journal of Consciousness Studies* 18: 233–256.

Devor, M., Rappaport, I., and Rappaport, H. (2015) Does the Golem feel pain? Moral instincts and ethical dilemmas concerning suffering and the brain. *Pain Practice* 15: 497–508.

Fisk, N.M., Gitau, R., Teixeira, J.M., Giannakoulopoulos, X., Cameron, A.D., and Glover, V.A. (2001) Effect of direct fetal opioid analgesia on fetal hormonal and hemodynamic stress response to intrauterine needling. *Anesthesiology* 95: 828–835.

Fitzgerald, M. (2005) The development of nociceptive circuits. *Nature Reviews Neuroscience* 6: 507–520.

Giannakoulopoulos, X., Sepulveda, W., Kourtis, P., Glover, V., and Fisk, N.M. (1994) Fetal plasma cortisol and β-endorphin response to intrauterine needling. *Lancet* 344: 77–81.

Gleeson, K. (2007) Persuading parliament: abortion law reform in the UK. *Australasian Parliamentary Review* 22: 23–42.

Halfmann, D. (2011) *Doctors and Demonstrators: How Political Institutions Shape Abortion Law in the United States, Britain, and Canada.* Chicago: University of Chicago Press.

Harris, D., O'Hare, D., Pakter, J., and Nelson, F.G. (1973) Legal abortion 1970–1971 – the New York experience. *American Journal of Public Health* 63: 409–418.

Hevner, R.F. (2000) Development of connections in the human visual system during fetal mid-gestation: a DiI-tracing study. *Journal of Neuropathology and Experimental Neurology* 59: 385–392.

Hindell, K. and Simms, M. (1971) *Abortion Law Reformed.* London: Peter Owen.

House of Commons (2007) *Science and Technology Committee: Scientific Developments Relating to the Abortion Act 1967,* vol. 1. London: Stationary Office.

Jeffcoate, T.N.A. (1960) Indications for therapeutic abortion. *British Medical Journal* (27 February): 581–588.

Kostović, I. and Jovanov-Milosević, N. (2006) The development of cerebral connections during the first 20–45 weeks' gestation. *Seminars in Fetal & Neonatal Medicine* 11: 415–422.

Lancet (1946) Medicine and the law: abortion for probable defects in the child. *Lancet* 1(6389): 208.

Lee, S.J., Ralston, H.J.P., Drey, E.A., Partridge, J.C., and Rosen, M.A. (2005) Fetal pain: a systematic multidisciplinary review of the evidence. *JAMA* 294: 947–954.

Leslie, C. (2010) The "psychiatric masquerade": The mental health exception in New Zealand abortion law. *Feminist Legal Studies* 18: 1–23.

Lowery, C.L., Hardman, M.P., Manning, N., Hall, R.W., and Anand, K.J.S. (2007) Neurodevelopmental changes of fetal pain. *Seminars in Perinatology* 31: 275–282.

Merker, B. (2007) Consciousness without a cerebral cortex: a challenge for neuroscience and medicine. *Behavioral and Brain Sciences* 30: 63–81.

Oberlander, T.F., Grunau, R.E., Fitzgerald, C., Ellwood, A.L., Misri, S., Rurak, D., and Riggs, K.W. (2002). Prolonged prenatal psychotropic medication exposure alters neonatal acute pain response. *Pediatric Research* 51(4): 443–453.

Pyn, B. (1973) The making of a successful pressure group. *British Journal of Sociology* 24: 451.

RCOG (Royal College of Obstetricians and Gynaecologists) (2010) *Fetal Awareness Review of Research and Recommendations for Practice: Report of a Working Party.* London: RCOG Press.

Robertson, J.A. (2015) Science disputes in abortion law. *Texas Law Review* 93: 1849–1883.

Spivack, C. (2007) To bring down the flowers: the cultural context of abortion law in early modern England. *William & Mary Journal of Women and the Law* 14: 107.

Sullivan, M.D. and Derbyshire, S.W. (2015) Is there a purely biological core to pain experience? *Pain* 156 (11): 2119–2120.

Tallis. R. (2005) *The Knowing Animal: A Philosophical Inquiry into Knowledge and Truth.* Edinburgh: Edinburgh University Press.

Terenghi, G., Sundaresan, M., Moscoso, G., and Polak, J.M. (1993) Neuropeptides and a neuronal marker in cutaneous innervation during human foetal development. *Journal of Comparative Neurology* 22: 595–603.

Tracey, I. and Mantyh, P.W. (2007) The cerebral signature for pain perception and its modulation. *Neuron* 55: 377–391.

Tuber, D.S., Berntson, G.G., Bachman, D.S., and Allen, J.N. (1980). Associative learning in premature hydranencephalic and normal twins. *Science* 210(4473): 1035–1037.

Ulfig, N., Neudorfer, F., and Bohl, J. (2000) Transient structures of the human fetal brain: subplate, thalamic reticular complex, ganglionic eminence. *Histology and Histopathology* 15: 771–790.

37

PAIN, MENTAL SUFFERING AND PHYSICIAN-ASSISTED DEATH

Daniel Weinstock

Many jurisdictions have in recent years eliminated blanket criminal prohibitions against physician-assisted death (hereafter PAD), and others seem set to follow suit.[1] This means that in a number of jurisdictions, the ethical and philosophical debate about PAD has moved from an initial phase, in which the question of the general permissibility or impermissibility of physicians aiding their very ill patients to die has been debated (Sumner 2011), to a second phase in which ethical questions to do with the setting-up of regulatory regimes surrounding the practice of PAD are being discussed.

It is moreover becoming increasingly obvious that the ethical and philosophical considerations that were deployed in order to frame the ethical issues in the first phase of the debate about PAD do not in and of themselves provide us with the intellectual resources needed to answer the very many questions that arise at the second phase. Thus, for example, much of the first phase of the debate surrounded the question of how the values of autonomy on the one hand, and of the inviolability of human life on the other, should be ranked (Sumner 2011; Somerville 2014). The terms of this debate do not provide us with the conceptual resources with which to address the question, for example, of what the specific medical conditions are that might qualify an individual to make the request for PAD. Nor do they help us in answering the question of the conditions under which physicians might be able to invoke the right to conscientious refusal when such a request is directed to them. Yet these questions, and others, are central to setting up a regulatory framework in which PAD will be administered, once it has been determined that the general objections to it do not ultimately defeat the general reasons for it.

This chapter will deal with just one of the many questions that will have to be addressed in setting up such regulatory frameworks. It will have to do with the status of mental and psychic suffering in the debate over the kinds of medical conditions that qualify or disqualify a person for PAD. Two questions will be central to my concern. First, I will address the issue of whether mental suffering unrelated to an underlying physical condition might qualify an agent for PAD (Sections I–II). Second, I will consider the question of whether such suffering might, in virtue of its impact on the agent's cognitive competence, *dis*qualify an agent from being able to request PAD (Section III).

1

One of the principal challenges that must be met in order to establish sensible regulatory frameworks for the administration of PAD has to do with the elucidation of the widely shared, but vague intuition that PAD should be a medical intervention of last resort (Miller et al. 1994), something that should be considered only in the case of patients with "incurable," "terminal" diseases, and who find themselves at the "end of life."

The problem with the intuition is that it seems to conflate a number of criteria that are only contingently related. One of these criteria has to do with proximity to death. Some people believe that the acceptability of PAD is tightly tied to its occurring only in cases in which death will occur imminently anyway, regardless of whether or not PAD is administered. For example, the legislative passage of the end of life law adopted in the Canadian province of Quebec in 2014, and which went into effect in early 2016, required that such a clause, restricting PAD to those at the "end of life," be added to the Bill at the last moment.

Taken as a sufficient condition for the administration of PAD, the "end of life" restriction is odd. To see this consider the following case: imagine a person who suffers from a rare disease that causes no pain or suffering, and that gives rise to a sudden, painless death before which the patient is completely free of any discomfort. Imagine, moreover, that the disease in question is one that allows physicians to determine the time of death with great precision (imagine for example that the only symptom associated with the disease is a discoloration that goes through a range of distinct shades at regular and foreseeable temporal intervals before death ensues).

Now imagine a person who finds himself twenty-four hours before his foreseen death. If anyone in the world is "terminal," or "at the end of life," this person is. Yet it is clear that in his case the question of the permissibility of PAD does not arise. He is well, though he will die tomorrow. There is thus no clinical reason for a physician to hasten his death, despite the fact that he will clearly die soon as a result of a fatal medical condition. Were he to make a request for PAD in these final twenty-four hours, this could justly be seen by the physician as an unreasonable request, since only loss of life would result from PAD, unredeemed by any benefit on the other side of the ledger.

There is another way to interpret the "end of life" requirement, one that interprets it not in a strictly temporal, but rather in a clinical manner. What I mean by this is that it could be that for some, "end of life" is taken to stand proxy for the idea that the medical condition with which a person suffers is "incurable" or "terminal." (Perhaps the conflation is invited by the idea that it is only in the final hours and days of a disease that it is possible to say that the probability of a person's condition improving is close to nil, either because there comes a point in the progression of a disease at which the likelihood of a person rallying is close to nil, or because the hope that a new kind of medical intervention might provide a cure lies too far in the future to make any difference to this particular patient.)

Let me first distinguish between these two ways of parsing the notion of "end of life." To say that a medical condition is "incurable" is to say that the medical condition cannot be eliminated by medical intervention. To say that it is "terminal" means that it will lead to the patient's death. Note that a condition can be "incurable" without being terminal, as is the case with many chronic medical conditions, while to say that it is terminal is not to imply that it is necessarily in all cases incurable. Some cancers can be cured, but are terminal in patients who do not respond to curative therapy that has succeeded in other cases.

Neither incurability nor the fact of being terminal is a sufficient condition for PAD. A medical condition can be incurable while giving rise to quite moderate symptoms, or to symptoms that can be managed through palliative means. What's more, we can adapt the example imagined above of the person whose inexorable and foreseeable path is toward death in such a way as to make plain that the simple fact that someone suffers from a medical condition that will lead to her death does not in and of itself qualify a person for PAD. The (perhaps medically improbable) example shows that there is a contingent, rather than a necessary, connection between the fact of being terminal and the properties that would have to be present in order for the request for PAD to be one that a physician might accede to.

Clearly, those conditions have to do with the pain and suffering that an individual is experiencing while in the grips of a medical condition. Now, pain and suffering are not in and of themselves sufficient conditions for the legitimacy of the request for PAD. After all, medicine aims at curing the medical conditions that underlie the pain and suffering that people experience, or at alleviating the pain and suffering even when it cannot cure the underlying condition. Thus, pain and suffering (which I am for the time being treating in an undifferentiated way as any kind of intensely negative subjective state, whether physical or mental) are necessary conditions for the admissibility of PAD, but they are only sufficient as part of a set of necessary and sufficient conditions that includes some other condition.

Might that condition be proximity to death? I don't see why this would be the case. Consider two patients, afflicted with different incurable medical conditions that give rise to exactly the same intensity of pain and suffering. One of the two will, according to the best clinical estimate, die in a day, while the second may very well live with this level of pain and suffering for months. It seems morally arbitrary to say that in virtue of his being closer to death, the first patient is entitled to PAD while the second is not. Defenders of the inviolability of human life will arguably not see much of a difference between violating that principle well before the predicted arrival of "natural death" and a slightly earlier violation of that principle. While consequentialists will, if anything, tend to see the alleviation of the pain of the individual whose suffering risks lasting the longest as the one of greatest ethical urgency.

Similarly, the idea that PAD can only be accepted when conjoined with a diagnosis of terminal illness must be rejected as well. Compare two patients whose pain and suffering are at any given moment identical. One of them suffers from a terminal disease, though one that will not cause his death in the immediate future, while the other suffers from a chronic disease unlikely to lead to death, though one that causes the same amount of pain and suffering. It seems morally arbitrary for the same reasons as those adduced above to say that a patient who will die anyway from his disease has the right to request PAD though the person who will not be killed by her disease but who experiences identical amounts of pain will be prevented from doing so.

The conclusion that is suggested by the foregoing sets of considerations is that pain and suffering justify the request for PAD but not in combination with the condition of imminent death or "terminalness." Rather, it seems that pain and suffering in the context of an incurable disease (whether chronic or terminal) justify the request for PAD.

However, palliative medicine has evolved to the point that it can manage pain and suffering associated with many medical conditions, even when it cannot eradicate the underlying medical condition. In order to arrive at a fuller characterization of the conditions justifying PAD, we must therefore add the condition that the pain and suffering associated with a medical condition not be such as to be managed to a sufficient degree by palliative medicine. The limits of the claim made on behalf of palliative medicine that it is capable of addressing virtually all cases of pain and suffering will be discussed in the following section, but for now, we have arrived at an at least provisionally plausible conclusion. A person qualifies for PAD when she suffers from an incurable medical condition, and when that medical condition causes pain and suffering that cannot be sufficiently mitigated by palliative medicine.

Now quite clearly this condition still leaves a number of questions open. For example, what does it mean to say that palliative medicine is not able to *sufficiently* mitigate pain and suffering? Who is to be the judge of the success or failure of palliative means? What's more, threshold questions still linger: What is the *level* of pain and suffering that is sufficient to trigger a justified request for PAD? And finally, what are the medical conditions that will be taken, by those who administer the regulatory apparatus through which requests for PAD are considered, to be *prima facie* candidates for PAD? In particular, can irremediable mental suffering associated with a mental illness unrelated to an underlying physical illness justify PAD?

2

Against the argument for allowing physicians to help their patients to die *if* the pain and suffering linked to their disease is untreatable, some critics of the legalization of PAD argue that this condition is in fact rarely, if ever, satisfied. Palliative care and pain management, they argue, have reached levels of sophistication that are such that the pain associated with their diseases can in the vast majority of cases be managed in a satisfactory manner through the administration of powerful analgesics (Emanuel 1999).[2] At the limit, they argue, those few patients whose pain is not manageable in this manner can be placed in a state of terminal sedation, in which pain is in effect managed through the extinguishment of consciousness.[3] Physicians who feel duty-bound to respond to their patients' requests to help them put an end to their pain can do so not by killing them, but by reaching into the tool kit of contemporary palliative care medicine (Rady and Verheijde 2015).

There can be no doubt about a number of claims. First, palliative care has in recent years considerably increased the range of treatments it has at its disposal in order to alleviate pain. Second, in many jurisdictions, funding for palliative care is insufficient, and leads to a situation in which not all patients can have reliable access to it (Wright 2008). The remediation of such a state of affairs is, where it exists, a moral imperative.

But these two observations do not foreclose the question of whether PAD can nonetheless be morally justifiable in a broad range of cases. This is the case for two principal reasons. First, many patients request PAD not because of the *pain* that they are in, but rather because of the *psychic or mental suffering* that their condition causes them. Thus, for example, some patients suffering from neurodegenerative diseases seek the right to PAD not because they are experiencing pain that might in principle be relieved by powerful analgesics, but because of the powerful negative mental states that they experience at the thought of their continued bodily degeneration. To illustrate this kind of situation, we can refer to the case of Gloria Taylor, whose case led to the Supreme Court of Canada's decision to strike down articles of the Criminal Code of Canada that made PAD a criminal offense in all cases. In her poignant testimony to the Supreme Court of British Columbia, she asserted: "I do not want the manner of my death to undermine the values that I lived my life in accordance with."[4]

The kind of mental suffering occasioned at the thought that one might be forced to continue to live in physical conditions that one deems unacceptable is clearly very distinct from somatic pain, and it is unclear that medical treatment can alleviate it. It is important to note that this kind of suffering is not alleviated even by the possibility of such extreme medical measures as terminal sedation, where a patient is made unconscious until death occurs. It is for Gloria Taylor the thought that she might be forced to end her life in a diminished physical state that causes her suffering, and palliative sedation does nothing to alleviate that thought. Indeed, the kind of condition she would be in were she terminally sedated is among the physical conditions that cause the negative mental states in question in the first place. Wrote Gloria Taylor about the prospect of an induced coma: "I do not want my last conscious thought to be worrying about what will happen – to my body and my family – once I am in the coma."[5]

Another difficult question arises however from the thought that someone may be justified in requesting PAD on the basis of her mental suffering. Once we accept that someone might be justified in requesting PAD on the basis of mental suffering occasioned by an underlying medical condition such as an incurable neurodegenerative disease, does it follow that that request is also justifiable when it is unaccompanied by such an underlying physical disease? To fix ideas, should we, for example, view requests for PAD that are formulated by patients suffering from severe treatment-resistant depression (TRD) as justified as well?

Let me recognize in a first instance that the question as I have framed it is badly formed. The dividing line between "physical" and "mental" illness is scientifically and clinically unsound.[6] First, mental illnesses are partly due to processes in the brain, in interaction with environmental determinants of various kinds. Second, a diagnosis of "depression," and *a fortiori*, of TRD, results from an exercise in clinical judgment, rather than in self-ascription, just as "physical" illnesses do.[7]

Once these clarifications have been introduced, there seems to be a strong *prima facie* case for allowing patients suffering from TRD to request PAD (Schuklenk and van de Vathorst 2015). After all, it is morally arbitrary to say that mental suffering qualifies someone for PAD, but to rule out some people because of the specific etiology of their suffering. Specifically, once we accept that irremediable mental suffering can be a valid reason to request PAD, what grounds do we have to deny it to those whose irremediable suffering (supposing it to be of the same intensity) is not caused by a medical condition located in the brain rather than in another part of the body?

An obvious response to this is to say that a diagnosis of TRD is more difficult to establish than is one of terminal metastatic cancer, or of ALS (Broome and de Cates 2015). A diagnosis of TRD is based on an inference made on the basis of the past resistance of a patient's depression to treatment, whereas a diagnosis of incurable cancer or ALS does not require such an inference from past to future, but is based rather on the evaluation of a patient's present state. In the case of illnesses such as cancer or ALS, it can be said with a fair degree of certainty that a patient's condition cannot be cured; in the case of a patient suffering from TRD, it can be said that her condition cannot be cured *yet*.

Is this distinction sufficient to rule TRD out as a condition qualifying an individual for PAD? Or, as libertarians argue, should it be considered equivalent to medical conditions that are more traditionally seen as qualifying conditions (Schuklenk and van de Vathorst 2015)? I don't think that it does. I want to suggest that the situation is not as simple as either conservatives (Miller 2015) or libertarians with respect to PAD have allowed.

Let us for the sake of the argument accept that there is a greater degree of certainty involved in a clinical diagnosis of ALS or of cancer than there is in the case of depression. This means that prognoses presented by physicians to patients suffering from clinical depression will always be presented probabilistically. It is neither the case that it is certain that a patient suffering from depression will recover nor is it certain that she will continue to experience the debilitating symptoms and suffering associated with deep depression. In delivering a prognosis to patients, medical professionals will base their diagnoses on past cases, and will present patients with diagnoses expressed in probabilistic terms. They will, for example, say to a patient that other patients who have been suffering from symptoms similar to hers, for similar lengths of time, and who have undergone treatment regimes similar to those that she has gone through, have experienced an amelioration of symptoms after a certain period of time in X percent of cases.

Now, on the view being defended here, it is when patients who have been diagnosed with an illness which medical science has failed to cure are experiencing suffering that cannot be alleviated in a manner acceptable to them that threshold conditions for the administration of PAD are met.

This set of criteria clearly rules out patients suffering from mental illnesses such as depression who have just received a diagnosis, or who are at very early stages of treatment. It would be unreasonable for them to request PAD (in a sense to be defined below), just as it would be morally unacceptable for a physician to accede to their request, since she could not plausibly claim that PAD was being administered only after every therapeutic option has been used.

But there comes a point at which, if symptoms persist for a sufficiently long period of time, if they are such as to occasion unremitting suffering, and if the probability, as assessed on the basis of inferences drawn from patients with similar symptomologies, of improvement is sufficiently low, then the request ceases to be unreasonable. That is, a patient may reasonably feel that the prognosis being probabilistically presented to her by the health-care professionals caring for her is unacceptable to her, and thus, that it would be reasonable for her to accept PAD.

Thus, if we admit subjective criteria among the conditions setting thresholds for admissibility to PAD, and if we accept that not just somatic pain, but also mental suffering, is among the criteria for admissibility, then it is on the face of it not more unreasonable for a patient suffering from TRD to request PAD rather than face a very low probability of alleviation of symptoms than it is for a victim of ALS to request it in the face of a prognosis of inexorable neurodegeneration over time.

Now, it is entirely possible that there might in some cases be reasonable disagreement between physician and patient on the question of whether PAD is advisable. That is, there may, given the probabilistic nature of the prognosis in the case of mental illness, be circumstances in which a physician believes that a therapeutic or palliative alternative is still possible, whereas the patient comes to form the view that it would not be unreasonable for her to refuse the odds presented to her by her physician. In such cases, the physician's right to conscientious refusal can certainly be invoked. I do not want to resolve these potential disputes in one way or another. What I want to have made at least plausible is the thought that there are cases in which it is reasonable for a patient suffering from severe TRD to refuse further treatment, and in which it is not unreasonable for a physician to accede to her demand for PAS.

The argument here raises two questions, only one of which I will be able to attend to in this chapter. The first has to do with the question of whether the kind of mental suffering involved in a mental illness such as depression doesn't paradoxically disqualify patients from competently requesting PAD in the first place. The second has to do with the reasonability condition which, I will argue, is implicitly built into any construal of qualifying conditions that attempts to combine objective and subjective criteria. Considerations of space require that I defer this second question to a future occasion.

3

The novel *Catch 22* by Joseph Heller is organized around the following paradox that bedeviled soldiers who attempted to get discharged from active military duty on the grounds of insanity. The "catch" was that the attempt to get discharged from the hell of war was if anything a mark of heightened sanity, one that proves that the solider is actually fit for battle.

A similar paradox is sometimes put forward by opponents of PAD (Downie and Lloyd-Smith 2015). Grant, they claim, that there may be some *ideal* cases in which PAD is morally justified. Those cases, the argument goes, are ones in which *competent individuals* suffering greatly because of some incurable medical condition make the fully informed request for PAD, in conformity with the doctrine that has become orthodox in medical ethics of free and informed consent. According to these arguments, the set of ideal cases is actually empty, because the kinds of medical conditions and psychic states that are present in these kinds of cases are incompatible, for robust contingent reasons, with the competent exercise of one's mental faculties.

Those who make the argument acknowledge that the connection between the kinds of medical conditions that *qualify* an individual for PAD, and the kinds of cognitive conditions that *disqualify* an individual from making a request for PAD, is contingent. That is, it is not part of the *definition* of competence that people are only competent when they are free from suffering, anxiety linked to disease, clouding of judgment linked to medication, and so on. Rather, the claim is that as a matter of fact, most, if not all people who find themselves in medical conditions so grave that they could trigger a morally legitimate request for PAD are probably to some degree diminished in their capacity to make medical decisions for themselves.

The argument can also be accompanied by the invocation of what is sometimes referred to as a "sliding scale" notion of competency (Buchanan and Brock 1990). The basic idea behind such a notion is that the requirements of competency and the stringency with which competency is verified vary depending on the stakes associated with a medical decision. The greater the stakes, the greater the requirement of competency, or so the argument goes. Now, clearly, there can be no more momentous a decision than that of ending one's life. And so, it would stand to reason, the cognitive requirements placed upon a patient who requests PAD should be very stringent indeed. It is likely, on this view, that very few medically plausible candidates for PAD will meet these stringent cognitive requirements.

The *prima facie* plausibility of this argument recedes, however, when we consider the impact that it would have on moral principles around which very little controversy exists in contemporary bioethics, and that are moreover central to the overall positions of conservatives with respect to PAD. While conservatives oppose PAD, they tend to follow the bioethical orthodoxy according to which patients should be allowed to refuse or to interrupt treatment, even when this decision risks shortening their lives. Indeed, it is a condition of the plausibility of their opposition to PAD that they not deny the right of patients to refuse treatment (Finnis 1995). Were they to deny that right, they could justly be accused of "life maximalism," the implausible view according to which the continuation of life matters more than does the person whose life it is, and whose judgments about her own well-being should guide her own decisions in the medical arena.

Now conservatives are at pains to deny that, from the point of view of physicians, there is any moral equivalency between the commission of a homicide and the fact of standing back and prescinding from administering medical care when a patient has refused such treatment. To revert to a standard distinction, they cleave to a sharp distinction (denied by some philosophers of consequentialist bent) between killing and letting die. According to this view, the physician acts in a morally culpable way when he kills (even when a patient has asked him for help in dying), but acts permissibly when he fails to treat a patient who has requested that treatment be interrupted (Keown 2012).

Forests have been felled in the attempt to determine whether the distinction between killing and letting die is ethically significant or not. But we can remain agnostic on this question for the purposes of this essay because while it may matter to the determination of the moral guilt or innocence of a physician, it does not matter to the criteria that must be put in place to determine the level of competence required of the patient making medical decisions. That is, from the point of view of the patient, both the choice to request PAD and the choice to ask for termination of treatment raise the highest possible medical stakes, namely whether the patient shall live or die. If we require of the patient that she exhibit a very high level of competence when making a request for PAD, one that she is unlikely to meet given the medical conditions that would qualify her for it, then, by parity of reasoning, we should require the same of patients who refuse life-saving or life-extending treatment. This would of course carry the risk that the range of cases in which it is morally acceptable to accede to a patient's wish for termination of treatment is as vanishingly small as the range of cases in which PAD is permitted. This is not a bullet that most conservatives are willing to bite. Thus, whatever the cognitive criteria that we put in place in order to determine the cognitive competency of candidates for PAD, it should not have as an effect the undercutting of what is after all one of the fixed points of contemporary clinical bioethics, that of recognizing the right of even grievously ill patients to refuse treatment.

4 Conclusion

I have not sought to settle any of the questions that arise in the context of the setting up of safe and humane regimes of PAD conclusively. I have sought to show how troubled the philosophical and ethical waters are that must be travelled in order to establish a safe and humane regime of PAD. In particular, I have sought to impress upon readers the urgency of thinking about the conditions for qualification of patients to PAD. I have urged reflection on the thorny question of whether irreducibly mental suffering, that is, mental suffering not associated with an underlying "physical" disease, can ever be among these qualifying conditions. I have delivered a qualified "yes" to this question, but have left open the question of the conditions under which it would be unreasonable for a patient in the grips of mental suffering due to a condition such as depression to request PAD from her physician.

Related topics

Chapter 18: Pain and consciousness (Pereplyotchik)
Chapter 13: Psychogenic pain: old and new (Sullivan)
Chapter 33: Pain management (Berryman, Catley, and Moseley)

Notes

1   The Supreme Court of Canada in the case of *Carter v. Canada (Attorney General)* recently struck down sections of the Criminal Code's blanket prohibition of assisted suicide. The legislature of Tasmania recently narrowly rejected a law that would have allowed PAD in a narrow range of cases.
2   For more on pain management, see Chapter 33, this volume.

3 See Chapter 18 of the present volume for a discussion of the connection between pain and consciousness.
4 Affidavit of Gloria Taylor to the BC Supreme Court, 25 August 2011.
5 Ibid.
6 For further criticism of this dichotomy, see also Chapter 13, this volume.
7 There is a great deal of scientific controversy concerning the etiology of major depressive disorder as well as concerning the possibility of arriving at a definitive clinical diagnosis of TRD. Obviously, my intention here is not to take sides on these debates in a definitive manner. For the purposes of this chapter, I will take TRD to fix ideas in the logical space occupied by medical conditions that give rise to grave mental suffering that is not accompanied by an underlying physical condition. For contending views on TRD, see Souery et al. 2006 and Little 2009.

References

Broome, M.R. and de Cates, A. (2015) Choosing death in depression. *Journal of Medical Ethics* 41(8): 586–587.

Buchanan, A. and Brock, D. (1990) *Deciding for Others: The Ethics of Surrogate Decision-Making*. Cambridge: Cambridge University Press.

Downie, J. and Lloyd-Smith, G. (2015) Assisted dying for individuals with dementia. In M. Cholbi and J. Varelius (eds.), *New Directions in the Ethics of Assisted Suicide and Euthanasia*. Pomona, CA: Spinger.

Emanuel, E. (1999) What is the great benefit of legalizing euthanasia or physician-assisted suicide?. *Ethics* 109(4): 629–642.

Finnis, J. (1995) A philosophical case against euthanasia. In J. Keown (ed.), *Euthanasia Examined: Ethical, Clinical and Legal Perspectives*. Cambridge: Cambridge University Press.

Keown, J. (2012) Against decriminalizing euthanasia, for improving care. In E. Jackson and J. Keown (eds.), *Debating Euthanasia*. Oxford: Hart Publishing.

Little, A. (2009) Treatment-resistant depression. *American Family Physician* 80(2): 167–172.

Miller, F. (2015) Treatment-resistant depression and physician-assisted death. *Journal of Medical Ethics* 41: 885–886.

Miller, F., Quill, T., Brody, H., Fletcher, J., Gostin, L., and Meier, D. (1994) Regulating physician-assisted death. *New England Journal of Medicine* 331(2): 119–123.

Rady, M. and Verheijde, J. (2015) Continuous deep sedation until death: palliation or physician-assisted death. *American Journal of Hospice and Palliative Medicine* doi:10.1177/1049909115609294.

Schuklenk, U. and van de Vathorst, S. (2015) Treatment-resistant major depressive disorder and assisted dying. *Journal of Medical Ethics*. doi:10.1136/medethics-2014–102458.

Somerville, M. (2014) *Death Talk: The Case against Euthanasia and Physician-Assisted Suicide*, 2nd ed. Montreal: McGill-Queen's University Press.

Souery, D., Papakostas, G., and Trivedi, M. (2006) Treatment-resistant depression. *Journal of Clinical Psychiatry* 67 (suppl. 6): 16–22.

Wright, M. (2008) Mapping levels of palliative care development. *Journal of Pain and Symptom Management* 35(5): 469–485.

INDEX

Note: page numbers in italic type refer to Tables; those in bold type refer to Figures.
As 'pain' is the major subject of the book, entries under this keyword have been kept to a minimum; readers are advised to look under more specific terms.

445

Printed in the United States
by Baker & Taylor Publisher Services